Computer simulation in brain science

Computer simulation in
brain science

Edited by

RODNEY M. J. COTTERILL

Division of Molecular Biophysics
The Technical University of Denmark

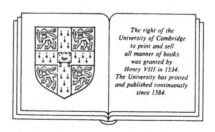

The right of the
University of Cambridge
to print and sell
all manner of books
was granted by
Henry VIII in 1534.
The University has printed
and published continuously
since 1584.

CAMBRIDGE UNIVERSITY PRESS

Cambridge

New York   New Rochelle

Melbourne   Sydney

CAMBRIDGE UNIVERSITY PRESS
Cambridge, New York, Melbourne, Madrid, Cape Town, Singapore, São Paulo

Cambridge University Press
The Edinburgh Building, Cambridge CB2 8RU, UK

Published in the United States of America by Cambridge University Press, New York

www.cambridge.org
Information on this title: www.cambridge.org/9780521341790

© Cambridge University Press 1988

First published 1988
This digitally printed version 2008

A catalogue record for this publication is available from the British Library

Library of Congress Cataloguing in Publication data
Computer simulation in brain science.
Includes index.
1. Brain—Mathematical models.   2. Neural circuitry—
mathematical models.   3. Computer simulation.
I. Cotterill, Rodney, 1933–   . [DNLM: 1. Brain—physiology.
2. Computer simulation. WL 300 C738]
QP376.C634 1988   612'82'0724   87-22430

ISBN 978-0-521-34179-0 hardback
ISBN 978-0-521-06118-6 paperback

CONTENTS

CONTRIBUTORS

Anninos, P. A.
Dept of Neurology, Medical School, University of Thraki, Alexandroupolis, Greece.

Anogianakis, G.
Dept of Physiology, Faculty of Medicine, University of Thessalonika, Greece.

Apostolakis, M.
Dept of Neurology, Medical School, University of Thraki, Alexandroupolis, Greece.

Barna, G.
Central Research Institute for Physics of the Hungarian Academy of Sciences, H-1525, Budapest, Hungary.

Bergman, Aviv
SRI International, 33 Ravenswood Ave., Menlo Park, CA 94025, USA.

Borg-Graham, Lyle J.
Center for Biological Information Processing and Harvard–MIT Division of Health Sciences and Technology, Massachusetts Institute of Technology, Cambridge, Massachusetts 02139, USA.

Caianiello, Eduardo R.
Dipartimento di Fisica Teorica e sue Metodologie per le Scienze Applicate, Università di Salerno, 84100 Salerno, Italy.

Chajlakhian, L. M.
Information Transfer Problems Institute, USSR Academy of Sciences, Moscow, USSR.

Changeux, J. P.
Institut Pasteur, 25 rue du Docteur Roux, 75724 Paris Cedex 15, France.

Clark, J. W.
Institute of Theoretical Physics and Astrophysics, University of Cape Town, Rondebosch 7700, Cape, RSA.
Permanent address: Dept of Physics and McDonnell Center for the Space Sciences, Washington University, St Louis, MO 63130, USA.

Cooper, Leon N.
Center for Neural Science and Dept of Physics, Brown University, Providence, Rhode Island 02912, USA.

Cotterill, Rodney M. J.
Division of Molecular Biophysics, The Technical University of Denmark, Building 307, DK-2800 Lyngby, Denmark.

Dammasch, Ingolf E.
Zentrum Anatomie, Universität Göttingen, Kreuzbergring 36, D-3400 Göttingen.

Dehaene, S.
Institut Pasteur, 25 rue du Docteur Roux, 75724 Paris Cedex 15, France

Diederich, S.
Institut für Theoretische Physik, Universität Giessen, Heinrich-Buff-Ring 16, 6300 Giessen, Federal Republic of Germany.

Dunin-Barkowski, W. L.
Information Transfer Problems Institute, USSR Academy of Sciences, Moscow, USSR.

Eckhorn, R.
Applied Physics and Biophysics, Philipps-University, Renthof 7, D-3550 Marburg, Federal Republic of Germany.

Efstratiadis, S.
Dept of Neurology, Medical School, University of Thraki, Alexandroupolis, Greece.

Érdi, P.
Central Research Institute for Physics of the Hungarian Academy of Sciences, H-1525, Budapest, Hungary.

Erdös, P.
Institute of Theoretical Physics, University of Lausanne, CH-1015 Lausanne, Switzerland.

Flyvbjerg, H.
The Niels Bohr Institute, University of Copenhagen, Blegdamsvej 17, DK-2100 Copenhagen Ø, Denmark.

Fukaya, M.
Dept of Electrical Engineering, University of Tokyo, 7-3-1, Hongo, Bunkyo-ku, Tokyo, Japan.

Harth, E.
Dept of Physics, Syracuse University, Syracuse, NY 13244-1130, USA.

an der Heiden, Uwe
Naturwissenschaftliche Fakultät, Universität Witten/Herdecke, D-5810 Witten, Federal Republic of Germany.

Henkel, R. D.
Institut für Theoretische Physik, Universität Giessen, Heinrich-Buff-Ring 16, 6300 Giessen, Federal Republic of Germany.

Hoffmann, Geoffrey W.
Depts of Physics and Microbiology, University of British Columbia, Vancouver, B.C., Canada V6T 2A6.

Hopfield, J. J.
Divisions of Chemistry and Biology, California Institute of Technology, Pasadena, CA 91125 and AT&T Bell Laboratories, Murray Hill, NJ 07974, USA.

Ingber, Lester
Dept of Physics – Code 61IL, Naval Postgraduate School, Monterey, CA 93943, USA.

Josin, Gary
Neural Systems Incorporated, 3535 West 39th Avenue, Vancouver, British Columbia V6N 3A4, Canada.

Kerszberg, Michel
Institut für Festkörperforschung der Kernforschungsanlage Jülich, D. 5170 Jülich, Federal Republic of Germany.

Kinzel, W.
Institut für Theoretische Physik, Universität Giessen, Heinrich-Buff-Ring 16, 6300 Giessen, Federal Republic of Germany.

Kitagawa, M.
Dept of Electrical Engineering, University of Tokyo, 7-3-1, Hongo, Bunkyo-ku, Tokyo, Japan.

Kohonen, Teuvo
Dept of Technical Physics, Helsinki University of Technology, Rakentajanaukio 2 C, SF-02150 Espoo, Finland.

Kürten, K. E.
Institut für Theoretische Physic, Universität zu Köln, 5000 Köln 41, BRD.

Larionova, N. P.
Information Transfer Problems Institute, USSR Academy of Sciences, Moscow, USSR.

Linsker, Ralph
IBM, T. J. Watson Research Center, Yorktown Heights, NY 10598, USA.

Littlewort, G. C.
Institute of Theoretical Physics and Astrophysics, University of Cape Town, Rondebosch 7700, Cape, RSA.

Marinaro, Maria
Dipartimento di Fisica Teorica e sue Metodologie per le Scienze Applicate, Università di Salerno, 84100 Salerno, Italy.

Matsumoto, Haruya
Dept of Instrumentation Engineering, Faculty of Engineering, Kobe University, Rokkodae, Kobe 657, Japan.

Mézard, M.
Ecole Normale Supérieure, 24 rue Lhomond, 75231 Paris Cedex 05, France.

Nadal, J. P.
Ecole Normale Supérieure, 24 rue Lhomond, 75231 Paris Cedex 05, France.

Niebur, E.
Institute of Theoretical Physics, University of Lausanne, CH-1015 Lausanne, Switzerland.

Okabe, Y.
Dept of Electrical Engineering, University of Tokyo, 7-3-1, Hongo, Bunkyo-ku, Tokyo, Japan.

Opper, M.
Institut für Theoretische Physik, Universität Giessen, Heinrich-Buff-Ring 16, 6300 Giessen, Federal Republic of Germany.

Pabst, M.
Applied Physics and Biophysics, Philipps-University, Renthof 7, D-3550 Marburg, Federal Republic of Germany.

Pandya, A. S.
Dept of Physics, University of Syracuse, Syracuse, NY 13244-1130, USA.

Pellionisz, András J.
Dept of Physiology and Biophysics, New York University Medical School, 550 First Ave, New York, NY 10016, USA.

Peretto, P.
CEN, Grenoble 85x, 38041 Grenoble Cedex, France.

Rafelski, J.
Institute of Theoretical Physics and Astrophysics, University of Cape Town, Rondebosch 7700, Cape, RSA.

Rall, W.
Mathematical Research Branch, NIDDK, National Institutes of Health, Bethesda, Maryland, USA.

Reitboeck, H. J.
Applied Physics and Biophysics, Philipps-University, Renthof 7, D-3550 Marburg, Federal Republic of Germany.

Roth, Gerhard
Naturwissenschaftliche Fakultät, Universität Witten/Herdecke, D-5810 Witten, Federal Republic of Germany.

Segev, I.
Mathematical Research Branch, NIDDK, National Institutes of Health, Bethesda, Maryland, USA.

Shaw, Gordon L.
Center for the Neurobiology of Learning and Memory, University of California, Irvine, CA 92717, USA.

Silverman, Dennis J.
Dept of Physics, University of California, Irvine, CA 92717 USA.

Toulouse, G.
Ecole Normale Supérieure, 24 rue Lhomond, 75231 Paris Cedex 05, France.

Travis, Bryan J.
Los Alamos National Laboratory, Los Alamos, NM 87545, USA.

Tsutsumi, Kazuyoshi
Division of System Science, The Graduate School of Science and Technology, Kobe University, Rokkodai, Kobe 657, Japan.

Unnikrishnan, K. P.
Dept of Physics, Syracuse University, Syracuse, NY 13244-1130, USA.

Vavilina, A. Ju.
Information Transfer Problems Institute, USSR Academy of Sciences, Moscow, USSR.

Winston, J. V.
206, Catalina, Fullerton, CA 92635, USA.

PREFACE

There has recently been a marked increase in research activity regarding the structural and function of the brain. Much of this has been generated by the more general advances in biology, particularly at the molecular and microscopic levels, but it is probably fair to say that the stimulation has been due at least as much to recent advances in computer simulation. To accept this view does not mean that one is equating the brain to an electronic computer, of course; far from it, those involved in brain research have long since come to appreciate the considerable differences between the cerebral cortex and traditional computational hardware. But the computer is nevertheless a useful device in brain science, because it permits one to simulate processes which are difficult to monitor experimentally, and perhaps impossible to handle by theoretical analysis.

The articles in this book are written records of talks presented at a meeting held at the Gentofte Hotel, Copenhagen, during the three days August 20–22, 1986. They have been arranged in an order that places more general aspects of the subject towards the beginning, preceding those applications to specific facets of brain science which make up the balance of the book. The final chapters are devoted to a number of ramifications, including the design of experiments, communication and control.

The meeting could not have been held without the financial support generously donated by the Augustinus Foundation, the Carlsberg Foundation, the Mads Clausen (Danfoss) Foundation, the Danish Natural Science Research Council, the Hartmann Foundation, IBM, the Otto Mønsted Foundation, NORDITA, the NOVO Foundation, and SAS. It is a pleasure to thank these philanthropic bodies, on behalf of all those involved in the enterprise.

Thanks are also due to John Clark and Uwe an der Heiden, for their moral support, in general, and specifically for their help in arranging the programme for the three days of tightly packed sessions.

It is also a pleasure to acknowledge our indebtedness to Carolyn Hallinger, the conference secretary, and to Ove Broo Sørensen and Flemming Kragh for their support with a host of technical matters.

Rodney Cotterill

1

Some recent developments in the theory of neural networks

LEON N. COOPER

A question of great interest in neural network theory is the way such a network modifies its synaptic connections. It is in the synapses that memory is believed to be stored: the progression from input to output somehow leads to cognitive behaviour. When our work began more than ten years ago, this point of view was shared by relatively few people. Certainly, Kohonen was one of those who not only shared the attitude, but probably preceded us in advocating it. There had been some early work done on distributed memories by Pribram Grossberg Longuet Higgins and Anderson. If you consider a neural network, there are at least two things you can be concerned with. You can look at the instantaneous behaviour, at the individual spikes, and you can think of the neurons as adjusting themselves over short time periods to what is around them. This has led recently to much work related to Hopfield's model; many people are now working on such relaxation models of neural networks. But we are primarily concerned with the longer term behaviour of neural networks. To a certain extent this too can be formulated as a relaxation process, although it is a relaxation process with a much longer lifetime.

We realized very early, as did many others, that if we could put the proper synaptic strengths at the different junctions, then we would have a machine which, although it might not talk and walk, would begin to do some rather interesting things. Kohonen has shown us some intriguing examples of such behaviour. We were soon confronted with a fundamental problem. Let us assume that you can form a network which will store memory, but which requires the adjustment of very large numbers of synaptic junctions. It is perfectly obvious that this cannot be done genetically, or at least not 100% genetically, if you believe that experience has anything to do with the content of your memory. So there must be some kind of rule, or set of rules, by which the synaptic strengths change.

Now, the use of the word 'synapse' may be something of a metaphor. The physiologists among us know that a synapse is a very complicated thing, and what we refer to as a synapse is really a logical grouping of large numbers of synapses, i.e. it is really a relation between inputs and outputs, and it is probable that what happens biologically is considerably more complex than any of the simple rules we write down. But the idea was that if we could write down a few rules which captured some of the qualitative properties, perhaps we would be on the right track.

Now it seemed to me that one of the things most lacking in this field, the thing required to convert it from the hand-waving stage to a field which was science as I understand it, was to construct pieces of theory that were well-defined and had a really rigorous structure, obviously highly over-simplified, but that could be brought into correspondence with serious experiment. Now that is not easy to do, and I am still not sure whether we have done it. Nevertheless this has been one of the dominating themes of our work for the last ten years. We chose a preparation, visual cortex, which may be the wrong starting point since it is a very complicated system, as compared to simpler systems like *Aplysia*. However, it is a system where interesting things seem to be happening, where experiments can be done, where there is a rich tradition of at least 20 years of experimentation, and where one has very robust effects. I cannot discuss all of these here, but those familiar with visual cortex and the history of the Hubel–Wiesel cells – the preference of the cells for certain orien-tations – know that there is a long history of experimentation in this area in which one can change the input–output relations of individual neurons by changing the visual experience of the animal. One reason this seemed so intriguing to us was that it appeared to be a situation in which one could observe changes in the neuron input–output behaviour almost as well as one could in hippocampus or *Aplysia*. I like to call this 'learning on a single-cell level', but am immediately thrown into conflict with some psychologists, who say learning is a much more complicated thing. However, when we learn something, there must be a change in the neural network; I believe that the origin of that change is what happens in individual cells in the network. And so one should be able to relate the large-scale properties to changes in individual cells. It is those changes that occur on a single-cell level that give us learning in a network level.

Experiments have been done in visual cortex that seem to indicate that the response characteristics of visual cortical cells depend on the visual environment of the animal. For example, if an animal is normally reared, the visual cortical cells will be sharply tuned and will be responsive to edges of one orientation, but not to edges of other orientations. This famous result is due to Hubel and Wiesel. It has been known for many years that if you raise animals in deprived environments, for example in the dark, the cells are not sharply tuned, but are broadly tuned. If you raise an animal with one eye open and the other eye closed, the cells will become responsive to the open eye, and sharply tuned to that eye, and they will lose their responsiveness to the closed eye, and so on. Large numbers of repeatable experiments have been done.

The question becomes: can one introduce a set of rules for synaptic change that will explain this behaviour? We have successfully introduced such a set of synaptic rules which involve what seem to be the variables that would provide the kind of learning we want on a network level. Let me describe this first on a single-cell level. Suppose you have a single cell with inputs from the external environment, and we introduce a modification procedure. What would be the necessary modification procedure to reproduce the experimental results? We were able to successfully reproduce what we call the 'classical' experimental results. In addition, we were able to show that there are some rather subtle new effects. Recent experiments do show these subtle effects. If they had been seen before, they had never been really explicitly pointed out or recognized.

One problem with this work is that, in addition to simplifying the synaptic junction, it made one assumption which was clearly not permissible, in that we considered the cortical synapses of the lateral geniculate nucleus to be capable of being both positive and negative. In other words, they could be both excitatory and inhibitory. Our recent work has solved this problem.

For our purposes, we can think of a set of inputs to a neuron, call them $d_1, \ldots, d_n$. Now the $d_1, \ldots, d_n$ is an n-dimensional vector; think of that n-dimensional vector as being a mapping of what is in the visual space. It is produced via the transduction cells of the retina, and so forth, so that for a particular image on the visual space you have a particular vector in this space. Now these inputs, measured in spikes per second, go through a set of synapses to the cortical cells. The cells integrate the electrical activity, so in effect the output of the cell is a non-linear monotonic function of $m \cdot d$. We are mostly concerned about the roughly linear region, though some of the other papers in these proceedings will take a different point of view and will try to make it as non-linear as possible. I am not going to insist on the virtue of one rather than the other. The point that we are making is that for the purposes of learning, the linearity is enough (Figs. 1.1 and 1.2).

To summarize, d is the input from the external world, and it changes as the image on the screen changes; m is a set of synaptic strengths that, if it changes at all, changes slowly with time. And it is m that contains the learning of the system. If one has a particular set of ms, with m thought of as a vector, a particular input that is parallel to it could give a large cell output. An input that is orthogonal to m would give zero output, so this set of ms, is, in a certain sense, already a memory because it distinguishes between one set and another set of inputs. Of course, for one cell one gets a rather limited memory, but if there are networks of these cells, all kinds of interesting things could occur.

Now the issue with which we are concerned is precisely how these ms change. Supposing you wish to 'teach' a single cell to recognize a vector. You could have a set of synaptic strengths that give a large response for one input and a very small one for another input. The cell will 'know' something. The question would then be: how do you design a rule so that the cell will learn to recognize a particular input? To correspond to the results in the visual cortex, you want the cell to learn to respond to one pattern and not to respond at all to others when in an environment with

Fig. 1.1. The inputs $d_1, \ldots, d_n$ from axons via *synaptic junctions* $m_1, \ldots, m_n$ produce local depolarizations $m_1d_1, \ldots, m_nd_n$ that are integrated in the cell body to produce a *firing rate*, c. The actual inputs and outputs are rapidly varying functions of time (spikes occur with durations of approximately 10^{-3}). Relevant time intervals for learning and memory are thought to be of the order of 0.5 s. We assume that for learning the relevant inputs and outputs are time averaged frequencies.

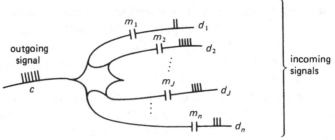

all patterns present. On the other hand, for non-patterned input, a cell's response should not prefer one pattern over another (Fig. 1.3).

Hebb originally proposed that if synaptic junctions change as a product of the output and input, they produce certain interesting correlation properties. It is now generally acknowledged that they cannot change in exactly this way. Still, one question is: is the post-synaptic variable involved? Some experimentalists say no, while every theoretician says yes. Yet there is good experimental evidence, particularly that obtained by Singer and others, which shows this variable must be implicated. If it is implicated, how? There are many other possibilities, particularly those involving what we call 'global' variables, for which there is good evidence.

We introduced a form of modification in which the change in m_j was a product of input d_j and a ϕ function. The properties of ϕ are that if for a given input the output is too low, the synaptic strength decreases in proportion to the input. On the other hand, if above this modification threshold the output is large enough, then the synaptic strength increases proportionally to the input. To explain the existing experimental results we need a negative and a positive region. In addition, to give the system the proper stability properties, it is required that the threshold move back and forth and that, to give it the most beautiful properties of all, it is required that it be a non-linear function of the average output of the cell. We always chose $\bar{c}^2$, but it could actually be $\bar{c}$ to any power that is larger than unity (Fig. 1.4).

Fig. 1.2. The cell output is a non-linear function of $m \cdot d$. In the linear region, we can write $c = \Sigma_{j=1}^{N} m_j d_j = m \cdot d$ where m_j is a somewhat idealized 'synaptic junction'.

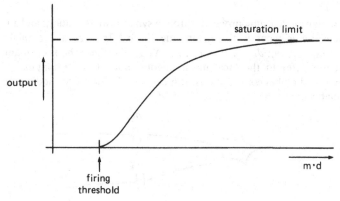

Let me describe the basic properties of the system. Suppose you have a two-dimensional system d^1 and d^2, that is, two inputs, so that the space of inputs can be spanned by these two vectors. You will then have four fixed points. One obtains a set of non-linear coupled differential equations. The non-linearity arises because all the ms are coupled to one another through the cs. If you have only two inputs d^1 and d^2, you look for fixed points in the space. Now the fixed points occur when ϕ is zero. Recall that ϕ is zero when the output is zero, or when the output is at threshold. If you count them up, this gives four fixed points for two dimensions. These four fixed points have different properties. We call m_1^* and m_2^* the selective fixed points. Why selective? It is because if the synapses acquire those strengths, they give you maximum output for one of the inputs and zero output for the other. And it is very easy to see geometrically, because if m_1^* lies perpendicular to d^2, when d^2 comes in you get zero. When d^1 comes in, you get a response. When m_2^* is perpendicular to d^1, you get zero for d^1 and a response for d^2. This is what Kohonen called an optimal mapping; d^1 and d^2 do not have to be orthogonal. In this respect it is a self-organizing optimal mapping. There is another fixed point, which is non-selective because it responds to both d^1 and d^2, and yet another fixed point at zero (in other words the cell does not respond at all). Now the interesting and important question is: which fixed points are stable? The answer is that the only stable fixed points are the selective fixed points. So that wherever you start in the synaptic space, if you keep putting in d^1s and d^2s you eventually end up at the selective fixed points.

Note that in order to get selectivity the synaptic strengths have both positive and negative values, but coming into the cortical cell from the eye, one encounters only excitatory synapses. If we limit synaptic

Fig. 1.3. Neuron learning proceeds through synaptic modification, and an important question is what is the magnitude of $\dot{m}_j$? In general we might write $\dot{m}_j = F(d_j, \ldots, m_j; d_k, \ldots, c; \bar{c}, \ldots; X, Y, Z)$ where the four quantities in parentheses refer to the local instantaneous; quasi-local instantaneous; time averaged; and global contributions, respectively. In the BCM modification, this equation becomes: $\dot{m}_j = \phi(c, \bar{c}; X, Y, Z) d_j - \varepsilon m$.

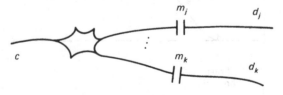

strengths to positive values, we would have partial but not complete selectivity. There are experimental results that show, if you shut off the inhibitory synapses by adding a chemical such as bicuculin, some of the selectivity is lost. This problem will be addressed later.

We can now model various experimental situations. We can have inputs from the left eye and the right eye, and then the output is a summation of left eye and right eye. We can have a normal environment in which we have patterned input to both eyes or, to contrast this, we can have monocular deprivation, patterns to one eye, noise to the other, and then we can run these simulations. We get results that correspond to the classical experimental results. For example, if in normal rearing, with both eyes open, the final stable state is at the selective fixed points in which the cells are binocular and selective, driven by the same pattern. If the eyes are closed, there is no development of selectivity (lid sutured or dark reared) and the cell is binocularly driven. For one eye open, the other eye closed – the very famous paradigm of monocular deprivation – selectivity develops to the open eye, while the closed eye is driven to zero. One instance in which the moving threshold is clearly necessary is in the situation of reverse suture. To get recovery, the threshold must move to a very low value.

In addition, there is a rather subtle connection between occular dominance and selectivity. How is it that, when both eyes are closed, the cell is not necessarily driven to zero, while when one eye is open and the other

Fig. 1.4. The modification threshold, θ_m, is a non-linear function of $\bar{c}$, the average output of the cell. We have used $\theta_m = (1/c_0)(\bar{c})^2$, but the precise form is not critical.

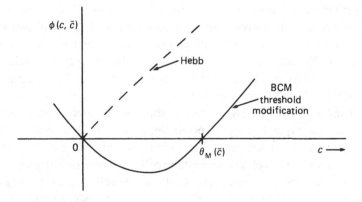

eye is closed, the response of the cell is driven to zero for the closed eye? From our point of view, the reason that it is not driven to zero when both eyes are closed is that the zero fixed point is unstable. But if one eye is closed and the other is open, once the open eye has become selective, the response of the cell is either close to zero or close to threshold. The ϕ function can be expanded close to zero and close to threshold and, depending on whether the input to the open eye is preferred or non-preferred, the appropriate expansion is at one point or the other. Now this expansion eventually results in a differential equation for the synapses between LGN and the closed eye that looks like this: $\dot{x}$ is plus or minus the noise squared times x, depending on whether the input to the open eye is preferred or non-preferred. Non-preferred inputs can only be achieved after the eye has become selective. In other words, before selectivity occurs, there is no driving of the closed eye to zero. And this gives you a correlation between ocular dominance and selectivity.

If one looks at some of the original results of Hubel and Wiesel, one can already see this correlation suggested. Recent experiments show a clear correlation between ocular dominance and selectivity, and this is precisely what the theory predicts.

This theory has been extended to include the situation in which there are many cells; in other words, where this is input from LGN to excitatory and inhibitory cortical cells and the excitatory and inhibitory cells are connected to one another via intracortical connections. We would like to restrict m, that is to say the inputs between LGN and the cortical cells, to positive values, since these synapses are excitatory.

The output of the jth cell is c_j, and we have an intracortical synapse L_{ij}. We should state that the cell firing rate involves not only being pushed through LGN by the inputs from the right eye and left eye, but also the intracortical connections; that of course is a rather complicated problem which was analysed by myself and a former student, Chris Scofield. We separated excitatory and inhibitory synapses and got some very nice, new predictions. The analysis was complex and we had to rely on extensive computer simulation. This led us to introduce what we call a 'mean field approximation' for the cortical network. Those familiar with theories of magnetism will immediately see where this comes from. The essential idea is that the typical cell gets specific input from LGN and also from large numbers of cortical cells. The other cortical cells are also often pushed by LGN. It is well known that the collaterals can be fairly long, so we replace the effect of many cortical cells on the cell we are watching by an average. In doing that, we simplify things enormously, and finally we get consistency conditions. The cell i is pushed by the LGN inputs, and then there is a kind of modulatory effect, an average field of the rest of the network. And this average field of the rest of the network is of course also pushed by the LGN inputs.

Very simply stated, previously we have $c = md$, whereas now we have $c = (m - \alpha)d$, and previously we said that m goes to certain fixed points m^*. The fundamental theorem that can be proved is that in the mean field theory, m goes to fixed points that are $m^* + \alpha$.

We can show that all the old fixed points are fixed points here, and that the stability of the fixed points is the same. Thus what was stable before is stable here. Recall that the problem previously was that in the m space one had to find a fixed point, which was inaccessible because of the necessity for negative components. Now, if α is sufficiently inhibitory, this effectively translates the co-ordinates, and all of the values of m^* are now available. So the fixed points will be available with excitatory synapses between LGN and cortical cells if the average inhibition of the network is sufficient.

A question that arises in learning theory is: do all synapses modify in the same way? We do not know the answer, of course, but we have been able to get away with assuming that we have modification between the LGN cortical synapses, and that there is no modification whatsoever among the inhibitory intracortical synapses. This makes the theory very beautiful and very easy to handle.

I would like to summarize some of these ideas. The first point I have already made: the fixed points of the old theory now becomes available, assuming only LGN-cortical excitatory synapses if the network is sufficiently inhibitory. We find that most learning can occur in the LGN cortical synapses. The inhibitory GABAergic cortical–cortical synapses need not modify at all. An experiment was done by Bear and Ebner, at Brown, testing how these GABAergic synapses change under severe conditions of monocular deprivation. They were disappointed to find no such changes. But this was a most welcome result; the fact that we can get away without much inhibitory modification opens the wonderful possibility that the major modification is just for the excitatory LGN cortical synapses. This makes it a much easier problem to treat, mathematically. Some non-modifiable LGN cortical synapses are required. An obvious candidate for these are the synapses onto the inhibitory cells, which go onto shafts rather than spines. It has been seen, in a preliminary experiment by Singer, that the synapses onto the shafts seem to be more resistant, as he put it, than those onto spines.

One of the interesting new results of this theory is that, in binocular deprivation zero is still an unstable fixed point, but the zero is now constructed in the following way: the zero output of the cell comes both from the LGN cortical synapses and from the network synapses which we have taken to be inhibitory. Suppose we suppressed the inhibitory network synapses; then we might expect that cells we could not previously see would suddenly emerge. Such a result has in fact been obtained. Freeman has also shown that an increase in excitability causes cells to appear where they weren't otherwise seen. One of the most interesting results occurs in monocular deprivation. Recall from the previous analysis, that in monocular deprivation the closed eye response goes to zero. And remember that α was previously zero, so that the closed eye result goes to zero only if the closed-eye LGN cortical synapses went to zero. In the mean field theory, the closed-eye response also goes to zero; however that means that the LGN-cortical synapses do not go to zero, but rather, go to α. Therefore, in this theory, we get the monocular deprivation results, but we get them without the LGN–cortical synapses going to zero. So that if inhibition is suppressed, we should get some response for the closed eye. This is in agreement with a result of Sileto and others in which they used bicuculin, which shuts off the inhibitory response, and found an increase in cells responsive to the closed eye. This could be further investigated by post-stimulus histogram, which reveals separate excitatory and inhibitory effects. This makes it possible, even in cells giving an average output of zero, to see excitatory and inhibitory effects, so one can separate the effects of excitatory and inhibitory cells.

In a molecular model we need, among other things, a candidate for the modification threshold, so that the synapses increase above θm, and decrease below θm. Further, θm must vary with the average activity of the cell. Such ideas are being developed actively now by Bear, Ebner and myself at Brown. We are pursuing the idea of using the distinction between the NMDA receptors and the non-NMDA receptors. On the post-synaptic membrane, the NMDA receptors are ones that allow calcium to enter. We are trying to link this with the threshold, θm, and are trying to determine if that threshold varies with the previous experience of the cell.

In summary, what I would like to say is that we propose that we have a theoretical account of the way a little piece of cortex can evolve with experience. There are some dramatic simplifications that would be wonderful, if true. The theory does seem to account for a large variety of the data that already exist and one of the exciting possibilities for the future is that we can find molecular models that underly these assumptions. If all comes together in this happy way, you can be sure I will be talking about this subject for a long, long time.

2

Representation of sensory information in self-organizing feature maps, and the relation of these maps to distributed memory networks

TEUVO KOHONEN

2.1 Is there enough motivation for a solid-state physics approach to the brain?

One of the salient features of the brain networks is that anatomical sections of a few millimetres width, taken from different parts of the cortex, look roughly similar by their texture. This observation might motivate a theoretical approach in which principles of solid-state physics are applied to the analysis of the collective states of neural networks. Such a step, however, should be made with extreme care. I am first trying to point out a few characteristics of the neural tissue which are similar to those of, or distinguish it from non-living solids.

Similarities. There is a dense feedback connectivity between neighbouring neural units, which corresponds to interaction forces between atoms or molecules in solids.

Generation and propagation of brain waves seem to support a continuous-medium view of the tissue.

Differences. In addition to local, random feedback there exist plenty of directed connectivities, 'projections', between different neural areas. As a whole, the brain is a complex self-controlling system in which global feedback control actions often override the local 'collective' effects.

Although the geometric structure of the neural tissue looks uniform, there exist plenty of specific biochemical and physiological differences between cells and connections. For instance, there exist some 40 different types of neural connection, distinguished by the particular chemical transmitter substances involved in signal transmission, and these chemicals vary from one part of the brain to another.

It is also difficult to see how the collective-state models could be applicable to the description of high-level intellectual functions or cognitive states, in which complex global experiences of the organism are reflected. For this reason I am rather suspicious about the applicability of the simplest models as such to problems in which concepts with a high level of coding and specificity, e.g., linguistic items, are applied. My personal view is that one has to look at the neural circuits as signal-processing stages, which decode and interpret concomitant signals gradually, in many steps. Most clearly such processing is visible in early sensory stages, whereas, although similar principles might be applied on higher levels, too, their interpretation with our present formalisms is very difficult.

Many experimentalists have criticized the theoretical models because they do not contain all the neural components that are known to exist in a particular area, or because high-level cognitive states are not demonstrated. This, on the other hand, is a fundamental misinterpretation of the modelling approach. For the understanding of the basic phenomena, modern science always aims at *idealized experiments* in which, for the study of one or a few factors at a time, the influence of the other factors ought to be eliminated. The theoretical model may also be simplified in its geometric structure or signal transformation function, if it is only regarded as a pure *case example* of an infinite number of its possible realizations.

In the network models discussed in this paper, a compromise between biological accuracy and theoretical clarity has been made. The main purpose has been to demonstrate a phenomenon that can be made to occur under certain conditions. These conditions seem to be fulfilled in many biological systems.

2.2 Physically motivated system equations for neurons

The first choice that one has to make in modelling concerns the geometric size of the section of a network to be taken into consideration. I do not consider any collective-network model referring to an area larger than, say, 5 mm in diameter as realistic. Then, however, one may be justified to neglect the differences in signal delays within the area in consideration. This then means that evoked potentials and brain waves cannot be demonstrated by such simplified models; the latter are regarded as macroscopic phenomena which arise from system properties. The observed wave-like dynamic phenomena very probably result from complex processing operations on signals during their passage between the thalamic nuclei and cortical areas, whereby they may not represent the most elementary processing functions at all.

The second requirement to be imposed on a model is clear definition of its input and output signals; the state of the network cannot simply be 'assumed'. The only reasonable definition of signal intensity is impulse frequency on an axon, which complies with the triggering frequency, or the 'activity' of a neural cell from which this axon emerges. Input to the network is connected through a set of afferent axons; if the size of the network is restricted to a few millimetres, it is not a poor approximation to assume that the input axons spread their signals to most, if not all, principal cells of this network. In addition to afferent axons, and the efferent axons which transmit signals to other system parts, the network further contains internal feedback connections (axon collaterals and feedbacks through interneurons). Each output is then a function of the inputs and other outputs; this seems to be a fundamental property of neural networks, and the transfer function of such a feedback system is not quite trivial.

Because of the global control actions of the brain, it is neither easy to measure or even define the transformation of signals in a neural cell, i.e., its *transfer function*. One of the biggest difficulties seems to be that the transfer parameters are not unique; the chemical state of the network may modulate them. Long-term changes, corresponding to learning effects, are superposed on the short-term modulation.

Traditionally, the neuron has been regarded as a thresholding device which somehow forms a weighted sum of its input signals and triggers an output signal. The input weights are thereby identified with the synaptic connectivities made by the afferent axons on the neuron. The output signal has been assumed zero if the sum remains below a certain threshold value, and one (or another constant) if the sum exceeds the threshold. I think it is time to abandon this view. Although the 'all-or-none' principle may hold for the triggering of individual pulses, it is the *impulse frequency* which defines the neural signal value. The neural impulses usually occur in sporadic bursts or volleys, and the averaged number of pulses generated by a neuron over any interval of time is a continuous positive function of the input signals. The output could only be regarded as binary if the impulse frequency would be flipped between its maximum value and zero, which is simply not true. If the output frequency, or triggering rate η_i of neuron i were related to the input pulse trains with frequencies ξ_j, respectively, then the transfer function of the neuron should be expressed as some continuous function

$$\eta_i = \eta_i(\xi_1, \xi_2, \ldots, \mu_{i1}, \mu_{i2}, \ldots), \tag{1}$$

where the μ_{ij} represent some coupling strengths of input signals to this neuron.

For the present discussion it is helpful to assume some analytical form for η_i, e.g.,

$$\eta_i = \sigma\left(\sum_{j=1}^{n} \mu_{ij}\xi_j - \theta_i\right), \tag{2}$$

where σ is a monotonically increasing scalar function ('sigmoid function'), with saturation limits at zero and some positive limit, and θ_i is a 'threshold' value. The scalar-product form in the argument of σ is not mandatory, as long as the neuron can somehow act as a *feature-sensitive unit*. Assume that $x = (\xi_1, \xi_2, \ldots, \xi_n)$ is the input vector, and $m_i = (\mu_{i1}, \mu_{i2}, \ldots, \mu_{in})$ is a parametric *weight vector* of neuron i. Any functional form, even a nonlinear one, for which μ_i is a maximum when x *matches best* with m_i will be acceptable for the 'transfer function' of the neuron.

Adaptation or *learning* in this network corresponds to changes in the μ_{ij} that are proportional to the occurring signals. According to the classical hypothesis of Hebb (1949), the connection strength between two cells increases if and only if the presynaptic activity (input signal) and post-synaptic activity (output of the neuron) are simultaneously high. In the traditional modelling notation, if, e.g., eqn (2) is taken to represent the transfer function, then

$$d\mu_{ij}/dt = \alpha\eta_i\xi_j, \tag{3}$$

where α is a 'plasticity parameter'. Obviously, this 'Hebb's law' needs some modification, first of all because it describes an irreversible effect; since both η_i and ξ_j are positive semidefinite, all the μ_{ij} will increase until the adaptable resources are exhausted. One modification of this law is to assume that the connectivity resources at a neuron are finite, and the incoming signals compete on them. Then, in effect (for details, cf., e.g., Kohonen, 1984), the factor ξ_j in Eqn (3) would be replaced by a term of the form $\xi_j - \xi_{jb}$, making changes in μ_{ij} positive or negative, i.e., reversible. In further analysis we may ignore ξ_{jb} if we rescale ξ_j; then we shall remember that the redefined ξ_j may attain positive or negative values. Another modification that is both natural and useful is inclusion of some *active, nonlinear forgetting* term to Eqn (3). Active forgetting means that this term is nonzero only if η_i is nonzero. For instance, we may write

$$d\mu_{ij}/dt = \alpha\eta_i\xi_j - \beta(\eta_i)\mu_{ij}, \tag{4}$$

where $\beta(\eta_i)$ is an otherwise arbitrary function, except that the constant term in its Taylor expansion shall be equal to zero. For many choices of the analytical form of β, Eqn (4) has been found to normalize the μ_{ij} such that the lengths of the vectors m_i will asymptotically tend to values which only depend on α and the serial coefficients of β, not on the signals. The latter result means that the comparison of x and m_i for the degree of their match can be based on the comparison of either inner products $m_i^T x$ or the lengths of the vectorial differences $\|x - m_i\|$.

2.3 Basic network structure for neural models

Perhaps the simplest nontrivial network organization in which rather complicated phenomena can already occur is depicted in Fig. 2.1. It may be interesting to compare this structure with a similar schematic representation of the cortical architectonics drawn by some neuroanatomists (cf., e.g., Braitenberg, 1974). In reality, the cells should be imagined to form a two-dimensional layer; in Fig. 2.1 this layer is drawn one-dimensional for clarity. The input lines (afferent axons) have been assumed to make connections with all the cells in this piece of network; such an assumption is not necessary in principle because similar effects are demonstrable with even randomly made input connections (e.g., Kohonen, 1982a). The regular input structure, on the other hand, represents a theoretical case

Fig. 2.1. The basic structure of neural circuits used in brain models.

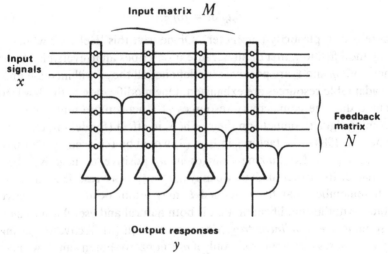

Input matrix M

Input signals x

Feedback matrix N

Output responses y

which allows a simpler mathematical treatment. Furthermore, in artificial devices (e.g., Kohonen, Mäkisara & Saramäki, 1984) such a complete connectivity matrix M has been found to yield the best signal processing accuracy, whereby it may be taken as the 'ideal case'.

The structure of the feedback network, denoted by matrix N in Fig. 2.1, may also be simplified in different ways for different purposes. We may assume, as made in the detailed example to be discussed below, that the matrix elements of N only depend on the distance between a pair of cells.

The dynamical behaviour of the system of Fig. 2.1 may be described by Eqns (5), (6) and (7). Let x be the vector of input signals, and y the vector of output signals, respectively; alternatively, y may be regarded as the set of activity states of the cells. Then

$$\mathrm{d}y/\mathrm{d}t = f(x, y, M, N) \qquad (5)$$

is a differential equation that describes the *relaxation of network activity* due to the feedback. If x were held constant, and if M and N were temporarily constant, too, then y should be stipulated to converge to some asymptotic state. Relaxation in neural circuits is a fast phenomenon, which will settle down in a few hundreds of milliseconds. The physical variables associated with relaxation consist of electrical potentials, ionic concentrations, and relatively simple organic chemicals such as neurotransmitters.

The parametric variables M and N which describe neural connectivities may change due to the occurring signals (cell activities), too, giving rise to *adaptive phenomena*. The differential equations relating to input and feedback connectivities, respectively, may be written

$$\mathrm{d}M/\mathrm{d}t = g(x, y, M) \qquad (6)$$

and

$$\mathrm{d}N/\mathrm{d}t = h(y, N). \qquad (7)$$

The physical changes associated with M and N correspond to changes in proteins and anatomical structures such as branching of the cells; accordingly, the time constants are much longer, on the average of the order of days or weeks. It is possible that there also exist simpler biochemical factors relating to M and N, which react to signals even faster, say, in seconds or minutes; such factors might then constitute the link between short-term and long-term memories. In this discussion, however, we shall ignore all the other adaptive phenomena except the long-term changes, and imagine that they primarily take place in the input matrix M.

2.4 Self-organizing feature maps

The brain is a collection of very different functions; these are as diverse as
the biological behaviour itself. Some of the neural circuits are needed for
the centralized control of the energy supply, i.e., cardiovascular functions, respiration, and metabolism; many emergency functions, in the
form of stimulus-response-relations, are probably also stored. However,
for the control of more complex behaviour it is necessary to imagine or
forecast sensory phenomena or other related occurrences, and this is not
possible without memory. The mental images must correspond to some
organized states of the brain, whereas it is self-evident that memory does
not store images in photographic form.

One has to realize that there are two different aspects in a discussion of
memory:

  (1) the internal representation ('coding') of sensory information in the
        brain networks;
  (2) the memory mechanism which stores and retrieves such represen-
        tations.

Physiological studies have indicated that the brain encodes sensory
information, at least in the primary sensory areas, in various geometrically organized 'maps'. One can find isolated areas on the cortex over
which, as it were, a two-dimensional coordinate system is defined. These
coordinates often correspond to well-defined dimensions of sensory
experiences such as topographic coordinates of the body, pitch of audible
tones, hue and saturation of colour, etc. Various feature-specific cells
exist everywhere in the brain, but a clear order along specified features
has only been found in the primary sensory areas. This does not exclude
the possibility that ordered maps would exist on higher levels, too;
however, the metric of such representations which defines the order may
be more complex.

In this presentation I shall demonstrate that the basic network model of
Fig. 2.1, with proper feedback connectivities and system equations,
automatically forms such geometric representations of feature dimensions of the input signals. This function seems to be independent of the
sensory modality, whereby even in artificial systems, many different
kinds of maps can be formed (e.g., Kohonen, 1982c). It seems that each
part of the map, in a certain optimal (nonlinear) way, seeks the dominant
parameters of the input signals and displays them on the map. We have
mostly dealt with two-dimensional maps on account of their easy visualization, whereas the method is readily generalizable to arbitrary topologies.

The structure of the self-organizing network is otherwise identical with that of Fig. 2.1, except that the cell layer is two-dimensional, and the feedback connectivity matrix N is assumed constant. In accordance with Eqn (1), the output of each cell is now described by a functional law of the type

$$\eta_i = \sigma\left(\sum_{j=1}^{n} \mu_{ij}\xi_j + \sum_{k \in S_i} \nu_{ik}\eta_k - \theta_i \right), \tag{8}$$

where S_i is the set of cells which have feedback connections to cell i. The weights ν_{ik} are assumed constant, with values which are often nicknamed the 'Mexican hat function': if cell k lies within a certain distance of cell i, then ν_{ik} is a function of this distance only, in a way depicted in Fig. 2.2.

Eqn (8), combined with Eqn (4), would then completely define the self-organizing process in which the set of values μ_{ij} will be optimally tuned to the feature coordinates. The mathematical discussion of this form, however, would be very cumbersome, and numerical computation based on these equations would also become heavy. For this reason we have significantly simplified this process, retaining only the most important functional dependencies in computation. At the same time the process became more effective!

One of the most central phenomena associated with self-organization is a clustering effect which strongly enhances the activity patterns over the network. We shall first demonstrate this effect in the 'relaxation approximation' whereby the parameters μ_{ij} in Eqn (8) are assumed constant. Their values may be assumed random, with a slight bias such that for any

Fig. 2.2. The 'Mexican hat' function.

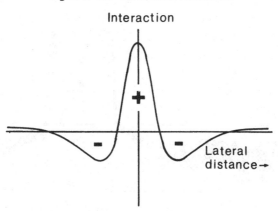

input x one may perceive a shallow maximum among the η_i. (Such a bias would be formed already during the first steps of the original adaptive process.) If, for simplicity again, we demonstrate this effect in a one-dimensional network, we can see how the particular feedback described by the 'Mexican hat function' will enhance the initial distribution of activity. With a temporarily stationary input x, an activity 'bubble' will be formed at a location where $m_i^T x$, the inner product of the input vector x and the weight vector of unit i, was roughly maximum (Fig. 2.3). The form of the 'bubble' is very stable, and only its location depends on x and the m_i. This fact is now used for the simplification of the process equations: we *postulate* the formation of a 'bubble', with fixed radius, at a location where $m_i^T x$ is maximum. However, taking into account the discussion in connection with Eqn (4), namely, that the adaptive process tends to normalize the vectors m_i to constant length, we can further simplify the algorithm, e.g., in the following form. Let us start with arbitrary, random initial values μ_{ij}. Let samples of input vector x be drawn from a defined statistical density function $p(x)$. For each sample we apply the following two computational rules:

(1) A stationary activity 'bubble' with some fixed radius is assumed to be formed in the network at a place where $\|x - m_i\|$ is minimum.

   If $\|x - m_c\| = \min_i \{\|x - m_i\|\}$, then N_c is defined as the set of cells corresponding to the active 'bubble'.

Fig. 2.3. Formation of 'bubbles' of activity over a one-dimensional network.

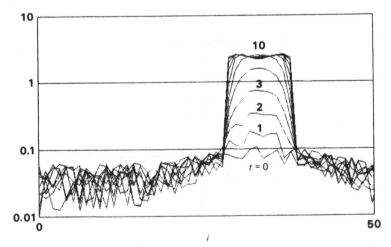

(2) If the μ_{ij} are changing according to Eqn (8), and if the activities η_i saturate to zero or high limits, then Eqn (8) can be written, with proper scaling, in two separate parts (notice that $\eta_i \in \{0, 1\}$ and $\beta(\eta_i) \in \{0, 1\}$):

$$\left.\begin{array}{ll} \mathrm{d}m_i/\mathrm{d}t = \alpha(x - m_i) & \text{for } i \in N_c \text{ (inside the bubble),} \\ \mathrm{d}m_i/\mathrm{d}t = 0 & \text{for } i \notin N_c \text{ (outside the bubble).} \end{array}\right\} \quad \text{(a)}$$

The above algorithm has been used in all practical simulations and self-organizing experiments. Even in this simplified form its mathematical treatment has been shown to be difficult. This is a Markov process, but due to the geometric constraints, its convergence conditions are very complicated. A few proofs for low-dimensional cases have recently been represented (e.g., Kohonen, 1982b; Kohonen & Oja, 1982; Cottrell & Forth, 1984, 1986; Ritter & Schulten, 1986).

2.5 Simulations

We have demonstrated by a number of different experiments (cf. Kohonen, 1982c; Kohonen, 1984; Kohonen *et al.*, 1984) that the above process is able to form two-dimensional 'maps' of the input signals x such that the most important feature dimensions that are present in the statistical distribution of x will be displayed as coordinates in the map. The following result is first used for illustration. The inner ear, as is well known, performs a frequency analysis of the acoustic waveforms and sends the result, an approximation of the spectrum, to the brain via a bundle of axons. By analogy, we collected samples of natural continuous speech, and each input vector x consisted of a 15-channel acoustic spectrum of the speech waveform, integrated over a 25.6-millisecond interval of time. The 15-dimensional vectors x were connected to a two-dimensional network model of the same type as Fig. 2.1 in parallel. The responses from the 'map' to different acoustic spectra were labelled according to the location of the centroid of the 'bubble' and the corresponding phoneme present in speech. The 'neurons' of the map were shown to learn the responses to the different phonemes in an orderly fashion (Fig. 2.4). (The 'neurons' in this demonstration were organized in a hexagonal lattice corresponding to the letters.) We have used such phoneme maps for the recognition of continuous speech, and practical microprocessor equipment has already been constructed (Torkkola & Riittinen, 1986).

The purpose of the next example is to demonstrate that a map of the environment of a subject can be formed in a self-organizing process whereby the observations can be mediated by very rude, nonlinear, and mutually dependent mechanisms such as arms and detectors of their bending angles. In this demonstration, two artificial arms, with two joints each, were used for the feeling of a planar surface. The geometry of the setup is illustrated in Fig. 2.5. The tips of both arms touched the same point which during the training process was selected at random, with a uniform distribution over the framed area. At the same time, two signals, proportional to the bending angles, were obtained from each arm; these signals (ξ_1, ξ_2, ξ_3, ξ_4), were led to a self-organizing array of the earlier type, and adaptation of its parameters took place.

The lattice of lines which has been drawn onto the framed area in this picture connects those points which represent *virtual images* of the weight vectors μ_{ij}, i.e., showing to which point on the plane each 'neuron' became most sensitive; each crossing thus corresponds to one cell of the neural network model. The lines are used to indicate which units are neighbours in the network. When a particular crossing point on the lattice is touched, the corresponding 'neuron' gives the maximum response. The resulting map was tested for both arms separately, i.e., by letting each of them touch the plane and looking at which point it had to be in order to cause the maximum response at a particular 'neuron'. These two maps coincided almost perfectly.

Fig. 2.4. Two-dimensional map of Finnish phonemes. The double labels mean mapping of different phonemes onto the same location.

a	a	a	ah	h	æ	æ	ø	ø	e	e	e
	o	a	a	h	r	æ	l	ø	y	y	j	i
o	o	a	h	r	r	r	g	g	y	j	i
o	o	m	a	r	m	n	m	n	j	i	i
l	o	u	h	v	vm	n	n	h	hj	j	j
	l	u	v	v	p	d	d	t	r	h	hi	j
.	.	u	v	tk	k	p	p	p	r	k	s
.	.	v	k	pt	t	p	t	p	h	s	s

2.6 Discussion

The first question, naturally, concerns the occurrence of 'maps' in the brain and their real form. Actually the name 'map' is used in brain physiology in two senses. Firstly, several kinds of *ordered* maps have been found in the primary sensory areas, and they very closely resemble the artificial maps reported in this paper. Secondly, there exist everywhere in the brain feature-selective cells that are scattered more or less randomly over a particular area, without clear topographic organization. It might happen, however, that even in the latter case the cells have been arranged according to some ultrametric order, although very little attention has been paid to this in physiological recordings.

One might ask for what purpose such maps are necessary. There is a clear answer to this: if the feature-selective functions are separated spatially and ordered according to some metrics, their responses become more logical and selective than if these functions were distributed among common neural units. Spatial separation is also advantageous for the control of motor functions which are organized in similar maps.

The most important and at the same time very difficult problem in the processing of sensory information seems to be how the neural system can optimally operate on the vague stochastic signals provided by the sensory organs. Among many alternatives for analyzing systems, we have found that the self-organizing maps described in this paper yield the best accuracy in simple recognition tasks. This is perhaps due to their ability to automatically allocate an optimal number of computing resources to the different feature dimensions, and due to the accurate nonlinear determination of the classification functions. The primary sensory areas of the

Fig. 2.5. Self-ordered mapping of the input plane of a feeler mechanism.

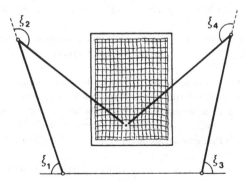

brain seem to be organized similarly, along various feature dimensions of the sensory signals.

There is some doubt about the same principle being applicable to higher-level information-processing in the brain. Although it is possible to demonstrate the formation of hierarchical data structures in the artificial maps, there is still no conclusive evidence about similar high-level maps occurring in the brain. It seems as if the higher cognitive states were more dynamic and not localizable; on the other hand, localized responses to certain perceived conceptual items have been found. Perhaps it would be safer to restrict these maps, at least in the beginning, to early sensory information processing and to relate them to experimental findings.

On the other hand, it might perhaps be too much to expect that small-sized models like these maps would already exhibit cognitive abilities. They should be regarded as the basic components in biological information processing, in a similar sense as logic circuits facilitate high-level abstract information processing in digital computers.

References

Braitenberg, V. (1974). 'On the representation of objects and their relations in the brain.' In *Physics and Mathematics of the Neurons Systems* (eds. Conrad, M., Güttinger, W., & Dal Cin, M.). Springer-Verlag, *Lecture Notes in Biomathematics*, Berlin, Heidelberg, New York, pp. 290–8.

Cottrell, M. & Forth, J. C. (1984). *Etude d'un processus d'auto-organisation*. Université de Paris-Sud, Report 84 T 57.

Cottrell, M. & Forth, J. C. (1986). 'A stochastic model of retinotopy: a self-organizing process.' *Biological Cybernetics*, 53, 405–11.

Hebb, D. (1949). *Organization of Behaviour*, Wiley, New York.

Kohonen, T. (1982a). 'Self-organized formation of topologically correct feature maps.' *Biological Cybernetics*, 43, 59–69.

Kohonen, T. (1982b). 'Analysis of a simple self-organizing process.' *Biological Cybernetics*, 44, 135–40.

Kohonen, T. (1982c). 'Clustering, taxonomy, and topological maps of patterns'. In *Proc. 6th Int. Conference on Pattern Recognition*, Munich, Germany, 19–22 October, 1982, pp. 114–28.

Kohonen, T. (1984). *Self-Organization and Associative Memory*. Springer-Verlag, *Series in Information Sciences*, Vol. 8, Berlin, Heidelberg, New York, Tokyo.

Kohonen, T., Mäkisara, K. & Saramäki, T. (1984). 'Phonotopic maps – insightful representation of phonological features for speech recognition'. In *Proc. 7th Int. Conference on Pattern Recognition*, Montreal, Canada, 30 July–2 August, 1984, pp. 182–5.

Kohonen, T. & Oja, E. (1982). *A Note on a Simple Self-Organizing Process*. Helsinki University of Technology Report TKK-F-A474.

Ritter, H. & Schulten, K. (1986). 'On the stationary state of Kohonen's self-organizing sensory mapping. *Biological Cybernetics*, **54**, 99–106.
Torkkola, K. & Riittinen, H. (1986). *A Microprocessor-Based Word Recognition System for Large Vocabularies*. Helsinki University of Technology Report TKK-F-A591.

3

Excitable dendritic spine clusters: nonlinear synaptic processing

WILFRID RALL and IDAN SEGEV

3.1 Passive cable properties of dendrites

The modeling of dendritic trees was carefully presented and discussed in earlier publications; only a few points will be summarized here. In Rall, 1962 it was shown how the partial differential equation for a passive nerve cable can represent an entire dendritic tree, and how this can be generalized from cylindrical to tapered branches and trees; this paper also showed how to incorporate synaptic conductance input into the mathematical model, and presented several computed examples. In Rall, 1964 it was shown how the same results can be obtained with compartmental modeling of dendritic trees; this paper also pointed out that such compartmental models are not restricted to the assumption of uniform membrane properties, or to the family of dendritic trees which transforms to an equivalent cylinder or an equivalent taper and, consequently, that such models can be used to represent any arbitrary amount of nonuniformity in branching pattern, in membrane properties, and in synaptic input that one chooses to specify. Recently, this compartmental approach has been applied to detailed dendritic anatomy represented as thousands of compartments (Bunow *et al.*, 1985; Segev *et al.*, 1985; Redman & Clements, personal communication).

Significant theoretical predictions and insights were obtained by means of computations with a simple ten-compartment model (Rall, 1964). One computation predicted different shapes for the voltage transients expected at the neuron soma when identical brief synaptic inputs are delivered to different dendritic locations; these predictions (and their elaboration, Rall, 1967) have been experimentally confirmed in many laboratories (see Jack *et al.*, 1975; Redman, 1976; Rall, 1977). Another computation demonstrated significantly different results at the soma for two different spatio-temporal patterns of synaptic input to the dendrites (i.e. the same amount of input produced a different output; see Fig. 7 of Rall, 1964). The distal-to-proximal sequence produced a larger voltage amplitude at the soma; given a suitable threshold, this input pattern could be discriminated. The proximal-to-distal sequence produced a longer lasting voltage of lower amplitude; this could be useful to bias the neuron to be fired by a small additional input. It may be noted that this theoretical prediction provided the basis for an interpretation of 'asymmetric' firing patterns in cochlear neurons by Erulkar *et al.* (1968). Other computations provided insight into the conditions for either linear or nonlinear combinations of the effects of synaptic inputs delivered to different dendritic locations, for both excitatory and inhibitory synaptic inputs (Figs. 8 and 9 of Rall, 1964). Further discussion and references can be found in Rall, 1964, 1967, 1977; Jack *et al.*, 1975; Redman, 1976; Rall & Segev, 1985, 1987.

Here Fig. 3.1 illustrates an idealized dendritic neuron consisting of six equal dendritic trees. Current is injected at a single branch terminal designated (I); this input branch is distinguished from its sibling branch (S), and its first and second cousin branches (C-1) and (C-2). The resulting steady voltage distribution in the various branches of the input tree (shown in this diagram) was computed from the general solution of this problem (Rall & Rinzel, 1973).

One noteworthy feature of these results is the contrasting decrement of voltage in the input branch and its sibling branch. Both branches have the same length and diameter in this idealized tree. However, the input branch is open to a large current flow into its parent branch; this permits a large flow of current along its cytoplasmic core resulting in a steep voltage decrement along the length of the input branch. In contrast, the sealed terminal of the sibling branch allows zero current to flow out of that end; also, little current flows across the high resistance of the cylindrical branch membrane; with so little current, this branch is almost isopotential. This contrast applies also to dendritic spines with interesting functional consequences (see below).

Another feature of these results is the contrast in input resistance values when the distal input location is compared with a central input location (at the soma). In this diagram, the dashed curve shows the lower voltage values obtained when the same amount of current is injected at the soma as that previously injected at the distal branch. In this example, the distal input resistance is 16 times larger than the somatic input resistance, and still larger factors can result from additional orders of

28   *W. Rall & I. Segev*

branching (Rall & Rinzel, 1973). This contrast in input resistance and its effect on voltage amplitude (i.e. local synaptic depolarization) is very important to the attainment of threshold conditions in excitable dendritic spines located on distal dendritic branches.

3.2 Dendritic spines and spine stem resistance

The existence of dendritic spines has been known for a hundred years, since the classical studies of Ramon y Cajal; however, the demonstration of synaptic contacts on spines was accomplished much later by means of electron microscopic observations (Gray, 1959). The variety in spine size and shape was demonstrated by Jones & Powell (1969) and by Peters & Kaiserman-Abramof (1970), as shown here in Fig. 3.2. Also included in

Fig. 3.1. Diagram of idealized neuron model composed of six dendritic trees, and plot of steady state voltage values for three different cases: current input at the soma (curve with short dashes), current input to a single distal branch terminal (input branch designated I; continuous curve), and the case of input divided equally among eight related branch terminals (I, S and cousins, C-1 and C-2; curve with long dashes). Modified from Rall & Rinzel (1973) which can be consulted for the mathematical statement and solution of this problem. The voltage scale is expressed relative to the product of the injected current and a reference input resistance (i.e. that of the dendritic trunk cylinder extended to semi-infinite length).

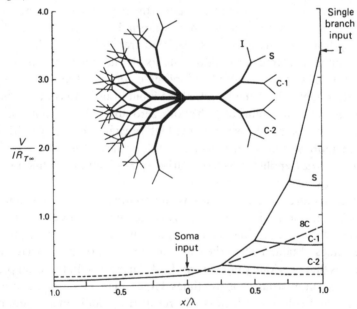

Fig. 3.2. Neuroanatomical montage prepared as slide in 1971 to introduce dendritic spines. Upper left shows dendritic branches covered with dendritic spines, from an 1897 study of cortical neurons by Berkley, following Ramon y Cajal. Upper right shows diagrammatic pyramidal cell together with enlarged drawings of spines and synapses, based upon electron microscopic observations, modified from Jones and Powell (1969). Lower left shows variety of dendritic spine shapes and sizes, modified from Peters and Kaiserman-Abramof (1970), while lower right gives our estimates (made in 1971) of the ranges of spine stem resistance values corresponding to the spines at left.

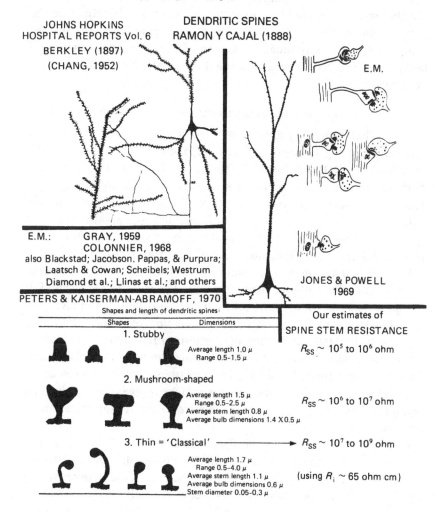

this diagram are our estimates of the electrical resistance to current flow inside the spine stem between the spine head and the spine base. These estimates depend on spine stem geometry and on the value of the intracellular resistivity, neither of which are known accurately; also, membranoùs inclusions within the spine stem cytoplasm may significantly increase the spine stem resistance (Wilson *et al.*, 1983; Miller *et al.*, 1985; Rall & Segev, 1987).

It was recognized by Chang (1952) that the high electrical resistance of the thin spine stem could be expected to attenuate the effect on the postsynaptic neuron of a synaptic input to a spine head. Because he expected significant attenuation, Chang concluded that summation of many synaptic inputs would be needed for effective excitation of such neurons.

3.3 Changing synaptic efficacy by changing spine stem resistance

The idea that changes in spine stem resistance values would change the relative weighting (synaptic efficacy) of many different synapses was introduced by Rall and Rinzel (1971*a,b*). At that time, they computed both steady state and transient responses for synaptic conductance input to a dendritic spine; this spine had only passive membrane, but a range of values was assumed for the amount of synaptic input and the values of spine stem resistance and other parameters (Rall, 1970, 1974, 1978; Rinzel, 1982; see also Diamond *et al.*, 1970; Jack *et al.*, 1975).

For steady state conditions, a simple Ohm's law argument can be used to explain the effect of spine stem resistance. This is illustrated by Fig. 3.3; the spine stem current is given by the intracellular voltage difference from spine head to spine base, divided by the spine stem resistance (this is true for both steady states and transients because more sophisticated analysis shows that negligible current crosses the membrane of the spine stem). This spine stem current times the input resistance (of the neuron at the branch input point where the spine is attached) gives the steady state voltage at this branch input point (relative to the resting intracellular reference potential).

Using physical intuition (or the algebra summarized in Fig. 3.3) one can see, for example, that the voltage at the spine base will equal exactly half that at the spine head for the special case where the spine stem resistance equals the branch input resistance; in other words, half of the total voltage drop occurs along the spine stem, while the other half occurs along the branches of the whole neuron (as illustrated in Fig. 3.1).

Both the graph and the equation in Fig. 3.3 show how the voltage ratio

Fig. 3.3. Diagram summarizing steady state implications of Ohm's law for the currents, voltages and resistances of one dendritic spine and the branch to which it is attached, also prepared as slide in 1971. The symbols, I_{SS} and R_{SS}, represent spine stem current and resistance; the voltages, V_{SH} and V_{BI}, are for the spine head and the spine base, which is also the branch input point having branch input resistance designated R_{BI}. The plot, at bottom displays the steady state ratio dependence defined by the equation above; it suggests an 'operating range' for adjustments of synaptic efficacy by changes of R_{SS} relative to R_{BI}.

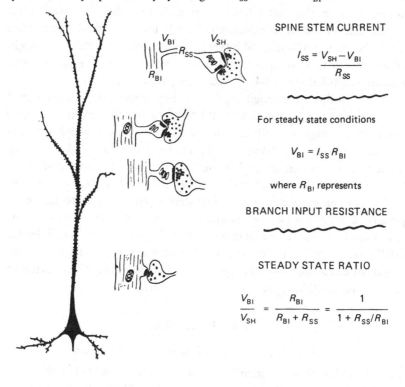

SPINE STEM CURRENT

$$I_{SS} = \frac{V_{SH} - V_{BI}}{R_{SS}}$$

For steady state conditions

$$V_{BI} = I_{SS} R_{BI}$$

where R_{BI} represents

BRANCH INPUT RESISTANCE

STEADY STATE RATIO

$$\frac{V_{BI}}{V_{SH}} = \frac{R_{BI}}{R_{BI} + R_{SS}} = \frac{1}{1 + R_{SS}/R_{BI}}$$

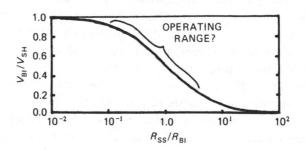

(spinebase–spinehead) depends on the ratio of spine stem resistance to branch input resistance; this illustrates the idea of an 'operating range' for changes in synaptic efficacy determined by changes in spine stem resistance (relative to branch input resistance). A qualitatively similar 'operating range' was found for transient responses to brief synaptic input, provided that the synaptic conductance input was sufficient for a large depolarization of the spine head. It may be noted that this did depend on nonlinearity in the spine head (approach to voltage saturation for depolarization due to conductance input); for very small inputs (that would be of no physiological interest) these nonlinear effects are negligible, as was later recognized also by others (Koch & Poggio, 1983; Kawato & Tsukahara, 1984; Turner, 1984; Wilson, 1984).

In view of this 'operating range' for changing spine stem resistance, it was suggested that evolution could have sacrificed maximal synaptic power in exchange for adjustability of relative synaptic weights. It was also pointed out that changes in the relative synaptic weights of large numbers of such synapses might contribute to neural plasticity underlying learning and memory (Rall & Rinzel, 1971a,b; Rall, 1974, 1978; Rinzel, 1982). This suggestion that the spine stem might be an important morphological locus for changes in synaptic weights did have an impact on anatomical studies; review of that literature is provided by Coss & Perkel (1985). Also noteworthy are the serial reconstructions of electron micrographs of dendritic branches, spines and synapses recently reported by Harris *et al.* (1985 and personal communication).

3.4 Excitable spines

3.4.1 Spines with excitable spine head membrane

The possibility that the membrane of dendritic spine heads might be excitable was assumed by Diamond *et al.* (1970). Although this possibility came up in various informal discussions at that time, it is noteworthy that Julian Jack analysed this possibility carefully and published an early and astute discussion (Jack *et al.*, 1975); he pointed out that for an optimal range of parameter values, an action potential at the spine head could result in amplification of the synaptic effect.

Not until 1983, to the best of our knowledge, did anyone carry out transient computations for the response of an excitable spine head to brief synaptic input; then two independent research groups reported preliminary results at a symposium of the Society for Neuroscience. To acknowledge this coincidence, we arranged to submit paired short papers, first to *Nature* and then to *Science* (only to be told that these results and insights were of insufficient interest to a wide audience); paired papers were finally published in *Brain Research* (Miller *et al.*, 1985; Perkel & Perkel, 1985). Since then various functional implications of excitable dendritic spines have been explored in collaborative discussions (with John Miller, John Rinzel, and Gordon Shepherd). Miller has focused more on the conditions under which excitable dendritic spine interactions could generate bursts of spikes (Malinow & Miller, 1984). Shepherd has focused more upon the possibility of saltatory propagation in distal dendrites, from one excitable spine head to another (Shepherd *et al.*, 1984). Our computations have focused on chain reaction effects in clusters of excitable spines (Rall & Segev, 1987).

3.4.2 Nonlinear dependence on spine stem resistance: excitable spines

Here Fig. 3.4 illustrates computed results for a single dendritic spine located on a dendrite having an input resistance of 262 megohms. A brief synaptic conductance input is delivered to the spine head and the resulting voltage transients are shown for the spine head (upper left) and for the spine base (lower left, with different amplitude scale); the solid lines are for excitable spine head membrane, while the dashed lines are corresponding controls for passive membrane. The left side of this diagram shows results for only two values of spine stem resistance: 630 megohms for (*a*) and 1000 megohms for (*b*). Comparing the two spine head action potentials at upper left, the shorter latency and greater amplitude of (*b*) indicate a secure spike, while the delay and the smaller amplitude of (*a*) indicate an insecure spike which barely succeeded under near threshold conditions. The reason case (*b*) is secure in that the larger spine stem resistance results in a steeper and larger depolarization of the spine head in response to the same synaptic input; this is shown best by the dashed curves which correspond to passive spine head membrane.

The right side of Fig. 3.4 summarizes results computed for 45 different values of spine stem resistance; a very strong nonlinearity is apparent. For spine stem resistance values less than 400 megohms (for this set of parameter values) the response of the excitable spine head membrane differs negligibly from the passive controls; when this resistance is increased from 400 to 600 megohms, some nonlinear deviation from the passive controls can be seen at the spine head; this is even more apparent at the spine base (see lower right). The greatest nonlinearity is over the range from 600 to 700 megohms; this clearly corresponds to conditions just below and just above threshold for generation of an action potential in the spine head membrane.

W. Rall & I. Segev

3.4.3 *Optimal range for maximal amplification*

Because the voltage delivered to the spine base (see lower right of Fig. 3.4) becomes smaller as spine stem resistance values increase above 700 megohms, it follows that maximal amplification of synaptic efficacy occurs for an optimal range of values near threshold; in this case, a

Fig. 3.4. Dependence on spine stem resistance values, computed for depolarizing voltages at spine head and spine base in response to brief synaptic conductance input to the spine head; shown for excitable spine head membrane (continuous curves) and for passive spine head membrane (dotted curves). See text for description and discussion. Computations assumed a spine head area of 1.5 square micra, of which ⅓ was assigned to the synaptic contact area and ⅔ was either passive membrane (with parameters given below) or excitable membrane with Hodgkin & Huxley (1952) kinetics adjusted to ten times the channel density for squid axon at 22 degrees, using the computer program described in Parnas & Segev (1979); synaptic excitatory conductance had a peak value of 0.37 nanosiemens, with a reversal potential of 100 mV, and a time course proportional to $t \cdot \exp(-t/p)$, where the peak time, $p = 0.035$ ms (with a 1.4-ms passive membrane time constant, this corresponds to a value of 40 for the usual alpha parameter); the dendrite was simplified to a 0.63-micron diameter cylinder extending one length constant in both directions (with sealed ends) and with parameters (Rm (membrane resistance) = 1400 ohm cm^2, Cm (membrane capacitance) = 1.0 microfarad per cm^2, Ri (internal resistance) = 70 ohm cm) implying an input resistance of 262 megohms.

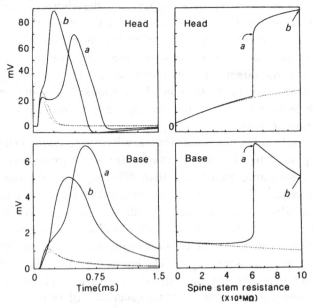

maximal amplification factor of about 6 occurs over an optimal range of about 630 to 670 megohms. An intuitive explanation of the reduced amplification computed for the larger spine stem resistance values can be achieved by noting that the areas under the two action potentials, (a) and (b) at upper left, are approximately the same, and that it is this time integral of spine head voltage (less spine base voltage) that drives the spine stem current and delivers charge to the neuron (at the spine base); thus, with approximately equal voltage drive, Ohm's law implies that the current and charge delivered to the neuron must decrease as the spine stem resistance is increased. Clearly, changes in other parameters which shift threshold conditions will change the optimal range for this parameter.

3.4.4 Distal branch arbors and spine clusters

The linear density of dendritic spines on distal dendritic branches has been reported as about two spines per micrometer of length (Wilson *et al.*, 1983); higher values can result when corrections are made for spines hidden from view (Feldman & Peters, 1979); the serial reconstructions of Harris *et al.* (1985 and personal communication) have yielded significantly higher densities for some neuron types. In any case, for distal branches of 25 micrometer length, it is quite conservative to allow 50 spines per branch. To simplify our computations, we idealized the distal dendritic arbors (Fig. 3.5) and assumed that every branch has exactly 50 spines, and that exactly five of these possess excitable spine head membrane.

The inset in Fig. 3.5 shows more detail for distal branches, A and B, together with their parent branch, C. The symbolic notation is meant to indicate a particular case in which synaptic input is delivered to two of the excitable spines belonging to branch A, and to three of the passive spines belonging to branch B, but to none of the spines belonging to parent branch C. This particular case is one of the five different cases presented next in Fig. 3.6.

3.4.5 Processing of different synaptic inputs

The use of symbols in Fig. 3.6 differs only slightly from Fig. 3.5. The left-hand column shows only those spines whose synapses are active in that particular trial; it is important to emphasize that the computation includes 45 passive spines and five excitable spines present on every branch for every trial. The middle column shows only those excitable spines that fired in response to that trial. The right-hand column shows only the resultant peak depolarization that reaches the neuron soma;

some of the computed voltage values in the branches will be mentioned in the text.

Case 1 shows a synaptic input delivered to only one distal excitable spine; only that one spine fires, generating a local voltage peak of 8.5 mV (at the middle of branch A); this delivers 24 microvolts to the soma, being

Fig. 3.5. Diagram for focus on one distal dendritic arbor of idealized neuron with six dendritic trees (of which five are represented by their equivalent cylinders; see Rall & Rinzel, 1973). Black spine heads are excitable, while those shown as open circles are passive; see text for further description and discussion of symbols and spine clusters. This idealized neuron was used for the computations summarized in Fig. 3.6. The branching is symmetric and satisfies the $\frac{3}{2}$ power diameter constraint for transformation to an equivalent cylinder (Rall, 1962, 1964, 1977); all branch lengths are set equal to 0.2 in dimensionless electrotonic length; here Rm was 2500 ohm cm^2, implying a 2.5-ms passive membrane time constant for the usual membrane capacity value; this Rm together with Ri of 70 ohm cm implies a 180-micron length constant for distal branches of 0.36 micron diameter; then the input resistance at the soma is 7.8 megohms, and with five orders of branching, Table I of Rall & Rinzel, 1973 shows that the distal branch input resistance must be about 50 times larger (here $L = 1.2$, $M = 5$ and $N = 6$). Computations for this model made use of the computer program, SPICE; see Vladimirescu *et al.* (1980), Bunow *et al.* (1985) and Segev *et al.* (1985). Excitable spine head membrane used Hodgkin & Huxley (1952) kinetics adjusted to five times the channel density for squid axon at 22 degrees.

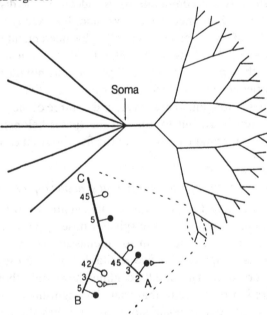

double the amount that would result from the same input to a distal passive spine. In this case, the excitable spine produces a small amplification of the response to the synaptic input, but there is no chain reaction between excitable spines. The same result would be expected for a single input to any one excitable spine on any of the terminal branches of this model.

Case 2 shows simultaneous synaptic inputs to two excitable spines on branch A; here the local depolarization of branch A is sufficient to reach the firing threshold of the other three excitable spines on branch A; this delivers an 84-mV peak depolarization at the soma. This result more than triples the result of Case 1; it is not five times as great for two reasons: three spines fire with a slight delay relative to the first two; also, the

Fig. 3.6. Excitable spine cluster firing contingencies; schematic summary for the five cases described and discussed in the text. Note that branches A, B and C represent the same distal dendritic arbor shown enlarged in Fig. 3.5. The computations were based on the information summarized in the legend of that diagram.

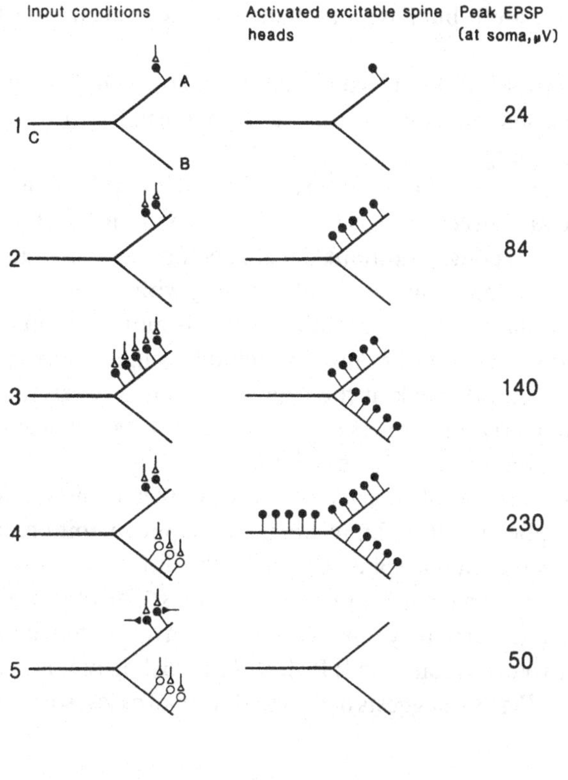

driving potential for synaptic current is reduced by the depolarization of branch A which peaks at 25.5 mV.

Several fascinating insights can be derived from this case. It is clear that the local depolarization is sufficient for the chain reaction to take place in branch A, but the 11.7-mV peak in branch B and the 8.6-mV peak in branch C are not quite sufficient to trigger chain reactions in the excitable spines of those branches. Note that the depolarization in branch B is larger than that in branch C; this was expected from an understanding of the asymmetric voltage attenuations in Fig. 3.1; this effect favors distally spreading chain reactions, and limits central spread. Cases 3, 4, and 5 show examples of the different results obtainable by adding a small amount of synaptic input to that of Case 2.

Case 3 shows simultaneous synaptic input to all five excitable spines belonging to branch A; here simultaneous firing of the five excitable spines of branch A produces sufficient local depolarization in branch B to fire (with slight delay) all five of its excitable spines; however, the local depolarization in parent branch C is not sufficient to fire its excitable spines (another example of the asymmetric decrement shown in Fig. 3.1). The result at the soma is less than twice that of Case 2 and less than ten times that of Case 1, but it is more than twice the control value for passive spines.

Case 4 shows a different combination of five simultaneous synaptic inputs with a significantly different result that can be attributed to more synchronous firing in branches A and B. The two inputs to branch A are the same as in Case 2, but here three additional simultaneous inputs are delivered to any three of the 45 passive spines of branch B; this additional input produces enough additional local depolarization in branch B to fire its five excitable spines almost simultaneously with those of branch A; the resulting depolarization in parent branch C is more than in Case 3, and here proved sufficient to fire its five excitable spines. Thus 15 spines fire producing a 230-mV peak at the soma; this is nearly ten times that for Case 1, and nearly three times that for Case 2; the amplification factor is close to four, relative to passive control.

Case 5 shows one of many possible examples of how effective and specific synaptic inhibitory input can be. Synaptic inhibition delivered to only one or two excitable spines can make the difference between success or failure in the firing of a large cluster of spines. The timing of inhibitory input relative to excitatory input can also be investigated along the lines previously explored (Rall, 1964; Jack *et al.*, 1975; Segev & Parnas, 1983).

Reviewing Fig. 3.6 suggests obvious additional cases, some of which we have already computed. If synchronous synaptic input is delivered to all five excitable spines of branch C, we find that all fifteen excitable spines on these three branches do fire; the voltage peak in A and B occurs 0.78 ms later than that in C. In this case, the amount of depolarization that spreads into the sibling arbor is significant, but not sufficient to fire those 15 excitable spines without some additional synaptic input to that arbor; with such an assist we would fire a cluster of 30 excitable spines in this pair of sibling arbors, but again, this could be blocked by very few strategically placed inhibitory synaptic inputs.

3.4.6 Brief discussion of excitable spine clusters

From the examples above it is clear that excitable spine clusters of different size can be fired, and that success or failure to fire depends upon a number of contingencies. This could provide a basis for logical processing of different synaptic input combinations, and for the realization of various computations and integrative functions. All of this depends very nonlinearly upon the various input parameters and system parameters, such as spine stem resistance. The spine stem resistance is still an attractive locus for changing synaptic weights (the effect is now more sensitive because of the steep nonlinearity displayed in Fig. 3.4); however, we do not suggest that this parameter represents the only one of importance. Also, it may be noted that the logical possibilities provided by the contingencies for the firing of various excitable spine clusters in distal dendritic arbors represents an updated version of an idea (about information processing in dendrites) that has been noted by several investigators over the years (Lorente de No & Condouris, 1959; Arshavskii *et al.*, 1965; Rall, 1970; Goldstein & Rall, 1974; also R. Fitz-Hugh, personal communication, and Y. Y. Zeevi, Ph.D. thesis and personal communication).

3.4.7 Significance of distal branch properties

Although this theoretical model can be made to work for different but inter-related ranges of parameter values, the importance of several insights noted with Fig. 3.1 can now be usefully reviewed. Without the large input resistance value found at distal dendritic locations, the local membrane depolarization produced by a few spine firings would be insufficient to fire other spines. The asymmetry of voltage decrement has several interesting consequences: (i) the local voltage of the distal branch spreads with negligible decrement into the spine heads of the nearby spines that did not receive synaptic input; if this were not true (if there were tenfold voltage decrement into these spine heads, as suggested by Diamond *et al.*, 1970, these other spines would not reach threshold) no chain reaction could occur; (ii) without asymmetry in the arbors, the chain reaction would travel centrally, enveloping the entire neuron in an 'all or nothing' response, which would destroy the richness made possible by distal cluster firings; (iii) with the asymmetry, fractionation into distal clusters of different size occurs naturally. In addition to these points, large values of spine stem resistance (plus branch input resistance) are needed in order to reach threshold depolarization of the excitable spine head when it receives a reasonable amount of synaptic input. In other words, a rather special set of circumstances makes distal dendritic locations particularly well suited for excitable dendritic spines.

3.5 Conclusion

For all of the above reasons, we suggest that evolution has placed voltage dependent ionic channels in the membrane of some distally located spine heads in sufficient number to make them excitable. Whether this suggestion is correct is not yet known; it is testable, in principle, by three different techniques, at least one of which can be expected to succeed in the next few years. These are (i) the use of antibodies to mark the locations of particular channels, (ii) the use of a patch clamp or a suction electrode to record from individual spines, and (iii) the use of voltage sensitive dyes to record voltage transients and perhaps also voltage decrements in distal dendritic branches and dendritic spines.

Acknowledgement

Dr Segev was a Fogarty Fellow at NIH; his present address is Department of Neuroscience, Institute of Life Sciences, the Hebrew University, Jerusalem, Israel. Some of the same results, figures, and insights have been presented at other symposia and may also appear in resulting publications.

References

Arshavskii, Y. I., M. B. Berkinblit, S. A. Kovalev, V. V. Smolyaninov & L. M. Chailakhyan (1965). 'The role of dendrites in the functioning of nerve cells.' *Dokl. Akademii Nauk SSSR*, **163**, 994–7. Translation in *Doklady Biophysics*, Consultants Bureau, N.Y.

Bunow, B., I. Segev & J. W. Fleshman (1985). 'Modeling the electrical behavior of anatomically complex neurons using a network analysis program: excitable membrane.' *Biol. Cybern.*, **53**, 41–56.

Chang, H. T. (1952). 'Cortical neurons with particular reference to the apical dendrites.' *Cold Spring Harb. Symp. Quant. Biol.*, **17**, 189–202.

Colonnier, M. (1968). 'Synaptic patterns on different cell types in the different laminae of the cat visual cortex. An electron microscope study.' *Brain Res.*, **9**, 268–87.

Coss, R. G. & D. H. Perkel (1985). 'The function of dendritic spines: a review of theoretical issues.' *Behavioural and Neural Biol.*, **44**, 151–85.

Diamond, J., E. G. Gray & G. M. Yasargil (1970). 'The function of the dendritic spines: an hypothesis.' In *Excitatory Synaptic Mechanisms*, P. Anderson & J. K. S. Jansen, eds., pp. 213–22, Universitetsforlaget, Oslo.

Erulkar, S. D., R. A. Butler & G. L. Gerstein (1968). 'Excitation and inhibition in cochlear nucleus. II. Frequency-modulated tones.' *J. Neurophysiol.*, **31**, 537–48.

Feldman, M. L. & A. Peters (1979). 'A technique for estimating total spine numbers on Golgi-impregnated dendrites.' *J. Comp. Neurol.*, **118**, 527–42.

Goldstein, S. S. & W. Rall (1974). 'Changes of action potential shape and velocity for changing core conductor geometry.' *Biophys. J.*, **14**, 731–57.

Gray, E. G. (1959). 'Axo-somatic and axo-dendritic synapses of the cerebral cortex: an electron microscopic study.' *J. Anat.*, **93**, 420–33.

Harris, K. M., Trogadis, J. & Stevens, J. K. (1985). 'Three-dimensional structure of dendritic spines in the rat hippocampus (CA1) and cerebellum.' *Abstracts*, Soc. for Neuroscience 15th Annual Meeting, 306.

Hodgkin, A. L. & A. F. Huxley (1952). 'A quantitative description of membrane current and its application to conduction and excitation in nerve.' *J. Physiol.* (Lond.), **117**, 500–44.

Jack, J. J. B., D. Noble & R. W. Tsien (1975). *Electric Current Flow in Excitable Cells*, Oxford Univ. Press, Lond.

Jones, E. G. & T. P. S. Powell (1969). 'Morphological variations in the dendritic spines of the neocortex.' *J. Cell. Sci.*, **5**, 509–19.

Kawato, M. & N. Tsukahara (1984). 'Electrical properties of dendritic spines with bulbous end terminals.' *Biophys. J.*, **46**, 155–66.

Koch, C. & T. Poggio (1983). 'A theoretical analysis of electrical properties of spines.' *Proc. R. Soc. Lond. (Biol.)*, **218**, 455–77.

Lorente de No, R. & G. A. Condouris (1959). 'Decremental conduction in peripheral nerve: integration of stimuli in the neuron.' *Proc. Nat. Acad. Sci.*, **45**, 592–617.

Malinow, R. & J. P. Miller (1984). 'Interactions between active dendritic spines could generate bursts of spikes.' *Soc. Neurosci. Abstr.*, **10**, 547.

Miller, J. P., W. Rall & J. Rinzel (1985). 'Synaptic amplification by active membrane in dendritic spines.' *Brain Res.*, **325**, 325–30.

Parnas, I. & I. Segev (1979). 'A mathematical model for conduction of action potentials along bifurcating axons.' *J. Physiol.* (Lond.), **295**, 323–43.

Perkel, D. H. & D. J. Perkel (1985). 'Dendritic spines: role of active membrane in modulating synaptic efficacy.' *Brain Res.*, **325**, 331–5.

Peters, A. & I. R. Kaiserman-Abramof (1970). 'The small pyramidal neuron of the rat cerebral cortex. The perikaryon, dendrites and spines.' *Am. J. Anat.*, **127**, 321–56.

Rall, W. (1962). 'Theory of physiological properties of dendrites.' *Ann. N.Y. Acad. Sci.*, **96**, 1071–92.

Rall, W. (1964). 'Theoretical significance of dendritic trees for neuronal input–output relations.' In *Neural Theory and Modeling*, R. Reiss, ed., pp. 73–97, Stanford Univ. Press, Stanford, CA.

Rall, W. (1967). 'Distinguishing theoretical synaptic potentials computed for different soma-dendritic distributions of input.' *J. Neurophysiol.*, **30**, 1138–68.

Rall, W. (1970). 'Cable properties of dendrites and effect of synaptic location.' In *Excitatory Synaptic Mechanisms*. P. Andersen & J. K. S. Jansen, eds., pp. 175–87. Universitetsforlaget, Oslo.

Rall, W. (1974). 'Dendritic spines, synaptic potency and neuronal plasticity.' In *Cellular Mechanisms Subserving Changes in Neuronal Activity*, C. D. Woody, K. A. Brown, T. J. Crow & J. D. Knispel, eds., *Brain Info. Service Res. Report*, **3**, 13–21.

Rall, W. (1977). 'Core conductor theory and cable properties of neurons.' In *Handbook of Physiology, Vol. 1, Pt. 1, The Nervous System, Cellular Biology of Neurons*, J. M. Brookhart, V. B. Mountcastle & E. R. Kandel, eds., pp. 39–97. American Physiological Society, Bethesda, MD.

Rall, W. (1978). 'Dendritic spines and synaptic potency.' In *Studies in Neurophysiology*, R. Porter, ed., Cambridge University Press, N.Y.

Rall, W. & J. Rinzel (1971*a*). 'Dendritic spines and synaptic potency explored theoretically.' *Proc. I.U.P.S.* (XXV Intl. Congr.), **IX**, 466.

Rall, W. & J. Rinzel (1971*b*). 'Dendritic spine function and synaptic attenuation calculations.' *Prog. and Abstr. Soc. Neurosci. First Ann. Mtg.*, 64.

Rall, W. & J. Rinzel (1973). 'Branch input resistance and steady attenuation for input to one branch of a dendritic neuron model.' *Biophys. J.*, **13**, 648–88.

Rall, W. & I. Segev (1985). 'Space clamp problems when voltage clamping branched neurons with intracellular microelectrodes.' In *Voltage and Patch Clamping with Microelectrodes*, T. G. Smith, Jr., H. Lecar, S. J. Redman & P. Gage, eds., pp. 191–215, American Physiological Society, Bethesda, MD.

Rall, W. & Segev, I. (1987). 'Functional possibilities for synapses on dendrites and on dendritic spines.' In *Synaptic Function* (eds. G. M. Edelman, W. E. Gall, and W. M. Cowan). John Wiley, N.Y. pp. 605–36.

Rall, W., G. M. Shepherd, T. S. Reese & M. W. Brightman (1966). 'Dendro-dendritic synaptic pathway in the olfactory bulb.' *Exp. Neurol.*, **14**, 44–56.

Redman, S. J. (1976). 'A quantitative approach to the integrative function of dendrites.' In *International Review of Physiology: Neurophysiology II, Vol. 10*, R. Porter, ed., pp. 1–36, University Park Press, Baltimore.

Rinzel, J. (1982). 'Neuronal plasticity (learning).' In *Some Mathematical Questions in Biology – Neurobiology, Vol. 15, Lectures on Mathematics in the Life Sciences*, R. M. Miura, ed., pp. 7–25, American Mathematical Society, Providence, RI.

Segev, I. & I. Parnas (1983). 'Synaptic integration mechanisms. Theoretical and experimental investigation of temporal postsynaptic interaction between excitatory and inhibitory inputs.' *Biophys. J.*, **41**, 41–50.

Segev, I., J. W. Fleshman, J. P. Miller & B. Bunow (1985). 'Modeling the electrical behavior of anatomically complex neurons using a network analysis program: passive membrane.' *Biol. Cybern.*, **53**, 27–40.

Shepherd, G. M. & R. K. Brayton (1979). 'Computer simulation of a dendrodendritic synaptic circuit for self- and lateral-inhibition in the olfactory bulb.' *Brain Res.*, **175**, 377–82.

Shepherd, G. M., R. K. Brayton, A. Belanger, J. P. Miller, R. Malinow, I. Segev, J. Rinzel & W. Rall (1984). 'Interactions between active dendritic spines could augment impact of distal dendritic synapses.' *Soc. Neurosci. Abstr.*, **10**, 547.

Turner, D. A. (1984). 'Conductance transients on dendritic spines in a segmental cable model of hippocampal neurons.' *Biophys. J.*, **46**, 85–96.

Vladimirescu, A., A. R. Newton & D. O. Pederson (1980). 'SPICE version 26.0.' *User's Guide*, EECS Dept., University of California, Berkeley.

Wilson, C. J. (1984). 'Passive cable properties of dendritic spines and spiny neurons.' *J. Neurosci.*, **4**, 281–97.

Wilson, C. J., P. M. Groves, S. T. Kitai & I. C. Linder (1983). 'Three dimensional structure of dendritic spines in the rat neostriatum.' *J. Neurosci.*, **3**, 383–98.

4

Vistas from tensor network theory: a horizon from reductionalist neurophilosophy to the geometry of multi-unit recordings

ANDRÁS J. PELLIONISZ

4.1 The brain and the computer: a misleading metaphor in place of brain theory

Contrary to the philosophy of *natural sciences*, the brain has always been understood in terms of the most complex *scientific technology* of man-made organisms, for the simple reason of human vanity. Before and after the computer era, the brain was paraded in the clothing of hydraulic systems (in Descartes' times), and in the modern era as radio command centers, telephone switchboards, learn-matrices or feedback control amplifiers. Presently, it is fashionable to borrow terms of holograms, catastrophes or even spin glasses. *Comparing brains to computers*, however, has been by far the most important and most grossly misleading metaphor of all. Its importance has been twofold. First, the early post-war era was the first and last time in history that such analogy paved the way both to a *model of the single neuron*, the flip–flop binary element, cf. McCulloch & Pitts, 1943, and to a *grand mathematical theory* of the function of the entire brain (i.e., information processing and control by networks implementing Boolean algebra, cf. Shannon, 1948; Wiener, 1948). Second, the classical computer, the so-called von Neumann machine, provided neuroscience with not only a metaphor, but at the same time with a powerful working tool. This made computer simulation and modeling flourish in the brain sciences as well (cf. Pellionisz, 1979).

The basic misunderstanding inherent in the metaphor, nevertheless, left brain theory in an eclipse, although the creator of the computers was the first to point out (von Neumann, 1958) that these living- and non-living epitomes of complex organisms appear to operate on diametrically opposite structuro–functional principles. The von Neumann-type *present-day computers are serially organized systems*, governed by a central clock, working through enormous sequences of operations which span great logical depths. They are processors of information in the well-defined Shannonian probability-theory sense, performing functions of mathematical logic and control. In contrast, future non-von Neumann processors ('Neuronal Computers', cf. Eckmiller, 1988), in order to be true to their other name of *brain-like machines, have to be massively parallel systems* with no clock, and having to do without the principle of simultaneity (cf. Pellionisz & Llinás, 1982). Their logical structure is extremely shallow, typically 3–7-step in depth, just as in the case of the living brain. These instruments are processors of multidimensional parameters. The signals admittedly carry 'biological information', yet the mathematical definition of this term is hitherto nonexistent (cf. Pellionisz, 1983). Moreover, the core of brain function is not the exertion of *logical* or *control* operations upon the outside word but its *representation* by an internal model (cf. Pellionisz, 1983).

In order to define general brain function, therefore, the emergence of a conceptually and formally homogeneous *representational brain theory* is required that is based on the most proper philosophy and axiomatic structure (cf. Palm & Aertsen, 1986; Pellionisz, 1986*b*).

4.2 Neurophilosophy: the place of reductionalist brain theory in natural science

The author's contribution to meeting the above challenges is manifested in tensor network theory, developed through the past decade (for review, see Pellionisz, 1986*e*, 1987*a*). After close to a decade of its development, this article sizes up its fundamental features and outlines the fields of its projected major applications in the future (see Fig. 4.1).

In its philosophy, tensor network theory is based on the conviction (see in detail in Churchland, 1986) that brain theory becomes more a part of natural sciences if it abandons the dogma of emulating the most advanced *technology*. Instead, it had better build its own theoretical structure on carefully laid axioms and utilize, of course, the most powerful *mathematical approach* available in the natural sciences to represent universal invariants (cf. Pellionisz, 1986*b*). *The specific concept and formalism in tensor network theory is that brain function is implemented by neuronal network transformations that represent physical objects by dual, sensory and motor-type multidimensional general vectors* (mathematically, these are covariant and contravariant tensors, cf. Bickley & Gibson, 1962; Pellionisz & Llinás, 1980). Based on such reductionalist predilection, tensor theory approaches the brain–mind structurofunctional entity from the viewpoint of multidimensional functional geometry, using it to build a geometrical representation theory. Thus, it is not by chance that the core of its mathematical apparatus is the one used in the unification of physical spacetime (theory of generalized reference-frame-aspecific vector-matrix operations, i.e., *tensor transformations*, as used, e.g., in. relativity; cf. Levi-Civita, 1926; Einstein, 1916). Therefore, tensor network theory is philosophically much more akin to the modern multidimensional superstring-theory of the universe (cf. Green, 1986), by elevating brain theory into the realm of the abstract natural sciences, than, e.g., to the overreductionalist brain-model offered by the quantitative descriptive apparatus of electronic gain-controlled amplifiers which, in effect, makes brain theory a chapter in control-engineering.

4.3 Tensorial approach to brain theory: representation of invariants by geometrical transformations of intrinsic coordinates

Mathematically, tensor network theory is based on the fact that the structure of the physical geometry of the organisms determines those natural coordinate systems that are intrinsic to the expression of their function. Therefore, adoption of the concept and formalism of coordinate-system-aspecific generalized vectors and matrices (tensors) enables and liberates one to deal with *any* frame of reference, in fact 'letting the brain speak in its own terms' (cf. Simpson & Graf, 1985). A characteristic example of coordinate

Fig. 4.1. Fields of research, potentially benefiting from a conceptually and formally homogeneous brain theory, such as Tensor Network Theory of the Central Nervous System.

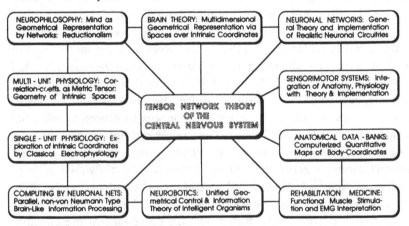

systems that are specified by the physical geometry of the body is shown in Fig. 4.2 concerning a head-stabilizing neuronal apparatus, the so-called vestibulo–collic reflex (see in detail in Pellionisz & Peterson, 1988).

Passively occurring head-movements are measured by the vestibular semicircular canal apparatus, and are compensated for by expressing the same movement (with opposite sign) by means of coordinated contractions of neck-muscles. It is physically obvious that the head contains built-in natural frames of reference for expressing its movements. As anatomically measured by Blanks, Curthoys & Markham (1972, see Fig. 4.2(*b*)) the three vestibular canals form an arrangement whose characteristic axes constitute a coordinate system that *resembles* the well-known Cartesian (3-axis, orthogonal) frame of reference. On the other hand, as anatomically established by Baker, Goldberg & Peterson (1985), the head-rotational-axes belonging to the pulling of neck muscles comprise a 30-axis arrangement (see Fig. 4.2(*c*)). Indeed, this neck-motor frame is one of the clearest examples of a highly non-orthogonal system of coordinates that is vastly overcomplete (since it uses ten times as many axes as the minimum required for expressing 3-dimensional rotations of a body around a center). Thus, this scheme demonstrates the possibility and importance of describing CNS function by means of transformations within and among *general coordinate systems*. While in the case of a few highly specialized systems (e.g. the vestibular canals) it is tempting to fall back on the use of Cartesian vectorial expressions, in most sensory and motor systems (let alone higher CNS functions) *the frames intrinsic to the neuronal expressions just simply cannot be taken for granted.*

Thus, when the CNS represents, e.g., head movements both in the sensory and motor manner, the question is not *if* the brain implements transformations of head-rotation expressed in vestibular frame into head-rotation expressed in the neck-motor frame, but *how* the CNS does it by its neuronal networks. Further, the question is *what group of neuroscientists* is up to the challenge of making use, for their own purposes, of those potent and general concepts and formalisms that are made available for quantitatively dealing with such general coordinate system transformations, both in sensorimotor neuronal operations and elsewhere in the CNS.

4.4 Neuronal networks: general theory of the structure and function of realistic neuronal circuits

While tensor network theory has been formulated to provide a conceptually and mathematically homogeneous *abstract* brain theory, it aims at

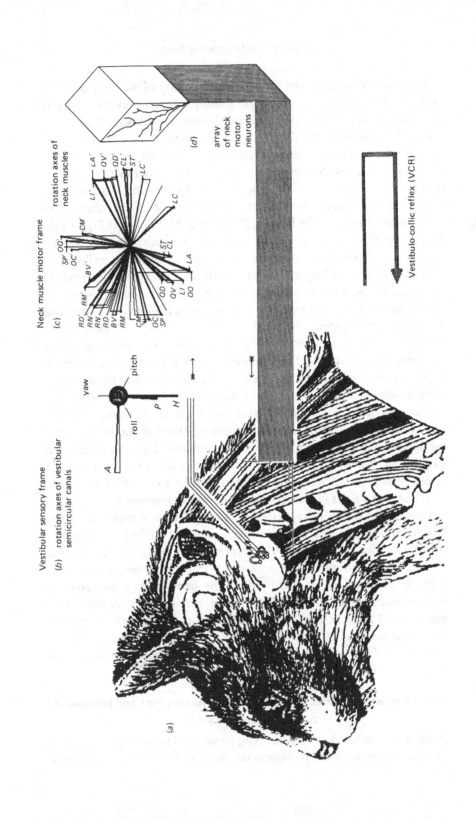

Vestibular sensory frame

(b) rotation axes of vestibular semicircular canals

yaw

pitch

roll

A

P

H

Neck muscle motor frame

rotation axes of neck muscles

(c)

LA'
QV'
QD'
CL'
ST'
LC'

LI'

CM'

SP' OO'
OC'
BV'

ST
CL

LC

LA

RD'
RN'
RN
RD
BV'
RM'

RM
CM
OC
SP
OO
LI
QV
QD

(d)

array
of neck
motor
neurons

Vestibulo-collic reflex (VCR)

(a)

never losing touch with the concrete neuroanatomical and physiological reality. By providing neuroscience with a *network theory*, it directly addresses those organizational properties which are inherent in and intrinsic to the physical organization of the brain. It has long been customary to mathematically represent the massively parallel neuronal networks of the CNS by *matrices*, which become here specific concrete implementations of the general reference-frame-aspecific *tensor operators* (cf. Pellionisz, 1986e). Availability of a general network theory may be significant, since it is a widely held view that *neuroscience must have a powerful enough concept and formalism that can be accepted as an abstract understanding of the function of specific quantitative neuronal networks*.

A particular elaboration of the above general features is shown in Fig. 4.3 (cf. Pellionisz & Peterson, 1988). The scheme illustrates one of the main difficulties posed by a general coordinate-system-transformation; i.e. the frames may be *overcomplete*. For example, the neck-motor system can produce the same movement using an infinite number of different patterns of muscle activation. The solution proposed by Pellionisz (1984) utilizes the difference between covariant and contravariant representations of the desired movement, both expressed in the motor frame as determined by the muscle geometry. The covariant representation can be uniquely established by projecting the movement vector upon each of the muscle axes. The problem is to find its unique inverse, the contravariant representation. In an overcomplete system the problem is not that this does not exist but that there are an infinite number of inverses. It has been proposed (Pellionisz, 1983, 1984) that the CNS chooses a unique solution, the Moore–Penrose generalized inverse of the covariant metric (Albert, 1972), which may be implemented by a network that could plausibly be constructed by developing nervous systems (Pellionisz & Llinás, 1985). Related models

---

Fig. 4.2. An example of implementing CNS function by transformations of general vectors among multidimensional, non-orthogonal coordinate systems. The frames of reference intrinsic to the vestibular-canal to neck-muscle sensorimotor reflex. (*a*) The head-stabilization sensorimotor reflex includes the vestibular semicircular canal sensory apparatus, and neck-muscle motor apparatus. (*b*) The vestibular apparatus is characterized by directions in the three-space belonging to A: anterior, P: posterior, H: horizontal semicircular canals (data from Blanks *et al.*, 1972). (*c*) The 30 major neck-muscles are characterized by rotational-directions (data from Baker *et al.*, 1985). (*d*) Motoneurons which generate rotations, expressed in the neck-muscle frame, have to receive signals transformed from the vestibular sensory frame in order to properly stabilize the head.

have been prepared for the vestibulo–ocular reflex (Simpson & Pellionisz, 1984), for the vestibulo–collic reflex (Peterson *et al.*, 1985) and for arm movements (Gielen & van Zuylen, 1986).

The solution in Fig. 4.3 is based on the three-step scheme of sensorimotor tensor transformation. The task is to change (a) the sensory frame into motor, (b) the measured, covariant type vector to an executable contravariant version, and (c) to increase dimensions from three to thirty. The central, covariant embedding tensor accomplishes both (a) and (c), simply by projecting the three sensory (*i* subscripts) upon the 30 motor axes (*p* subscripts), mathematically expressed as

$$c_{ip} = s_i \cdot m_p, \qquad (1)$$

where **s** and **m** are the coordinates of the (normalized) sensory and motor axes, and each matrix-element of c_{ip} is the inner (scalar) product of the vectors of coordinates of the *i*th and *p*th axis.

Fig. 4.3. Tensor network model of the three-step vestibulo-collic head-stabilization sensorimotor reflex (cf. Pellionisz & Peterson, 1988). Transformation from sensory coordinates to a motor frame (where the latter may be of higher dimensions) can be accomplished by a three-step tensorial scheme. The vestibular sensory metric tensor, vestibulo-collic sensorimotor tensor and contravariant neck motor tensor transformations can be expressed verbally, by abstract reference frame aspecific tensor-symbolism (see in text) or by matrix- (patch-) and network-diagrams. Here, the three matrices are shown, for the particular vestibular and oculomotor frames of the cat (cf. Fig. 4.2) by patch-diagrams only, and by a quantitative visualization of the corresponding neuronal networks that can accomplish such transfer. Network diagrams illustrate the massively parallel architecture of the CNS, where convergences and divergences are the rule, and separated point-to-point connections rarely, if ever, characterize the structure.

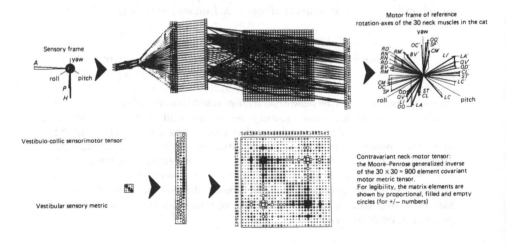

The reason that the c_{ip} covariant embedding tensor is necessary but not sufficient is that c_{ip} is a *projective* tensor. It turns a physical-type (contra-variant) input vector into an output that is provided in its projection-components (covariants). However, our case is the opposite; the available sensory input is covariant, while the output required is contravariant. This is why the other two conversions are necessary; the vestibular sensory metric tensor g^{pr} that converts covariant sensory reception into contravariant sensory perception, and the contravariant neck-motor metric g^{ie} (the large 30×30 matrix in Fig. 4.3) that turns covariant motor intention into contravariant motor execution. This general function of transforming covariant non-orthogonal versions into contravariant ones by a metric tensor can be accomplished for any given set of axes by a matrix of divergent-convergent neuronal connections among primary and secondary vestibular neurons and among brain-stem premotor neurons and neck-motoneurons (Baker *et al.*, 1984). The required con-travariant metric tensor g^{pr} is the inverse of the covariant metric tensor g_{pr}:

$$g^{pr} = (g_{pr})^{-1} \qquad (2)$$

where components g_{pr} are the inner (scalar) products of the vectors of coordinates of the (normalized) axes s_i:

$$g_{pr} = s_i s_i \qquad (3)$$

The question of how CNS neuronal networks can arrive at a unique covariant-to-contravariant transformation led to the proposal of a metaorganization principle and procedure which utilizes the Moore–Penrose generalized inverse (Pellionisz, 1983, 1984; Pellionisz & Llinás, 1985). This solution is based on arriving at the eigenvectors of the system (those special vectors whose covariant and contravariant expressions have identical directions) by a reverberative oscillatory procedure (muscle proprioception recurring as motoneuron output, setting up stabilizing tremors). The eigenvectors would imprint a matrix of neural connections that can serve as the proper coordination-device (e.g. cere-bellar neuronal circuit). The unique inverse of g^{ie} can be obtained from the outer (dyadic matrix) product (symbolized by $><$) of the eigenvectors E_m, weighted by the inverses of the eigenvalues λ_m (the inverse is 0 if $\lambda_m = 0$, cf. Albert, 1972):

$$g^{ie} = \sum_m 1/\lambda_m \cdot (E_m >< E_m). \qquad (4)$$

The tensor network model of the vestibulo-collic reflex emerges from the quantitative data of Fig. 4.2 in the form shown in Fig. 4.3. Each of the three matrices in the model is represented by a patch-diagram in which the size and sign of each matrix element are indicated by filled (positive) and open (negative) circles. Four columns represent canal inputs (**H,A,P**, at the left side of the network-diagram), motor nerve outputs (**LC . . .**, at right side) and two intermediate neural stages.

Another rendering of the tensor network model of the vestibulocollic reflex is shown in Fig. 4.4. This presentation is basically a neuromorphological elaboration of the tensorial scheme of Fig. 4.3. First, the transformation-matrices are not represented here by visually difficult-to-comprehend complex sets of interconnections (used in the top part of Fig. 4.3), but by so-called 'tensor modules' (cf. part of Fig. 4.4, marked 'cerebellar nuclei'). In such a module, the input vector arriving by the incoming axons is transformed by the synaptic interconnection-set into an output vector (the connections are shown by patches, cf. bottom part of Fig. 4.3). A single dendritic tree of the output neurons is drawn to symbolize cells which implement the transformation. A second difference in Fig. 4.4 in comparison with Fig. 4.3 is the detailed elaboration of the cerebellar embodiment of the motor metric tensor. In Fig. 4.3, the third and last transformation is shown by a one-step network. This conversion, however, does not occur in a simple 'throughput-type' network, but is performed by the cerebellar 'add-on-type' network (cf. Pellionisz, 1984).

The 'add-on' structurofunctional architecture of the cerebellum (probably a result of its character as 'an evolutionary afterthought') enables

---

Fig. 4.4. 'Tensor modules' in a network model of the vestibular-neck motor head-stabilization reflex, involving the cerebellum. In all, the 3-dimensional vestibular signals, expressed by covariant components, are transformed by the vestibulo-cerebellar neuronal network into 30-dimensional neck motor signals, expressed by contravariant vectorial components. This rendering of the tensor-matrices utilizes tensor-modules (see, e.g., the module marked 'cerebellar nuclei'), where the n-dimensional input vector is shown by a strip of n incoming axons, the n-dimensional output vector is by a strip of n outgoing axons. The dendritic trees of output neurons are shown only by a representative single cell, and the synaptic connectivities among input and output neurons are shown by an $n \times n$ matrix, illustrated by a patch-diagram. The basic 3-step transformation is implemented in the vestibular and cerebellar nuclei. The cerebellum serves as an add-on circuit, which turns the covariant motor intention into a contravariant motor execution. The accessory optic system and olivary system serve the role of reporting the misperformance of the head-compensation reflex thus the climbing fibers generate an ongoing modification of the cerebellar metric tensor (Simpson *et al.*, 1979). AOS: accessory optic system, CF: climbing fibers, CN: cerebellar nucleofugal path, GC: granule cells, ME: motor execution signals, MF: mossy fibers, PC: Purkinje cells, PF: parallel fibers.

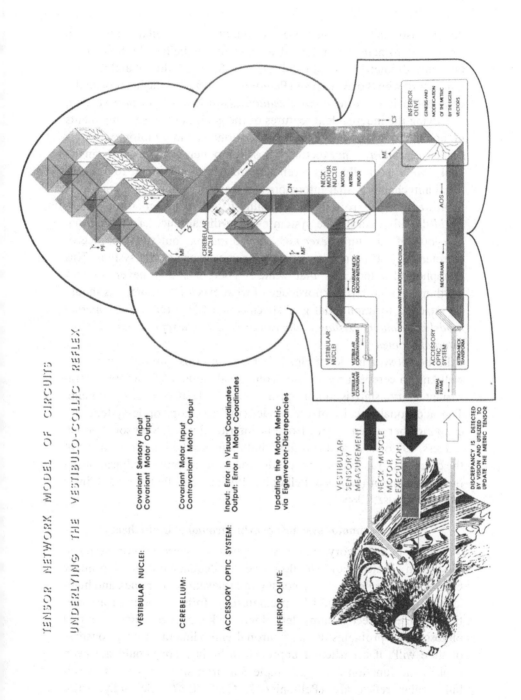

TENSOR NETWORK MODEL OF CIRCUITS

UNDERLYING THE VESTIBULO-COLLIC REFLEX

VESTIBULAR NUCLEI: Covariant Sensory Input
Covariant Motor Output

CEREBELLUM: Covariant Motor Input
Contravariant Motor Output

ACCESSORY OPTIC SYSTEM: Input: Error in Visual Coordinates
Output: Error in Motor Coordinates

INFERIOR OLIVE: Updating the Motor Metric
via Eigenvector-Discrepancies

VESTIBULAR
SENSORY
MEASUREMENT

NECK MUSCLE
MOTOR
EXECUTION

DISCREPANCY IS DETECTED
BY VISION AND UTILIZED TO
UPDATE THE METRIC TENSOR

direct sensorimotor operations even *without* any cerebellar contribution (motor performance is retained in case of cerebellar ablation but it becomes 'dysmetric'; cf. Bloedel *et al.*, 1985). The 'add-on' architecture is in accord with the hypothesis (Pellionisz, 1985*b*) that the function of the cerebellum is to turn *motor intentions* (which are *covariant* vectors, specifying the independent features of the goal, but whose components do not add up to properly make the performance) into motor *executions* (which are *contravariant* vectors, whose components actually perform the goal). Metaphorically, this cerebellar architecture is similar to a 'secretarial antechamber' that intercepts and transforms the *intentional commands* emanating from the boss' main office. For his 'good intentions' *could* directly operate the system even in the absence of the 'add-on' side-loop of secretarial *executive transformation*, but such absence of secretaries typically results in 'ataxic' performance of the system. This metaphor also indicates that while a good secretary never initiates anything, a 'secretarial' knowledge of what executive commands should be attached to intentional goal-specifications does require *an internal model of relations existing in the external system; a representation of the external geometry*.

In the network model of Fig. 4.4 which conforms with the structure of well-known cerebellar nets, the geometrical model of covariant-contravariant relationships is comprised in the 'cerebellar nuclei' tensor module. The additional circuits of the model (the accessory optic system and climbing fiber system arising from the inferior olive, cf. Simpson, Soodak & Hess, 1979) serve as a corollary that monitors the misperformance of the cerebellar transformation, yielding ongoing adaptive modifications of the metric tensor (Llinás & Pellionisz, 1985; cf. also Pellionisz & Llinás, 1979; Pellionisz, 1986*a*).

4.5 Sensorimotor systems: proving ground of brain theory

Tensorial brain theory was first applied to sensorimotor systems. Firstly, any brain theory should prove its adequacy on simple primary CNS operations before being considered relevant for complex and high-level CNS tasks. It would be premature to forge theories of associations, pattern recognition, let alone tackling such almost purely philosophical problems as the neuronal embodiment of consciousness or 'free will', if a particular approach in brain theory could not even explain the function of, e.g., simple 3-neuron structures as the vestibulo-ocular reflex arc (Pellionisz & Graf, 1987). Secondly, since sensorimotor operations are measurable and describable by physical means, it is possible to put forward, in case of sensorimotor transfer, not merely an abstract brain theory but also its quantitative elaboration. This should, in turn, result in direct experimental comparison of experimental measurements with theoretical predictions (Peterson *et al.*, 1985; Gielen & van Zuylen, 1986).

Thirdly, as will be shown below, any theoretical understanding gained from the knowledge of sensorimotor systems lends itself to direct utilization not only in the immediate fields relating to motor systems, such as kinesiology and rehabilitation medicine, but also in the biologically related fields of robotics (*neurobotics*, cf. Pellionisz, 1983) and of the technology of brain-like computers (*neuronal computers*; cf. Eckmiller, 1988). An eventual co-evolution of *brain theory* with some of the most important *technological challenges* of our time may prove to be of substantial benefit both for constructing intelligent robots and brain-like computers, assuming that brain theory is not an epigon of the technology but can put forward its own mathematical foundation (Pellionisz, 1987*b,c*, 1988*a*).

4.6 Data-banks for quantitative anatomy: computerized maps of body-coordinates

Looking beyond the basic challenge of creating and formulating a geometrical approach in brain theory, the first requirement towards its quantitative elaboration is the availability of morphological data that specify the coordinate systems intrinsic to the physical geometry of living organisms. Quantitative morphological specification of sensorimotor systems began about a century ago by Helmholtz' (1896) measurements of the extraocular musculature. This field has experienced a rapid growth in the past decade (Blanks *et al.*, 1972; Ezure & Graf, 1984; Simpson *et al.*, 1986; Daunicht & Pellionisz, 1986). The data-sets should ideally be obtained in a manner in which they are compatible with one another as well as with the theoretical requirements. Also, it would be useful to make them widely and conveniently available for the research community. Therefore, it is expected that the field will soon support the establishment of data-banks to gather, hold and disseminate the findings of the rapidly emerging discipline of quantitative computerized anatomy. The data-banks could serve as nodes of a computer network. With the widespread availability of today's economical graphic work-stations, linked by telephone network-connections, quantitative sensorimotor research and its applications will no doubt experience a quantum jump of efficiency. As outlined below, such a modernized approach to reveal the

structure of living organisms is expected to have a major impact on a
range of fields of research and applications.

4.7 Rehabilitation medicine and kinesiology: functional muscle stimulation and EMG-motor unit interpretation

The main contribution of the tensorial approach to the sensorimotor field
may be that of providing with a quantitative theory (e.g. by offering a
general solution for the coordination of overcomplete musculature, cf.
Simpson & Pellionisz, 1984; Peterson *et al.*, 1985; Gielen & Zuylen,
1986). Nevertheless, potential use of its elements, e.g. the Moore–Penrose generalized inverse, can be illustrated even in such simple structures
of anatomy as the *skeleton* of the neck-motor apparatus (Fig. 4.5(*a*)).

  The most rudimentary physical geometry underlying motor performance is the skeletal structure. Once the position and the measurements of
the vertebral column of the cat's neck is established (cf. Vidal, Graf &
Berthoz, 1986), it is possible to use the quantitative tensor model to
predict the nature of the constraints that the Moore–Penrose generalized
inverse would impose on head-movements executed with the use of this
overcomplete joint-structure. The intrinsic system of coordinates for the
2-dimensional displacement of the head (specified by displacement of the
cat's eye) can be calculated from the x,y coordinates of the vertebral
rotation-joints. As shown in Fig. 4.5(*a*), given a motor intention-vector,

---

Fig. 4.5. Coordination of an overcomplete skeleto-motor system. Predictions are
calculated by the Moore–Penrose generalized inverse of the covariant metric
tensor of the coordinates intrinsic to the 8 cervical joint–7 neck muscle motor
apparatus (programming by: A. Pellionisz & J. Laczkó, anatomy by:
F. Richmond, J. Baker, P. Vidal & W. Graf, tensor model by A. Pellionisz &
B. Peterson). (*a*) Tensor model of constraints of movements inherent in the
overcomplete skeletal apparatus composed of 8 cervical joints. The coordinate-
axes of the displacement of the head are determined by the joint rotation-points.
A movement intention (see arrow) is decomposed into covariant intention
components and transformed into contravariants by the Moore–Penrose inverse.
(*b*) Pulling of each of the 7 representative muscles determine a displacement of
the head (in case of multiarticular muscles, the knowledge of the relative stiffness
of joints is required). (*c*) Movement intention, similar to that in A, will produce a
head-shift, with almost all movement at C1/C2 and C7. Predicted muscle-
activations *correspond to* EMG signals, thus could be a basis for functional
stimulation and EMG interpretation. (*d*) Model, *identical* to that in C, producing
a markedly different movement-pattern for a 'look-up' motor intention. Movement is almost exclusively C1/C2 rotation, without neck-tilt ('EMG'-pattern is
also different). Different 'motor strategies' may arise from a single model.

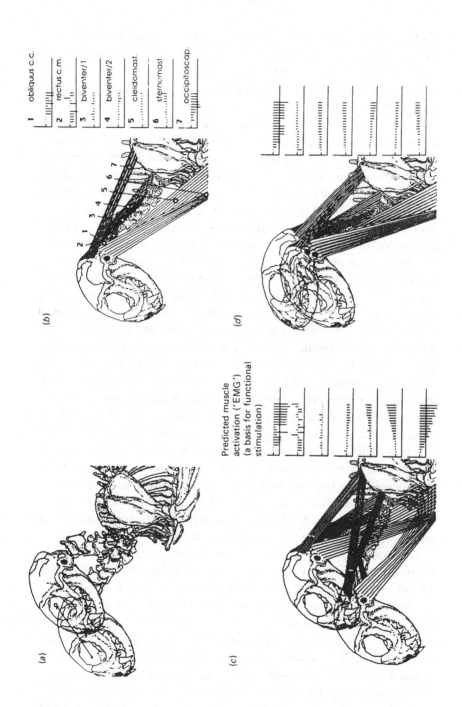

(a)

(b)

1 obliquus c.c.
2 rectus c.m.
3 biventer/1
4 biventer/2
5 cleidomast.
6 sternomast.
7 occipitoscap.

(c)

Predicted muscle
activation ('EMG')
(a basis for functional
stimulation)

(d)

the Moore–Penrose generalized inverse of the covariant metric tensor of the intrinsic frame will determine a characteristic movement-pattern of the head, in which the cervical column remains a rigid body and almost all of the movement is generated by rotation around C1/C2 and C7 joints (cf. Vidal & Berthoz, 1986).

While it is important to study the fundamental physical constraints of motor performance imposed by the skeleton, movements are controlled by the CNS not in a rather low-dimensional, nonetheless overcomplete, *joint-coordinate space*, but in very high dimensional *neuronal* coordinate space. Between these two extremes of dimensionality is the *muscle-space*, spun over the coordinates intrinsic to the pulling of the individual muscles. Fig. 4.5(*b–d*) shows a preliminary study of the motor control of a musculoskeletal system from the *muscle space*. As seen, even though the apparatus is *overcomplete* since 2-dimensional displacements of the eye-center are determined by eight joints and seven muscles, the tensorial approach can predict, with the use of the Moore–Penrose generalized inverse, a unique execution of movement. It is a characteristic feature of the model that the pattern of movement differs greatly on the motor intention (specified by the displacement of the eye-center). For example, Fig. 4.5(*c*) shows a head-movement similar to one in Fig. 4.5(*a*). However, if the intention is to look up (Fig. 4.5(*d*)) the *identical* model will display a movement-pattern where practically all rotation occurs at C1/C2 and the neck will not tilt. This model suggests, therefore, that the 'different strategies' occurring in motor performance (Nashner, 1977) may be an epiphenomenon of one underlying model and might not invoke a set of different mechanisms to choose from. The model in Fig. 4.5(*b–d*) goes beyond the skeletal model only in the sense that in the case of multiarticular muscles the calculation of the intrinsic coordinate system (establishing the axes that belong to the pull of individual muscles) also necessitates an assumption of the relative stiffness of the joints.

The study shown in Fig. 4.5 can predict an activation-pattern of an overcomplete number of muscles in case of a coordinated movement. This illustrates the potential use of the tensorial approach in the fields of prothestics (Mann, 1981), and functional neuromuscular stimulation (FNS, cf. Kralj & Grobelnik, 1973; Mauritz, 1986; Gruner, 1986 in Pellionisz, 1987*b*). In these applications a central problem is to arrive at a biologically realistic algorithm which can generate the unique set of an overly large number of muscle activation components that are necessary to make an intended movement. The tensorial analysis could also prove to be useful for the interpretation of large numbers of EMG and motor unit measurements (cf. Loeb & Richmond, 1986), where the problem is, again, on what theoretical grounds to conceptually unify and interpret the multiple sets of quantitative experimental data. The problem of interpreting multi-unit EMG and motor unit signals also relates to the question discussed in the last section of this paper.

4.8 Neurobotics: unified geometrical theory of intelligent organisms

Treating motor control problems in terms of multidimensional geometry (with the use of general coordinates) may have an importance in a wider context. Namely, it could lead to a generally applied formalism that yields the means for the unification of fields that are as closely related to sensorimotor research as kinesiology, sports medicine and ergonomy (both in civilian and other applications) and also with those that presently seem to be beyond the realm of the biological sciences. As discussed elsewhere (Pellionisz, 1983, 1985c; Loeb, 1983) by adopting, *both* in *robotics* and *neuroscience*, a common language, e.g. the formalism of generalized vectorial expressions (not just those expressed in Cartesian 3-dimensional, orthogonal frames) these fields could be united by their common language. Finally, in the widest context, the question of how the CNS may exert communication, control and command operations on a most complex (living) organism, in terms of multidimensional geometry and by means of massively parallel computation, is not without the interest of c^3 theorists (cf. Ingber in this volume).

4.9 Computing by neuronal networks: the nature of computation and the structure of the networks

Presently, there is a rapidly growing interest in computing by neuronal networks (cf. this volume; also Eckmiller, 1988). Thus, the question may arise how the tensorial approach relates to this unfolding trend. First of all, while other approaches aim at interpreting the function of imaginary neuronal networks that lack any specific structure (characterized by a set of 'everything-to-everything' interconnections), the tensor approach deals with *existing, not arbitrary, neuronal networks* (such as vestibulo–ocular, vestibulo–collicular and cerebellar networks). Further, this approach provides formal means of handling both their structure (cf. the 'tensor module' above) and their function, in terms of transformation of general vectorial expressions. Perhaps the most important difference is, however, that the tensor formalism defines the *intrinsic mathematical nature of computation*: stating that the calculations performed by networks are transformations of generalized vectors that are expressed in intrinsic coordinates (Pellionisz, 1986d). Thus, in case of the cerebellum, for example, it is possible to state the general function of specific cerebellar circuits (e.g. in different species), i.e., that all individually different cerebellar circuits implement a general covariant-contravariant metric tensor transformation. As a matter of course, it can be reasonably expected that by adopting the axiom of general coordinates, a large part of the research done in the field of associative memories and intelligence will gain new dimensions in the not-so-far-future.

4.10 Single cell electrophysiology: exploration of intrinsic coordinates

Lowering our sights from the distant vistas to present-day possibilities and necessities, a practical and immediate question is how the inherently *multidimensional* theories may relate to data-procurement by classical and widely available *single-cell* recordings. Since it is not the actually utilized technique that determines the fundamental merits of a scientific project but the potency of the *underlying scientific hypothesis*, it is therefore proposed here that by adopting a multidimensional *concept* even single-cell recordings may quickly gain new significance. An example of this may be the exploration of coordinates intrinsic to neuronal function in the CNS. In case of sensorimotor systems, sensory detectors (e.g. primary vestibular neurons) must, by definition, use the frame intrinsic to the structure of sensory mechanism (the vestibular canals). On the other hand, motor effectors (e.g. oculo-motor or neck-motor neurons) must utilize the frame intrinsic to the musculature. Thus, when detecting direction-sensitive firings of neurons *in the middle of a sensorimotor apparatus* (e.g. brain-stem saccadic bursters, or neurons of the motor cortex; cf. Georgeopoulos, Schwartz & Kettner, 1986), an immediate question is whether these neurons use the sensory or the motor frame or *something other*. In fact, based on available data (Simpson *et al.*, 1986) it has already been proposed that these cells may use a coordinate system that is neither the sensory nor the motor frame, but the *eigenvector-frame* of the extraocular muscle apparatus (Pellionisz, 1986c, 1988b). Since eigenvector-frames have been calculated for several species (Pellionisz, 1985a; Pellionisz & Graf, 1987; Pellionisz, 1986c; Daunicht & Pellionisz, 1986), quantitative predictions are already available to be tested in a comparative manner, since predictions of the eigendirections are different in various species. These theoretical predictions could be verified or rejected by means of experimental investigations *using only classical single-unit recordings*.

4.11 Multi-unit physiology: correlation coefficients as metric tensor: exploring the geometry of functional CNS hyperspaces defined over multi-unit signals

Although, for technical reasons, classical electrophysiological methods have been developed for *single units* it has been evident to most workers that, given the axiom that the CNS is a massively parallel system, sooner or later experimental methods needed to be invented to access a multitude of neurons simultaneously (see the review in Llinás, 1974). Such, so-called multi-unit recording techniques have, indeed, been pioneered through the past decades (cf. Freeman, 1975; Gerstein *et al.*, 1983; Reitböeck, 1983; Bower & Llinás, 1983). Partly because establishing, mastering and honing such techniques is an exceedingly demanding endeavor, attention has only recently been focussed on the further, and equally excruciating question of how to theoretically interpret the vast arrays of data made available by such parallel methods. At first, the mere visualization of such parallel recordings is satisfactory (Bower & Llinás, 1983), since it represents the long-awaited fullfilment of the dream by Sherrington (1906), who envisioned the massively parallel brain function in the form of the dynamic flickerings of myriads of neurons as an 'enchanted loom'.

The classical quantitative analysis of multi-unit data is the cross-correlation technique (cf. review in Gerstein *et al.*, 1983). This method concludes in establishing $n \times n$ tables of cross-correlogram coefficients among n signals. One of the many advantages of this stochastical approach is the availability of software for this conventional quantitative computer analysis. The most important shortcoming inherent in correlograms is, however, that they have hitherto been the end-product of the analysis. The interpretation and evaluation of the $n \times n$ tables of cross-correlograms (in case of n data source) is, however, a source of frustration for the neuroscience community (cf. Kruger, 1982).

Another, more recent fundamental concept of interpreting multi-unit recordings is the massive data-compression of n recordings along time into the movement in time *of a single point in a functional n-space*. This extremely powerful concept, which was pioneered by Aertsen, Gernstein & Johannesma (1986), is depicted in Fig. 4.6.

In such an approach, the individual activities in the multi-unit recording represent at every time-point an ordered set of quantities; a mathematical vector. The coordinates are, then, taken as representing a point in the *n*-space. Although this concept would open the way to comprehensive geometrical interpretation of multi-unit recordings, such as calculation of distances, directions, trajectories, center of mass, gravitational clustering and similar geometrical features, *such calculations are possible only in the case where the geometry of the n-dimensional hyperspace is known*. As it has often been pointed out (see, e.g., the note added in proof in Pellionisz & Llinás, 1985, #2), however, a central problem of brain theory is that *there is absolutely no assurance that the CNS functional hyperspaces are limited to either simple Euclidean or even to Riemannian geometry*.

Fig. 4.6. The functional geometry inherent in CNS hyperspaces defined over multi-unit signals is not a matter of convenient assumption of an Euclidean metric. On the contrary; establishment of the metric tensor of the unknown geometry is the goal of multi-unit experimentation. (*a*) multi-unit recording symbolized by $n = 3$ signal sources. (*b*) 'Point in the n-space' concept (Aertsen *et al.*, 1983) of interpreting the recorded activities (e.g., firings of neurons). (*c*) Convenient, but unsupported assumption of an Euclidean 'flat' geometry in the *n*-space permits calculation of geometrical features, but the working hypothesis that the Kronecker delta serves as the metric tensor is untenable. (*d*) The concept of a proposed approach to multi-unit recordings: The functional geometry of the *n*-space is unknown, it is to be established by determining its metric tensor.

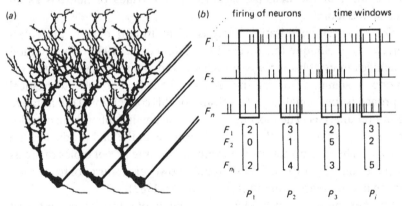

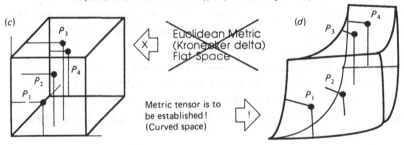

When postulating a functional hyperspace over activities of multi-units, the problems with arbitrarily assumed geometries become painfully obvious. The first question is whether the space is spun over *discrete* or *continuous* variables of coordinate components. While most workers operate with the tacit assumption that neuronal activities represent 'continuous' variables (e.g., frequencies), moreover, that the manifold is derivable, 'smooth' (Aertsen, Gernstein & Johannesma, 1986), even this working hypothesis is not universal. Assumptions of a discrete space, spun over 0, +1 (or −1, +1) binary values of neuronal activity-variables can still be found, possibly because of the remnants of the 'Computers = Brains' McCulloch–Pitts school (where neurons were considered as flip–flop binary units, just like computer-elements). Postulation of such discontinuous, thus non-derivable (non-smooth) manifold is particularly questionable in case of interpretations of multi-unit recordings from the cerebellum (Carman, Rasnow & Bower, 1986). Operations of this organ, throughout evolution, centered around *vestibulo*–cerebellar transformations. The vestibulo–cerebellar apparatus, however, is well-known to employ a frequency-coding (see, e.g., Bloedel *et al.*, 1985), resulting in a reasonably smooth and continuous functional space. A further questionable assumption is the postulation of a highly specific structure of CNS multidimensional functional manifold (e.g. invoking a geometry with Hamming-distances; Carman *et al.*, 1986), since there is absolutely no guarantee that such geometry, indeed, is manifested by CNS function. In most approaches, in fact, the simplest and most parsimonious assumptions are introduced, such that the functional multidimensional hyperspace is *continuous* and 'smooth', moreover, that it is endowed with a position-independent 'flat' *Euclidean geometry* (cf. Aertsen *et al.*, 1986). While most workers are keenly aware of the provisionary nature of such initial postulates (which only serve technical convenience), one cannot overemphasize the stopgap nature of this compromise, lest some followers might be led to the mistaken belief that the geometry of CNS functional spaces is truly known.

In contrast, as depicted in Fig. 4.6, the nature of the geometry of CNS functional hyperspaces is not a matter of convenient assumption, but represents the very challenge that neuroscience must, at some time, squarely face and properly meet. In fact, neuronal functional manifolds may well be endowed with complex geometries that are characterized by a metric tensor which is position-dependent (the space being curved), the axes could be non-orthogonal, non-rectilinear (curvilinear) or even only locally linear. Further, the distinct possibility exists that some CNS hyperspaces (e.g., cognitive neocortical spaces in infants) may not have, at an early developmental stage, an explicit structured geometry at all. It is possible, that 'learning', defined here as the structuring of the geometry of the functional space, may start with amorphic, 'chaotic' spaces with no metric tensor at all. While the above arguments are tacitly accepted in general, it often presents an irresistible temptation that the assumption of a Euclidean metric, even if it is false, permits swift calculations of distances, directions, trajectories, etc., in the CNS manifolds. In contrast, an acknowledgement that the geometry is, indeed, unknown would keep such activities on an uncertain hold until methods for establishing the unknown metric were made available.

In an attempt to break through the above impasse and to contribute to further fruition of the seeds inherent in the above-mentioned existing techniques, an approach is proposed as in Fig. 4.7 (announced in the Soc. Neurosci. Convention, 1986), which in effect could synthesize the 'table-of-cross-correlograms' stochastical interpretation with the 'point-in-the-*n*-space' geometrical analysis. Such unification may open a new way to reveal features of the metric tensor of the geometry of the functional *n*-dimensional hyperspace. The proposal hinges on the consideration that

Fig. 4.7. Concept of the proposal, that the table of cross-correlation coefficients (**r**) of the activity of *n*-signal sources approaches the table of covariant metric tensor components (**g**). Both the coupling of covariant (projection-type) vectorial components (**r**), and the angle between the axes (**g** = cos (ϕ)) expresses the same measure: 'how close are *a* and *b*?

Correlation coefficients
($n \times n$ table for n neurons)

r

Pellionisz' proposal:

r = g

Covariant metric tensor
($n \times n$ table for n axes)

g

Statistical measure of the coupling between *a,b* values of individual points as judged from $i (= 4)$ number of samples

Geometrical measure of the interdependence of general coordinates in the *a,b* *n*-space, judged by $n (= 2)$ axes

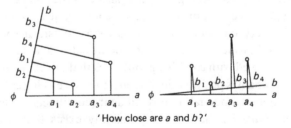

'How close are *a* and *b*?'

if the points in the *n*-space are viewed as expressed in a general, non-orthogonal frame (which, however, we may not know) then the *n* × *n* correlation coefficient table contains *statistical measures of the coupling between the separate coordinates* (e.g., *a, b* components) belonging to the points. If the (unknown) axes were perfectly aligned, the *a* and *b* values would be identical (coupled by coefficient 1), whereas in case of an orthogonal set of axes the *a* and *b* values would be independent (the coupling would be 0). Thus, the *correlation-coefficients*, by expressing the degree of how close are *a* and *b*, are directly related to the *angle between the coordinate-axes*, therefore correlograms may help us establish the relation of the unknown axes.

The above conceptual intuition has been mathematically explored in the study shown in Fig. 4.8. For demonstration purposes, a two-axis

Fig. 4.8. Quantitative elaboration of the proposal. Comparison of the covariant metric tensor and the cross-correlation-coefficient **r**, calculated for four randomly selected points in a two-axis frame (the angle of axes incremented by 5°). (*a*) Comparison of **r** and **g** reveals a similarity of these measures, even if only four data-points are considered. (*b, c*) Two-axis frame with four data points. Covariant vector components are closely coupled (close to 1) if the cosine of the angle of axes is near 1, whereas the coupling is loose (close to 0) if the cosine is nearing 0. Formulae at bottom show the conventional method of calculating correlogram-coefficients, and the covariant metric tensor.

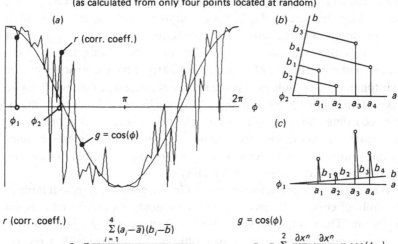

Covariant metric tensor $g = \cos(\phi)$ compared to the correlation-coefficient r, (as calculated from only four points located at random)

r (corr. coeff.)

$$r_{ab} = \frac{\sum\limits_{i=1}^{4}(a_i-\bar{a})(b_i-\bar{b})}{\{\sum\limits_{i=1}^{4}(a_i-\bar{a})^2 \cdot \sum\limits_{i=1}^{4}(b_i-\bar{b})^2\}^{\frac{1}{2}}}$$

$g = \cos(\phi)$

$$g_{ab} = \sum\limits_{n=1}^{2}\frac{\partial x^n}{\partial y^a} \cdot \frac{\partial x^n}{\partial y^b} = \cos(\phi_{ab})$$

frame of reference was investigated, with a varying ϕ angle between them (see Fig. 4.8(b) and (c)). For four randomly selected points, the covariant (projection-type) a and b components were established. Visual comparison of Fig. 4.8(b) and (c) shows, that the a and b components are very close to one another if the ϕ angle is small (Fig. 8(c)), while the a and b components are rather different (e.g., for points 2 and 4) if the ϕ angle is close to perpendicular (Fig. 4.8(b)). The visual impression is borne out by mathematical analysis, where the cross-correlogram coefficient ($\mathbf{r}$) and the covariant metric ($\mathbf{g}$) are calculated by the conventional formulae below (where the covariant metric yields the cosine of the angle of axes): (5,6)

$$r_{ab} = \frac{\sum_{i=1}^{4} (a_i - \bar{a})(b_i - \bar{b})}{\{\sum_{i=1}^{4} (a_i - \bar{a})^2 \cdot \sum_{i=1}^{4} (b_1 - \bar{b})^2\}^{1/2}} \tag{5}$$

$$g_{ab} = \sum_{n=1}^{2} \frac{\partial x^n}{\partial y^a} \cdot \frac{\partial x^n}{\partial y^b} = \cos(\phi_{ab}) \tag{6}$$

Plotting $\mathbf{r}$ and $\mathbf{g} = \cos(\phi)$ in Fig. 4.8(a) reveals that even in case of only four (different) randomly selected points in each two-axis frame (where ϕ was changed by five-degree increments), the $\mathbf{r}$ and $\mathbf{g} = \cos(\phi)$ values are, indeed, close enough to warrant further studies.

It has to be emphasized, that the cross-correlogram method is an inherently statistical stochastic measure, while the geometrical measure of the closeness of the axes (the cosines of the angles between them) yields a single deterministic value of ϕ. Since in case of stochastical analysis the size of the statistical sample is crucial, therefore the calculation of $\mathbf{r} = \mathbf{g}$ has been implemented in Fig. 4.9 for a varying, much larger number than four randomly selected points, in order to ascertain the convergence of $\mathbf{r} = \mathbf{g}$ with the increase of the number of points. Comparison of the precision of $\mathbf{r} = \mathbf{g}$ in case of 4, 10, 100 or 1000 points clearly shows that for a customary 3–5% biological precision the statistical sample need not be larger than about 100 measurement-points. Given the fact that in multi-unit recordings firing of units can usually be obtained during protracted time (with literally thousands of unitary activities either in extracellular spiking, motor unit or EMG activities), the required number of sampling should pose no insurmountable difficulty.

The proposal for the convergence of the correlation coefficient table to the table of covariant metric tensor components appears to be a useful beginning. The road, however, is long towards synthesizing the classical statistical correlogram-analysis of multi-unit recordings with a recent, multidimensional geometrical interpretation. However, in the proposed approach *the geometry (the metric tensor) of the multidimensional functional hyperspace is not taken for granted*, but the very purpose of the analysis is to establish the unknown metric tensor. Thus, one can foresee that with enough time and investment new types of functional geometries of the CNS will be revealed, such that we have very little knowledge (or even imagination) about at the present time.

In order to provide a glimpse of the future possibilities, an arbitrary example is shown in Fig. 4.10, to illuminate how one would go about conceptually and formally treating large $n \times n$ tables of cross-correlogram components.

Suppose that a 30×30 table of cross-correlogram coefficients were experimentally established in a 30-electrode-recording. It is visible in the left-side plotting in Fig. 4.10, that the off-diagonals of the cross-correlogram component table are non-zeroes. This means that the activities of the measured units are not independent of one another, but they are coupled. This could be the result of the activities arising from a

Fig. 4.9. Convergence of the correlation coefficient **r** to the covariant metric tensor **g** if the size of the statistical sample increases (from $n = 4$ to $n = 10$, $n = 100$ and $n = 1000$). A sample-size in the range of 100 is deemed sufficient for biological precision of 3–5%.

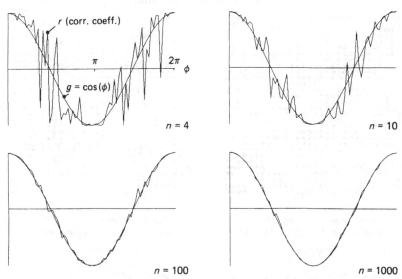

Convergence of the correlation-coefficient r to the covariant metric tensor $g = \cos(\phi)$ by increasing the number of points (n) in the statistical sample

András Pellionisz

coordinate system with non-orthogonal (non-independent) axes (in fact, in the given arbitrary example the coupled 'recordings' originated from the neck-muscle axes, shown in Fig. 4.2). The two questions that an investigator may ask are as follows: (a) is it possible to reconstruct the set of coordinate axes which yielded the given table? (b) without the knowledge of the axes, is it possible to understand the functional geometry inherent in such recordings?

A positive answer to question (a), in many cases, is not altogether impossible. If the firings arise, e.g., from motoneurons, which are connected to a set of muscles (as in the case of this exemplary demonstration shown in the left plotting in Fig. 4.10), then measurement of the physical geometry of the muscular arrangement could directly reveal

Fig. 4.10. Demonstration of a table of cross-correlogram-coefficients considered equal to the covariant metric tensor, and calculating its dual contravariant metric tensor. The calculation uses the Moore–Penrose formula, yielding a proper inverse if the space is complete, and a generalized inverse if the space is overcomplete. With measurement of correlograms (left), and calculation of the dual metric (right), both metric tensors are available, thus the geometry of the functional space is determined. This enables one to calculate geometrical features of eigenvectors, distances, angles, geodesic trajectories, etc. (In this arbitrary demonstration the cross-correlograms were *not* taken from multi-unit measurements, but originated from the set of neck-motor axes shown in Fig. 4.2.)

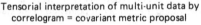

Tensorial interpretation of multi-unit data by
correlogram = covariant metric proposal

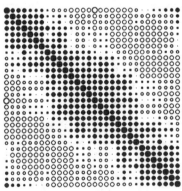
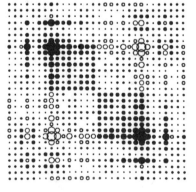

Correlogram coefficients (*r*)   Non-Euclidean contravariant
of an array of *n* neurons (*n* × *n*)   metric tensor of neuron *n*-space

Proposal: $g^{a,b}$

$r_{a,b} = g_{a,b}$ Calculated as the Moore-Penrose
(Corr. coefficients = covariant metric)   generalized inverse of $g = r$)

these axes. However, in most cases, e.g. when dealing with units deep inside a neuronal (e.g. non-sensorimotor) apparatus, it might prove to be beyond our means to ever establish the underlying frames. Such may be the case, e.g., when dealing with olfactory space (cf. Freeman, 1975), where the individual 'axes' of detecting odors may never be physically established in the manner of how the muscle rotational axes or the vestibular canals can be visualized. Nevertheless, if according to this proposal the table of cross-correlogram coefficients is taken as the covariant metric tensor, its dual tensor (the contravariant metric) can be established either by its regular inverse, or by the Moore–Penrose generalized inverse.

Answering question (b), a knowledge of *both metric tensors* (also called fundamental tensors, cf. Einstein, 1916) comprises a knowledge of the geometry of the *n*-space from which practically every geometrical property of the space can be calculated *without knowing the axes themselves*. One example, well worth mentioning here, is the calculation from the metric tensor of the functional eigenvectors, which lead to direct and feasible experimental hypotheses. Mathematical spaces in the CNS, e.g. the one used in this chapter in which the contravariant metric tensor is the Moore–Penrose generalized inverse of the covariant metric tensor, do not even have names at this point of time. Yet, mathematical specification of the dual metric tensors would already enable one to properly calculate trajectories (e.g. geodesic lines), directions, distances, angles, center of gravity, gravitational clustering and many other geometrical features that we have just started to contemplate.

The above survey of the vistas from Tensor Network Theory, although exhausting, is by no means exhaustive. It is expected that since any formally and conceptually coherent brain theory might exert a conglomerating and unifying effect on a wide range of disciplines, the significance of brain theory, that we have barely begun to appreciate, will only increase in the future.

Acknowledgements

This work was supported by grants NS 22999 and NS 13742 from NINCDS.

References

Aertsen, A., Gerstein, G. & Johannesma, P. (1986) From neuron to assembly: neuronal organization and stimulus representation. In *Brain Theory: Proceedings of the First Trieste Meeting on Brain Theory*, 1–4 October, 1984, eds. G. Palm & A. Aersten, Berlin: Springer Verlag, pp. 7–24.

Albert, A. (1972). *Regression and the Moore–Penrose Pseudouniverse*. New York: Academic Press.

Baker, J., Goldberg, J. & Peterson, B. (1985) Spatial and temporal response properties of the vestibulocollic reflex in decerebrate cats. *J. Neurophysiology*, **54**, 735–56.

Baker, J., Goldberg, J., Wickland, C. & Peterson, B. W. (1984). Spatial and temporal properties of vestibulo-neck reflex EMG. *Society for Neuroscience Abstracts*, **10**, 162.

Bickley, W. G. & Gibson, R. E. (1962) *Via Vector to Tensor*. New York: John Wiley & Sons.

Blanks, R. H. I., Curthoys, I. S. & Markham, C. H. (1972). Planar relationships of semicircular canals in the cat. *American J. of Physiology*, **223**, 55–62.

Bloedel, J. R., Dichgans, J. & Precht, W. (1985). *Cerebellar Functions*. Berlin: Springer Verlag.

Bower, J. & Llinás, R. (1983). Simultaneous sampling of the responses of multiple, closely adjacent Purkinje cells responding to climbing fiber activation. *Society for Neuroscience Abstracts*, **9**, 607.

Carman, G. J., Rasnow, B. & Bower, J. M. (1986). 'Analysis of the dynamics of activity in ensembles of neurons recorded simultaneously in cerebellar cortex'. *Society for Neuroscience Abstracts*, **12**, 1417.

Churchland, P. S. (1986). *Neurophilosophy: Towards a Unified Science of the Mind–Brain*. Cambridge, Massachusetts: MIT Press.

Daunicht, W. & Pellionisz, A. (1986). 'Coordinates intrinsic to the semicircular canals and the extraocular muscles in the rat'. *Society for Neuroscience Abstracts*, **12**, 1089.

Eckmiller, R. and C. von Malsburg, eds. (1988). *Neuronal Computers*. Proceedings of the Nat. Adv. Lab. Workshop in Düsseldorf, Springer Verlag.

Einstein, A. (orig. 1916). 'The foundation of the general theory of relativity'. In *The Principle of Relativity* (1952), pp. 111–64, ed. A. Sommerfeld, New York: Dover.

Ezure, K. & Graf, W. (1984). 'A quantitative analysis of the spatial organization of the vestibulo-ocular reflexes in lateral and front-eyed animals'. *Neuroscience*, **12**, 85–93.

Freeman, W. J. (1975). *Mass Action in the Nervous System*. New York: Academic Press.

Georgeopoulos, A. P., Schwartz, A. B. & Kettner, R. E. (1986). Neuronal population coding of movement direction. *Science*, **233**, 1416–19.

Gernstein, G. L., Bloom, M. J. K., Espinosa, I. E., Evanczuk, S. & Turner, M. R. (1983). 'Design of a laboratory for multineuron studies. *IEEE Systems, Man & Cybernetics*, **13**, 668–76.

Gielen, C. C. A. M. & van Zuylen, E. J. (1986). 'Coordination of arm muscles during flexion and supination: application of the tensor analysis approach'. *Neuroscience*, **17**, 527–39.

Green, M. B. (1986). 'Superstrings'. *Scientific American*, Sept., pp. 48–60.

Gruner, J. A. (1986). 'Considerations in designing acceptable neuromuscular stimulation systems for restoring function in paralyzed limbs'. *Central Nervous System Trauma*, 3(1), 37–47.

Helmholtz, H. L. F. (1896). *Handbuch der Physiologischen Optik*. Zweite Auflage. Leipzig: Voss.

Ingber, L. (this vol.). 'Applications of biological intelligence to command, control and communication'.

Kralj, A. & Grobelnik, S. (1973). 'Functional electrical stimulation – a new hope for paraplegic patients?' *Bulletin of Prosthesis Research*, **10–20**, 75–102.

Kruger, J. (1982). 'A 12-fold microelectrode for recording from vertically aligned cortical neurons'. *J. Neuroscience Methods*, **6**, 347–50.

Levi-Civita, T. (1926). *The Absolute Differential Calculus (Calculus of Tensors)*. New York: Dover.

Llinás, R. (1974). 'Motor aspects of cerebellar control'. *Physiologist*, 17, 19–46.

Llinás, R. & Pellionisz, A. (1985). 'Cerebellar function and the adaptive feature of the central nervous system. In *Adaptive Mechanisms in Gaze Control. Facts and Theories*. Reviews in Oculomotor Research, V. 1., eds. A. Berthoz & G. Melvill-Jones. Amsterdam: Elsevier, pp. 223–32.

Loeb, G. E. (1983). 'Finding common ground between robotics and physiology'. *Trends in Neuroscience*, 5, 203–4.

Loeb, G. E. & Richmond, F. J. R. (1986). 'Synchronization of motor units in and among diverse neck muscles during slow movements in intact cats'. *Society for Neuroscience Abstracts*, 12, 687.

Mann, R. W. (1981). 'Cybernetic limb prosthesis. *Annals of Biomedical Engineering*, 9, 1–43.

Mauritz, K. H. (1986). 'Restoration of posture and gait by functional neuromuscular stimulation (FNS)'. In *Disorders of Posture and Gait*, eds. W. Bles & T. Brandt, Amsterdam: Elsevier, pp. 367–85.

McCulloch, W. S. & Pitts, W. (1943). 'A logical calculus of the ideas immanent in nervous activity'. *Bulletin of Mathematical Biophysics*, 5, 115–33.

Nashner, L. M. (1977). 'Fixed patterns of rapid postural responses among leg muscles during stance'. *Experimental Brain Research*, 30, 13–24.

Palm, G. & Aertsen, A. (1986). *Brain Theory: Proceedings of the First Trieste Meeting on Brain Theory*, 1–4 October, 1984. Berlin–Heidelberg–New York–Tokyo: Springer Verlag.

Pellionisz, A. (1979). 'Modeling of neurons and neuronal networks'. In *The Neurosciences: IVth Study Program*, eds. F. O. Schmitt & F. G. Worden, Boston: MIT Press, pp. 525–46.

Pellionisz, A. (1983). 'Brain theory: connecting neurobiology to robotics. Tensor analysis: utilizing intrinsic coordinates to describe, understand and engineer functional geometries of intelligent organisms. *J. Theoretical Neurobiology*, 2(3), 185–211.

Pellionisz, A. (1984). 'Coordination: a vector-matrix description of transformations of overcomplete CNS coordinates and a tensorial solution using the Moore–Penrose generalized inverse'. *J. Theoretical Neurobiology*, 110, 353–75.

Pellionisz, A. (1985a). 'Tensorial aspects of the multidimensional approach to the vestibulo–oculomotor reflex and gaze', In *Reviews of Oculomotor Research. I. Adaptive Mechanisms in Gaze Control*, eds. A. Berthoz & G. Melvill-Jones, Amsterdam: Elsevier, pp. 281–96.

Pellionisz, A. (1985b). 'Tensorial brain theory in cerebellar modeling'. In *Cerebellar Functions*, eds. J. Bloedel, J. Dichgans & W. Precht, Heidelberg: Springer, pp. 201–29.

Pellionisz, A. (1985c). 'Robotics connected to neurobiology by tensor theory of brain function'. *Proceedings of IEEE International Conference on Systems, Man & Cybernetics*, pp. 411–14.

Pellionisz, A. (1986a). 'David Marr's theory of the cerebellar cortex: a model in brain theory for the "Galilean combination of simplification, unification and mathematization"'. In *Brain Theory*, eds. G. Palm & A. Aertsen, Berlin–Heidelberg–New York: Springer Verlag, pp. 253–7.

Pellionisz, A. (1986b). 'Old dogmas and new axioms in brain theory. Commentary to "Cortical connections and parallel processing: Structure & function: by D. H. Ballard"'. *Behavioral and Brain Sciences*, 9, 103–4.

Pellionisz, A. (1986c). 'Tensorial relationship found for structural and functional reference frames of brain function: Saccade neurons in monkey utilize frames composed of the eigenvectors of the frame of extraocular muscles'. *Society for Neuroscience Abstracts*, 12, 1186.

Pellionisz, A. (1986d). 'Tensor network theory and its application in computer modeling of the metaorganization of sensorimotor hierarchies of gaze'. In *Proc. 'Neuronal Networks for Computing'*, AIP 151, New York: American Institute of Physics, pp. 339–44.

Pellionisz, A. (1986e). 'Tensor network theory of the central nervous system and sensorimotor modeling'. In *Brain Theory: Proceedings of the First Trieste Meeting on Brain Theory*, 1–4 October, 1984, eds. G. Palm & A. Aertsen, Berlin: Springer Verlag, pp. 121–45.

Pellionisz, A. (1987a). 'Tensor network theory of the central nervous system'. *Encyclopedia of Neuroscience*, ed. G. Adelman, Boston: Birkhauser.

Pellionisz, A. (1985a). 'Tensor network theory of the central nervous system'. *Encyclopedia of Neuroscience*, ed. G. Adelman, Boston: Birkhauser, pp. 1196–8.

Pellionisz, A. (1987b). 'Tensor geometry: mathematical brain theory for neurocomputers and neurobots. A parallel algorithm for functional neuromuscular stimulation'. In *Proc. 9th Annual Conf. of IEEE/Engineering in Medicine and Biology Society*, Boston

Pellionisz, A. (1987c). 'Sensorimotor operations: a ground for the co-evolution of brain theory with neurobotics and neurocomputers'. In *Proc. IEEE 1st Ann. Internatl. Conf. on Neural Networks*, San Diego.

Pellionisz, A. (1988a). 'Tensor geometry: a language of brains and neurocomputers. Generalized coordinates in neuroscience and robotics'. In *Neural Computers'*, Springer Verlag (ed. R. Eckmiller).

Pellionisz, A. (1988b). 'Tensorial aspects of the multidimensional massively parallel sensorimotor function of neuronal networks'. In: *Vestibulospinal Control of Posture and Movement*. Progress in Brain Research (ed. by Allum, J. H. J. and Powpeiano, O.). Elsevier.

Pellionisz, A. & Graf, W. (1987). 'Tensor network model of the "Three-neuron vestibulo-ocular reflex arc" in cat. *J. Theoretical Neurobiology* 5, 127–31.

Pellionisz, A. & Llinás, R. (1979). 'Brain modeling by tensor network theory and computer simulation. The cerebellum: distributed processor for predictive coordination. *Neuroscience*, 4, 322–48.

Pellionisz, A. & Llinás, R. (1980). 'Tensorial approach to the geometry of brain function: cerebellar coordination via metric tensor'. *Neuroscience*, 5, 1125–36.

Pellionisz, A. & Llinás, R. (1982). 'Space–time representation in the brain. The cerebellum as a predictive space-time metric tensor'. *Neuroscience*, 7, 2949–70.

Pellionisz, A. & Llinás, R. (1985). 'Tensor network theory of the metaorganization of functional geometries in the CNS'. *Neuroscience*, 16, 245–74.

Pellionisz, A. & Peterson, B. W. (1988). 'A tensorial model of neck motor activation'. In *Control of Head Movement*, eds. B. W. Peterson & F. Richmond, Oxford: Oxford University Press, pp. 178–86.

Peterson, B. W., Baker, J., Wickland, C. & Pellionisz, A. (1985). 'Relation between pulling directions of neck muscles and their activation by the vestibulocollic reflex: tests of a tensorial model'. *Society for Neuroscience Abstracts*, 11, 83.

Peterson, B. W. & Pellionisz, A. J. (1986). 'A tensorial model of the kinematics of head movements in the cat. *Society for Neuroscience Abstracts*, 12, 684.

Reitboeck, H. J. P. (1983). 'A 19-channel matrix drive with individually controllable fiber micro-electrodes for neurophysiological applications'. *IEEE Transactions on System, Man & Cybernetics*, SMC-13, 5, pp. 676–82.

Shannon, C. (1948). 'A mathematical theory of communication'. *Bell System Technology J.*, **27**, 3–4.

Sherrington, C. (1906). *The Integrative Action of the Nervous System*. New York: Scribner.

Simpson, J. I. & Graf, W. (1985). 'The selection of reference frames by nature and its investigators'. In *Adaptive Mechanisms in Gaze Control. Facts and Theories*. Reviews of Oculomotor Research, V. 1, eds. A. Berthoz & G. Melvill-Jones, Amsterdam: Elsevier, pp. 3–20.

Simpson, J. I. & Pellionisz, A. (1984). 'The vestibulo–ocular reflex in rabbit, as interpreted using the Moore–Penrose generalized inverse transformation of intrinsic coordinates. *Society for Neuroscience Abstracts*, **10**, 909.

Simpson, J. I., Rudinger, D., Reisine, H. & Henn, V. (1986). 'Geometry of extraocular muscles of the rhesus monkey'. *Society for Neuroscience Abstracts*, **12**, 1186.

Simpson, J. I., Soodak, R. E. & Hess, R. (1979). 'The accessory optic system and its relation to the vestibulo-cerebellum'. In *Reflex Control of Posture and Movements, Progress in Brain Research*, vol. 50, eds. R. Granit & O. Pompeiano, Amsterdam: Elsevier, pp. 715–24.

Vidal, P. P., Graf, W. & Berthoz, A. (1986). 'The orientation of the cervical vertebral column in unrestrained awake animals'. *Experimental Brain Research*, **61**, 549–59.

von Neumann, J. (1958). *The Computer and the Brain*. New Haven: Yale University Press.

Wiener, N. (1948). *Cybernetics, or Control and Communication in the Animal and the Machine*, Cambridge: MIT Press.

5

Neurons with hysteresis?

GEOFFREY W. HOFFMANN

5.1 Introduction

In the last few years we have learnt an enormous amount about how the immune system functions. We now have at least the outline of an immune system network theory that seems to account for much of the phenomenology (Hoffmann, 1980, 1982, Hoffmann *et al.* 1988). The many similarities between the immune system and the central nervous system suggested the possibility that the same kind of mathematical model could be applicable to both systems. We found that a neural network theory analogous to the immune system theory can indeed be formulated (Hoffmann, 1986). The basic variables in the immune system network theory are clone sizes; the corresponding variables in the neural network theory are the rates of firing of neurons. We need to postulate that neurons are slightly more complex than has been assumed in conventional neural network theories, namely that there can be hysteresis in the rate of firing of a neuron as the input level of the neuron is varied.

The added complexity of the hysteresis postulate is compensated by a new simplicity at the level of the network; the network can learn without any changes in the synaptic connection strengths (Hoffmann, Benson, Bree & Kinahan, 1986). Learned information is associated solely with a state vector; memory is a consequence of the fact that due to the hysteresis associated with each neuron, the system tends to stay in the region of an N-dimensional phase space to which its experiences have taken it. A network's stimulus–response behaviour is determined by its location in that space.

5.2 Neurons with hysteresis

On the basis of presently available neuro-physiological data, it seems feasible that at least some neurons exhibit hysteresis at the single cell level. Such hysteresis could, theoretically, occur through a variety of biochemical mechanisms, and we will see that there is experimental evidence for one mechanism. I will first describe two theoretical models; one that involves just a single allosteric enzyme, and another due to Lisman (1985), that involves three enzymes, one of which acts autocatalytically on itself. I will then briefly review a model that involves both allostery and autocatalysis, and that has been formulated by Miller & Kennedy (1986) on the basis of experimental studies of an important brain enzyme.

5.2.1 A model based on an allosteric enzyme

Let X be a key metabolite that controls the rate of firing of neurons, such that the rate of firing is (say) proportional to the concentration of X. The concentration of X is assumed to be affected by a second substance Y that reflects the net level of inhibitory signals the cell receives. We consider the following simple reaction scheme:

$$A \to X,$$
$$X \to B \text{ (slow)},$$
$$X \to B \text{ (catalysed by } Y),$$
$$\text{Excess } X \text{ inhibits } Y.$$

Now X is produced at a constant rate from A; X is broken down by two processes, one of which is slow and is independent of Y. The second breakdown process involves Y as an enzyme or the activator of an enzyme. High levels of X inhibit the enzymatic breakdown of X by Y. This phenomenon (substrate inhibition) can occur when an enzyme has two binding sites for the substrate, and requires that the enzyme have two forms with different activities. This is known in biochemistry as 'allostery'. If we denote the concentrations of X and Y in neuron i by x_i and y_i, respectively, an appropriate differential equation for x_i as a function of time can have the form

$$\dot{x}_i = 1 - x_i - \frac{x_i y_i}{1 + \alpha x_i^2}, \tag{1}$$

where α is a constant. The inhibitory input y_i is given by

$$y_i = \sum_{j=1}^{N} \beta_{ij} x_j, \tag{2}$$

where β_{ij} is the synaptic connection strength from neuron j to neuron i. The β_{ij} correspond to the T_{ij} of Hopfield, except that learning can occur with the β_{ij} fixed (see below).

There can be three steady-state values for each x_i, two of which are stable (A and C, Fig. 5.1), and one of which is unstable (B in Fig. 5.1).

Geoffrey Hoffmann

With N neurons, each of which can be in either a high x_i or a low x_i steady state, the number of attractors can be almost 2^N (Hoffmann, 1986). The number of unstable steady states in the system can be close to 3^N.

5.2.2 The Lisman model: a model based on autocatalysis

Lisman (1985) described a biochemical model with properties that are similar to those of the above model, and which is based on enzymes that are known to exist in neurons. The Lisman model involves autocatalytic phosphorylation of a kinase enzyme, and dephosphorylation by a phosphatase enzyme. Denoting the unphosphorylated kinase by A, the phosphorylated enzyme by X, and a phosphatase enzyme by P, the main reactions are:

$A \rightarrow X$ catalysed by X, with adenosine triphosphate (ATP) as a
second substrate ('forward reaction'),

Fig. 5.1. Kinetics in a hypothetical model based on allostery. The rate of change in the rate of firing of a neuron, $\dot{x}_i$, as a function of x_i for three different values of the input y_i: low ($y_i = y_L$), intermediate ($y_i = y_I$), and high ($y_i = y_H$). For $y_i = y_I$ the neuron has two stable steady state rates of firing, $x_i = A$ and $x_i = C$.

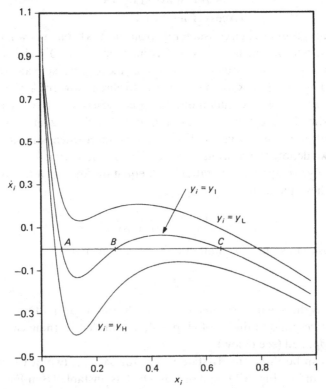

$X \rightarrow A$ catalysed by P, releases phosphate ('reverse reaction'),
with the constraint that

$$[A] + [X] = \text{constant} = [A_0]$$

(conservation of the total amount of the kinase). The square brackets
denote 'concentration of', and we will again denote the concentration of
X in neuron i by x_i. The 'reverse reaction' is not exactly the reverse of the
'forward reaction'; this is a dissipative system, with ATP being utilized to
provide the necessary free energy to drive the forward reaction, while no
ATP is generated in the reverse reaction. Assuming conditions that result
in mass-action kinetics for the forward reaction and Michaelis–Menten
kinetics for the reverse reaction, the net rate of the production of X in
neuron i, $\dot{x}_i$, is given by

$$\dot{x}_i = \text{forward rate} - \text{reverse rate},$$

$$= k_1([A_0] - x_i)x_i - \frac{k_2[P]x_i}{K_\mathrm{M} + x_i}, \tag{3}$$

where k_1 and k_2 are rate constants and K_M is a Michaelis–Menten
constant. The forward rate is the difference between a quadratic term and
a linear term in x_i, resulting in an inverted parabola as shown in Fig.
5.2(*a*). This curve can intersect the curve for the reverse reaction at three
places as is also shown in Fig. 5.2(*a*). For appropriately chosen values of
the parameters this model then results in a form for $\dot{x}_i$ versus x_i that is
similar to that obtained with model 1 (Fig. 5.2(*b*), compare Fig. 5.1).
Lisman suggests that input to this bistable system can be mediated via a
third enzyme that is also a kinase (a phosphorylating enzyme).

5.2.3 The Miller–Kennedy model: autocatalysis and allostery in real brains

An exciting recent development is that biochemical evidence supporting
a 'Lisman plus allostery' model has been obtained by Miller & Kennedy
(1986). This work involves the most abundant protein kinase in the brain,
Type II Ca^{2+}/calmodulin-dependent protein kinase. This enzyme constitutes about 1% of brain protein, and is most highly concentrated in a
region of the brain that is believed to be involved in long-term memory
(Erondu & Kennedy, 1985). It has autocatalytic phosphorylating activity,
and is dephosphorylated by brain phosphatases. It is a large protein with
a molecular weight of about 600 000, and can be multiply phosphorylated,
up to a level of about 30 phosphate groups per enzyme molecule. The
autocatalytic activity can be regulated by incoming electrical activity via
calcium ions. When it has very few or no phosphate groups attached to it,
the autophosphorylation is calcium-dependent. When more than about

three to four phosphate groups are attached to the enzyme it seems to exist in a different allosteric form, and the autocatalytic phosphorylation then occurs in the absence of calcium. An allosteric change seems to be necessary for the enzyme to work as the basis of a bistable system, since the autocatalytic phosphorylation is intra-molecular, rather than inter-molecular as was assumed in the Lisman model.

5.3 Network dynamics

We have shown that the dynamics of N-dimensional systems like the system (1) can be conveniently displayed on a phase plane (Hoffmann *et*

Fig. 5.2. Kinetics in the Lisman model, a model based on some known biochemical autocatalytic processes. (*a*) The velocities of the forward (kinase) and reverse (phosphatase) reactions as a function of the concentration of the kinase that is phosphorylated, x_i. The concentration x_i is expressed as a fraction of the total kinase concentration. (*b*) The net reaction rate (forward rate minus reverse rate) $\dot{x}_i$ as a function of x_i. Note the similarities between Figs. 5.1 and 5.2(*b*). (Fig. 5.2 adapted from Lisman, 1985.)

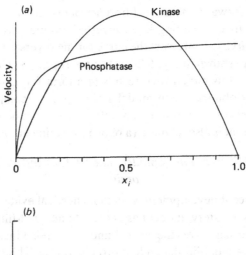

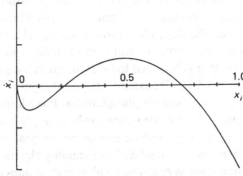

al., 1986). Equation (1) with $\dot{x}_i$ set equal to zero defines an S-shaped curve in the x_i, y_i plane. If a neuron has a steady firing rate, its values of x_i and y_i must lie on that S-shaped curve, which is a locus of equilibrium. The curve consists of three branches: two stable branches separated by an unstable branch. When the system is at equilibrium, each of the neurons has a pair of coordinates in the x_i, y_i plane that is located somewhere along the two stable branches of the locus of equilibrium. Small transient stimuli cause neurons to leave the locus of equilibrium, and return to it in a way that is characteristic of the initial state and the particular stimulus. If the system starts in a particular stable steady state, its responses are qualitatively independent of the magnitude of the applied stimuli up to a certain threshold level. Larger stimuli cause some neurons to switch from the low firing rate stable branch of the equilibrium curve to the high firing rate branch or vice versa, and the system can then converge towards a new equilibrium state, where its stimulus-response behaviour can be slightly different. There can be close to 2^N different ways of distributing the neurons between the two stable branches. These are the stable steady states mentioned above. The system can make a large number of different responses to a correspondingly large number of different stimuli, and unless the amplitudes of the stimuli exceed the threshold level, the system stays in the same region of the phase space.

Such networks have been shown to be capable of producing arbitrary outputs, provided N is sufficiently large (Hoffmann, 1986). A particular output is produced if the system has an initial condition that can lead to that output. The hysteresis associated with each neuron tends to keep the system as a whole in a restricted region of the N-dimensional phase space, and this is the basis for memory in the theory. The particular region in that space where the system is located depends on the set of stimuli to which it has been subjected. In contrast to conventional neural network models, the formation of memories does not need to involve changes in the synaptic strengths, β_{ij}.

5.4 Teaching

These networks can be taught to exhibit prespecified stimulus-response behaviour (Hoffmann, Benson, Bree & Kinahan, 1986). We systematically perturb the network until it reaches a region of phase space where it gives the desired stimulus-response behaviour. The idea is that a brain is moved around in the N-dimensional phase space by the stimuli that it receives, until it reaches a point in that phase space such that it is no longer strongly perturbed by the stimuli.

In our training algorithm we simply apply stimuli and observe responses. There is no 'twiddling' of the synaptic connection strengths. Only the various stimuli themselves are used to move the system around in the N-dimensional phase space until a satisfactory region in that space is found. If at some point a satisfactory response to a stimulus is not obtained, the stimulus is reapplied and can intensify. A wrong response means the system was in an unsatisfactory region of the phase space. Applying the same stimulus again takes the system further away from the region of phase space that did not give the correct response. If a good response is obtained, we pass on to another stimulus. This algorithm presumes to mimic the way real brains learn by experience. The system automatically keeps being changed until a functional complementarity between the stimulus and the response is obtained. If we are exposed to a stimulus and respond to it appropriately, our response can lead to the elimination of, or escape from, the stimulus. If we do not respond appropriately, the stimulus can persist, and possibly intensify, independently of whether the stimulus is being provided by a teacher or other aspects of the individual's environment. We have trained networks consisting of 20 neurons to respond to stimuli in prespecified ways using an algorithm based on these ideas. The correct responses were defined in a binary fashion, so that untrained networks had a 50% chance of making individual correct responses. Our degree of success in training these networks has so far been modest. In one series of experiments, we achieved an average accuracy of 73% when we were training for a particular response to a single stimulus, 70% when there were two stimuli, 66% with three stimuli, and 59% when there were four stimulus–response pairs being taught. Recent results indicate that networks with random non-negative, unsymmetrical β_{ij} can learn just as well as the networks with symmetric β_{ij} that we used initially.

5.5 Convergence problems?

Many important questions concerning the neurons-with-hysteresis theory are unresolved. Can our teaching strategy converge for a large number of different stimuli and responses and, if so, how fast can the convergence be? What neural architectures optimize the probability of convergence and the rate of convergence? Convergence might be slow for large systems with many stimulus–response pairs. We need to remember that the amount of processing done by our brains is huge; it has been said that while we would need a million brains (or so) to do the computation performed by a single Cray computer, we would also need a million Crays (or so) to simulate what is performed by a single brain. Each device is so different from the other that it is intrinsically very difficult for them to simulate each other's operations

There is a big difference between the brain and the immune system with respect to the convergence problem. The design of the immune system ensures that each response is automatically complementary to the stimulus that evokes it, so that a response is automatically tailored to be appropriate for just the corresponding stimulus. This is not the case for the brain. In the analogy between the two systems, clones of lymphocytes in the immune system correspond to single neurons in the brain, and x_i in the immune system is the size of the clone i (Hoffmann, 1986). When the immune system receives a stimulus, something foreign (an antigen) stimulates just those clones to divide that have receptors that recognize the foreign entity. These clones can then produce antibodies with precisely the same shapes (variable regions or 'V-regions') as the receptors that recognized the foreign material. The production of these antibodies constitutes the main aspect of the response of the system, since the antibodies eliminate the stimulus. The complementarity at the molecular level between antigen and the receptors of the selected antibody-producing clones ensures that a suitable new region in the N-dimensional phase space can be found quickly. The part of the network that is most strongly perturbed by something foreign is automatically the part of the network that is most appropriate to respond. In the case of the brain there is no automatic complementarity between the applied stimulus and the appropriate response of the system. It follows that for the brain the finding of an appropriate region of phase space, such that a response to a particular stimulus is 'correct', has to involve trial and error.

If we wish to quantitatively compare the rates of learning of the immune system and the central nervous system, it is appropriate to define units of time that are 'natural units' for each of the systems, and then express the time taken to learn something in terms of these natural units. A suitable natural unit would be the minimum time required for one of the x_i variables to double in magnitude. In the case of the immune system this is of the order of 10^5 s, and in the case of the central nervous system it is of the order of about 10^{-3} s. The immune system typically makes an appropriate response to something completely foreign within a small number of its natural time units. A brain typically takes a much larger number of its natural time units to learn to make an appropriate response to a completely new stimulus (that is, a stimulus unlike anything experienced previously by the brain). In this sense the immune system learns much faster than the brain.

5.6 Pain and joy

The problem of how to interpret pain and joy in terms of neural networks is not often addressed. We have speculated on a possible interpretation in terms of the above theory (Hoffmann & Benson, 1986). I will now review those ideas and expand on them a little.

The above teaching method is a brute force approach, that might be viewed as being based on using only 'pain'. (If the response is incorrect, we increase the magnitude of the stimulus.) The efficiency of our teaching could presumably be much greater if we could add something to the algorithm equivalent to joy. A speculative neural interpretation of pain and joy is in terms of familiar and unfamiliar regions of phase space. Perhaps pain is associated with stimuli that take one away from familiar regions of phase space (as most random strong stimuli could be expected to do), and joy results from stimuli that are special in the sense that they move one back towards more familiar regions. When a brain has developed a set of memories, it presumably spends most of its time in a relatively small section of the total phase space. In an environment with a restricted number of dominant stimuli we would expect some of the neurons to become firmly established close to either the high or the low stable steady-state x_i values. If, for instance, even just one in 1000 of the neurons were to become permanently established in either the high or the low x_i state, this would imply the restriction of a system of 10^{10} neurons to a fraction $2^{-10\,\text{million}}$ (approximately $10^{-3\,\text{million}}$) of the total phase space. In fact the fraction of the phase space to which a brain is restricted seems likely to be even much smaller than this, due to correlations in the firing rates of other neurons as well, which also reflect correlations in the stimuli and the limited number of different stimuli that are received from the environment. Specific stimuli that the brain receives periodically (for instance specific stimuli experienced as a result of consuming food) would be expected to play an important role in keeping it in that particular limited region of phase space. Stimuli that cause pain are normally not received periodically, and they are likely to be more random in nature. There are many directions in phase space away from a restricted (familiar) region, and only a small number of directions back towards the most familiar regions if one is removed from them. Thus this idea would account for the fact that a limited set of specific stimuli can impart joy, while a broad range of relatively nonspecific stimuli can impart pain. New stimuli could move one back towards familiar regions of phase space if they are somehow correlated (in the context of the wiring diagram of our brains) with other stimuli with which we are familiar. If this idea is correct, we might be able to simulate joy by making a network accustomed to a certain set of stimuli during its 'ontogeny'. Stimuli that are correlated with the early set might then be used as rewards for correct responses in a training algorithm.

A skeptic might object that the phenomena of boredom and our appetite for novel experiences are difficult to accommodate in this pain and joy theory. In order to see how this potential problem might be resolved, we have to introduce a distinction between strong stimuli and weak stimuli. Twisting someone's arm is a strong stimulus in an unfamiliar direction, and immediately causes pain. Putting someone in a prison cell is a relatively weak unfamiliar stimulus (the perception of the four walls). A weak stimulus applied for an extended period of time can be similar to a strong stimulus applied for a short time (with respect to the way that a network is perturbed), and such a stimulus is similarly likely to take the subject to an unfamiliar region of phase space. (In the long term, the prison environment can of course become familiar, and some long-term convicts become more comfortable inside than outside.) In contrast, a variety of weak stimuli, provided they are of low intensity, move one in a variety of directions, and therefore not so quickly away from a familiar region. The difference between the boring and the interesting experience in this context is similar to the difference between a directed walk and a random walk with small steps. The random walk typically does not take one very far compared to the directed walk. A variety of stimuli both keeps one within (or close to) a more familiar region of phase space, and is likely to include some movement that is towards more familiar regions. In a directed walk, all the steps are soon away from the familiar region, even if they start by being towards the familiar region. A full explanation of entertainment and boredom might be more complicated than these simple ideas, and might have to include roles for hormones such as adrenalin. Be that as it may, our preference for variety and our aversion to boredom are not paradoxes in the context of the theory.

These ideas can be tested at two levels. Firstly we can see whether they work at the level of our computer model, that is, whether they prove useful in the development of more successful teaching algorithms. Secondly, the concept predicts that the periodic application of a specific stimulus to an animal during its early ontogeny could lead to the animal becoming addicted to that stimulus. That is, if such an animal were then given control over the application of the stimulus, it might learn to apply the stimulus to itself, and then continue to apply the stimulus with roughly the same periodicity.

5.7 Self and non-self; familiar and unfamiliar

I have previously listed 15 similarities between the immune system and the brain (Hoffmann, 1986). There is another analogy between the two systems that is worthy of consideration. When we are surrounded by many objects that are almost always present in a particular well-known environment, together with a single unfamiliar object, the unfamiliar object typically captures our attention. We are consequently likely to remember things about the unfamiliar object, and to remember very little about the familiar objects. That is, unfamiliar objects initiate changes in the brain to a much greater extent than familiar objects. Constantly present objects can be thought of as being part of psychological 'self'. Just as we do not react immunologically to self components, so are our brains relatively unperturbed by parts of the environment that do not change. We will see in the next section that this property leads to support for the neurons-with-hysteresis theory, in preference to the Hebb theory of learning.

5.8 Problems with the Hebb postulate

Most other models of learning (see, for instance, Hopfield, 1982) involve modifiable synaptic connections T_{ij}, that are postulated to change according to correlations such as

$$\Delta T_{ij} = [x_i(t)x_j(t)]_{\text{average}}, \tag{4}$$

where the average is calculated over some optimally chosen time period. This concept is due primarily to Hebb (1949). There is, however, no provision in the Hebb theory that would lead to a brain being more affected by non-familiar objects than familiar objects. By contrast, a network of neurons that exhibit hysteresis is automatically more affected by unfamiliar than familiar stimuli. This can be seen from the way that stimuli cause long-term changes in this theory. Sufficiently large stimuli switch some neurons from a low firing rate to a high firing rate or vice versa. Familiar stimuli will already have switched many of the neurons that they could possibly switch; novel aspects of the environment are therefore automatically more effective than familiar stimuli in changing the state of the system significantly.

Another problem with the Hebb theory is that it does not provide an explanation for the functional complementarity between stimuli and responses that brains can exhibit. As we will see in the next section, problems have been solved recently using networks with adjustable synaptic T_{ij} values by setting the values in *ad hoc* ways, that do not seem to pretend to imitate the ways in which modifications occur biologically.

5.8 Neural networks and computing

People who are interested in neural networks have two goals in mind. One goal is to understand how the brain works, and the other goal is to find ways of eventually doing interesting and/or useful computations with massively parallel computing machines. Progress towards achieving one of these goals does not automatically imply progress towards achieving the other. As an example, we consider the recent very interesting progress made by Hopfield & Tank (1985) in computing with neural nets. These authors showed that the travelling salesman problem can be solved using a Hopfield neural network (Hopfield, 1982, 1984). The travelling salesman problem (TSP) consists of finding the shortest closed route for visiting each of N cities just once. A TSP with N cities is solved using a neural network consisting of exactly N^2 neurons. The neurons are arranged in a square matrix, in which each row corresponds to one of the cities, and each column corresponds to a position in the solution path (first city, second city, etc.). Hopfield & Tank formulate an energy function that has a minimum corresponding to the solution to the TSP. The energy function is not particularly simple. It contains three triple summation terms and one double summation. Quadratic terms in the energy function define a neural network connection matrix, and linear terms define input biases to the network. The dynamics of the neural net result in the energy function automatically being minimized, and the energy function is constructed in a way that ensures that at the end of the calculation just one neuron in each row and one in each column is in the 'firing' state. The solution of the TSP can then be read out as a sequence from those final values. This work is impressive as an example of massively parallel computation; a solution to the problem is quickly found by the network. But as a theory for problem-solving by real brains it leaves important questions unasked, let alone answered. For instance, how could the Hebb postulate (see equation (4) above) lead to the formation of a set of T_{ij} (synaptic strengths) that result in the complex energy function used by the authors? How would being confronted with a TSP lead to the appropriate modifications in synaptic connection strengths of precisely N^2 neurons? Even if a set of neurons with the appropriate set of connection strengths for a particular TSP exist, how can they be specifically addressed when the subject is confronted with a particular TSP? How would these neurons be isolated from the perturbing influences of the rest of the network while they do their computation? These seem to be fundamental problems that make it difficult to accept the model as a theory for computation by real, biological neural networks.

On the other hand, will a network consisting of neurons that each exhibit hysteresis be useful for computations? The teaching algorithm we have used so far (with 'pain' only) is perhaps unlikely to be practical for solving complex and interesting problems. Including 'joy' in the algorithm as suggested above might help to achieve more impressive results. Alternatively, it may be possible to devise much more efficient artificial algorithms, that do not necessarily presume to imitate the way that real brains learn, for locating points in the N-dimensional phase space that have interesting stimulus–response behaviour. If appropriate architectures and algorithms can be found, the resulting theory could be both physiologically realistic and useful. These are challenges for future analytic and computational work.

Note added in proof

Recent work has shown that energy functions can be used with this type of network to find points in the N-dimensional phase space that exhibit prespecified stimulus response behaviour. See 'Learning by selection using energy functions' by P. Stolorz and G. W. Hoffmann, in *Systems with Learning and Memory Abilities*, J. Delacour and J. C. S. Levy, editors, Elsevier, North Holland, in press.

Acknowledgements

This research was financed by the Natural Sciences and Engineering Research Council of Canada, Grant No. A-6729.

References

Erondu, N. E. and Kennedy, M. B. (1985). 'Regional distribution of type II Ca^{2+}/calmodulin-dependent protein kinase in rat brain. *J. Neurosci.*, **5**, 3270–7.

Hoffmann, G. W. (1980). 'On network theory and H-2 restriction'. *Contemporary Topics in Immunobiology* vol. 11, ed. N. Warner, pp. 185–226. Plenum Press.

Hoffmann, G. W. (1982). 'The application of stability criteria in evaluating network regulation models'. *Regulation of Immune Response Dynamics* C. DeLisi & J. Hiernaux, eds., pp. 137–62, CRC Press, Boca Raton, Florida.

Hoffmann, G. W. (1986). 'A neural network model based on the analogy with the immune system'. *Journal of Theoretical Biology*, **122**, 33–67.

Hoffmann, G. W., Benson, M. W., Bree, G. M. & Kinahan, P. E. (1986). 'A teachable neural network based on an unorthodox neuron'. *Physica* **22D**, 233–46.

Hoffmann, G. W. & Benson, M. W. (1986). 'Neurons with hysteresis form a network that can learn without any changes in synaptic connection strengths'. In *Neural Networks for Computing*, J. Denker, ed., *American Institute of Physics Conference Proceedings*, vol. 151, pp. 219–26.

Hoffmann, G. W., Kion, T. A., Forsyth, R. B., Soga, K. G. and Cooper-Willis, A. (1988) The *N*-dimensional network, in *Theoretical Immunology*, A. S. Perelson, ed., Addison-Wesley Publishing Company.

Hopfield, J. J. (1982). 'Neural networks and physical systems with emergent collective computational abilities'. *Proceedings of the National Academy of Sciences (USA)*, **79**, 2554–8.

Hopfield, J. J. (1984). 'Neurons with graded response have collective computational properties like those of two-state neurons'. *Proceedings of the National Academy of Sciences (USA)*, **81**, 3088–92.

Hopfield, J. J. & Tank, D. W. (1985). 'Neural Computation of Decisions in Optimization Problems'. *Biological Cybernetics* **52**(3), 141–52.

Lisman, J. E. (1985). 'A mechanism for memory storage insensitive to molecular turnover: a bistable autophosphorylating kinase'. *Proceedings of the National Academy of Sciences (USA)*, **82**, 3055–7.

Miller, S. G. & Kennedy, M. B. (1986). 'Regulation of brain type II Ca^{2+}/calmodulin-dependent protein kinase, by auto-phosphorylation: a Ca^{2+}-triggered molecular switch'. *Cell*, **44**, 861–70.

6

On models of short- and long-term memories

P. PERETTO

6.1 The equations of motions

Due to the existence of synaptic noise and to the incommensurability of transmission delays the dynamics of neuronal activity must appeal to a probabilistic description (P. Peretto & J. J. Niez, 1986a). Let $\varrho(I, n)$ be the probability for a system comprising N neurons to be in state I at time n:

$$I = \{S_i\} \in [-1, 1]^N.$$

S_i is the state of neuron I, $S_i = -1$ for silent neurons, $S_i = +1$ for firing neurons. We assume that the process is Markovian. The probability $\varrho(I, n)$ is therefore given by:

$$\varrho(I, n) = \sum_J W(I|J) \cdot \varrho(J, n - 1),\tag{1}$$

where $W(I|J)$ is the probability for the system to jump from state J to state I in one time step, it is given by (see P. Peretto & J. J. Niez, 1986b).

$$W(I|J) = \frac{1}{2N} \cdot \left[1 - \mathrm{erf}\left(\frac{\Sigma_j C_{ij} S_j(J) - h_i}{B} \right) \right].\tag{2}$$

In eqn (2) I and J are identical except for the state of neuron i; C_{ij} is the efficacy of the synapses linking the neuron j to the neuron i; h_i is a polarizing field (which includes eventually the effect of a threshold) created on neuron i by afferent, say sensory, fibres. Finally, B is a noise parameter.

The activity of neuron i at time n, i.e. its relative instantaneous frequency, is given by:

$$\langle S_i \rangle_n = \sum_I \varrho(I, n) \cdot S_i(I).\tag{3'}$$

The correlated activity between neurons i and j is given by a similar formula:

$$\langle S_i \cdot S_j \rangle_n = \sum_I \varrho(I, n) \cdot S_i(I) \cdot S_j(I). \tag{3''}$$

From eqns (1), (2) and (3) the following rigorous equations are derived:

$$\frac{d\langle S_i \rangle}{dt} = -\frac{1}{T} \cdot \left[\langle S_i \rangle - \left\langle \text{erf} \left(\frac{\Sigma_j \, C_{ij} \cdot S_j - h_i}{B} \right) \right\rangle \right],$$

$$\frac{d\langle S_i S_j \rangle}{dt}$$

$$= -\frac{1}{T} \cdot \left[\langle S_i S_j \rangle - \frac{1}{2} \left\{ \left\langle S_j \, \text{erf} \left(\frac{\Sigma_k \, C_{ik} S_k - h_i}{B} \right) \right\rangle + \left\langle S_i \, \text{erf} \left(\frac{\Sigma_k \, C_{jk} S_k - h_j}{B} \right) \right\rangle \right\} \right]. \tag{4}$$

The time constant T scales as T_r/N where T_r is the refractory period.

The first equation which drives the neuronal activities can be solved using the mean field approximation provided, obviously, that this approximation is valid. Then, and in the limit of large Ts, it is equivalent to the dynamic equation proposed by J. J. Hopfield (1984) (for a proof see the appendix).

The mean field approximation amounts to neglecting the fluctuations of stochastic observables with respect to their mean values. It is justified when the synaptic efficacies are Hebbian. It is not justified when the efficacies are random (even symmetrical) variables.

Let us now turn to the description of the synaptic dynamics. The synaptic dynamics is a result of a competition between a driving term which tends to modify the synaptic efficacies according to the present activity of the network and a saturation term which limits the growth of the efficacies. It is assumed that the driving term obeys the general principle enacted by Hebb (1949) which states that the synaptic changes follow the correlated activities of the neurons, the corresponding synapses link. In its most simple form the dynamic equation for the synaptic efficacies is therefore:

$$\frac{dC_{ij}}{dt} = \frac{1}{T_e} \langle S_i S_j \rangle - R(C_{ij}). \tag{5}$$

We emphasize that the equation driving the synaptic dynamics involves the correlated activities of neurons which cannot be reduced to a product of neuronal activities unless the mean field theory is valid. When the starting synaptic efficacies are random or, more generally, when they generate frustrated states, the mean field approximation cannot be used and there are no analytical solutions to the problem of learning. Monte-Carlo methods have then to be used. It must also be stressed that the correlations between neuronal activities cause the neural tissue to develop

P. Peretto

spontaneous organizations in epigenetic models. Correlations have also been invoked by C. von der Malsburg and E. Bienenstock (1986) as an organizing principle for engrams in the cortex.

6.2 Learning is an unstable process

We consider a simple system made of fully interconnected neurons (Fig. 6.1). Every neuron is polarized by a sensory signal and the system is to learn a single pattern. Therefore,

$$h_i = h \cdot S_i: \quad (S_i = \pm 1). \tag{6}$$

We also assume that the efficacies vanish at origin time ($C_{ij} = 0, i, j$). Finally, we suppose that saturation arises from a weak constraint which compels the synaptic resources to satisfy:

$$\sum_j |C_{ij}| = N \cdot C^s. \tag{7}$$

Fig. 6.1. A fully connected network comprising only 'open' neurons.

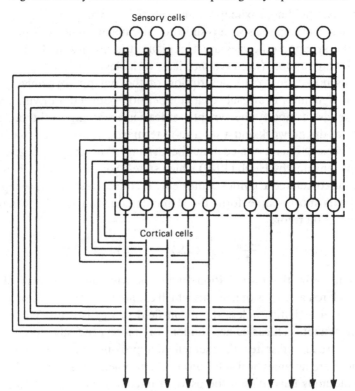

Sensory cells

Cortical cells

It can be shown that the saturation process takes the form of a relaxation term:

$$R(C_{ij}) = \frac{1}{T_0} \cdot C_{ij},\tag{8}$$

where the relaxation 'time' T_0 depends on the learning protocol. As in the case of the strong constraint given by

$$|C_{ij}| \leq C^s,\tag{9}$$

which has been studied by J. P. Nadal *et al.* (1986), this saturation mechanism is not a passive one. The old patterns are erased by new configurations and not by the effect of time.

This model is one of the few which can be studied using the mean field approximation because it does not contain any frustration effects. Using the reduced variables:

$$x = \langle S_i \rangle \cdot \text{sgn } (S_i^0)$$

and $\hspace{11cm}$ (10)

$$y = C_{ij} \cdot \text{sgn } (S_0^i) \cdot \text{sgn } (S_j^0).$$

The equations (4) and (5) become:

$$\left. \begin{array}{l} \dfrac{dx}{dt} = -\dfrac{1}{T} \cdot \left[x - \text{erf} \left(\dfrac{Nxy + h}{B} \right) \right], \\[4mm] \dfrac{dy}{dt} = +\dfrac{1}{T_e} x^2 + \dfrac{y}{T_0}. \end{array} \right\} \tag{11}$$

The fixed points of the dynamics are given by:

$$x^* = \text{erf} \left[\frac{1}{B} \cdot \left(\frac{NT_0}{T_e} x^{*3} + h \right) \right] = \text{erf } [\alpha x^{*3} + \beta].\tag{12}$$

For a given 'learning parameter' α and variable 'polarization parameter' β, we observe two regimes (Fig. 6.2).

(1) For low values of β, depending on the starting neuronal activity, the synaptic efficacies either saturate to values close to their maximum value

$$C_{ij} = S_i^0 \cdot S_j^0,\tag{13}$$

or remain close to zero.

(2) For β larger than some transition value $\beta(\alpha)$, the synaptic efficacies always stick to their maximum given by eqn (13).

This all-or-nothing behaviour suggests that learning is an unstable process. Let us assume, for example, that an activity fluctuation brings a part of the system above the transition polarization. All synapses belonging to this part will saturate, giving rise to large inhomogeneities among synaptic efficacies.

Let us now turn to the learning of several patterns. The dynamics is simulated using a Monte-Carlo algorithm. Figs. 6.3 and 6.4 show some examples of a simulation carried out on a sample of 32 neurons experiencing five orthogonal patterns. We recall that the neuronal activities of a network with synaptic efficacies given by the 'Hebbian' rule

$$C_{ij} = \sum_{\mu=1}^{M} S_i^\mu \cdot S_j^\mu \tag{14}$$

(which is the most efficient local rule for storing patterns) are conveniently described by a set of order parameters defined by:

$$q^\mu = \frac{1}{N} \cdot \sum_i \langle S_i \rangle S_i^\mu. \tag{15}$$

Fig. 6.2. Equilibrium activities in a fully connected network experiencing one pattern. From top to bottom the various curves correspond to increasing polarizing signals ($\beta = 0, 0.05, 0.10, 0.15, \ldots$). Those parts of curves with positive slopes are stable whereas the parts with negative slopes are unstable.

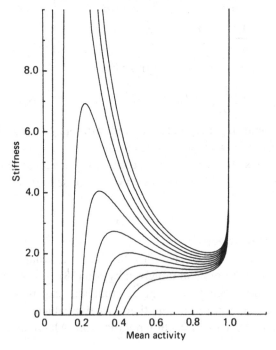

Fig. 6.3. Time evolution of the five learning parameters Q^{μ} ($\mu = 1, \ldots, 5$) in a system of 32 neurons learning five orthogonal configurations, $\alpha = 4.6$: (*a*) Regime 1: $\beta = 0.20$. No learning. (*b*) Regime 2: $\beta = 0.50$. The four first patterns are efficiently imprinted in the network. So is a fifth configuration which the system experiences from $t = 115$ (*MCS/N*) on. (*c*) Regime 3: $\beta = 0.50$. The fifth configuration is learned alone from $t = 115$ (*MCS/N*) on. It replaces all the previously imprinted patterns.

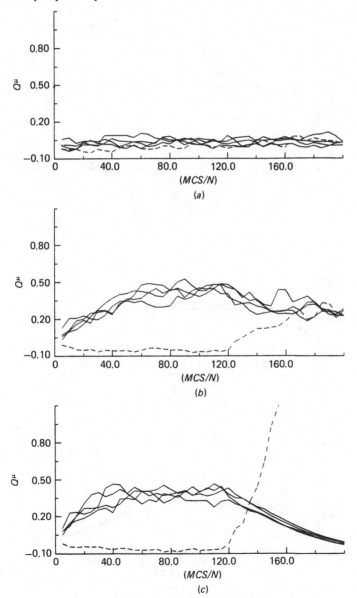

Fig. 6.4. Time evolution of the five learning parameters Q^μ ($\mu = 1, \ldots, 5$) in a system of 32 fully connected neurons learning five orthogonal configurations (as in Fig. 6.3), $\alpha = 6.4$: (a) Regime 3: $\beta = 0.50$. The system starts learning the four first patterns correctly but at $t \simeq 60$ (MCS/N), the learning process destabilizes and finally only one configuration is imprinted. (b) Regime 4: $\beta = 0.90$. All patterns, including the fifth, are correctly imprinted. (c) Regime 5: $\beta = 0.90$. The fifth pattern replaces the four previously stored configurations.

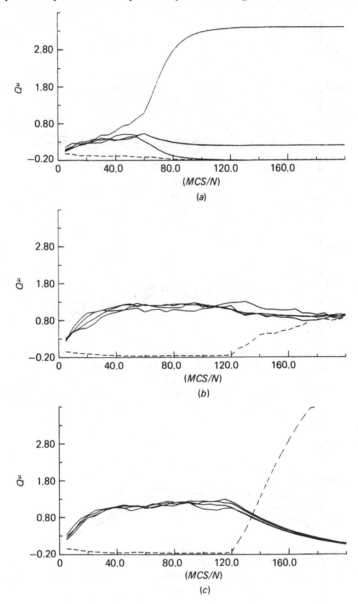

(a)

(b)

(c)

Similarly, the efficiency of learning is most easily monitored using a new set of order parameters given by:

$$Q^\mu = \frac{1}{N^2} \sum_{ij} \cdot C_{ij} S_i^\mu S_j^\mu. \tag{16}$$

If the synaptic efficacies satisfy eqn (14) the M order parameters Q^μ are equal and maximum.

We use several protocols of learning. The first is to learn the patterns in turn during equal times. We observe four regimes.

(1) At low polarization level no pattern can be learned at all.

(2) For larger values of β, the patterns are learned evenly ($Q^\mu = Q$; $\forall\mu$). The learning process is therefore efficient even though the synaptic efficacies are far from reaching their maximum values, due to the effect of noise.

(3) As the polarization parameter increases, the system becomes unstable with respect to the learning of one or several patterns ($Q^\mu = Q^{\mu'}$, $Q^{\mu''} = 0$, for example). The learning process therefore loses a part of the available information.

(4) At still larger polarizations the patterns are again evenly stored. This is easy to understand since the polarization is so strong that the activities of neurons are clamped along the sensory signals.

The ranges of polarizations β giving rise to the various regimes depend on the learning parameter α. Large αs tend to widen the range of regime 3 at the expense of all other regimes. For example, very large αs prompt the system to spontaneously polarize in one random state, even in the absence of any external polarization ($\beta = 0$).

In other protocols M patterns are learned for a while and afterwards the system starts learning an extra pattern, either together with the previous patterns or alone. In the first procedure the extra pattern is stored with those already imprinted in regime 2 and 4. It is not stored in regimes 1 and 3. In the second procedure the extra pattern progressively erases and replaces the already imprinted pattern in regimes 2 and 4. It has no effect in regimes 1 and 3 (see Figs. 6.3 and 6.4).

Finally, we have considered systems with hidden units which are neurons not directly connected to sensory fibres (see T. Sejinowsky & G. Hinton, 1985) (Fig. 6.5). The computer simulations are carried out using 64 fully connected neurons 32 of which are polarized by external signals h_i. We find that the open neurons behave in a way similar to that which has been described above. The hidden neurons, however, always behave as in regime 1 (no learning) or in regime 3 (occurrence of one or several irreversible stored states).

6.3 A general framework to model memory

The results yielded by computer simulations are rather disappointing. They reveal pathological behaviours which have to be cured. More specifically:

(a) The system either displays irreversible behaviours (in regime 3 for example) or fully reversible behaviour (in regimes 2 and 4). It does not show the mixture of behaviours which is observed in real neural systems.

(b) The system has no internal dynamics of its own: once in an equilibrium state, it stays there for ever. This is to be contrasted with the ceaseless activity of real networks. In irreversible regimes the simulation shows that these steady states are even insensitive to external inputs. The system is, so to speak, obsessed by one or a few patterns. This is especially true for hidden units.

Fig. 6.5. An example of a fully connected network with 'hidden' units.

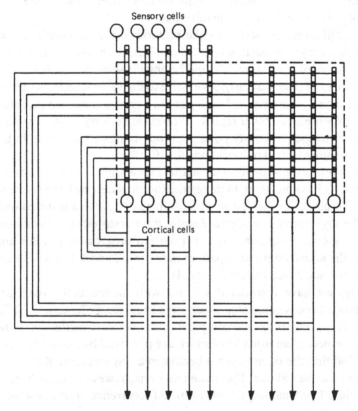

(c) It is unable to store temporal correlations between learned patterns, whereas these correlations must play a central role in a number of phenomena, such as classical conditioning, for example.

(d) In the ranges of parameters which allow learning, the storage heavily depends on the learning protocol. A pattern experienced for too long erases all the previously stored information. Therefore, the model so far used cannot account for long-term memory.

We now propose some possible cures:

The coexistence of reversible and irreversible processes in neural networks can be guaranteed by the cooperation of two biological mechanisms working at the synaptic level. In other words, we assume that the synaptic efficacies are a superposition of two contributions called short- and long-term efficacies respectively.

$$C_{ij} = C_{ij}^s + C_{ij}^l. \qquad (17)$$

These terms first differ in the way they saturate; the saturation process is a reversible one as in Nadal (1986) for short-term efficacies. It is irreversible as in Linsker (1986), for long-term efficacies.

Moreover, to avoid the trapping of the dynamics in steady states we introduce delay effects which can even reverse the sign of the short-term learning procedure. This is similar to the anti-learning mechanism proposed by J. Crick (1983) to account for the role of dream sleep in the reorganization of (long-term) memory. This process destabilizes the states which should show tendencies to become stationary. It also introduces temporal correlations between the imprinted patterns.

Finally, a simple exogenous (not at the synaptic level) mechanism is proposed which renders the long-term storage insensitive to the learning protocol.

6.4 Short-term memory

It has been shown (J. P. Changeux & TY. Heidmann, 1986) that the dynamics of synaptic efficacies involve delay effects. It is natural to take them into account in the driving term of eqn (5). These phenomena can be located in either side of the synaptic cleft or in both sides. If one assumes that presynaptic delays are dominant, the dynamic equation of synaptic efficacies are:

$$\frac{dC_{ij}^s}{dt} = \int_0^\infty \langle S_i(t) \cdot S_j(t - t') \rangle \cdot r^s(t') \, dt' - R^s(C_{ij}^s), \qquad (18)$$

where $r^s(t)$ is the short-term delay function. The saturation term R^s is supposed to obey the weak reversible constraint introduced in Section

P. Peretto

6.2. The shape of $r^s(t)$ is displayed in Fig. 6.6(a). It passes through zero at time T_m. Possible experimental evidences that the delay function changes sign can be found in the phenomenon of habituation or low-frequency depression (D. Lloyd & V. Wilson, 1957). Moreover, we assume that

$$\int_0^\infty r(t)\, dt = -\lambda; \quad \lambda \geqslant 0. \tag{19}$$

The introduction of the delay function has several profitable consequences. It avoids the trapping of the system in steady states. Obsessional states are erased. This leaves the network in a naive state but makes it possible for it to store new patterns. Likewise a pattern to which the system is submitted for too long is erased.

As a consequence the range of parameter which allows a faithful storing of configurations in regime 2 is widened at the expense of regime 3, provided the learning time for each pattern is shorter than T_m.

Fig. 6.6. Short-term and long-term delay functions of the driving force of the dynamics of short-term and long-term efficacies.

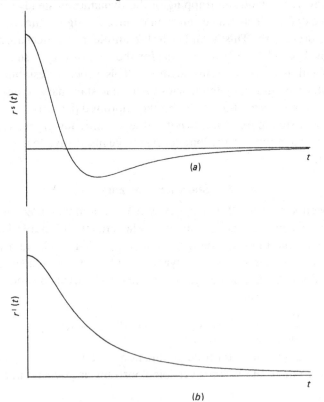

Also, a pattern which is learned in p steps, each lasting a time τ, is better stored than the same pattern which is learned for a time p, τ.

Moreover, couplings between temporally correlated configurations are now stored in synaptic efficacies. Instead of the Hebbian formula eqn. (14), the efficacies are:

$$C_{ij} = \sum_{\mu, \nu} \Gamma_{\mu\nu} S_i^\mu S_j^\nu. \qquad (20)$$

It must be stressed that the matrix Γ is generally non-symmetrical and therefore the synaptic efficacies are also non-symmetrical.

6.5 Long-term memory

The memory dynamics of long-term efficacies obeys the same part of the equations as those driving the short-term efficacies, except that the saturation term R^l is irreversible and that the shape of the corresponding delay function $r^l(t)$ is different (see Fig. 6.6(b)). In the strong constraint hypothesis for example, this means that the synaptic efficacies must keep the extrema values $+C^l$ or $-C^l$ once they reach the limits.

We argue now that long-term memory needs another control mechanism to be efficient. Indeed, the long-term memory resources are limited: the long-term memory storage capacity is no larger, for a network of given size, than the short-term memory capacity. But long-term storage is irreversible and the resources cannot be wasted. It is necessary that the significant configurations are stored. On the other hand, the contribution of a significant configuration to the long-term synaptic efficacies must not grow too much even though the system experiences this configuration several times. Otherwise, this would hinder the storage of forthcoming configurations. However, this significant configuration also must not be erased by the anti-learning process, as it would be if the driving terms of short and long-term efficacies were similar.

To satisfy those seemingly contradictory constraints we propose that the long-term storage process is under the control of a novelty filter. The role of the filter is to deliver a strong inhibitory signal when the neural network is in an already learned state and no signal when the network experiences a novel pattern. The inhibitory signal would stop the long-term memory process using some diffuse (non-local) biochemical reactions. It is easy to devise a novelty filter. The interesting thing is that an analogue of such a filter could eventually be found in the limbic system, in the hippocampus in particular.

Let us assume that fibres stemming from the system make axo-axonal contacts of the type observed by E. Kandel (1976), or hetero-junctions similar to those proposed by D. Marr (1969) in his model of cerebellum on the dendrites of a set of cells k (Fig. 6.7).

After the learning of a number of patterns the efficacies of the hetero-junctions are

$$C_{ijk} = -K \sum_{\mu} S_j^{\mu} \cdot S_i^{\mu}; \quad (i, j \in \text{cortex}; K > 0). \tag{21}$$

Let the network experience a familiar configuration. The membrane potentials V_k of cells k are then strongly negative

$$V_k = \sum_{ij} C_{ijk} \cdot S_i \cdot S_j \simeq -K \cdot N^2, \tag{22}$$

and the long-term memory mechanism remains idle. On the contrary it is active as long as a novel pattern has not left its trace in the hetero-

Fig. 6.7. A network with a feed-back circuit controlling long-term memory.

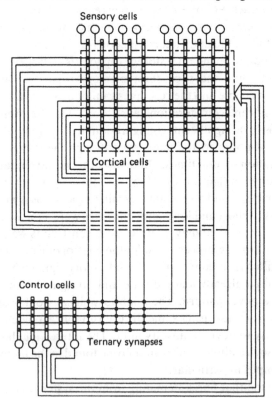

junctions. The dynamics of long-term memory therefore can be modelled by

$$\frac{dC_{ij}^l}{dt} = g(t) \cdot \int_0^\infty \langle S_i(t) \cdot S_j(t - t') \rangle \cdot r^l(t') \, dt' - R^l(C_{ij}^l), \qquad (23)$$

where the function $g(t)$ embeds the effect of the filter.

We propose tentatively that the hippocampus could be this novelty filter. The role of the hippocampus as a comparator has already been proposed by O. S. Vinograda (1975) and L. Nadel (1975). Its function is not very specific. So is the mechanism we propose here which only carries out the logical function NAND. Its destruction hinders new long-term storage but does not impair the old imprints. Finally, it is known that hippocampus has strong inhibitory effects on the cortex, that this inhibition is carried through acetylcholine neurotransmitters, and that the acetylcholine molecules are especially abundant in the hippocampus (D. Campbell & L. Raskin, 1978; D. Blozovski & J. Bachevalier, 1975). Acetylcholine, therefore, could be the chemical agent which has been evoked above.

6.6 Summary and conclusions

We have shown that simple learning rules are unable to account for the most simple memory properties displayed by natural neural networks. In particular, the models built on these simple assumptions behave either reversibly or irreversibly, whereas reversibility and irreversibility manifest themselves simultaneously in natural systems by short-term memory and by long-term memory respectively. This compels us to propose that the synaptic efficacies are made of two contributions, namely short- and long-term efficacies. The two contributions differ by their saturation processes and the delay functions of their driving mechanisms, in the framework of a saturation process due to the strong constraint mechanism, the short-term synaptic efficacies cannot exceed the limits $+C^s$ or $-C^s$ but they are free to leave the limits provided they stay in the allowed range. On the contrary, the long-term synaptic efficacies must stick to their limit values $+C^l$ or $-C^l$ once they reach the limits.

We also introduce delayed learning algorithms for both types of efficacies. This yields a number of interesting features. The most important, in our opinion, is that the network never remains idle in steady states. The activity does not result from cycling behaviours associated, for example, with asymmetrically connected noiseless synchronous networks, but it is always relaxational. Delays also induce correlations between temporal strings of patterns. Using the revised algorithms we have been able, in particular, to retrieve temporal sequences of patterns (Peretto & Niez 1986b).

Finally, we argue that an efficient long-term memory storage process needs yet another control mechanism. This mechanism is a novelty filter and a possible implementation of this filter is proposed. It is tentatively suggested that the limbic system, especially the hippocampus, could fulfil this function.

We now imagine the landscape of the phase space of neural networks as made of a hard background dug with holes corresponding to long-term memorized patterns, and superposed to it a soft, continuously moving material with temporary depressions corresponding to the recent experiences, i.e. to short-term memory. If the limits C^s of reversible processes are larger than the limits C^l of irreversible processes the recently memorized patterns can overflow the deeply imprinted configurations, but they are swiftly forgotten and the long-term memorized patterns can reappear.

Obviously, the present approach of a constructive theory of memory is rather speculative. Also, many crucial questions have been left aside. To cite only one we could wonder how the hidden units organize and whether they are able to build representations of the activities of the open units. This has not been explored yet. It is probable that a gross architectural organization, such as the columnar partition of the cortex, is necessary to achieve an efficient organization of knowledge. The concept of 'modular self-adaptative networks' of R. Linsker (1986) could be of great help.

Appendix

We start from eqn (4). Let

$$T_{ij} = C_{ij}/B, \qquad h_i = 0, \qquad \mathrm{erf}\,(x) = g(x). \tag{1}$$

This transforms the equation into

$$T \cdot \frac{d\langle S_i \rangle}{dt} + \langle S_i \rangle = g\!\left[\sum_j T_{ij} \cdot \langle S_j \rangle \right]$$

$$\sum_j T_{ij}\langle S_j \rangle = g^{-1}\!\left[\langle S_i \rangle + T\frac{d\langle S_i \rangle}{dt} \right] \simeq g^{-1}[\langle S_i \rangle] + T \cdot \frac{d\langle S_i \rangle}{dt} \cdot g^{-1'}(\langle S_i \rangle). \tag{2}$$

Using $\langle S_j \rangle = V_j$; $V_i = g(u_i)$ or $u_i = g^{-1}(V_i) = g^{-1}(\langle S_i \rangle)$, we obtain

$$\frac{du_i}{dt} = \frac{d\langle S_i \rangle}{dt} \cdot g^{-1'}(\langle S_i \rangle), \tag{3}$$

and, finally,

$$\sum T_{ij} \cdot V_j - u_i = T \cdot \frac{du_i}{dt},\qquad(4)$$

which is the equation proposed by J. J. Hopfield (1984).

References

Amit, D., Gutfreund, H. & Sompolinsky, H. (1985). *Phys. Rev. Lett.*, **55**, 1530.

Blozovski, D. & Bachevalier, J. (1975). *Rev. Psychobiol.*, **8**, 97.

Campbell, B. A. & Raskin, L. A. (1978). *J. Comp. Physiol. Psychol.*, **92**, 176.

Crick, F. & Mitchinson, G. (1983). *Nature*, **304**, 111.

Changeux, J. P. & Heidmann, T. (1986). In *New Insights into Synaptic Function*, G. Edelman, W. Gall & W. Cowman, eds. Wiley, N.Y.

Hebb, O. (1949). *The Organization of Behaviour*. Wiley, N.Y.

Hopfield, J. J. (1982). *Proc. Natl. Acad. Sci., USA*, **79**, 2554.

Hopfield, J. J. (1984). *Proc. Natl. Acad. Sci., USA*, **81**, 3088.

Kandel, E. (1976). *Cellular Basis of Behavior. An introduction to Behavioral Biology*. Freeman, SF.

Kohonen, T. (1984). *Self Organization and Associative Memory*. Springer Verlag, Berlin.

Linsker, R. (1986). To appear in *Proc. Acad. Sci. USA*.

Lloyd, D. & Wilson, V. (1957). *J. Gen. Physiol.*, **40**, 409.

Marr, D. (1969). *J. Physiol.*, **202**, 437.

von der Malsburg, C. (1973). *Kybernetik*, **14**, 85.

von der Malsburg, C. & Bienenstock, E. (1986). In *Disordered Systems and Biological Organization*, E. Bienenstock, F. Fogelman & G. Weisbuch, eds., NATO ASI Series, vol. 20.

Nadal, J. P., Toulouse, G., Changeux, J. P. & Dehaene, S. (1986). *Europhys. Lett.*, **1**, 535.

Nadel, L. (1975). *Behav. Biol.*, **14**, 151.

Peretto, P. & Niez, J. J. (1986a). *IEEE Trans.,. Syst. Man. Cybern.*, **16**, 73.

Peretto, P. & Niez, J. J. (1986b). In *Disordered Systems and Biological Organization*, E. Bienenstock, F. Fogelman & G. Weisbuch, eds., NATO ASI Series, vol. 20.

Sejinowsky, T. & Hinton, G. (1985). In *Vision, Brain and Cooperative Computation*, M. Arbib & A. Hanson, eds. MIT Press, Cambridge, USA.

Vinograda, O. S. (1975). *Hippocampus*. Plenum Press, vol. 2.

7

Topology, structure and distance in quasirandom neural networks

J. W. CLARK, G. C. LITTLEWORT and J. RAFELSKI

7.1 Introduction

Computer simulation of the activity of complex neural networks representing substantial portions of the brain is limited by a number of practical considerations, notably the capacity of existing computers and the finite human resources available for analysis of a proliferating output. Whatever the specific model chosen, whether operating in discrete or continuous time, and whether involving the firing states or the firing rates of neurons as the basic dynamical variables, there will arise the possibility that 'edge effects' seriously diminish the relevance of the simulation to the behavior of the actual biological system. Such effects may arise, principally, from the fact that the number of neuronal elements in the simulation is too small, or, secondarily, from the fact that the numbers of synaptic inputs to given elements are inappropriate.

In this contribution we shall make an attempt to quantify edge effects in terms of a simple conception of interneuronal distance, reasoning that the asymptotic autonomous behavior of neural models will hinge critically on the topological properties of the net. This will be especially true of the repertoire of cyclic modes (Clark, Rafelski & Winston, 1985) of an assembly of N binary threshold elements operating syncronously in discrete time. As a first approximation to a meaningful definition of the distance d_{ki} from neuron i to neuron k in such models, one may use simply the minimum number of synaptic junctions which information must traverse in going from i to k. This definition ignores the differential strengths of synapses as well as the influence of 'longer paths' from i to k involving more synaptic jumps. Rather, the emphasis is justifiably placed on the (assumed) existence of a universal delay time τ for signal transmission from presynaptic to postsynaptic neuron. We note, further, that this definition generally implies that the 'metric matrix' d_{ki} will be asymmetric, since the least number of synaptic steps from k to i, in the direction of information transfer, may differ considerably from the number of steps required to get from i to k. It is expected that the notion of interneuronal distance introduced here, albeit primitive, captures some of the novel features of the topology of the brain which are essential to its dynamical behavior as an assembly of interacting neurons. An obvious shortcoming is that no distinction is made between excitatory and inhibitory synapses lying along the shortest path from i to k.

As a first exemplification of our definition of distance in neural systems, we consider the case of randomly assembled networks with homogeneous structure. In Section 7.2, theoretical formulae are derived which give the statistical distribution of distances in such systems, as a function of the number N of neurons and the density m of connections. Edge effects are prominent at small N and low m. In Section 7.3, we compare the distances found in actual model nets used in simulations, with the 'ideal' statistical distribution. For nets with putatively homogeneous structure ('unstructured nets'), the deviations, which may be attributed to deficiencies in the random-number generators chosen as well as statistical fluctuations, are minimal. For sample nets with imposed structure (designed as systems of netlets with relatively dense internal connections and relatively sparse internetlet connections, or as ring-like assemblies) the average distance shows, in general, a significant enhancement over the statistical prediction for unstructured nets. We close with some qualitative remarks concerning the implications of large average distances for the dynamical behavior of the system and cite some estimates of average distances in living nets, especially the neocortex.

7.2 Distances in unstructured random networks

As in various models (Clark *et al.*, 1985; Hopfield, 1982, 1984; Kürten & Clark, 1986; and references cited therein), it is convenient to introduce a connection matrix (V_{ij}) formed from the strengths of the synaptic couplings between neurons. Here the real number V_{ij} represents the net strength, or efficiency, assigned to the synapses through which neuron j acts directly upon neuron i. If V_{ij} is zero, there is no coupling from j to i, while a positive [negative] value implies that j acts in an excitatory [inhibitory] manner on i.

In one class of models which has received much study, the individual neuronal states are represented by a binary variable π_i which takes on the value 1 if neuron i is firing and 0 if it is not. A given neuron i fires at the decision time t if the total stimulus it feels, computed as $\Sigma_j V_{ij}\pi_j(t - \tau)$, equals or exceeds the threshold value V_{0i}; otherwise it assumes (or remains in) the inactive configuration. The traditional dynamical law (McCulloch & Pitts, 1943) is that at discrete times t separated by a universal delay τ, neuron i updates its state synchronously with all the other neurons. In another popular dynamical model (Hopfield, 1982), τ is set zero and each neuron is allowed to update its state at random times, thus breaking synchronism in an extreme manner. The following considerations, however, are strictly independent of such detailed assumptions regarding the rules for dynamical evolution of the network.

The essential line of argument resumes with the observation that the connectivity matrix (V_{ij}) is not known in detail for neural systems (e.g. cortical structures) of substantial complexity. Retreating to a state of almost complete ignorance, we consider a network of N neurons connected up randomly, subject to the minimal specification that the probability that any particular neuron j provides an input link to neuron i is given by m, where $0 < m < 1$. The connection probability m will be referred to as the connectivity. Networks constructed according to this prescription are said to belong to the class of unstructured random nets. In this section we are concerned with the properties of a statistical ensemble of such networks, while the next section presents corresponding results for distances in actual simulation nets realized through the use of a random-number generator.

An additional specification might be that each neuron is assigned exclusively excitatory or inhibitory character, in its effect on neurons to which it sends connections, the inhibitory option being selected with probability h, where $0 \leq h \leq 1$. Moreover, individual strengths V_{ij} may be chosen for the non-zero couplings, again randomly, say between some specified limits for excitatory and inhibitory cases. But these details will not affect the ensuing formal arguments, since the key question is whether or not neuron j has an efferent connection to neuron i, of whatever strength and sign.

Consider now an ensemble of networks, each assembled randomly according to the minimal prescription above, for given N and m. In a generic member of this ensemble, each neuron has, on average, $M = Nm$ inputs and the same number M of outputs. Focusing on a particular neuron, called A, we would like to determine the number $n(d)$ of neurons lying at distance d (a positive integer) from A in the typical net. To circumvent ambiguity, we assume that all distances in the assembly are finite, i.e., information can pass from any neuron in the net to any other neuron in the net by some sequence of synapses. This is generally the case for the actual model networks used in the simulations of Clark *et al.* (1985) and Littlewort (1986). Let $q(d)$ be the number of neurons at distances from A greater than d. Then, clearly,

$$q(d) = N - \sum_{r=1}^{d} n(r). \qquad (2.1)$$

Strictly, both $n(d)$ and $q(d)$, as determined here, are to be interpreted as ensemble averages. On average, each neuron has Nm output lines, so we have, trivially,

$$n(1) = Nm. \qquad (2.2a)$$

The number of neurons left over is $N - Nm$ and hence

$$q(1) = N(1 - m). \qquad (2.2b)$$

Now pick arbitrarily one of the neurons, say B, which receives one of the Nm outputs from A. On average this neuron will itself have output lines going to Nm neurons. As indicated schematically in Fig. 7.1, we must expect that some neurons of this latter group are in fact reached after only one step from neuron A; the rest are at distance two from A. More precisely, outputs from B reach a fraction m of the $q(1)$ neurons left over after one step. This leaves a smaller pool of unreached neurons numbering $q(1) - mq(1) = N(1 - m)(1 - m)$. But neuron A has Nm target neurons like B, each of which reduces the pool of left-overs by a factor $1 - m$. Hence there are

$$\begin{aligned} q(2) &= q(1)(1 - m)^{Nm} \\ &= q(1)(1 - m)^{n(1)} \end{aligned} \qquad (2.3)$$

neurons unreached after two steps. In this manner we arrive at the

Fig. 7.1. Schematic representation of overlapping sets of target neurons of selected neurons A and B.

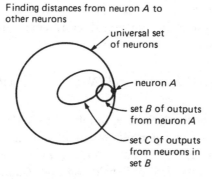

Finding distances from neuron A to other neurons

universal set of neurons

neuron A

set B of outputs from neuron A

set C of outputs from neurons in set B

following recursion relations for the function $n(d)$, where $d \geq 1$:

$$q(d + 1) = q(d)(1 - m)^{n(d)},$$
$$n(d + 1) = q(d) - q(d + 1)$$
$$= q(d)[1 - (1 - m)^{n(d)}]. \qquad (2.4)$$

These relations are initiated by eqns. (2.2a) and (2.2b). In the trivial limiting case that every neuron synapses on every other neuron, i.e., $m = 1$, we verify that $n(1) = N$ and $q(d) = 0$ for all d.

Since $n(d)$ is, by definition, the number of target neurons at distance d from a given source neuron in a generic net of the ensemble (or more strictly the ensemble average of the number of neurons at distance d), the probability distribution of neuron-to-neuron distances is simply $n(d)/N$. Proper normalization of this distribution is guaranteed by

$$1 = \sum_{d=1}^{d_{max}} n(d)/N, \qquad (2.5)$$

where d_{max} is the maximum allowed distance in the network, some number $\leq N$. We may then express the average interneuronal distance, quite generally, as follows:

$$\langle d \rangle = \sum_{d=1}^{d_{max}} w(d)\, d\, n(d)/N, \qquad (2.6)$$

where a distance weighting function $w(d)$ has been inserted to emphasize the fact that more elaborate notions regarding distance measure in neural systems might be implemented at this point. (For example, we might want to weight more heavily those d values which are achieved by numerous distinct pathways from source to target neuron, or to assign weights in accordance with the mix of excitatory and inhibitory connections involved in traveling to a given d, etc.) However, we shall restrict our analysis to the case of uniform weights, $w(d) = 1$ for all d, corresponding to the primitive notion of synaptic distance introduced above. It will be found that even this simplest of all cases leads to new insights. In this case explicit appeal to the initializing equations (2.2) and to the recursion relations (2.4) produces the rearranged series representation

$$\langle d \rangle = 1 + \sum_{d=1}^{d_{max}} q(d)/N$$
$$= 2 - m + q(2)/N + q(3)/N + \ldots + q(d)/N + \ldots. \qquad (2.7)$$

We observe that for fixed, finite m unrelated to N, $\langle d \rangle$ is asymptotic to $2 - m$ at large N, which again reduces to unity in the trivial case of full connectivity, $m = 1$. This follows since $q(d)$ is arbitrarily small for $d \geq 2$ at large enough N, if m is held constant. Caution is in order in seeking limiting behaviors with respect to m, especially small m, since the above derivation strictly applies only when m is such that $Nm = M$ (the average number of inputs or outputs of a sample neuron) is a positive integer. In fixing m and letting N increase without limit, we are assuming that M increases linearly with N. In general, one may suppose that M scales like N^p. Instead of taking $p = 1$ we can study the case $p = 0$, which means that M remains fixed at some finite value M while N grows. In this case the average distance cannot saturate asymptotically, as may be seen from the fact that the minimum number of steps needed to cover the net is N/M and the average distance must be larger. (Non-saturation follows immediately from the series representation (2.7) if we invoke the first recursion relation of (2.4). The latter implies that asymptotically $q(d + 1) = q(d) = N$, so all of the terms of the series in the first line of (2.7) contribute equally.) We note that this second asymptotic scenario might correspond to considering an ever greater sample of cortical tissue, where the number of inputs per neuron remains roughly constant at something like 100. In the general case $M \propto N^p$ the innocent-looking recursion relations (2.4) have elusive properties necessitating delicate analysis.

Figs. 7.2 and 7.3 present the results for the dependence of $\langle d \rangle$ upon m

Fig. 7.2. Average distance $\langle d \rangle$ as a function of connection probability m in randomly assembled networks of various sizes N. The solid curves are calculated from eqn (2.7), derived for a statistical ensemble, while the crosses show actual mean distances in representative sample nets without intentionally imposed structure.

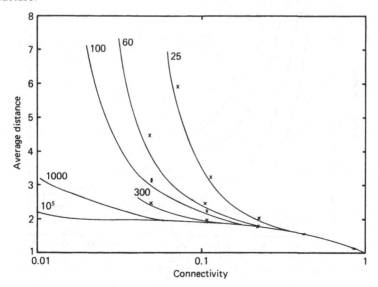

and upon M, respectively, determined from the expansion (2.7) for chosen values of N ranging from 25 (essentially the lowest value used in simulations), through 100–300 (typical choices in simulation), to the values $10^4 - 10^5$ characteristic of a cortical column. These diagrams provide revealing views of edge effects. Fig. 7.2 shows that the mean interneuronal distance in nets of size 100–300 (commonly used in simulation studies) diverges markedly from that of nets of size 10^5 (judged large enough to neglect edge effects in the indicated m domain) as m drops below 0.1. We are reminded in quantitative terms of the importance of using large nets when looking at sparse connectivity. Fig. 7.3 suggests the beginning of the unlimited growth of the average distance as the number of neurons increases while keeping fixed the mean number of inputs M. This process is especially rapid at small M. As M increases, the discrepancies between adjacent N curves diminish somewhat, but remain unacceptably large at small N.

The messages conveyed by Figs. 7.2 and 7.3 regarding edge effects are complementary: Fixing m, average distances are artificially *long* in nets of small N, if the aim is to simulate nets of large N. But fixing M, small-N nets have average distances which are artificially *short*.

Fig. 7.3. Average distance $\langle d \rangle$ as a function of mean number of inputs per neuron M in randomly assembled networks of various sizes N, calculated from eqn (2.7).

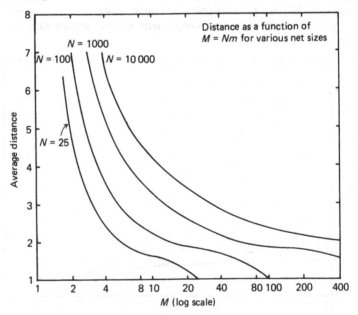

An interesting feature which is visible in Fig. 7.2, but, more importantly, also easily recognizable in Fig. 7.3, is the presence of distance plateaus. Focusing on Fig. 7.3, we see that for a given value of N there is a range of M for which the average distance changes little. It may be inferred that this range of M is of special importance for setting up simulation experiments, as it seems that (a) fringe effects associated with too sparse or too dense connectivity are minimized in a useful sense, and (b) the relevant topological properties are least sensitive to statistical fluctuations associated with finite net size. It is intriguing that the conditions in a cortical column ($N \sim 10^{4-5}$, $M \sim 10^2$) put it in or near a 'minimum-sensitivity domain', and one might speculate that such domains have some intrinsic biological significance.

7.3 Unstructured and structured sample networks

A random-number generator was used to obtain a collection of definite connection matrices (V_{ij}) and thus a set of sample networks belonging to the class of unstructured quasirandom nets characterized by given N and connection probability (or connectivity) m. Such model networks have been used in a large number of dynamical simulation studies, the results of which are summarized elsewhere in these proceedings (Littlewort, Clark & Rafelski, 1988). The distribution of distances in these systems is found by appealing to the fact that if the distance from neuron l to neuron k is d, then the klth element of the dth power of the matrix (V_{ij}) will be non-zero, while that element of all lower powers will vanish. Thus we may simply compute successive powers of the connection matrix, and, by counting the number of elements that change from zero to a non-zero value at each stage, arrive at the distance distribution $n_s(d)$ in the sample net. From this distribution we may determine the corresponding average distance $\langle d \rangle_s$. The resulting average distances for a number of putatively unstructured sample nets are plotted in Fig. 7.2 (crosses). Agreement with the curves derived theoretically for a statistical ensemble is reasonably good, but deteriorates at smaller connectivity and/or smaller net size, where fluctuations are naturally larger. Deviations from the theoretical curves are due in part to the fact that the random-number generator does not produce a purely random sequence, as well as to the fact that in actual nets the numbers of inputs (outputs) of a given neuron will in general deviate from the ensemble-average M. Results for the distance distributions in some sample nets are provided in Figs. 7.4 and 7.5. In Fig. 7.4 the net size is kept fixed at $N = 100$ and several connectivities are considered, the actual values for the average numbers of input lines per neuron being

22.2, 10.8 and 5.0. In Fig. 7.5 the connectivity m is kept fixed at 0.05 while the net size is varied from 300 down to 25. Corresponding results derived from the recursion relations and expansion of Section 7.2 are plotted for comparison. (For Fig. 7.4, the m values 0.222, 0.108 and 0.05, respectively, are inserted into the relevant formulas.) The predicted distance distribution naturally spreads toward larger d as m is decreased for given N; also, the distribution flattens out as N is decreased for given m. The results for the sample nets follow these trends, although there are seen to be appreciable deviations from the ensemble-based curves, for the reasons cited above. For the set of results in Fig. 7.4, these deviations become less noticeable for higher connectivity, as expected.

In view of the highly structured (e.g., layered) nature of living neural networks, it is of great interest to examine cases where (in place of a prescribed uniform connection probability m) some form of structure, or 'architecture', is imposed on an otherwise randomly connected neuronal assembly. Such architecture may (or may not) be prominently reflected in

Fig. 7.4. Upper set of dashed curves: distance distributions in sample nets of size $N = 100$, for three values of connectivity. (Note dashed curve is indistinguishable from solid curve in the case with average number of inputs 22.2.) Lower set of dashed curves: distance distributions in sample networks of size $N = 100$ with imposed netlet structure, for three choices of average connectivity and local emphasis L. Solid curves: corresponding statistical predictions for purely random nets, determined by recursion relations (2.4).

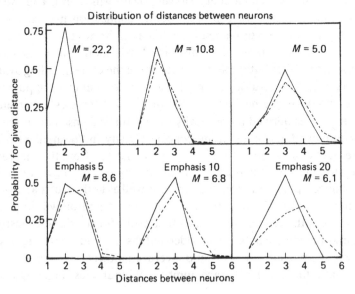

the appearance of the connection matrix (V_{ij}). Two of the more obvious cases are represented schematically in Fig. 7.6. Both of these involve connectivity prescriptions with local emphasis, i.e., higher probability for connections with 'near neighbors.' (The quotes acknowledge the fact that in neural systems such neighbors need not actually be in close proximity in ordinary space, and that it is the prescribed non-uniform connectivity which really determines the distance in the sense considered here. This reminds us that the concept of distance being explored is a topological property of the net and not a metrical property as would usually be implied by the term.) The two examples shown correspond on the one

Fig. 7.5. Distance distributions for various values of net size N at constant connectivity $m = 0.05$. Solid curves: statistical predictions for purely random nets, determined by recursion relations (2.4). Dashed curves: results for sample nets without intentionally imposed structure. Solid curves: corresponding statistical predictions for purely random nets, determined by recursion relations (2.4).

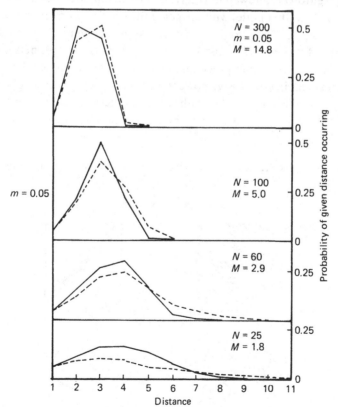

hand to a grouping of neurons into netlets with relatively large internal and relatively small external connection densities, and on the other to a situation in which the connections form the system into a sort of ring structure, for the purposes of information processing. The former type of structure (division into netlets) is achieved by emphasizing connectivity in diagonal blocks of the connection matrix, wherein non-zero values of the elements are more common than otherwise. The latter (ring or cylinder or toroid) structure is created by emphasizing appropriate off-diagonal matrix elements at the expense of others.

Most of our explicit studies of random networks with imposed structure dealt with nets consisting of 'weakly interacting' netlets, constructed as follows. The set of N neurons was arbitrarily divided into g groups (netlets) each containing N/g neurons. The intranetlet connections were formed in the same manner as for the unstructured nets considered above, with a specified probability m_{int} that an arbitrary neuron i in the netlet will receive an input line from an arbitrarily chosen neuron j of the netlet. Neuron i is allowed to receive a connection line from an arbitrary neuron j in another netlet with the generally smaller probability m_{ext}. We take the ratio $L = m_{int}/m_{ext}$ as a measure of local emphasis in structured networks of this type. The distribution $n_s(d)$ for such sample nets may be determined by the same procedure as in the case of unstructured nets, i.e., by calculating successive powers of (V_{ij}). Results for particular nets, all with $N = 100$ and $g = 4$, but with varying choices of local emphasis, viz. $L = 5, 10$ and 20, are shown in Fig. 7.4. The corresponding average

Fig. 7.6. Network architecture as reflected in the character of the connectivity matrix (V_{ij}).

Connection matrices with local emphasis

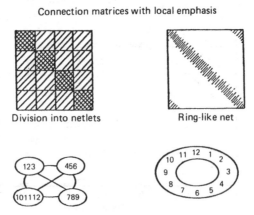

Division into netlets   Ring-like net

numbers of input lines per neuron prevailing in these nets are 8.6, 6.8 and 6.1. Curves for the statistical ensemble, computed at m values 0.086, 0.068 and 0.061, are included for comparison. It is seen that the distribution is skewed toward larger distances in the structured nets, the effect becoming more pronounced as the emphasis L increases. However, even for an emphasis as large as 20, the peak of the distribution is only shifted to the right by one unit (and the average distance only rises by about one), so the introduction of longer distances by the imposed netlet architecture is hardly dramatic. At local emphasis 5 with 4 netlets (which means that in a statistical ensemble of such structured nets there would be 5 internal to every 3 external connections to a given neuron), the distribution is in practice indistinguishable from that of ordinary, unstructured sample nets having the same average number of inputs per neuron. These findings indicate that even rather small differences of the distance distribution from the corresponding reference distribution for unstructured nets may be symptomatic of sharply different topological character and distinctive neural architecture. Although we have not yet considered nontrivial choices of the weights introduced in eqn (2.6), we suspect that the effects of structure on the mean-distance measure can be amplified by a suitable prescription for $w(d)$.

Some more limited investigations were carried out for nets with imposed ring-like structure. The recipe adopted in this case for constructing connection matrices is that, after an arbitrary numerical labeling $1, \ldots, N$ of the neuronal elements, V_{ij} is taken to be non-zero only if $i - j \leqq L'$, where L' is the chosen number of 'near neighbors'. If this condition is met, then the connection probability from j to i is a specified value m. Choices of L' range in practice from 3 to 20, with m ranging from 0.2 to 0.8 (the larger m values being associated with fewer near neighbors). For small L', average distances are large compared to those in the other sample nets studied – as expected. The distance distributions for ring-structured nets tend to be rather flat.

Results for the average distance in a number of sample networks, structured and unstructured, are collected in Fig. 7.7. All these examples refer to net size 100, and statistical curves are included to allow assessment of edge effects and the enhancement of average distance by structure.

7.4 Conclusions

Quantitative information concerning edge effects in neural network simulation experiments has been gained through the introduction of a simple definition of neuron-to-neuron distance as the least number of synaptic junctions which must be passed in going from the first neuron to the second. Concentrating on randomly assembled nets without intrinsic structure, we have constructed plots of average distance versus connectivity (connection probability) m and versus mean number of inputs per neuron $M = Nm$, for specified neuron number N. Inspection of Figs. 7.2 and 7.3 shows that there are significant edge effects in nets of the typical simulation size $N = 100$. These diagrams provide complementary views of such effects. For example, Fig. 7.2 tells us that if we fix the connectivity, or density of connections, at $m = 0.1$, the average distance for $N = 100$ *exceeds* by less than half a unit the mean distance appropriate to a random net of cortical-column size $(N = 10^{4-5})$. On the other hand, Fig. 7.3 tells us that if we fix the average number of incoming connections per neuron at $M = 10$, the mean distance in a net of size 100 is *too short* by nearly two units, in comparison with a net of $N = 10^4$ neurons.

Fig. 7.7. Representative results for average distance in unstructured and structured sample networks, all with $N = 100$. Solid and dashed curves give ensemble-based statistical predictions calculated from eqn (2.7), for comparison. The numbers beside the points for overtly structured sample nets denote local emphasis measure L or L', as appropriate.

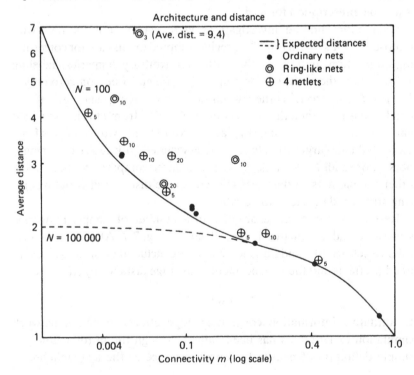

Methods for detecting structure in seemingly random nets have been proposed, based on the above topological concept of (minimum) synaptic distance. We furnish an explicit prescription for the evaluation of the distribution of distances from source to target neurons in a net with specified connection matrix (V_{ij}). The result can be compared with that derived for an ensemble of truly random nets. In more vivid language, we offer a means for detecting 'spatial' order in an otherwise apparently random 'gas' of neurons. Within the context of neural model simulations, such order may be an accident of the network generation process or it may correspond to an overt imposition of structure. Ordering might also take place upon implementation of one or another of the plasticity algorithms considered by Clark *et al.* (1985) and Littlewort (1986), which envision temporal alteration of the synaptic efficiencies depending on correlations in recent network activity. However, this possibility lies outside the scope of our present treatment. Since, ordinarily, the plasticity algorithm adopted will not alter the zero or non-zero character of the V_{ij}, but only their absolute strengths, it becomes essential to introduce a more refined definition of distance. As a step in this direction one may invoke a non-trivial choice of the weights $w(d)$ in the average distance defined by eqn (2.6).

Within the context of a particular network model, including a rule for updating the state of the system, the nature of the neuron-to-neuron distance distribution defined here should have important dynamical implications. However, this matter has not yet been investigated systematically. Intuitively, one might expect that in the discrete-time model explored by Clark *et al.* (1985) and many other authors, a large average distance tends to promote the occurrence of terminal cycles of large period and complex reverberatory composition, and possibly also long transients. This expectation may be contrasted with recent analytic results of Kürten (1988a,b), based on the thermodynamic limit and assuming equal numbers of excitatory and inhibitory synapses: it is found that a 'chaotic regime' (characterized by large periods and extreme sensitivity to initial conditions) exists only above $M = 2$ (cf. Fig. 7.3).

Turning to biological nerve nets, neuroanatomically measured distance distributions, when compared with our theoretical result for a purely random net of corresponding size and connectivity, would give some indication of the degree of randomness and specificity in neural tissue. It is worth noting in this regard that Szentagothai (1978) (cf. also Uttal (1978)) has estimated that the minimum number of synapses which must be traversed in the cerebral cortex in progressing from one neuron, arbitrarily selected, to another neuron, arbitrarily selected, is on the average something like 5–10. Among our sample nets such average distances were only achieved in cases corresponding to imposed ring-like structure.

Acknowledgements

Research support from the Foundation for Research Development, RSA, and from the Condensed Matter Theory Program of the Division of Materials Research of the U.S. National Science Foundation, under Grant No. DMR-8519077, is greatly appreciated.

References

Clark, J. W., Rafelski, J. & Winston, J. V. (1985). 'Brain without mind: Computer simulation of neural networks with modifiable neuronal interactions.' *Physics Reports*, **123**(4), 215–73.

Hopfield, J. J. (1982). 'Neural networks and physical systems with emergent collective computational abilities.' *Proc. U.S. Nat. Acad. Sci.*, **79**, 2554–8.

Hopfield, J. J. (1984). 'Neurons with graded response have collective computational properties like those of two-state neurons.' *Proc. U.S. Nat. Acad. Sci.*, **81**, 3088–92.

Kürten, K. E. & Clark, J. W. (1986). 'Chaos in neural systems.' *Physics Letters*, **114A**, 413–18.

Kürten, K. E. (1988*a*) 'Transition to chaos in asymmetric neural networks'. In *Condensed Matter Theories*, eds. J. Arponen, E. Pananne & R. F. Bishop. New York: Plenum.

Kürten, K. E. (1988*b*) 'Critical phenomena in model neural networks'. Submitted to *Physics Letters*.

Littlewort, G. C. (1986). Phase Transitions in Neural Networks. M.Sc. Thesis, University of Cape Town.

Littlewort, G. C., Clarke, J. W. & Rafelski, J. (1988). 'Transition to cycling in neural networks'. These proceedings, pp. 345–56.

McCulloch, W. S. & Pitts, W. (1943). 'A logical calculus of the ideas immanent in nervous activity.' *Bull. Math. Biophys.*, **5**, 115–37.

Szentagothai, J. (1978). 'Specificity versus (quasi-) randomness in cortical connectivity. In *Architectonics of the Cerebral Cortex*, eds. M. A. B. Brazier & H. Petsche. New York: Raven Press.

Uttal, W. R. (1978). *The Psychobiology of Mind*. New York: Halsted Press.

8

A layered network model of sensory cortex

BRYAN J. TRAVIS

8.1 Introduction

I am the set of neural firings taking place in your brain as you read the set of letters in this sentence and think of me.

(D. Hofstadter, *Metamagical Themas*)

Neurobiological systems embody solutions to many difficult problems such as associative memory, learning, pattern recognition, motor coordination, vision and language. It appears they do this via massive parallel processing within and between specialized structures. The mammalian brain is a marvel of coordinated specialization. There are separate areas for each sense modality, with massive intercommunication between areas. There are topographic maps, many specialized neuron types, and quasi-regular small-scale structure (columns and layers) which vary from area to area to accommodate local needs, and plasticity in connections between neurons. Feedback occurs on many levels. This complexity is apparently necessary for the kind of multi-mode processing that brains perform, but it's not clear how much of this structure is necessary to perform isolated tasks such as vision or speech recognition; nor do we know if nature's solutions are optimal. (See chapter 8 of Oster & Wilson (1978), for example, for an interesting discussion of optimization in biology.)

Regardless of whether the brain represents the optimal structure for cognitive processes, it is the only successful one we know of. By analyzing it and modeling it, we may learn the principles on which it operates, and presumably be able to apply these principles to computer technology.

Our knowledge of neural systems originates with experimental studies. Experimental data should lead to conceptual models, ultimately to computational theories, which can be implemented through well-defined algorithms (Marr, 1982). These provide a tool for high-level information processing whose worth can be evaluated explicitly. If one is interested in their biological or psychological validity, model predictions can be tested with further biological measurements. This usually leads to new theories and algorithms.

No comprehensive computational theory of the brain has been established at present, although some interesting work in this direction is developing (Pellionisz, 1984). There is a great deal of data on the hardware the brain uses; namely, its anatomy and its physiology. There is also some understanding of the algorithms (transformations) that the brain employs on sensory input. The fuzziest area of our knowledge of the brain concerns exactly what the brain is computing and why.

Models of cognitive processing are, at present, highly idealized and simplified. Nevertheless, they show the rich behavior that neural systems are capable of.

In the area of learning and pattern recognition, a fruitful theoretical approach has been the study of neural networks. Much of the work in this field has focused on the mathematical properties of nets with varying degrees of realism (Clark, Rafelski & Winston, 1985). Recently, the minimum energy theory (Hopfield, 1982) has led to a breakthrough in the ability of networks to perform cognitive functions. Capacity has increased as structure increases from symmetric neural connections (Ackerly, Hinton & Sejnowski, 1985) to non-symmetric (Lapedes & Farber, 1986) to high-order correlation (Chen *et al.*, 1986) models. Another viewpoint that promises to be very powerful is the application (Hogg & Huberman, 1984, 1985) of concepts from dynamical systems theory to neural networks.

These studies: (1) generally look at neural nets in isolation; that is, without simulating the kind of sensory input that real neural systems operate on; (2) do not attempt to implement the actual structure of parts of the nervous system, such as cortex, that presumably are necessary for recognition, memory, etc. One recent study (Krone *et al.*, 1986) does incorporate some of the detail of mammalian cortex, but still makes many simplifications with regard to neuron types and their connectivity. Also, no plasticity was allowed in synaptic strengths (an important process, as shown, e.g., by Buhmann & Schulten, 1986); and the processing of sensory data that occurs in subcortex structures was omitted. (Even so, several interesting features were seen in that model's behavior.)

The goal of the project described in this paper is to build a biologically valid model of a sensory system, which integrates what is known both structurally and physiologically at several levels, from the peripheral sense organ to the midbrain nuclei to the cortex. Despite the complexity of these systems, there is a great deal of data available at each level to permit a fairly realistic model for some sensory systems (vision, hearing, and olfaction), although simplifications in scale must be made especially at the cortex level to remain within present computer memory and speed limits. Attractive features of such a model are that it: (1) includes more structure (and presumably more processing capacity) than previous models; (2) provides each subsystem with the kind of input that the biological counterpart receives (to understand what the brain is doing requires a clear description of the data it operates on); (3) emphasizes the dynamic or time dimension; and (4) provides a means of testing theories about sensory perception. In the remainder of this article, the structure of the cortex and subcortical nuclei are discussed in the context of a particular sensory system, the auditory. A computational model is presented, and results of an application of the model are shown.

8.2 Layered neural systems

A great deal of experimental work over the last hundred years has slowly revealed the intricacies of the structure of the mammalian brain. Input from the periphery reaches the brain either through the spinal cord or special cranial nerves. These neural signals pass through a variety of midbrain nuclei (large groups of neurons) before they finally reach the cortex (outer surface of the brain). The cortex is actually a collection of fairly well-defined cortical regions (Fig. 8.1), each of which is dedicated to a specific cognitive function, such as visual processing. Massive communication occurs between most of these regions.

Although our knowledge of the cortex is still incomplete, many features are well established. The cortex consists of several (generally six) layers of neurons (see Fig. 8.2), each layer having a characteristic composition of specific neuron types (Truex & Carpenter, 1969). (The nuclei of the lower brain are also layered structures.) The number and thickness of layers varies in different regions of the brain (Fig. 8.3), presumably reflecting differences in function. The upper layers of the cortex are fairly recent in the evolutionary development of the mammalian brain. These layers are especially rich with neurons in man. Neural activity follows a generally vertical pattern; signals from the periphery enter mainly in layer 4, pass to the upper layers and then to the lowest layers, and then back up. Neurons in the upper layers also project to other cortical areas, and neurons in the lower layers also project to subcortical nuclei. In addition to the layered structure a vertical columnar organization has been established through physiological measurements. These columns are roughly 0.5 mm in diameter and contain several thousand cells. Cells within a column generally exhibit the same sensitivity to sensory stimuli. Considerable lateral interaction between columns is now known (Imig & Morel, 1983) to occur.

Fig. 8.1. Map of functional areas of brain cortex (Brodman, 1909).

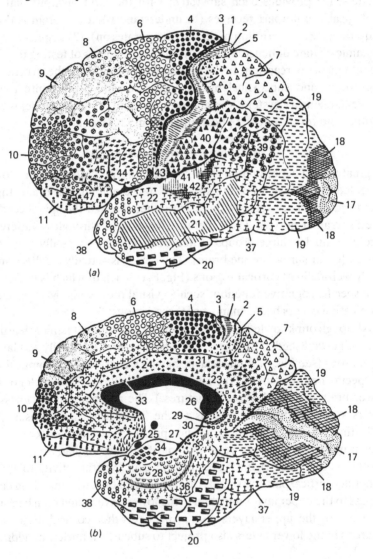

Neurons are very complex structures. They receive input on their dendrites, a collection of branch-like processes which radiate from the soma (body) of the neuron for many microns to millimeters. Input signals from other neurons travel down the dendritic branches, decaying as they travel towards the soma where they are summed. If the membrane potential is raised sufficiently, an action potential will travel down the neuron's axon. Axons can extend for considerable distances, up to millimeters in the cortex, to meters in the periphery. Axonal projections frequently branch, sending collaterals to several layers. Transmission from one neuron to another occurs at synaptic junctions via chemical transmission (in almost all cases). A large number of transmitter molecules have been identified. Some transmitters produce an inhibitory effect on the receiving neuron, while others are excitatory; the nature of the effect depends on the type of receptors on the receiving neuron. Each neuron usually receives input from many (up to thousands) of other neurons; each neuron typically transmits to many neurons.

The neurons found in the cortex layers come in a great variety of forms. Roughly, nine or ten types of cortical neurons have been identified with many subtypes recognized. Cortical neurons are not arranged haphazardly. Certain neuron types are found in certain layers and not

Fig. 8.2. Layered structure of neocortex (Brodman, 1909).

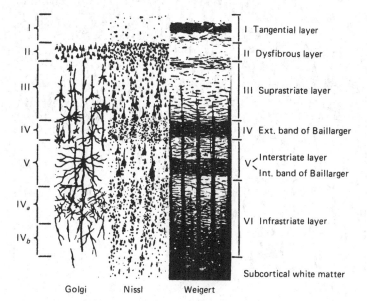

others. Some neurons, such as basket cells, synapse only on one or two types of neurons. Axonal projections are fairly specific as to the layers they reach. Two commonly found cortical neurons are shown in Figs. 8.4 and 8.5.

8.3 Structure of the auditory system

The sensory system considered in this paper is the auditory. The comprehension of sound and speech begins with transduction of sound waves into transient motions of the basilar membrane of the cochlea in the inner ear (Figs. 8.6, 8.7, and 8.8). Displacements of the basilar membrane lead to discharge of hair cells in the organ of Corti and generation of action potentials in auditory nerve fibers. A particular frequency will cause peak displacement at a characteristic location along the basilar membrane. The dynamics of the organ of Corti is still a subject of great interest (Hudspeth, 1985). Details of cochlear structure and function are given by Pickles (1982).

Fig. 8.3. Variations in cortex structure, showing five cortical types: (1) agranular; (2) frontal; (3) parietal; (4) polar; (5) granular (von Economo, 1929).

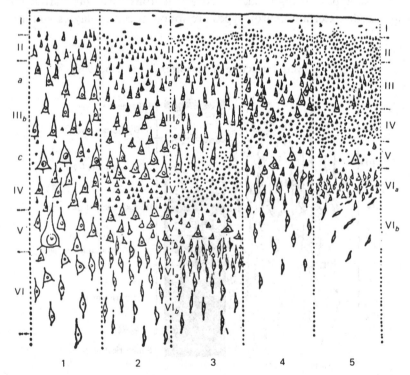

Fig. 8.4. A pyramidal cell in layer 2. Note branching of axonal process (Gilbert & Wiesel, 1979).

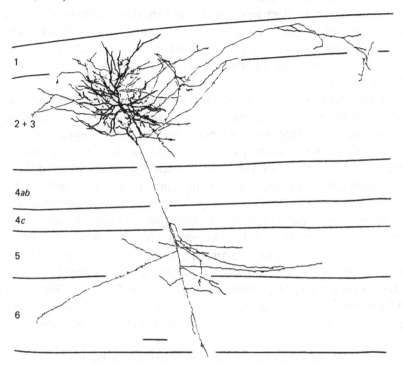

Fig. 8.5. A pyramidal cell in layer 5. Apical and basal dendritic regions are visible. Note the very large horizontal extension of axonal collaterals (Gilbert & Wiesel, 1979).

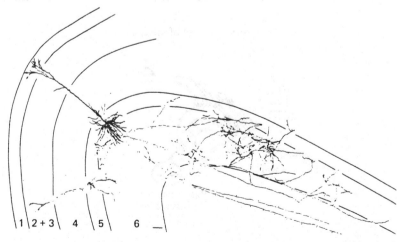

The auditory nerve bundle feeds into several nuclei in the lower brain and midbrain regions before the cortex is reached (Fig. 8.9). Some of these nuclei use auditory input to initiate behavior such as head turning and other reflex actions. Others serve to sharpen auditory input and to integrate input from each ear. Fibers from all these nuclei converge onto the auditory cortex. More details are given in the review article by Imig & Morel (1983).

In the auditory system, the cortex surface is organized into several tonotopic maps. In a tonotopic map, a particular point on the cochlear basilar membrane (representing a particular frequency) maps to a specific strip of tissue in the auditory cortex. At least four are known in the cat brain (Fig. 8.10); two are very specific maps, the other two are diffuse. This multiplicity of frequency maps also appears in various nuclei of the medial geniculate body. The tonotopic map is conserved throughout the auditory system, but mappings onto isofrequency strips are both divergent and convergent (Fig. 8.11). Association fibers connect isofrequency curves from each map onto the corresponding isofrequency curves in the other maps. Along an isofrequency curve, each ear is represented by alternating clusters of neurons. It is believed (Merzenich, Jenkins & Middlebrooks, 1984) that this second dimension of the auditory cortex map is used with the frequency map to accomplish spatial localization of sound.

Little is known about processing of auditory data at higher levels of the brain, except that neural activity extends outward from the primary auditory area to associational areas and is integrated with other sense modalities. There is of course a strong interaction with the speech generation areas (Wernicke and Broca). Most of the experimental work

Fig. 8.6. Gross structure of the cochlea.

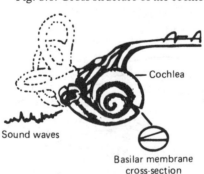

Fig. 8.7. Cross-section of cochlea, showing the three chambers and detailed picture of basilar membrane and organ of Corti (Allen, 1977).

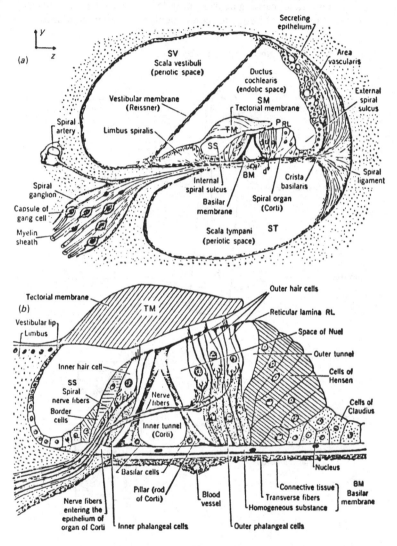

Bryan J. Travis

Fig. 8.8 (*a*) Properties of basilar membrane vary rapidly. Innervation of inner hair cells is fairly specific; that of outer hair cells is diffuse. (*b*) Traveling wave moves along basilar membrane, causing peak amplitude at a location corresponding to input frequency. (*c*) Map of frequency components for two simple sounds.

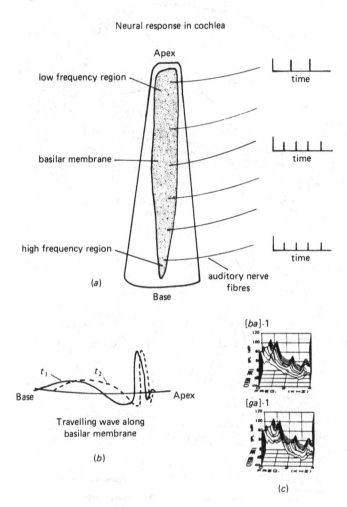

Fig. 8.9. Series of midbrain nuclei in the auditory pathway. Each consists of two
or three layers with very regular structure (Truex & Carpenter, 1969).

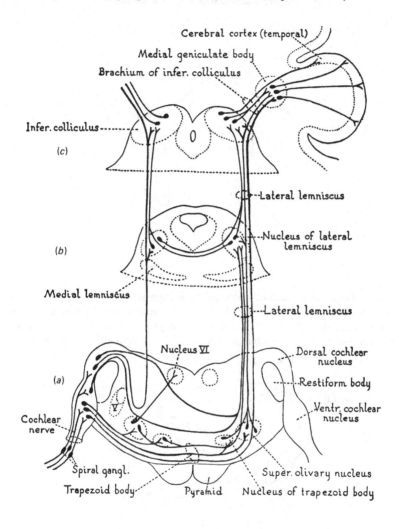

Fig. 8.10. Multiple tonotopic maps in cat auditory cortex.

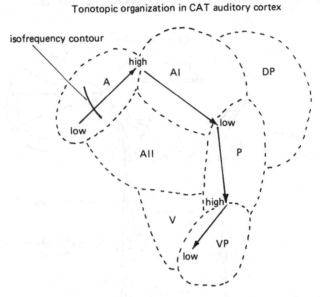

Tonotopic organization in CAT auditory cortex

Fig. 8.11. (*a*) Each point on the cochlear partition is represented on a strip of cortical tissue in cortex areas A, AI, P, VP. Association fibers connecting, for example, map A with map P, connect neuron groups of essentially the same frequency, but with considerable divergence in the isofrequency direction (*b*).

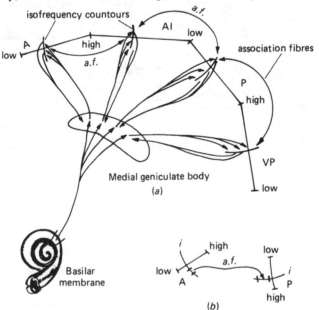

has used cats, with some measurements in owls and monkeys. Recently, the human auditory cortex has become accessible via the magneto-encephalographic (MEG) technique.

8.4 The model

A three-part mathematical model of the auditory system has been developed. It includes a hydromechanical model of the cochlea with hair cell innervation for studying transduction of sound into basilar membrane motion and then into neural signals. This model is similar to others (Allen, 1977; Holmes, 1982) that have been studied, but attempts to treat the temporal dimension more realistically. Output from this portion of the auditory model can be, and is being, compared to auditory nerve recordings. The second portion applies layered neural networks to simulate auditory processing in nuclei such as the dorsal cochlear nucleus. Several of these nuclei have a relatively simple structure (two or three layers with feed forward only) and, based on recent studies, (Shamma, 1985*a,b*) use lateral inhibition to sharpen the auditory signal train. The medial geniculate nucleus (MGN) has a more complex structure involving feedback within itself and with the cortex to which it projects. The third part of the model attempts to simulate neural activity in the auditory cortex, including feedback to the midbrain nuclei. Because of the extremely large number of neurons and interconnections between neurons in the brain, only a very small portion of the cortex (roughly a few square millimeters) can be modeled in great detail, and even then certain aspects, such as connection to other cortex areas, will be difficult or impossible on present computers. Alternatively, a coarser-grained model can be used to approximate an 'average' structure of larger cortex regions. Even these crude models may contain enough structure to have cortex-like dynamics. The emphasis in this paper is on the application of this third part of the model to auditory processing.

A general neural network model is used to simulate cortex-like structures. The model, a computer code called LCM, operates in discrete time (a continuous time version is under development). It allows a variable number of layers, number of neurons and neuron types. The composition of each layer is determined by the user. For each layer, the types of neurons are specified, as well as the spatial density (number/unit area) for each type, radii of influence (distance over which a neuron's axonal projections and dendrites extend in each direction in each layer), refractory periods and the excitatory or inhibitory character of each type. The effect of electrotonic transport from the point of synaptic junction to the

Table 8.1. *Distribution of dendrites and axons of primary excitatory neurons*

Neuron type	Layer containing cell body	Layers for apical dend.	Layers for basal dend.	Layers for axonal proj.
Pyramidal	2	1	2	2,3,5,6
Pyramidal	3	1	3	2,3,5,6
Spiny stellate	4	1,4	4	2,3,5,6
Pyramidal	5	1,4,5	5	2,3,5,6
Spindle	6	1,4	6	2,3,4,5,6

cell body is included via space constants. Neurons can send axonal projections into multiple layers and dendrites can extend beyond a single layer. Within radii of influence, actual connections between neurons are determined on a probabilistic basis. Two- or three-dimensional structures can be created. Input stimuli to a network can be simple or time-dependent and can be fed in as a topographic map and in a 'dual' manner to simulate input from multiple sources, e.g. binaural input. Special routines are used to simulate peripheral sensory organs – the retina for vision and the cochlea for hearing, with options to present realistic stimuli, such as a bar moving across the retinal field, or a word's sound train entering the cochlea. Super networks can be created which consist of layered neural networks that communicate with one another. In this way, different sense modalities can be coupled, and thalamic nuclei and cortex can communicate in both directions. The state of each neuron at each time step is determined by summing inputs from all other neurons, subtracting its threshold value and then, if the neuron is not in a refractory state, using the Fermi probability to calculate whether the neuron fires an action potential. It is assumed that plasticity in connectivity is governed by a differential Hebbian rule (Kosco, 1986) in which connection strength depends on previous activity (increases with use, decreases with disuse), with the restrictions that the sign (excitatory or inhibitory) of a connection cannot change and that connection strength is bounded.

To demonstrate the LCM model, a six-layer, two-dimensional simulation of cortex containing the neuron types (Imig & Morel, 1983; Pickles, 1982; Gilbert, 1983; Kolb & Whishaw, 1985; Shepherd, 1979) described in Tables 8.1–8.3 was constructed. It has been assumed that neuron types

Table 8.2. *Distribution of dendrites and axons of two excitatory intracortical neurons*

Neuron type	Layer containing cell body	Layers for dendrites	Layers for axons
Horizontal cell	1	1	1
Martinotti cell	2	2	1
Martinotti cell	3	3	1,2
Martinotti cell	4	4	1,2,3
Martinotti cell	5	5	2,3,5
Martinotti cell	6	6	2,3,5,6

Table 8.3. *Common inhibitory neurons in the cortex*

Neuron type	Layer containing cell body	Layers for dendrites	Layers for axons
Golgi II	1	1	1
Golgi II	2	2	2
Chandelier	2	2	1,2
Golgi II	3	3	3
Basket	3	3	3
Chandelier	3	3	1,2,3
Golgi II	4	4	4
Basket	4	4	4
Double bouquet	4	4	1,2,3,4, 5,6
Golgi II	5	5	5
Basket	5	5	5
Golgi II	6	6	6

in the auditory areas are approximately the same as those found in other cortex areas. Input stimuli are directed into layer 4. The flow of neural activity is then up into layers 2 and 3 (and 1), then down to layers 5 and 6. Activity flows from layers 5 and 6 back up to 4 and the upper layers, creating an iterated loop. Pyramidal cells in layers 2, 3, and 6 are assumed to represent output units. Input vectors were constructed to represent approximately the frequency and temporal patterns seen for words and syllables in auditory nerve recordings (Sinex & Geisler, 1984) in animals and voice spectrographs in humans.

Figs. 8.12 and 8.13 show connectivity for two neurons obtained on one simulation involving 600 neurons. In Fig. 8.13, a particular spindle cell in layer 6 (indicated by 'x') receives input from many neurons in layer 5 (remember the long range of pyramidal cell axons in layer 5 shown in Fig. 8.5) as well as pyramidals in layers 2 and 3. Apical dendrites extend into layer 1 where they receive input from the horizontal cells. Fig. 8.12 shows neurons which connect to a layer 2 pyramidal cell. Note the essentially vertical structure. The set of neurons connecting to each neuron will vary even within the same neuron type because of the randomness factor used in determining connections.

An input stimulus was directed into layer 4. This stimulus had a repeat rate of 20 ms and components at four frequencies corresponding to

Fig. 8.12. Connectivity to a pyramidal cell in layer 2.

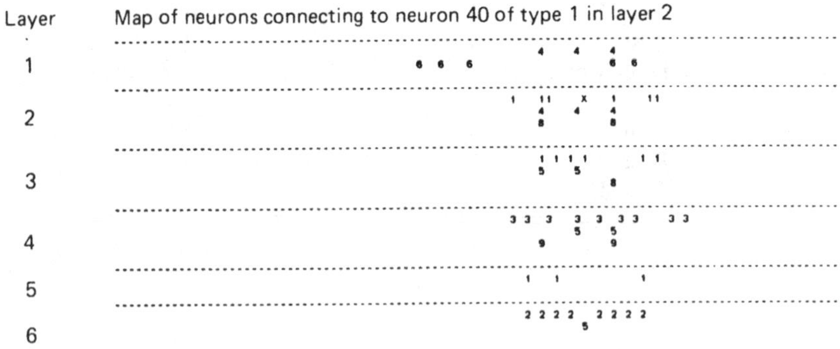

Layer   Map of neurons connecting to neuron 40 of type 1 in layer 2

Key:
1. pyramidal cell   6. horizontal cell
2. spindle cell   7. basket cell
3. spiny stellate cell   8. chandelier cell
4. Golgi II   9. double bouquet
5. Martinotti   X. cell receiving input from others shown

locations at $x = 183$–267, $x = 333$–383, $x = 450$–500, and $x = 670$–750 in Fig. 8.14. Fig. 8.14 shows contours of activity in the cortex model at 100 ms. The x-axis represents distance along the cortex in the direction of increasing frequency (topographic map). The y-direction represents vertical position, i.e., $y = 0$ is the bottom of the deepest layer, while $y = 5000$ μm represents the top of the cortex. The columnar nature of the activity is immediately apparent. In addition, activity is segregated vertically into three regions – high activity in the upper layers (layers 2 and 3), moderate to high activity in the lower layers (5 and 6), and low or inhibitory activity in layer 4 (about $y = 2000$ in Fig. 8.14). At later times (several hundred ms), layer 4 is strongly inhibited, as though the cortex were trying to turn off or ignore a constant input signal. Total activity shows a definite decrease around 50–60 ms after introduction of the input signal. This may represent the time required for the cortex model's processing to be effected. The overall pattern of behavior is very much like that proposed by Edelman & Finkel (1984).

Activity in individual neurons varies greatly. Figs. 8.15 and 8.16 show spike trains from two model pyramidal cells. For one, the input triggers a rapid burst of activity for 50 ms, followed by a silent period until a little over 100 ms, with renewed activity thereafter. For the other, not much activity occurs until after 50 ms, and activity varies. Connection strength can also show interesting behavior. In Fig. 8.17, the total strength of all connections to a particular pyramidal cell oscillates in time in a sawtooth fashion. Another neuron (Fig. 8.18) shows a more erratic evolution.

Fig. 8.13. Connectivity to a spindle cell in layer 6.

Layer	Map of neurons connecting to neuron 20 of type 2 in layer 6
1	.... • .... • • • • ... • ... • .... • ....
2	.... ı ıı ıı ı ....
3	.... ıı ıı ....
4	.... 4 .. 4 .. 4 ....
5	ı .. ı .. ı .... ıı ı ..... ıııı ı .... ı .. ıııı ....
6	.... ₈²² ˟ ˢ²ₛ² ....

Key:
1. pyramidal cell
2. spindle cell
3. spiny stellate cell
4. Golgi II
5. Martinotti
6. horizontal cell
7. basket cell
8. chandelier cell
9. double bouquet
X. cell receiving input from others shown

These small fluctuations in connectivity strength allow the model cortex to modulate its activity on the basis of past experience.

A method of characterizing the behavior of a layered network with the structure described is required. The overall activity of the system can be plotted. Activity vs. time of individual neurons, and connection strength between any two neurons can be generated. Contour plots of activity on any vertical or horizontal plane through the system can also be generated. These output forms can be compared to physiological measurements to validate the model as well as to visualize the global or local behavior vs. time of the net. However, to get a handle on what the model is doing, to quantify its capacity for learning or discriminating, some additional function is needed. The concept of iterated maps may provide the needed metric.

Fig. 8.14. Contours of activity at 100 ms. The y-axis represents depth, the x-axis is in direction of increasing frequency.

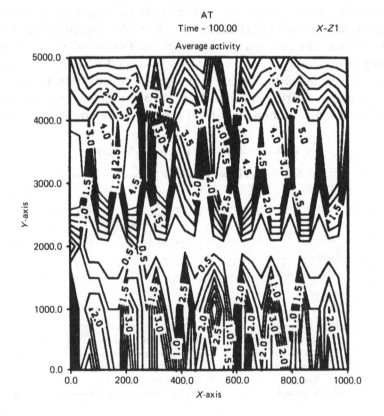

8.5 Cortex dynamics and iterated maps

An iterated function $f^n(x)$ is defined as

$$
\left.
\begin{aligned}
f^n(x_0) &= x_n = f(x_{n-1}), \\
x_{n-1} &= f(x_{n-2}), \dots, x_1 = f(x_0),
\end{aligned}
\right\} \tag{1}
$$

i.e., $\quad f^n(x) = f\{\dots f[f(x)] \dots\}$ where f is applied n times.

Non-linear functions allow a rich variety of behavior under iteration (Feigenbaum, 1980; Peitgen & Richter, 1985). Stable points may exist which act as attractors. The iterated function maps a set of points $X(i)$, the basin of attraction, into the attractor point y. For a system evolving in time, the membership of basins of attraction may change as well as the attractor set.

Fig. 8.15. Activity of a pyramidal cell from the model simulation.

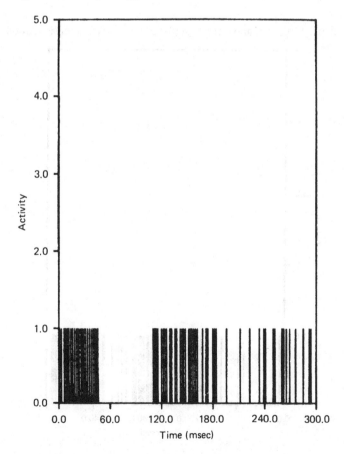

Our multi-layered model of the cortex is an iterated function. The looping from middle to upper to lower to middle layers provides the iteration and the all-or-none firing of model neurons provides the non-linearity. Plasticity in the connection strengths allows for modifications of attractor points and basins of attraction.

In the auditory system, a word can be recognized despite differences in intensity, frequency shifts, and time duration. In the model this behavior is approximated when

$$f^n(ax_{i+m}^j(bt)) \rightarrow f^n(\underline{x}_i^j(t)), \tag{2}$$

for an appropriate range of (a, b, m), where $x_i^j(t)$ is the rate of firing of input neurons corresponding to frequency i (or location i because of the topographic mapping) for input pattern j, subscript m represents a shift in frequency, a corresponds to a change in intensity or rate of firing, b effects a time dilation. The underbar indicates a reference point, i.e., $\underline{x}^j(t) =$

Fig. 8.16. Activity of another pyramidal cell from the model simulation.

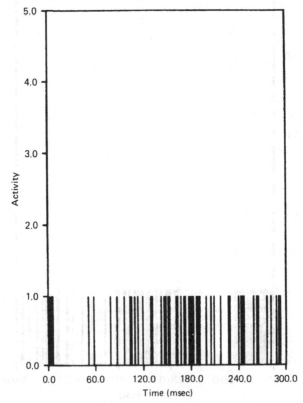

$(x_1^i, x_2^i, \ldots, x_n^j)$ is the input vector at a reference intensity, time duration and frequency. The arrow in eqn (2) means that the iterated map of the transformed pattern reaches the same limit point as the iterated map of the reference pattern after a sufficient number of iterations.

Iterated maps are the subject of intense research activity in the field of dynamical systems theory. The maps represented by cortical activity involve many degrees of freedom and display a stochastic quality. The theory for such systems is still far from well developed. However, there are strong suggestions that they are capable of having extremely large numbers of attractors and can converge very rapidly, two features that cortex seems to have. Studies of eqn (2) in the context of the auditory system are in progress, but results will not be presented here.

Fig. 8.17. Connection strength history for a model pyramidal neuron.

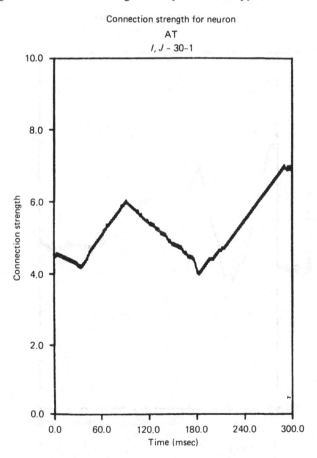

Connection strength for neuron
AT
I, J – 30–1

8.6 3-D application

A three-dimensional model has been constructed based on an hypothesis
(Merzenich *et al.*, 1984) for spatial localization of sound. This would also
provide a mechanism for separating simultaneous sound inputs. A strict
tonotopic mapping is preserved throughout the auditory system. Several
maps are recognized in auditory cortex; for each region, a well-defined
tonotopic (frequency) mapping defines one of the two surface spatial
dimensions. The other spatial dimension represents a combination of
input from both ears, arranged in alternating strips, labeled EE and EI
(Fig. 8.19). In an EE strip, binaural stimulation produces more excitation
than monaural stimulation. In EI strips, binaural stimulation results in

Fig. 8.18. Connection strength history for another model pyramidal neuron.

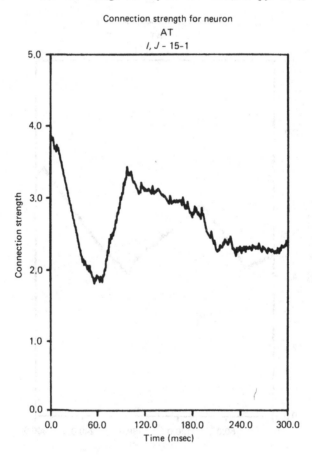

less excitation than monaural. The contralateral ear in EI and EE is excitatory, the ipsilateral is inhibitory or excitatory.

Intensity and timing differences between the input from the two ears are somehow used by the cortex together with some subcortical auditory nuclei to determine spatial location of sounds simultaneously with the cortex analyzing the informational content of sounds. The spatial location function probably involves the 'binaural' dimension of auditory cortex. An interesting feature of this dimension is its alterability throughout life. A possible mechanism of spatial location would simply involve mapping of a sound onto different coordinates of the binaural dimension of auditory cortex, as shown in Fig. 8.20.

The model has the same layered structure previously described, but the input to layer 4 is modified. In the x-direction, a strict tonotopic map is maintained. In the y-direction (the other horizontal direction) radii of influence are considerably larger for input neurons, and input from each ear is alternated so as to form the EE and EI strips. Also, the number of

Fig. 8.19. Two-dimensional map into auditory cortex. In one direction, a well-defined frequency-to-location map is maintained. In the orthogonal direction, alternating bands of excitatory-excitatory and excitatory-inhibitory bands are found, integrating input from the two ears.

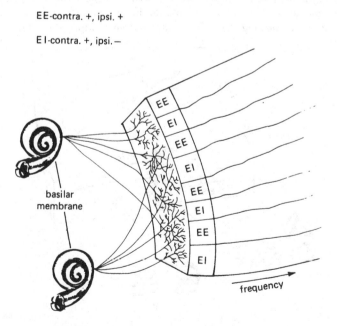

EE-contra. +, ipsi. +

EI-contra. +, ipsi. −

EE

EI

EE

EI

EE

EI

EE

EI

basilar
membrane

frequency

neurons has been increased to 20 160 and the total number of interconnections has increased strongly, to about 0.77 million. On average, each
neuron receives input from about 40 other neurons. Two input trains are
directed into the cortex model, one train is slightly shifted in intensity
from the other. The resulting activity pattern in the cortex at 100 ms is
shown in Figs. 8.21–8.24. The calculation was repeated with the input
patterns from the ears switched, representing a shift in spatial location of
the sound source. The activity pattern generated by this switched input
signal was subtracted at each time step from the field generated in the
previous simulation. Figs. 8.25 and 8.26 show contours of this difference
field for layers 3 and 5 at 100 ms. The differences are organized roughly
into bands. The same sound maps into different cortical patterns when the
binaural input balance changes.

This analysis has many limitations; for example, it does not yet fully
represent the processing that occurs in subcortical nuclei, nor does it
couple several cortical topographic maps, nor does it include connections
to other cortical regions. Also, although it contains a lot of neurons, it is
still several orders of magnitude from the actual structure. Nevertheless,
it is sufficiently realistic to use in exploring the dynamics of neurophysiological systems.

Fig. 8.20. Intensity and timing differences between signals from the right and the
left ear may lead to unique representation in auditory cortex as a function of
spatial location, allowing separation of inputs from multiple sound sources.

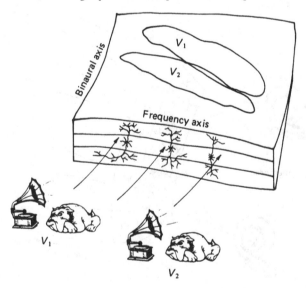

Fig. 8.21. Contours of neural activity in layer 1 at 100 ms.

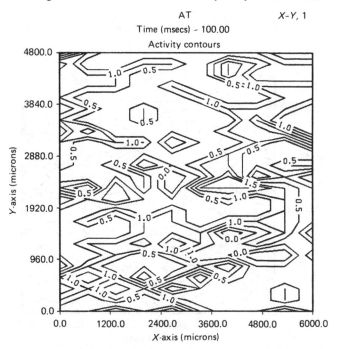

Fig. 8.22. Contours of neural activity in layer 3 at 100 ms.

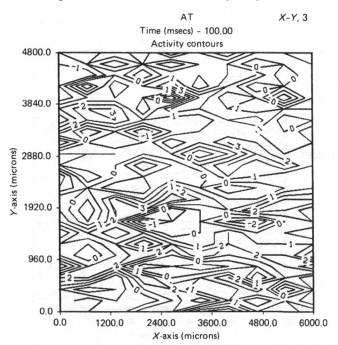

Fig. 8.23. Contours of neural activity in layer 5 at 100 ms.

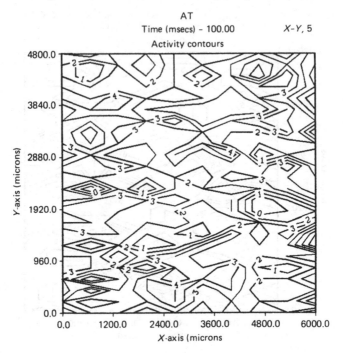

Fig. 8.24. Contours of neural activity in layer 6 at 100 ms.

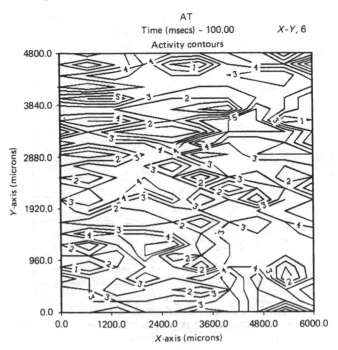

Fig. 8.25. Contours of differences in activity resulting from intensity shift in binaural input, for layer 3 at 100 ms.

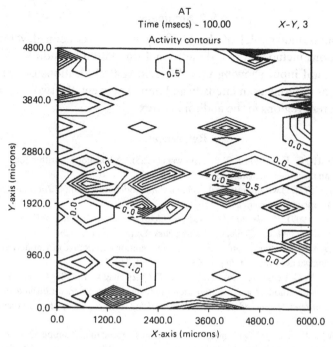

AT
Time (msecs) - 100.00   X-Y, 3
Activity contours

Fig. 8.26. Contours of differences in activity resulting from intensity shift in binaural input, for layer 5 at 100 ms.

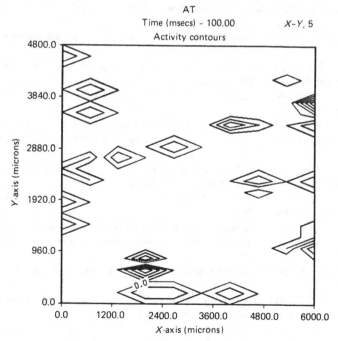

AT
Time (msecs) - 100.00   X-Y, 5
Activity contours

146   *Bryan J. Travis*

8.7 Summary

A computational model of the auditory system has been developed. Applications include a three-dimensional simulation of auditory cortex with binaural input showing that different spatial locations of sounds, encoded as differences in intensity and timing between the two ears, map into different regions in the auditory cortex.

References

Ackerly, D. H., G. E. Hinton & T. J. Sejnowski (1985). 'A learning algorithm for Boltzmann machines.' *Cognitive Science*, **9**, 147–69.

Allen, J. B. (1977). 'Two-dimensional cochlear fluid model: new results.' *Journal of the Acoustical Society of America*, **61**, 110–19.

Brodman, K. (1909). *Vergleichende Lokalisationlehre der Grosshirnrinde in ihren Prinzipien dargestellt auf Grund des Zellenbaues*, Leipzig: J. A. Barth.

Buhmann, J. & K. Schulten (1986). 'Associative recognition and storage in a model network of physiological neurons.' *Biological Cybernetics*, **54**, 319–35.

Chen, H. H., Y. C. Lee, G. Z. Sun, H. Y. Lee, T. Maxwell & C. L. Giles (1986). 'High order correlation model for associative memory.' New York: *American Institute of Physics, Conference Proceedings No. 151, Neural Networks for Computing, Snowbird, Utah, 1986*, pp. 86–99.

Clark, J. W., J. Rafelski & J. V. Winston (1985). 'Brain without mind: computer simulation of neural networks with modifiable neuronal interactions.' *Physics Reports* (Review Section of Physics Letters), **123**, 215–73.

Edelman, G. H. & L. H. Finkel (1984). 'Neuronal group selection in the cerebral cortex.' Chapter 22 in G. H. Edelman, W. E. Gall & W. M. Cowan, eds. (1984), *Dynamic Aspects of Neocortical Function*. New York: John Wiley & Sons.

Feigenbaum, J. (1980). 'Universal behavior in nonlinear systems.' *Los Alamos Science*, **1**, 4–27.

Gilbert, C. & Wiesel, T. (1979). 'Morphology and intracortical projections of functionally characterised neurones in the cat visual cortex'. *Nature*, **280**, 120–5.

Gilbert, C. (1983). 'Microcircuitry of the visual cortex.' *Annual Review of Neuroscience*, **6**, 217–47.

Hogg, T. & B. A. Huberman (1984). 'Understanding biological computation: reliable learning and recognition.' *Proceedings of the National Academy of Sciences, USA*, **81**, 6871–5.

Hogg, T. & B. A. Huberman (1985). 'Attractors on finite sets: the dissipative dynamics of computing structures.' *Physical Review A*, **32**, 2338–46.

Holmes, M. H. (1982). 'A mathematical model of the dynamics of the inner ear.' *Journal of Fluid Mechanics*, **116**, 59–75.

Hopfield, J. J. (1982). 'Neural networks and physical systems with emergent collective computational abilities.' *Proceedings of the National Academy of Sciences, USA*, **79**, 2554–8.

Hudspeth, A. J. (1985). 'The cellular basis of hearing: the biophysics of hair cells.' *Science*, **230**, 745–52.

Imig, T. J. & A. Morel (1983). 'Organization of the thalamocortical auditory system in the cat.' *Annual Review of Neuroscience*, **6**, 95–120.

Kolb, B. & I. Q. Whishaw (1985). 'Principles of neocortical organization.' Chapter 8 in *Fundamentals of Human Neuropsychology*. New York: W. H. Freeman and Co.

Kosco, B. (1986). 'Differential Hebbian learning.' New York: *American Institute of Physics, Conference Proceedings No. 151, Neural Networks for Computing, Snowbird, Utah, 1986*, pp. 277–82.

Krone, G., H. Mallot, G. Palm & A. Schüz (1986). 'Spatiotemporal receptive fields: a dynamical model derived from cortical architectonics.' *Proceedings of the Royal Society of London B*, **226**, 421–44.

Lapedes, A. S. & R. M. Farber (1986). 'Programming a massively parallel, computation universal system: static behavior.' New York: *American Institute of Physics, Conference Proceedings No. 151, Neural Networks for Computing, Snowbird, Utah, 1986*, pp. 283–298.

Marr, D. (1982). 'The philosophy and the approach.' Chapter 1 in *Vision*, San Francisco: W. H. Freeman & Co.

Merzenich, M. M., W. M. Jenkins & J. C. Middlebrooks (1984). 'Observations and hypotheses on special organizational features of the central auditory nervous system.' Chapter 12 in G. H. Edelman, W. E. Gall & W. M. Cowan (eds.), *Dynamic Aspects of Neocortical Function*. New York: John Wiley & Sons.

Oster, G. F. & E. O. Wilson (1978). 'A critique of optimization theory in evolutionary biology.' Chapter 8 in *Caste and Ecology in the Social Insects*. Princeton, N.J.: Princeton University Press.

Peitgen, H.-O. & P. H. Richter (1985). *Frontiers of Chaos*. Universität Bremen: Forschungsgruppe Komplexe Dynamik.

Pellionisz, A. J. (1984). 'Coordination: a vector-matrix description of transformations of overcomplete CNS coordinates and a tensorial solution using the Moore–Penrose generalized inverse.' *Journal of Theoretical Biology*, **110**, 353–75.

Pickles, J. O. (1982). *Introduction to the Physiology of Hearing*. Orlando: Academic Press.

Shamma, S. A. (1985a). 'Speech processing in the auditory system. I: The representation of speech sounds in the responses of the auditory nerve.' *Journal of the Acoustical Society of America*, **78**, 1612–21.

Shamma, S. A. (1985b). 'Speech processing in the auditory system. II: Lateral inhibition and the central processing of speech-evoked activity in the auditory nerve.' *Journal of the Acoustical Society of America*, **78**, 1622–32.

Shepherd, G. M. (1979). *The Synaptic Organization of the Brain*. New York: Oxford University Press.

Sinex, D. G. & C. D. Geisler (1984). 'Comparison of the responses of auditory nerve fibers to consonant-vowel syllables with predictions from linear models.' *Journal of the Acoustical Society of America*, **76**, 116–21.

Truex, R. C. & M. B. Carpenter (1969). 'The cerebral cortex.' Chapter 22 in *Human Neuroanatomy*. Baltimore: Williams & Wilkins.

Von Economo, C. (1929). *The Cytoarchitectonics of the Human Cerebral Cortex*. London: Oxford University Press.

9

Computer simulation of networks of electrotonic neurons

E. NIEBUR and P. ERDÖS

9.1 Introduction

The fundamental aim of simulation of neural nets is a better understanding of the functioning of the nervous system. Because of the complexities, simplifying assumptions have to be introduced from the beginning. In many frequently used models these assumptions are:

Each model neuron can be in one of few discrete states (e.g. 'on', 'off', 'refractory').

The totality of interactions between neurons is treated summarily by specifying few parameters, often just one 'synaptic strength', which is determined randomly, or by a deterministic algorithm, or by a combination of both.

The information processing by a neuron consists of comparing the value of a certain parameter, which is determined by incoming signals from other neurons, with some threshold. Essentially, when the value of this parameter exceeds the threshold, the neuron transits to another one of its possible states. A typical example for this parameter is the membrane potential at the axon hillock, which is determined by summing the action potentials impinging on this neuron during a certain time and whose value determines whether the neuron 'fires' or not.

The hypothesis that individual neurons can be described in a simple way makes the simulation of networks containing many model neurons possible. On the other hand, there are important parts of nervous systems, where model neurons simplified to the extent described above have little in common with reality. One of the reasons for the failure of this simple description is that the summation of synaptic inputs on a neuron occurs by means of graded ('electrotonic') potentials that spread along its dendrites. Therefore, the dependence of the voltage at the axon hillock on the spatiotemporal pattern of the synaptic input may be much more complicated than a simple time-weighted summation (Rall, 1964, 1977).

Even the concept of a neuron as a threshold element (i.e., an element that undergoes an important change when some parameter passes a certain value) is not applicable for certain parts of neural circuitry. More and more examples are found where the output of a neuron is a continuous function of its membrane potential. In these examples, graded potentials are used not only to collect and modify synaptic input in the interior of one neuron, but also for communication between neurons. This has been observed in systems which never show all-or-nothing spikes, and in others consisting of neurons communicating both by spikes and by graded potentials (see, e.g., Shepherd, 1978; Reese & Shepherd, 1972; Schmitt, Dev & Smith, 1976; Burrows, 1985).

Obviously, simulation using model neurons with the simplified features described above are not well suited for modeling neural nets communicating via electrotonic interactions. In the sequel, we shall present a model using neurons which show a much more realistic, complicated behavior than the simplified neurons described previously.

The organization of the paper is as follows: In the second part, we summarize the basic ideas of cable theory for dendrites and define the concept of networks of electrotonic neurons and its components. In the third part, we will describe the nervous system of nematodes. We show that modeling by means of electrotonic neural nets may be appropriate for nematodes. In the fourth part, we give some results of this approach.

9.2 Electrotonic neural networks

Let us suppose that the voltage differences along a neural process* are much larger than those between points inside the process in a plane perpendicular to the axis, and that the extracellular voltage is constant. Under these quite general assumptions, the following partial differential equation holds for the transmembrane voltage along a neural process:

$$\frac{d}{4R_i} \frac{\partial^2 V}{\partial x^2} - c_M \frac{\partial V}{\partial t} = j_M, \tag{2.1}$$

where t = time, x = space coordinate along neural process, V = voltage across cell membrane, R_i = volume resistivity of cytoplasm, d = diameter

*A neural process is an extension of the neuron cell body.

of neural process (cylindrical shape assumed), c_M = capacitance per unit area of membrane, j_M = transmembrane current.

(Rall (1977) treats the underlying assumptions in detail.)

In dendrites with purely passive conduction and without synapses, $j_M = g_R(V - V_R)$, where V_R is the resting potential and g_R the resting conductivity. We can take possible synaptic input into account by defining synaptic conductivities g_{exc}, g_{inh} and synaptic voltages V_{exc}, V_{inh}. They are all independent of V, and g_{exc} (g_{inh}) is identically zero, except at the location of an excitatory (inhibitory) synapse and while the latter is excited. Hence we put

$$j_M = g_{exc}(V - V_{exc}) + g_{inh}(V - V_{inh}) + g_R(V - V_R). \qquad (2.2)$$

In contradistinction to the Hodgkin–Huxley model, where the conductivities are determined by a set of voltage-dependent differential equations, here the synaptic conductivities do not depend on V: Instead, they are fixed by the synaptic input.

This model was introduced by W. Rall (Rall 1964, 1977) and used (often in modified form) by many workers since then, mostly for the investigation of the dependence of signalling properties on synaptic location on the dendrites. Usually, eqns (2.1), (2.2) are written in the form

$$\lambda^2 \partial^2 V/\partial x^2 - \tau \partial V/\partial t = (V - V_R) + E(V - V_{exc}) + I(V - V_{inh}), \qquad (2.3)$$

where $\lambda^2 = d/(4R_i g_R)$ = characteristic length, $\tau = c_M/g_R$ = characteristic time, $E = g_{exc}/g_R$, $I = g_{inh}/g_R$.

The use of cable theory for dendrites and the assumption of membrane conductivities changing with synaptic input have to be augmented by more ingredients in order to model a network of *electrotonic neurons* (as we will call neurons communicating by graded potentials). This ingredient is the synaptic coupling between neurons. In early work, attention was focused on the response of a neuron (or a part of it) on synaptic stimulation. Later, Shepherd & Brayton (1979) used a model for a chemical synapse in which the postsynaptic conductivity change was controlled by the voltage in the presynaptic nerve process. Such a model synapse, which establishes a relation between the input (presynaptic voltage) and the output (postsynaptic conductivity) of a synapse, makes it possible to treat the coupling of neurons forming a neural network.

9.2.1 Components of a model neuronal network

(a) *Nerve processes.* The main 'hardware' components of a nervous system are nerve processes (in a wide sense, i.e., including soma, dendritic spines, etc.) and connecting synapses, together with devices for input and output (sensory cells, neuromuscular junctions (NMJ), etc.).

We use eqn (2.3) as a model for a dendritic process which propagates only passively spreading potentials. For parts of the dendritic process where active properties of the membrane are supposed to be important, a more complicated expression than (2.2) for the calculation of j_M may be used (Perkel & Perkel, 1985; Miller, Rall & Rinzel, 1985 and references therein).

(b) *Chemical synapses.* We use as a model for the functioning of an excitatory (inhibitory) synapse a localized change in the excitatory (inhibitory) conductance g_{exc} (g_{inh}) in eqn (2.2), which has a sigmoidal dependence on the presynaptic voltage (see Fig. 9.1). Variation of the parameters (which may be different for each synapse in the system) models important special cases of synaptic transmission, for instance $V_{thr} < 0$ and $g_{min} < 0$ models a tonically transmitter-releasing synapse, whose output conductance depends linearly on the input voltage within a certain range of the latter.

The time dependence of the conductances g_{exc} and g_{inh} may be taken as complicated as is necessary for the particular situation. The simplest possibility is that the conductance is changed simultaneously with the presynaptic voltage change. A simple way to take into account the synaptic delay t_{del} is to set $g(t) = F[V_{pre}(t - t_{del}) - V_R]$, where F is the sigmoidal function shown in Fig. 9.1. Changes in the properties of the synapses, like facilitation (apart from the facilitation effect introduced by the membrane capacitance), fatigue or, on a longer time-scale, synaptic

Fig. 9.1. Characteristic curve of a chemical model synapse, showing the post-synaptic conductance $g(t')$ at time t' vs. the presynaptic voltage V_{pre} at time t. V_{thr} and V_{sat} are the threshold and saturation presynaptic voltages. g_{min} and g_{sat} are the minimum and saturation conductivities. In general, $t' = t + t_{del}$, where t_{del} is the synaptic delay.

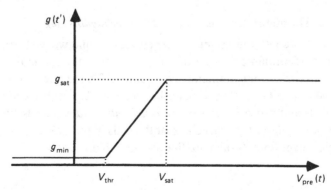

plasticity, may be incorporated by multiplying the conductance change by a factor, whose value depends on the history of the synapse.

(c) *Electrical synapses.* To model electrical synapses, i.e., gap junctions, it is simplest to assume a time-independent ohmic resistance in the area of the junction. If a gap junction exists between the neurons i and j, then this corresponds to adding the term

$$g_g(V_i - V_j) \tag{2.4}$$

to the right-hand side of eqn (2.2) for the two neurons in question; g_g is the conductance of the gap junction. While a chemical model synapse is by construction unidirectional, the gap junctions so defined are reciprocal. However, Bennett (1972) has shown that by an appropriate choice of parameters this model allows also unidirectional operation, as is observed experimentally in some instances.

9.2.2 *Constructing a network*

Given a neural system to be modelled, we represent the functioning of each of its processes by an equation of type (2.3) or, if necessary, of the more general type (2.1). As a rule, boundary conditions assuming vanishing current leaking out of the ends of neural processes are adequate. Coupling between these equations is introduced by terms representing the synapses. The equations are solved by division of the nerve processes into sequential compartments, each of which may have different parameters according to the physiological situation to be modelled (e.g. greater diameter for the soma than for dendrites). Mathematically, this corresponds to an approximation of the system of coupled partial differential equations by a system of coupled ordinary differential equations. These are solved numerically by standard procedures on a computer.

9.3 The motor nervous system of *Caenorhabditis elegans*

The fact, that the nervous system of nematodes (round worms) consists exclusively of identifiable neurons of very simple morphology, makes this system most suitable for systematic investigations. This was recognized as early as 1908 when Goldschmidt published a complete reconstruction of all nerve cells and process tracts of *Ascaris lumbricoides* (Goldschmidt, 1908, 1909). Because of the large size of the cells in this animal, electro-physiological experiments on it are likewise possible.

Fig. 9.2. Structure of a typical motoneuron (DB3) in the ventral cord of *Caenorhabditis elegans*. Chemical synapses are indicated by arrows, together with the name of their synaptic partners*. The direction of the arrow (out of or into the neuron) indicates the flow of information, i.e., which neuron is pre- and post-synaptic, respectively. Gap junctions are represented by the symbol ⊢⊣. The process in the dorsal cord is drawn on a larger scale and only the first part of it is shown (after J. G. White, personal communication).

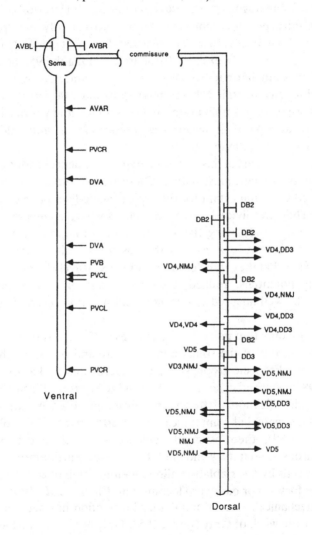

*Neurons are given names consisting of a few alphanumeric characters.

Another property of nematodes is, that to a large extent, the nervous systems of different species are similar. All classes of motoneurons of the somatic musculature in *Ascaris* have analogues with similar morphology in the free living nematode *Caenorhabditis elegans*, despite the difference in size of these species (length 300 mm for *Ascaris l.* and 1 mm for *C. elegans*). Furthermore, the same type of neurotransmitter has been identified for analogous cell classes in both animals (Stretton *et al.*, 1985; S. L. McIntire, personal communication). Since recently, the structure of the complete nervous system of *C. elegans* is known at the electron-micro-scopic level. There are exactly 302 neurons among the 959 nongonadal cells of an adult hermaphrodite *C. elegans*, connected by about 5000 morphologically identified chemical synapses and 2000 gap junctions. All neurons are of very simple morphology with few, if any, branching (see Fig. 9.2) and make their synapses *en passant* (White *et al.*, 1976; J. G. White, personal communication).

An interesting part of this system consists of the neurons controlling the activity of the somatic musculature. There are 69 motoneurons which are considered to be important for the typical snake-like locomotion of the animal. They are divided into seven classes whose members are distri-buted rather evenly along the ventral cord. An important property of these motoneurons in *Ascaris* is the absence of all-or-nothing spikes, which means that they transfer information exclusively by decrementally spreading potentials. Indeed, their membrane properties have been shown to be well adapted to this mode of operation (Davis & Stretton, 1982).

There are only four pairs of interneurons in *C. elegans* that synapse on the motoneurons of the somatic musculature and run along the whole ventral cord. From electrophysiological experiments on *Ascaris* (Stretton *et al.*, 1985; Walrond *et al.*, 1985; Walrond & Stretton, 1985*a,b*), as well as from identification of the neurotransmitters used by the cells (S. L. McIntire, personal communication; Stretton *et al.*, 1985; Johnson & Stretton, 1980), there is good evidence for a classification of the motoneurons in excitatory and inhibitory classes. Furthermore, selective killing of cells by laser ablation allows identification of cells responsible for either forward or backward locomotion (Chalfie *et al.*, 1984).

The mechanical base of undulatory locomotion has been elucidated mainly by the work of Gray (Gray, 1953; Gray & Lissmann, 1964), who observed the forces exerted by a creeping snake on its support. It is beyond the scope of this chapter to go into the details of the mechanical problems involved in this motion. Gray proved that the snake uses a certain pattern of muscle activity for its undulatory creeping progression. We will assume that the efficient locomotion of the nematode is due to the same output pattern of its motor nervous system. It consists of alternating zones of tense and relaxed muscles whose spatial distribution rests constant relative to the wave-like path described by the body. In the frame of reference of the moving worm, this corresponds to alternate contractions of muscles on the left and right side. These zones of muscle activity travel along the body contrary to the direction of locomotion (see Fig. 9.3).

9.3.1 Models for locomotion

(a) *Previous work.* There have been several attempts to explain the formation of the muscle waves mentioned in the preceding section. For higher animals, one would probably expect a mechanism called 'instructive model', i.e., the detailed control of every muscle group by an interneuron. In nematodes, this possibility is practically ruled out by the morphological structure.

Another simple mechanism is the 'one-spike, one-wave' model, assuming that an excitation travelling along the interneurons evokes a muscle contraction at the position where it is just passing by (Crofton, 1971). A somewhat related (called 'neurocratic') model assumes that the propa-

Fig. 9.3. *Caenorhabditis elegans* in typical, wave-like posture. The shaded areas indicate the parts of the body musculature which must contract to produce a locomotion in the specified direction. *L* denotes the length of the wave which the body forms.

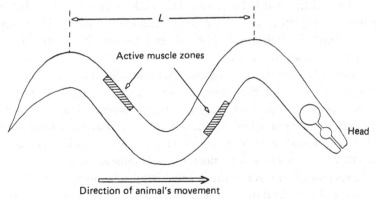

gation of the waves is due to travelling electrical activity in the *muscle* and that the only function of the nervous system is to switch this mechanism on and off. This model is compatible with the observation that muscle cells are coupled electrically to each other.

Recently, Stretton *et al.* proposed a model in which the motoneurons of each of the five similar segments of the body of *Ascaris* are arranged functionally in a closed loop (Stretton *et al.*, 1985). The overlap between segments could convey the phase information for the synchronization of activity in adjacent segments.

(b) *Present model.* R. L. Russell (pers. comm.) has pointed out that some synapse-free parts of the motoneuron dendrites in *C. elegans* lying anteriorly or posteriorly to the regions with NMJs might function as stretch receptors. Electrotonic stretch receptors have been observed in other systems (Bush, 1981). This led us to suppose that in the resting animal the voltage in all motoneurons is under the threshold for muscle excitation. If now the 'brain', i.e., the set of neurons in the cephalic ganglia and the neurophile in the nerve ring, 'decides', e.g., that the worm is to go forward, the voltage in the corresponding interneuron is increased by synaptic input from the nerve ring. The excitation spreads down the ventral cord along the process of the interneuron and is passed to the coupled motoneurons, which are responsible for forward movement.

If this were the only input to the motoneurons, the effect of the 'decision' would be a shrinking of the body over its whole length, because all somatic muscles contract simultaneously. Now consider the additional influence of stretch receptors: Let L be the length of the body wave. It is required, that a region of NMJs should be activated then and only then, when there is a curve in the body towards the same side on which the NMJ is located at a distance of $L/4$ in front of the NMJ, or there is a curve in the body towards the other side at the same distance behind the NMJ (see Fig. 9.3). This information could be delivered by stretch receptors lying anterior or posterior to the NMJs.

This model has the merit to be the only one among those presented which is compatible with the following simple experiment (R. Durbin & E. Niebur, unpublished): If a *C. elegans* is kept in water in a glass capillary of a diameter smaller than twice the amplitude of the wave which the body usually forms, it rests for a long time in a typical posture, which is a helix formed by the whole body. The most plausible muscle excitation pattern for the explanation of this posture is a unilateral contraction. This is just what one would expect if the postulated stretch receptors were excitatory on compression or inhibitory on stretch, or both.

9.4 Simulation

9.4.1 Forward locomotion network

Simulation on a computer of the neural network described in Section 9.3 may decide if the hypotheses presented in that section describe reality. This simulation is a concrete example of how the components described in Section 9.2 can be combined to model an existing neural network. Out of the neurons in *C. elegans* which control the somatic musculature, we choose those thought to be responsible for forward locomotion. These are the excitatory motoneurons VB and DB, the inhibitory motoneurons VD and DD, and the interneuron AVB (for the notation used see Chalfie *et al.*, 1984). The only other neuron class that has been shown to be involved in forward locomotion, the interneuron PVC, seems not to be essential, because animals lacking it can move forward normally (Chalfie *et al.*, 1984). (These neurons, however, are important for touch sensitivity) Fig. 9.4 shows the resulting network, where the synaptic connections

Fig. 9.4. Network of neurons responsible for forward locomotion in *Caenorhabditis elegans*. The AVB-process (thick black line) continues anteriorly and posteriorly in the ventral cord, while the shape of the other neurons is as sketched; they do not extend further. The arrows of the chemical synapses point in the direction of information flow. NMJ = neuromuscular junction.

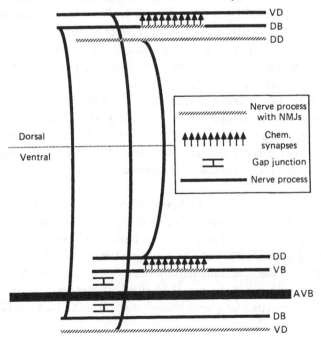

are introduced according to the electron-microscopic reconstruction of C. elegans (J. G. White, personal communication).

9.4.2 Choice of parameters

The parameters in eqn (2.1) are the diameter of the neural process d, the capacitance of the cell membrane c_M and the resistance of the cytoplasm R_i. For the model synapses, we must furthermore specify the transmembrane conductance g_R for the resting membrane and those for all excitatory, inhibitory, and electrical synapses there are in the system.

Because of the simple morphology of the neurons in nematodes, the *diameter* of the dendrites can be obtained rather accurately from the electron-microscopic pictures. We assume throughout a cylindrical form with constant diameter. Another relatively well known parameter is the *capacitance* of the cell membrane. This seems to be nearly a biological constant and its value of about 1 μF/cm^2 is just what is obtained by elementary considerations of the physics of a lipid bilayer (see, e.g., Hobbie, 1978). A third parameter whose value is rather uncritical is the *resistance of the cytoplasm* in nerve cells. It is between 0.5 Ωm and 1 Ωm.

On the other hand, an enormous range of values has been reported for the *transmembrane conductance*. For instance, Bush (1981) stated values between 10 kΩ^{-1} m^{-2} and 500 kΩ^{-1} m^{-2} for different parts of the *same* nerve process (the S-fiber of the mud-crab *Scylla*). These variations in g_R are due to the greatly varying lengths over which electrotonic signals have to be transmitted. The characteristic length, over which a passively spreading signal decays, augments with smaller g_R (see definition after eqn (2.3)). Indeed, the unusually low value of g_R in the *Scylla* S-fiber is an adaptation to the necessity to transfer electrotonically a sensory input over a length of several millimetres. An analogous situation occurs in the *Ascaris* motoneurons. Those parts of the neurons which are postsynaptic to interneurons are centimetres away from the region presynaptic to NMJs. The observed characteristic length is 6.3 mm (Davis & Stretton, 1982).

The price to pay for a low transmembrane conductance is a great characteristic time τ (see eqn (2.3)) which determines the time needed for an appreciable voltage change. It is probable that the transmembrane conductance adapts itself (e.g., by changing the density of ion channels) in order to meet the functional requirements of the particular neuron. So, whenever we do not have more detailed information, we assume a membrane resistivity that gives a characteristic length λ (see eqn (2.3)) of

Table 9.1. *Parameters of model neurons*

	C. elegans interneuron	C. elegans motoneuron	Ascaris motoneuron
d	10^{-6} m	0.33×10^{-6} m	16×10^{-6} m
R_i	0.5 Ωm	0.5 Ωm	0.5 Ωm
c_M	10^{-4} μF m^{-2}	10^{-4} μF/m^{-2}	10^{-4} μF m^{-2}
g_R	0.5 Ω^{-1} m^{-2}	1 Ω^{-1} m^{-2}	15×10^{-2} Ω^{-1} m^{-2}
V_R	−70 mV	−70 mV	−70 mV

the order of the process length. The values used in the simulation of the circuit described in *C. elegans* are given in Table 9.1.

Finally, we have to insert values for the *synaptic conductances*. In our case we have only gap junctions, whose areas may be estimated from the electron-microscopic pictures. The order of magnitude of the resistance of gap junctions was given as 10^{-4} Ωm^2 by Bennett (1977). Again, we will assume that this determines just the order of magnitude, but that the animal may tailor the resistance of a particular gap junction to its needs.

9.4.3 Results of simulation

A simulation of the whole circuit (see Fig. 9.4) has not yet been achieved. At present, questions related to subsystems are being treated.

First, we investigate whether the 'one-spike, one-wave' model described in Section 9.3 is a hypothesis which can explain the propagation of the muscular waves. For this it is necessary that the velocity of an excitation travelling in a neuron comes close to that of a muscular wave. The latter can be determined experimentally; it is approximately 2 mm s^{-1} for *C. elegans* swimming in water and $\frac{1}{3}$ mm s^{-1} for creeping on agar. Similar values have been observed for other nematodes of comparable size (Gray & Lissmann, 1964).

Now we turn to the simulation of a travelling excitation in the interneurons of the ventral cord of *C. elegans*. The interneuron is represented by a neural process with the parameters given in Table 9.1. The excitation by its presynaptic partners is modelled by setting the voltage in the anterior part (which is presumed to be in the nerve ring) of the interneuron for a certain time interval t_{NR} equal to a value V_{NR} greater than the resting potential. We define the propagation velocity of the excitation as the velocity with which the maximum of the resulting voltage distribution travels down the process. This velocity was found to be approximately 10 cm s^{-1} and quite independent of t_{NR} and V_{NR}. This is by a factor 50 greater than the observed velocity of the fastest muscle wave observed in *C. elegans*. We conclude that the muscular waves in *C. elegans* are *not* the result of an electrotonically propagated excitation travelling along the body with the same velocity as the muscle wave.

It is interesting to perform the same calculation for *Ascaris* motoneurons (parameters in Table 9.1). We obtain a propagation velocity of the excitation of about 22 cm s^{-1}, which lies in the range of the experimentally measured values of 21–38 cm s^{-1} (Johnson & Stretton, 1980; Walrond & Stretton, 1985*b*). Again, the excitation travels much faster than the muscular waves in that animal.

Having ruled out the 'instructive' model and the 'one-spike-one-wave' model, we are left with those models in which the interneurons switch on and off some activity for the body as a whole. We may ask the question whether this can be accomplished by just one of the four interneuron classes or whether the cooperation of more than one of them is necessary? In other words: Is a single interneuron capable of evoking a significant

Fig. 9.5. Voltage vs. time in one of the two AVB interneurons and in the coupled motoneuron DB3 caused by excitation of the interneuron in the nerve ring. The interneuron voltage is plotted at the gap junction to DB3, the motoneuron voltage in the neuromuscular junction region in the dorsal cord. The motoneuron DB3 is the one depicted in Fig. 9.2, and the interneurons AVB are connected to it at the gap junctions AVBL and AVBR, respectively, on the top left of Fig. 9.2.

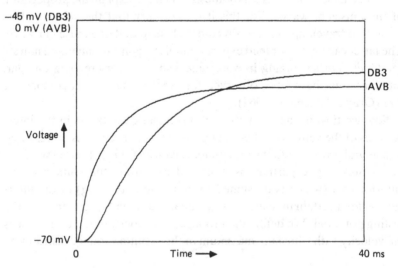

voltage change at the NMJs of its postsynaptic motoneurons? By a 'significant' change we understand a change of some millivolts; this has been shown to elicit transmitter release and ensuing voltage change in muscle cells postsynaptic to the NMJs in *Ascaris* (Stretton *et al.*, 1985).

The motoneurons VB and DB are coupled to the interneurons AVB by gap junctions (see Fig. 9.4). From the electron-microscopic pictures we obtain their lengths (about 2 μm) and their positions relative to motoneurons and interneurons. We assume that their specific resistance is 10^{-4} Ωm^2 and use the values given in Table 9.1 for the parameters of the model neurons AVB, DB, and VB. Fig. 9.5 shows the result of a computer simulation using the equations of Section 9.2. Shown is the voltage in the region near the NMJs of the motoneuron DB, when the part of AVB in the nerve ring is excited from the assumed resting potential of -70 mV to zero potential, i.e., by 70 mV. Both motoneurons show a clear voltage-rise in this region (the curve for VB is similar to that of DB). We may conclude that excitation of a single interneuron in the nerve ring is sufficient for an excitation of the muscles postsynaptic to VB and DB.

9.5 Conclusion

We described the beginnings of a computer simulation of the electrotonic nerve network of a worm. This network is responsible for locomotion. The experimentally known parameters used in conjunction with the model described here lead to encouraging preliminary results.

Acknowledgements

We are grateful to Dr J. G. White for the communication of unpublished material. One of us (E.N.) thanks Dr J. G. White and R. Durbin for their hospitality at the Laboratory of Molecular Biology of the Medical Research Council, Cambridge. The support of the Swiss National Science Foundation through Grant number 2.683-0.85 is gratefully acknowledged.

References

Bennett, M. V. L. (1972). 'Comparison of electrically and chemically mediated synaptic transmission.' In G. D. Pappas & S. D. Waxman, eds., *Structure and Function of Synapses*. Raven Press, New York.

Bennett, M. V. L. (1977). 'Electrical transmission: a functional analysis and comparison to chemical transmission.' In E. R. Kandel, ed., *Handbook of Physiology*, vol. 1, Amer. Physiol. Soc., Bethesda, MD, pp. 39–98, 357–416.

Burrows, M. (1985). 'Nonspiking and spiking local interneurons in the locust.' In Selverston, A. I., ed., *Model Neural Networks and Behavior*. Plenum Press, New York.

Bush, B. M. H. (1981). 'Non-impulsive stretch receptor in crustaceans.' In A. Roberts & B. M. H. Bush, eds., *Neurons without Impulses*, Cambridge University Press, pp. 147–76.

Chalfie, M., Sulston, J. E., White, J. G., Southgate, E., Thomson, J. N. & Brenner, S. (1984). 'The neural circuit for touch sensitivity in *Caenorhabditis elegans*. *J. Neurosci.*, 5(4), 956–64.

Crofton, H. D. (1971). 'Form, function and behavior.' In B. M. Zuckermann, W. F. Mai & R. A. Rohde, eds., *Plant Parasitic Nematodes*. Academic Press, New York.

Davis, R. E. & Stretton, A. O. W. (1982). 'Motorneuron membrane constants and signaling properties in the netmatode *Ascaris*.' *Soc. Neurosci. Abstr.*, 8(2), 685.

Goldschmidt, R. (1908). 'Das Nervensystem von *Ascaris lumbricoides* und *Ascaris megalocephala* I. *Ztsch. Wiss. Zool.*, 90, 73–136.

Goldschmidt, R. (1909). 'Das Nervensystem von *Ascaris lumbricoides* und *Ascaris megalocephala* II.' *Ztsch. Wiss. Zool.*, 92, 306–57.

Gray, J. (1953). 'Undulatory propulsion.' *Quart. J. Micr. Sci.*, 94, 551–78.

Gray, J. & Lissmann, H. W. (1964). 'The locomotion of nematodes.' *J. Exp. Biol.*, 41, 135–54.

Hobbie, R. K. (1978). *Intermediate Physics for Medicine and Biology*. John Wiley, New York.

Hodgkin, A. L. & Huxley, A. F. (1952). 'A quantitative description of membrane current and its application to conduction and excitation in nerve.' *J. Physiol.*, 117, 500–44.

Johnson, C. D. & Stretton, A. O. W. (1980). In B. M. Zuckermann, ed., *Nematodes as Biological Models*, vol. 1. Academic Press, New York, pp. 159–95.

Miller, J. P., Rall, W. & Rinzel, J. (1985). 'Synaptic amplification by active membrane in dendritic spines.' *Brain Res.*, 325, 326–30.

Perkel, D. H. & Perkel, D. J. (1985). 'Dendritic spines: role of active membrane in modulating synaptic efficacy.' *Brain Res.*, 325, 331–5.

Rall, W. (1964). 'Theoretical significance of dendritic trees for neuronal input–output relation.' In R. F. Reiss, ed., *Neural Theory and Modelling*, Stanford University Press, Palo Alto, pp. 73–97.

Rall, W. (1977). 'Core conductor theory and cable properties of neurons.' In E. R. Kandel, ed., *Handbook of Physiology*, vol. 1, Amer. Physiol. Soc., Bethesda, pp. 39–98.

Reese, T. S. & Shepherd, G. M. (1972). 'Dendro-dendritic synapses in the central nervous system.' In G. D. Pappas and S. D. Waxman, eds., *Structure and Function of Synapses*. Raven Press, New York.

Schmitt, F. O., Dev, P. & Smith, B. H. (1976). 'Electrotonic processing of information by brain cells.' *Science*, 193, 114–20.

Shepherd, G. M. (1978). 'Microcircuits in the nervous system.' *Sci. Am.*, 238, 93–103.

Shepherd, G. M. & Brayton, R. K. (1979). 'Computer simulation of a dendrodendritic synaptic circuit for self- and lateral-inhibition in the olfactory bulb.' *Brain Res.*, 175, 377–82.

Stretton, A. O. W., Davis, R. E., Angstadt, J. D., Donmoyer, J. E. & Johnson, C. D. (1985). 'Neural control of behavior in *Ascaris*.' *Trends Neurosci.*, June 1985, pp. 294–300.

Walrond, J. P., Kass, I. S., Stretton, A. O. W. & Donmoyer, J. E. (1985). 'Identification of excitatory and inhibitory motoneurons in the nematode *Ascaris* by electrophysiological techniques.' *J. Neurosci.*, 5(1), 1–8.

Walrond, J. P. & Stretton, A. O. W. (1985a). 'Reciprocal inhibition in the motor nervous system of the nematode *Ascaris*: Direct control of ventral inhibitory motoneurons by dorsal excitatory motoneurons.' *J. Neurosci.*, **5**(1), 9–15.

Walrond, J. P. & Stretton, A. O. W. (1985b). 'Excitatory and inhibitory activity in the dorsal musculature of the nematode *Ascaris*, evoked by single dorsal excitatory motoneurons.' *J. Neurosci.*, **5**(1), 16–22.

White, J. G., Southgate, E., Thomson, J. N. & Brenner, S. (1976). 'The structure of the ventral cord of *Caenorhabditis elegans*.' *Phil. Trans. R. Soc. Lond. Ser., B.*, **275**, 327–42.

10

A possible role for coherence in neural networks

RODNEY M. J. COTTERILL

10.1 Introduction

This article addresses a well-defined issue: does coherent firing of several neurons play a role in the function of the cerebral cortex? Its main purpose is to present the results of a computer simulation of a neural network in which the exact timing of impulses is indeed of paramount importance. And it is demonstrated that such a network would have potentially useful powers of discrimination and recall.

It is reasonably clear that the timing of the arrival of nerve impulses at a given neuron cannot be a matter of total indifference. The voltage across a neural membrane relaxes back towards its resting value, once a stimulus has been removed, so it is easy to envisage situations in which incoming impulses will fail to provoke a response unless they can act in unison by arriving simultaneously, or nearly so, at the somatic region. And there is a considerable corpus of evidence that the timing of incoming impulses is important. In the human auditory system, for example, small temporal offsets between impulse trains in the two cochlear nerves is exploited to locate sound sources, while the relative timing of impulses in the same nerve appears to be essential for the correct functioning of speech discrimination (Sachs, Voigt & Young, 1983). There is also evidence that the timing of sensory stimulation, down at the ten-millisecond level, is critically important for classical conditioning (Sutton & Barto, 1981). And on the clinical side, one sees an extreme example of neuronal synchronization in the case of epilepsy, which apparently arises from mutual excitation between neurons (Traub & Wong, 1982).

Evidence of the importance of timing, albeit indirect, also comes from psychophysical experiments, such as those of Zemon & Ratliff (1984), in which visual evoked potentials were tied to summation effects of excitatory and inhibitory postsynaptic potentials originating in the visual cortex. The South American electric fish, *Eigenmannia virescens*, even appears to have phase-sensitive neurons in its midbrain, capable of discrimination around the millisecond level (Bastian & Heiligenberg, 1980).

The wherewithal to probe the extent of correlated neural firings should soon be at hand. A number of centres have recently developed facilities which permit simultaneous recording from several neurons (Gerstein, Bloom, Espinosa, Evanczuk & Turner, 1983; Reitboeck, 1983; Kuperstein & Eichenbaum, 1985), and there has already been some discussion of the interpretation of the voluminous data which these set-ups will no doubt produce (Knox & Poppele, 1977; Gevins, Doyle, Cutillo, Schaffer, Tannehill, Ghannam, Gilcrease & Yeager, 1981; Gerstein, Perkel & Dayhoff, 1985). We should soon know whether correlated trains of impulses do occur in the cortices of alert experimental animals, under the influence of appropriate stimuli.

Meanwhile, one must resort to simulations of the type described in this article, which is divided up in the following manner. The necessary neural background is presented in the next section, and there then follows a discussion of the concept of coherence and correlation, in the neural context. The computer model is then described, and separate sections are devoted to the discussion of possible applications to memory and autism. The article closes with a general discussion of the issue of coherence.

10.2 Biological background

The brain consists of approximately one hundred thousand million nerve cells which are called neurons. A typical neuron has a shape not unlike that of a leguminous plant (see Fig. 10.1). It has a reasonably well-defined body, referred to as the soma, and a large number of extended protuberances, known as processes. These latter, extending outwards from the body like numerous tentacles, are of two types. There are the dendrites, which are patterned rather like the limbs and branches of a tree, and these carry signals towards the soma. They are known as the afferent processes. Then there is a single process extending from the soma over a distance that is often many times the diameter of the latter. This is the axon, which usually terminates in a similar branching pattern. It is referred to as an efferent process, and it transmits signals emanating at the soma, onwards towards other cells. The connections between nerve cells, the synapses, can be excitatory or inhibitory. Synapses are small regions of near-con-

Fig. 10.1. The pyramidal cell, sketched here, is one of the prominent types of neuron found in the cortex. It takes its name from the shape of its soma, or cell body. Information, in the form of electrochemical waves, flows along the dendrites, towards the soma. If the voltage at the latter exceeds a certain threshold value, an electrochemical impulse is passed out along the axon. This signal, with its relatively high velocity (about 20 ms^{-1}) and all-or-nothing character, differs markedly from the slower, graded, and attenuated signals observed in the dendrites.

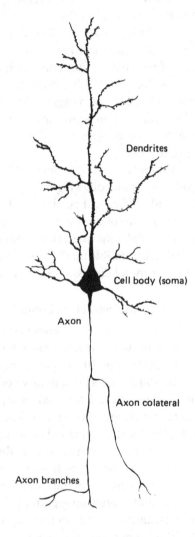

tact, in which the signal from one cell to another is passed chemically, and is mediated by molecules known as neurotransmitters. Within a given nerve cell, the transmission of information from the dendrite towards the soma is electrochemical in nature and is transmitted with an attenuation which is dependent upon distance and time. A typical time constant for dendrite attenuation lies around 10 ms (Shepherd, 1979; Kawato, Hamaguchi, Murakami & Tsukahara, 1984). The transmission of a signal from the soma out along the axon is, on the other hand, of the all-or-nothing type known as an action potential, or nerve impulse. This signal propagates without appreciable attenuation, at a speed of approximately 20 ms^{-1}, the duration of the impulse lasting about 1 ms or so (Hodgkin & Huxley, 1952). Once the soma has given out such an impulse, it cannot be stimulated to generate a further impulse until a certain minimum time has elapsed, and this is referred to as the refractory period, which is approximately 10 ms in duration.

A given nerve cell can make upwards of a thousand synaptic contacts with neighbouring cells, so that the total number of synapses in the entire brain may be as high as 10^{14} or 10^{15}. The time taken for the neurotransmitter molecules to diffuse across the synaptic gap is generally taken to be about 1 ms or so, and this is referred to as the synaptic delay (Kuffler & Nicholls, 1976). In practice there are several processes contributing to this mechanism, the first of these being the fusion of the small membrane-bounded sacks, which contain the neurotransmitter and which are referred to as vesicles, with the presynaptic membrane. This causes the liberation of the neurotransmitter into the synaptic gap, and after the molecules have diffused across they dock with receptor molecules which are able to generate the further electrochemical response in the dendrites referred to by the adjective electrotonic. These stages are shown in Fig. 10.2 for an idealised dendritic spine.

Anatomical observations of the microstructure have revealed that many different types of neurons are present in the brain, and that they are linked up in a manner rather suggestive of electronic circuitry. The cells do thus not bear a relationship to the whole as do, for example, the atoms in a crystal. It is important to emphasize this in view of the recent emergence of spin-glass models of the brain (Hopfield, 1982), which take no account of the observed variety of cell types. The cerebral cortex, or neocortex as it is also called, consists of sheets of cells roughly 3 mm thick, and it is highly convoluted to permit its accommodation within the skull. There are indications of a subdivision within these sheets, groups of cells being lined up in columns of approximately 0.5 mm in diameter, lying perpendicular to the cortical surface. The density of synaptic contacts between the cells in a given column is rather high, whereas there are somewhat fewer synaptic junctions between the various columns, which are observed to make up a loose mosaic. It was this latter arrangement which suggested the structure for the model described in this paper.

10.3 Coherence and correlation in the neural context

The central idea in this article is that the exact timing of the arrival of nerve impulses at the extremities of a given neuron is critically important. The docking of neurotransmitter molecules with receptors on the post-synaptic membrane touches off the electrotonic wave which flows down the dendrite towards the soma. But this wave is attenuated in both space and time and if it is to make a contribution to the collective influence of all incoming waves, at the soma, it must arrive at approximately the same time as waves which have travelled along other dendrites. If waves arrive

Fig. 10.2. The neurons in the brain are not in direct contact with one another, and the passage of information between these cells is a chemical process rather than an electrochemical one. The transfer occurs non-instantaneously at synapses, which are primarily formed between an axon branch and the terminal region of a dendrite (although axonal–somatic and dendro–dendritic synapses are also encountered). When the impulse arrives at the tip of the axon branch, it provokes fusion of vesicles (which are membrane-bounded packets containing neuro-transmitter molecules) with the presynaptic membrane. The vesicles thereby release their contents into the synaptic cleft, which is typically about 20 nm wide, and the neurotransmitter molecules drift across to the postsynaptic membrane and dock with receptor molecules. This initiates the graded electrochemical wave in the dendrite: the electronic response. The sequence of stages is here indicated from left to right.

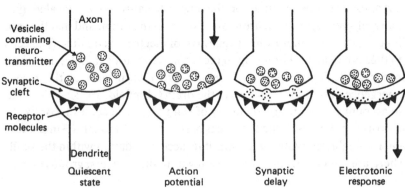

out of phase with one another, their potential for raising the somatic voltage above its threshold value will not be realized.

There are actually three time constants to be considered, in connection with this issue, and we may take them in the order they are encountered as information flows from one soma, out along the axon and axonal branch, across the synapse, and finally along the dendrite towards the next soma. It is a common fallacy to imagine the first of these steps as occupying an appreciable amount of time; in one's mind's eye, the impulse is seen as a well-defined blip travelling out along the axon, not unlike a soliton wave. This is quite misleading, as the following little calculation will demonstrate. The duration of an action potential pulse is about 1 ms, and the pulse travels at very roughly 20 ms^{-1} (though actually faster or slower than this depending upon the degree of myelination). The spatial extent of the pulse, measured between its leading and trailing edges is thus about 20 mm. But a typical axon, in the cortex, might be a mere 0.5 mm, so the trailing edge of the impulse will not even have left the soma by the time the leading edge has reached the extremities of the axon branches; using a visual analogue, we could imagine the entire axon and its branches as 'glowing' simultaneously.

The other two time constants are appreciably longer, and it is through them that pulses initially coherent with each other can get out of phase. This is true of the synaptic delay, with its approximately 1-ms duration, and it is true to an even greater extent of the electrotonic delay, which is typically ten times longer.

It is possibly quite significant, in this context, that some synapses connect axon branches directly with somatic regions (Shepherd, 1979). These axonal–somatic synapses would enable one soma to pass information on to another soma without the dendritic delay intervening, and this could permit the presynaptic neuron to act as a sort of pacemaker, as discussed later in this article.

It is possible that the classic observations of Hubel & Wiesel (1962) can be taken as support for the idea that correct functioning in the brain is dependent on coherent excitation of various neurons. Our reasoning, here, will build on qualitative concepts already put forward by Barlow & Levick (1965). The observations in question were made on cells in the visual cortex of cats, using microelectrodes that were so fine that the activity of a single cell could be measured. The cats were anaesthetized with their eyes open, the controlling muscles having been temporarily paralysed so as to fix the stare in a specific direction. Hubel and Wiesel discovered that a given cortical cell can be specifically sensitive to a bar of light moving across a particular region of the cat's visual field, but only if the bar has a certain specific orientation and is moved in a certain direction.

These observations have been explained by assuming certain patterns of synaptic connections to the relevant cells in the lateral geniculate nucleus (Hubel & Wiesel, 1962), the latter being a small knee-shaped region in the thalamus, part of which acts as a sort of relay station in the visual pathway. Of particular interest here is the fact that Hubel and Wiesel observed that there is a particular velocity of the moving light bar which gives the maximum response at the corresponding cell in the visual cortex. This most favourable velocity lies at around $5°$ s^{-1}. From the geometry of the situation it is reasonably straightforward to show that the speed of the image of the bar across the retina is equivalent to approximately one cell diameter during a time interval of about 10 ms. This is a rather suggestive value, because it is comparable to typical electrotonic response times over typical dendritic lengths (Shepherd, 1979). Indeed, these characteristic dimensions and times become even more interesting when we look at the underlying structure of the retina (see Fig. 10.3).

There are five distinct cell types in this part of the eye: the receptor cells, which are responsible for converting the energy of the incoming photons into electrical activity; the horizontal cells; the bipolar cells; the amacrine cells; and finally the ganglions, which have a highly elongated shape, with their axons actually constituting the first part of the optic nerve. The receptor cells have their long axes lying normally to the surface of the retina, whereas the horizontal cells lie in the plane of the retina, and indeed form contacts between the receptor cells. These horizontal cells are rather special in that they have no well-defined directionality, and there is indeed no clear differentiation into dendritic and axonal extensions. It thus seems rather unlikely that these horizontal cells display action potential activity. Their responses are more likely to be of the electrotonic type, with the longer time constants associated with that type of function.

Let us suppose that the role of a particular horizontal cell is exclusively excitatory. We imagine that the moving bar of light falls first on one of the receptor cells, and then travels on in the direction of the next receptor cell down the line. Illumination of the first receptor cell elicits a response, which is passed along the plane of the retina by the horizontal cell. Because the electrotonic time constant of the latter is comparable to the above-stated 10 ms, this electrotonic response will have precisely the timing required to produce reinforcement of the reaction of the second receptor cell, and so on. Because the response of the horizontal cell is certainly unilateral, this provides a mechanism which could underlie the directionality observed by Hubel and Wiesel. It can, in fact, be looked upon as evidence supporting the idea of coherent excitation.

10.4 The new computer model

We will now describe a recently constructed computer model which aims at testing the idea of coherence, and at elucidating possible consequences of this mode of action. The model comprises a series of layers, each consisting of the same number of cells, and with all possible combinations of the cells in two adjacent layers having unidirectional synaptic contacts. A single axonal input is assumed to feed into each synapse, and the latter is assumed to be followed by a single dendritic pathway to the subsequent

Fig. 10.3. Anatomical studies have established that the mammalian retina has an orderly structure composed of five different types of cell. In this schematic picture, these types are indicated by letters: R, for the receptors, which convert the energy of incident light photons into an electrochemical response; H, for the horizontal cells; B, for the bipolar cells; A, for the amacrine cells; and G for the ganglion cells, the axons of which collectively form the optic nerve. The structure of the retina is somewhat surprising in that the incident light must pass the numerous cells of the other four types before it reaches the receptors (i.e. the light enters from below, in the diagram).

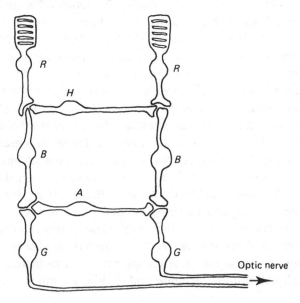

somatic region. Because of the unidirectionality, an input pattern to the first layer, consisting of action potential pulses or a lack of these, will give rise to further patterns of firings and failures to fire, travelling down through the model layer by layer. Whether a particular synapse is excitatory or inhibitory is chosen by a random number generator, and this type of choice is also applied to the initial synaptic strengths, to their maximum values, and also to the time constants and maximum amplitudes of the electrotonic responses in the associated dendritic regions. Finally, the random number generator is also used to select a distributed set of values for the synaptic delays.

At any time t, the input voltage at the soma of the jth cell in the ith layer will be given by

$$V_{j,i}(t) = \sum_k \Phi_{k,i-1}(t) S_{j,i,k,i-1} D_{j,i,k,i-1}(t),$$

where the k summation is over the n neurons in layer $i - 1$, and $\Phi_{k,i-1}(t)$ is the output voltage of the kth neuron in that layer. This output voltage can take only the (normalized) values of 1 or 0, depending on whether or not the input voltage to that cell reached the threshold value θ. The factors S are measures of the current synaptic strengths, while the terms $D(t)$ take account of the temporal variation of the dendritic voltages. At each time step the value of $V_{j,i}(t)$ is compared with θ, and the corresponding output voltage $\Phi_{j,i}(t)$ is set at 1 or 0 depending upon whether that threshold has or has not been exceeded.

With the model functioning according to the above rules, and with between about half and all the synapses chosen to be excitatory, trouble is encountered in the form of an avalanche effect. The system is critically poised between collapse to a state in which no signals are able to get through to the lower layers, on the one hand, and what could be called 'blow-up', with all cells firing in each of the lower levels irrespective of how few cells are caused to fire in the first layer. This effect is illustrated in Fig. 10.4, and it can be readily overcome by adopting a feed-back procedure. It is well known that interneurons are frequently present in a neural assembly, and that their efferent synapses are often inhibitory. A case in point occurs in the mossy fibre – CA3 pyramidal cell – basket cell complex of the hippocampus (Mackey & an der Heiden, 1984). If each of these cell types is imagined as being lumped into a single cell, the dynamics of the system displays alternating periods of oscillation and quiescence because of the negative feed-back from the basket cells. But if, on the contrary, these interneurons are permitted to influence the system through well-distributed inputs and feed-back outputs, they will be able to control the neural assembly in a quite subdued fashion. Taking this system as a lead, one introduces an extra negative term to the right-hand side of the above equation, namely $-\alpha F_{i-1}$, where F_{i-1} is the number of cells in layer $i - 1$ which are currently firing or in their refractory period, and α is a variable feed-back factor. Introduction of this term, and adjustment of α eliminates the blow-up effect, as desired.

A study of the properties of this system, by computer simulation, has revealed several interesting modes of behaviour, one of which was certainly quite unexpected. The natural time-constant of such a system is determined by the minimum possible time lapse between successive pulses generated in a given cell, that is to say by the refractory period. A periodic input is given to the first layer of the system, and one then studies

Fig. 10.4. This computer model consists of 15 topological layers, each comprising 32 cells. Synaptic contacts are made between each cell in a given layer and all 32 cells in the following layer. (There are thus 1024 synapses between each pair of adjacent layers.) The transmission of information is unidirectional, from top to bottom, and the state of each cell is indicated by a 0, for the quiescent state, * for the moment of firing off an action potential, and a dot (.) is used if the cell is in its refractory period, which is of a standard length of 20 computational time steps. The electrotonic time-constants were randomly selected, and uniformly distributed in the interval 1–75 time steps, while the synaptic delays were in this case all a standard single time step. The synapses were either excitatory or inhibitory, this being chosen at random. The periodic input pattern consisted of simultaneous firings of every other cell in the first layer, with a period of 60 time steps. In real time, one time step is about 0.5 ms. The picture shows two separate waves of activity, one near the upper region, and one further down. The latter has gone into what has been referred to as the blow-up regime, in which all cells in a given topological layer fire roughly simultaneously. This effect can be obviated by the introduction of negative feed-back.

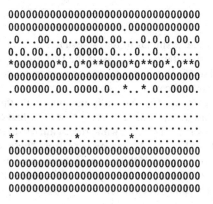

```
00000000000000000000000000000000
000000000000000000.000000000000
.0...00..0..0000.00...0.0.0.00.0
0.0.00..0..00000.0...0..0..0....
*0000000*0.0*0**0000*0**00*.0**0
00000000000000000000000000000000
.000000.00.0000.0..*..*.0..0000.
................................
................................
................................
*.........*........*...........
00000000000000000000000000000000
00000000000000000000000000000000
00000000000000000000000000000000
00000000000000000000000000000000
```

the successive generation of impulses in cells in the lower layers. If, for instance, some of the cells in the first layer are given impulses which are coincident with one another, it is found that there is a periodic generation of impulses in the lower layers, at the same frequency as the input frequency. But if cells in the first layer are given impulses which are temporarily offset from one another, a new phenomenon is observed, namely that after an initial transient period, it appears to be impossible for the cyclic state to maintain itself beyond a certain level in the system. This has been given the tentative name 'pinch-out', and the phenomenon is illustrated in Fig. 10.5. It is observed for all phase offsets lying in the approximate range 150–210°, for the particular conditions of this investigation.

It is interesting to speculate on the possible advantage, to the brain, of such a phenomenon. It could indicate that signals are unable to penetrate to higher regions of the cortex, unless there is the requisite degree of synchronization between the various inputs to the first layer of cells. This, in turn, could mean that the appropriate regions act as a sort of coherence discriminator. Indeed, there is the suggestion that one could have a piece of cerebral hardware designed to respond to correlations between various inputs.

It is natural to speculate as to whether this type of circuitry could have relevance to what was stated earlier in connection with the primary visual processes at the retina. The general idea here would be that unless the signals were generated by the receptor cells at just the right time, no signal would ultimately reach the corresponding cells in the visual cortex. And because the correct synchronization of these signals from the receptor cells would be dependent upon the light stimulus occurring at precisely the right time, this would give the velocity sensitivity accounted for in the previous section.

Fig. 10.5. (*a*) This model is similar to that shown in Fig. 10.4. The periodic input pattern consisted of simultaneous firings of the first and eighth cells in the first layer, with a period of 60 time steps. As can be seen from the situations at these twelve different instants, the network achieves a cyclic state, the period of which matches that of the input. (*b*) An antiphase input to the model shown in Fig. 10.5(*a*) gave a dramatically different response. The first cell in the first layer is made to fire at times 1, 61, 121, . . . , while the eighth cell in that layer is made to fire at times 31, 91, 151, ... As can be seen from these selected situations, information is able to reach the 15th layer only during an initial transient period. Thereafter, despite continuation of the input, nothing is able to penetrate beyond the eleventh layer. This phenomenon has been dubbed 'the pinch-out effect'.

continued

1

```
*000000*
00000000
00000000
00000000
00000000
00000000
00000000
00000000
00000000
00000000
00000000
00000000
```

8

```
.000000.
000000*0
00000000
00000000
00000000
00000000
00000000
00000000
00000000
00000000
00000000
00000000
```

14

```
.000000.
000000.0
0*000000
00000000
00000000
00000000
00000000
00000000
00000000
00000000
00000000
00000000
```

20

```
.000000.
000000.0
0.000000
00000000
00000000
00000000
00000000
00000000
00000000
00000000
00000000
00000000
```

21

```
00000000
000000.0
0.000000
00000000
00000000
00000000
00000000
00000000
00000000
00000000
00000000
00000000
```

61

```
*000000*
00000000
00000000
0.0000.0
.00000..
.00000...
..0..00..
..0...000
*00..0000
000..0000
00000000
00000000
```

82

```
.000000.
000000.0
0.0000000
00000000
0.0000.0
.0000...
.0...0*0
..0...000
00.*000.0
00000000
00000000
00000000
```

200

```
.000000.
000000.0
0.000000
00000000
0.0000.0
.0000...
00..000.
000..0000
000.*.00
00.0..0.
.00.00.0
```

421

```
*000000*
00000000
00000000
0.0000.0
.0000...
00..000.
000*0000
000.00.0
000...00
00.0..0.
*00.00.0
```

436

```
.000000.
000000.0
0.000000
00000000
0.0000.0
.0000...
00..00.
000.0000
000.00.0
000000..
.00.00.0
```

781

```
*000000*
00000000
00000000
0.0000.0
.0000...
00..000.
000*0000
000.00.0
000...00
00.0..0.
*00.00.0
```

961

```
*000000*
00000000
00000000
0.0000.0
.0000...
00..000.
000*0000
000.00.0
000...00
00.0..0.
*00.00.0
```

(a)

(b)

10.5 Possible application to a pathological condition

Any model which claims to reflect reality must win its spurs by explaining reality's exceptions and idiosyncrasies. The question thus arises as to whether a model of the type described in this article has anything to say about pathological conditions. It has been suggested that autism, which usually manifests itself during a patient's first four years of life, might be caused by unduly long synaptic delays (Cotterill, 1985). Synaptic delays are a parameter in the present model, so this issue could indeed be investigated.

The autistic child is most often quite free from physical abnormality, and the chief symptom is a gross reticence or inability to interact with the environment. The patient appears apathetic to both people and objects, and in the early stages this can be mistaken for contentment. The condition apparently has an organic aetiology (Da Masio, 1978; Piggott, 1979) with hereditary origins (Folstein & Rutter, 1979). Possibly the strongest recent endorsement of the organic view comes from the widely observed, but inadequately documented, fever effect (Sullivan, 1980). When autistics have a moderate fever, they invariably display dramatically more normal behavioural patterns, including a greater desire or ability to communicate. The effect appears to reach a maximum for fevers of around 2 °C. It seems unlikely that such a modest rise could appreciably influence the rates of either the metabolic processes or the molecular diffusion involved in neural function. But temperature changes of as little as 1 °C can markedly alter the fluidity of membranes (Träuble, Tuebner, Wooley & Eibl, 1976), such as those which form the synapses and the neurotransmitter-charged presynaptic vesicles.

An increase in the fluidity of these membranes would lower the vesicle–synapse fusion time, and thereby decrease the synaptic delay. We have already seen how this latter quantity might control what could be called the neural coherence length, which is a measure of the degree of interneuron cooperativity. Lower synaptic delays would increase this length, and one could speculate whether the autistic fever effect indicates that there is a connection between coherence in the behavioural sense and actual physical coherence at the neural level. Equally intriguing is the possibility that autism stems from a neural lipid composition profile which departs from the ideal.

It is clear that these issues would be amenable to investigation with the aid of computer models of the type described in this paper, and such studies have recently produced some most interesting results. The model had 32 cells in each of its 15 topological layers, in this case, and the parameter of interest was, of course, the synaptic delay. Fig. 10.6 shows the dramatic result of changing the mean value of the latter from 0.5 milliseconds to 2.0 milliseconds. For the longer synaptic delay, the pinch-out effect is again observed.

This is a most intriguing result because it offers a particularly direct explanation of what might lie at the heart of the autistic syndrome. At normal body temperature, the patient's faulty lipid profile gives the synaptic delays that are too long and information is not able to traverse some critical part of the brain because of the pinch-out effect. During a sufficiently high fever, the increased synaptic membrane fluidity gives lower synaptic delays: the pinch-out effect disappears, the information gets through, and the patient appears to recover almost dramatically, only to go back into his or her invisible shell once the fever subsides.

10.6 Memory

We must now discuss the applicability of the present model to an obviously central issue in brain science, namely memory. It has been implicit in what has been advocated that we endorse the idea, apparently first promulgated by Hebb (1949), that memory traces are stored via the agency of modifiable synapses. Because of its dependence on our central theme, coherence, the holographic theory of memory (Longuet-Higgins, 1968; Gabor, 1968a,b; Westlake, 1970) is of special interest, even though

Fig. 10.6. The pinch-out effect can also be induced by increasing the spread in the synaptic delays. The mean delay in the model was a single time unit for the situation shown at the left, in which information is clearly able to penetrate to the lower layers. But an increase of the mean synaptic delay to four time units gives pinch-out, as seen at the right. The model comprised 15 layers, each with 32 neurons, and both pictures correspond to the situation at 800 time steps.

```
00000000000000000.0.0.0.0.0.0.0.      00000000000000000.0.0.0.0.0.0.0.
0000.000000000000000000000*00.0       0000000000000000000000000.0..0
00000000000000000000000000000.00      000000000000000.000000000000000
00000000.00000000000000000000000      000000000.000000000000000.000000
00000000000000000000000000000000      00000000000000000000000000000000
00000000000000000000000000000000      00000000000000000000000000000000
00000000000000000000000000000000      00000000000000000000000000000000
00000000000000000000000000000000      00000000000000000000000000000000
00000000000000000000000000000000      00000000000000000000000000000000
000000.,00000000000000.000000000      00000000000000000000000000000000
.00.0000...00.00000.000..000.000      00000000000000000000000000000000
00..0*0.0000.0.00.00..000.0...00      00000000000000000000000000000000
000..0..000000...0000.....*..00.      00000000000000000000000000000000
00000000..0000......0..0.*0..000      00000000000000000000000000000000
0.0.0.00000.000.00.0.000000.0...      00000000000000000000000000000000
```

one recent article in this area (Nobili, 1985) accords prime of place to the glial cells rather than the synapses.

As normally employed (Soroko, 1980), the recording of a hologram occurs when the beam scattered from an object interferes with a plane reference wave, to give a standing wave pattern. Subsequent viewing of the holographic recording illuminated by the reference wave alone reveals an image of the object. One of the great attractions of the holographic process, in the context of memory, is that the entire object can be imaged in this way, albeit at a lower resolution, if only a fraction of the hologram is used. This is reminiscent of Lashley's observation of similar apparent total recall in ablated animal brains (Lashley, 1963).

It is actually implicit in the analysis of the holographic process that the reference wave is not really required. There is an alternative mechanism, even though it is not normally practicable (Kohonen, 1984). It arises in the following way. Let us imagine the object as being composed of two parts A and B. Illumination of the composite, AB, with coherent light produces interference, and the resultant standing wave pattern can be recorded in the usual way, to produce a hologram. If that hologram is now illuminated only by the light being scattered from A, an image of B will be seen, at least in principle. But this would be very difficult to achieve in practice because the wave emanating from A would not be plane, and the slightest displacement of A would preclude the desired reconstruction. In the case of a system of neurons, however, the dendrites and axons function in a manner analogous to optical fibres, and there is no marked vulnerability to such disturbance.

Now a good argument could be made for the proposition that the primary function of some areas of the neocortex is to record correlations. This is probably not the case for the primary visual and hearing areas, but it is almost certainly true of the speech area, for example (see Fig. 10.7). Perhaps the neural modifications, be they in the synapses or the glial cells, are analogous to AB correlations in the above-described mode of holography. If that is the case, the system would have the highly desirable property that stimulation of the appropriate region of the neocortex by input A would elicit a memory recall of B, and vice-versa.

This issue, too, has proved eminently amenable to study by the present computer model, and some insight has even been gained into the question of why there are so many synaptic contacts per neuron.

The model was further stretched out to include 128 neurons in each of the ten topological layers. The synchronously applied pattern consisted of action potentials to every other cell in the first layer, the 64 other cells remaining quiet. There is of course no geometrical significance to such a pattern because all cells in a given layer are connected to all cells in the following layer, but the choice of this alternating sequence has the advantage of being easily recognizable. Now because there are, by definition, no prior connections before any of these cells are encountered, any convenient division of them can be looked upon as giving independent groups of cells which could play the roles of the portions A and B discussed above. Let us, for example, consider the 64 cells lying to the left of the mid-point of the first topological layer as belonging to part A, and the 64 cells lying to the right as constituting part B.

The composite pattern AB, namely the above-described firing of every other cell, was injected into the first layer and the consequent firing pattern in the second layer was monitored. Hebbian learning (Hebb, 1949) was introduced by strengthening those synapses lying between cells which showed correlated firings, and weakening those involved in anti-correlations (Hopfield, 1982). After a suitable learning period, the model was then subjected to only a portion of the first input, namely what has been referred to as part A. As can be seen in Fig. 10.8, the resultant firing pattern in the second layer was remarkably similar to that which was previously observed for an AB input. To be specific, the original AB input caused 60 of the 128 cells in the second layer to fire, while the postlearning A input provoked firing of 42 cells in the second layer. Moreover, with the

Fig. 10.7. The pinch-out effect (see Fig. 10.5) might be particularly important in the primary areas, such as those devoted to vision and hearing. The association mechanism illustrated in Fig. 10.8 would probably be limited to such secondary areas as that responsible for word recognition.

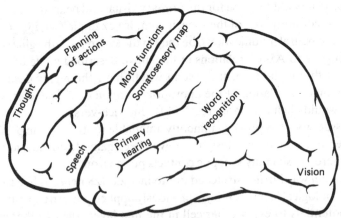

exception of just one cell, all the postlearning firings in layer two occurred in cells which also fired before and during learning.

The learning and recall effects demonstrated by these computations are, of course, caused by the phase discrimination in the model, and it is not difficult to account for the disparity between the 60 prelearning firings and the 42 postlearning firings. The firing of a second-layer cell requires the simultaneous arrival of electrotonic pulses from a number of first-layer cells. These latter can of course lie either in portion A or portion B of the

Fig. 10.8. Four different situations are depicted here, in the order in which they occurred. The model has been further stretched out, and now comprises ten layers, each with 128 neurons. The top picture shows the initial output (which has been designated AB in the text). The response in the second layer is shown in the second part of the diagram, Hebbian learning having been in force during the intervening period. When only half the original input is now injected (designated A in the text), as seen in the third part of the figure, the second-layer response (bottom part of the figure) bears a striking resemblance to that earlier observed for the full AB input. The network is thus functioning like a hologram.

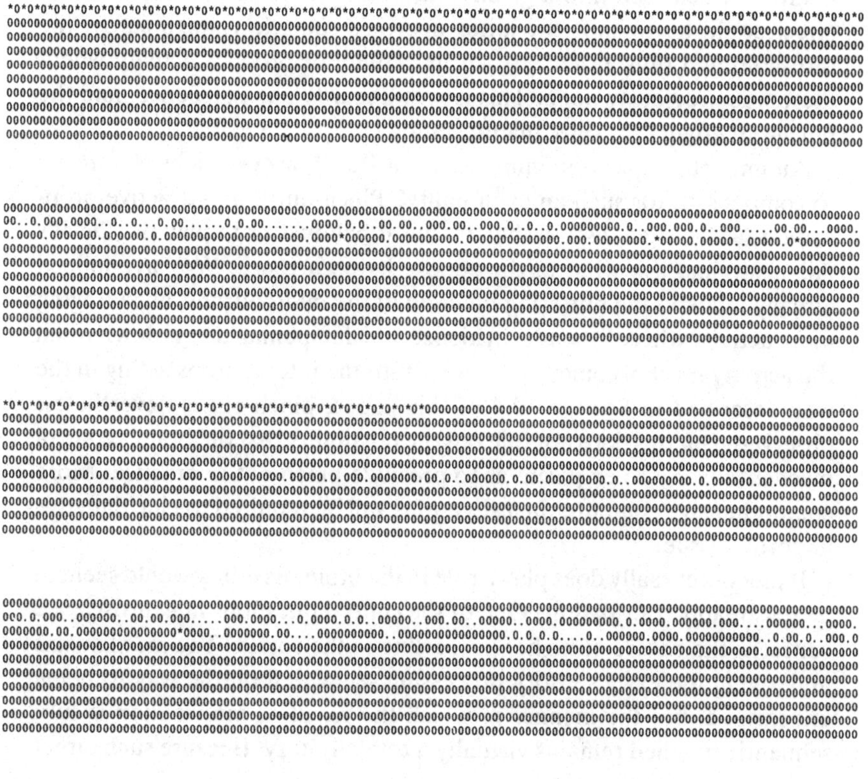

first layer. Although the most likely situation will correspond to a fairly even distribution of contributions from A and B, there will be some cases where a disproportionately large number of cells in just one half of the first layer cause a second-layer firing. Such lop-sided distributions will become progressively less common as the number of synaptic contacts per cell increases.

10.7 Discussion

One of the main results of the present study is, of course, the observation of what has been provisionally called the pinch-out effect. Its discovery was serendipitous, but in retrospect its existence might have been anticipated, particularly if the key role of non-linearity in life's processes had been properly appreciated. One has only to contemplate the intricacies of tissue differentiation, for example, to see how abrupt changes of regime are so central to an organism's structure and function. In the case of the neuron, the regime in question is its firing state, and the action potential threshold sets the watershed for the two totally different modes of behaviour. And although the changes in the firing patterns of those other neurons which feed into a given neuron might appear minor, their net effect could be to shift the latter neuron's somatic voltage across the threshold and thus either quench its activity or produce activity where there was previously none. This is non-linearity par excellence, and the pinch-out effect is its stark manifestation.

An important question immediately arises, however: does Nature try to compensate for such an eventuality? Pinch-out is an attractive proposition, as we shall discuss shortly, but it behoves us to play the Devil's Advocate and ask what might oppose its occurrence. We have indeed already invoked the buffering function of the interneurons, encouraging more activity where little is in evidence and dampening things down when the activity level becomes excessive. With the interneurons acting in the way described in Section 10.4 of this paper, pinch-out is nevertheless observed. But this does not rule out the possibility that the brain's control mechanisms are so exquisite as to preclude pinch-out in practice. More comprehensive computer investigations will be required to elucidate this important issue.

If pinch-out really does play a role in the brain, its utility would seem to be reasonably transparent. One of the central questions in neuroscience concerns the nature of higher processing in the cortex. The mechanisms underlying the early sensory processing seem well on the way to being understood, but the manner in which the resulting information is subsequently handled remains virtually a total mystery. Because such target structures as the muscles and the glands have to be informed whether or not they are to respond to a given set of sensory inputs, the task of the brain's higher processing will, in the final analysis, be one of passing on or not passing on information, and this suggests an important mandate for the pinch-out effect: to provide a mechanism whereby brain components discriminate between information to be transmitted to target structures and information to be blocked or ignored.

If the brain wants to exploit the regulatory possibilities inherent in coherence discrimination, it has the necessary circuitry at its disposal. We have already noted that the dendritic delay is avoided when an axonal branch synapses directly onto the somatic region of the following cell, and the point can now be made that the presynaptic cell in such a case acts like a pace-maker. Consider, for instance, the situation in which neither the depolarization of the target cell's somatic membrane by the incoming dendritic waves nor that due to the incoming signal across the conjectured axonal–somatic synapse is sufficient, by itself, to exceed the threshold. If, however, their combined effect is such as to provoke a supercritical depolarization, the result will be not merely an output pulse but one whose timing is dictated by the signal arriving via the axonal–somatic synapse. Indeed, if a cell makes axonal–somatic synapses with a number of target cells it will, like the sergeant on a parade ground, keep all the latter in step. A highly schematic layout of such a situation is depicted in Fig. 10.9.

Fig. 10.9. A hypothetical (and highly schematic) layout for forced synchronous firing of a number of cells in a topological layer. The thin straight lines are dendrites, and the thick straight lines are axon branches. The large circles are somatic regions, while the small circles and their associated crescents indicate synapses. The pace-maker cell could be a spontaneous emitter of action potential bursts, but it could also be collectively driven by the cells from the layer preceding those shown in the diagram.

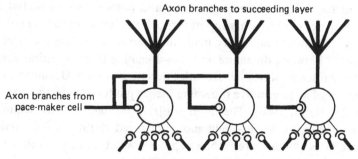

But pace-maker neurons, even if they exist, can only be part of the story; we must ask about their location with respect to the sensory input. Two possibilities suggest themselves. One is that the pace-makers are independent and spontaneous emitters of bursts of action potential impulses. It is worth emphasizing, in fact, that recent evidence points to an intracellular origin of such bursts, rather than cyclic patterns due to feed-back effects in an assembly of neurons (Russell & Hartline, 1978). The most obvious alternative would place the pace-maker in a topological position analogous to that of an interneuron. This would be particularly intriguing; it implies that the approaching rabble of haphazard signals, in the various input cells, collectively waken the sleeping sergeant, who responds to the reveille by getting the troops into step.

It might appear that the intercellular coherence generated by the hypothetical pace-maker cells would preclude phase differences occurring, but it must be borne in mind that phase differences will also arise because of dendritic path differences, and that these, in turn, will be linked to different input patterns. The induced coherence would thus serve to provide an invariant base-line, against which the various phases would be revealed and distinguished.

Although a number of other models do not require coherence (Pellionisz & Llinas, 1982; Clark, Rafelski & Winston, 1985), they are at least not in conflict with the concept. This appears not to be the case with the spin-glass approach (Hopfield, 1982), however, where asynchronous firings seem to be an essential feature. In this connection it is interesting to consider the recent surge of interest in the dreaming state. Crick & Mitchison (1983) suggest that we dream in order to rid our minds of spurious memories, and Hopfield, Feinstein & Palmer (1983) report a decrease in the accessibility of the spurious memories which actually occur in a spin-glass model, by subjecting the latter to a process called unlearning. This unlearning involves reversing the way in which synapses normally change their strength, subject to the degree of correlation between the firings of the presynaptic and postsynaptic cells, but no anatomical or physiological support for such a reversal was presented.

The Crick–Mitchison theory made no attempt to explain the regular alternation between dreaming and non-dreaming periods during sleep. This intermittency, which occurs with a period of around 90 minutes, was the subject of an alternative dreaming theory put forward by the present author (Cotterill, 1986). The latter conjectured that recently acquired memories become increasingly more impaired during non-dreaming sleep, and it postulated a refreshment process which corrects for this. The impairment was suggested to arise from random fusions of presynaptic vesicles with the presynaptic membrane, and the correction process was supposed to take the form of injection of a blank wave to neurons on the input side of the memory cortex. It was argued that the cortex would not be able to tolerate more than a certain degree of impairment, and hence the need for periodic refreshment, since the degeneration is presumably as inevitable as it is inexorable. It was also implicit in this new theory that some of the brain's processes are so automatic that the mere injection of the hypothetical blank wave is sufficient to produce trains of thought which, lacking the feed-back controls presumably present during wakefulness, have the bizarre characteristics which are the hallmark of the dreaming state.

Our task here is to establish the relevance of coherence in the context of these new ideas on dreaming, but we will first propose an improvement to the theory. Although the random vesicle fusions are amenable to a quantitative analysis which is actually capable of accounting for the 90-min interdream period, we now suggest that a more plausible impairment process is the relaxation of certain proteins associated with synapses. The point is that it has been established that the types of protein which underlie the mechanism of muscle contraction are also present in dendritic spines, just beneath the postsynaptic membranes. This is certainly true of actin, and it is probably also true of myosin (Fifkova & Daley, 1982). This has given rise to the suggestion that dendritic spines change their dimensions as a consequence of nervous activity (Bradley & Horn, 1979; Brandon & Coss, 1982; Crick, 1982; Fifkova, 1985), and this in turn could physically modify the associated synapses and change their effectivity. (It is interesting to find that, at the neuronal level at least, mind and muscle are perhaps not so distinct as has usually been assumed; brain and brawn might not be the mutually exclusive attributes they have traditionally been taken to be.) If the passage of an electrochemical signal from the postsynaptic membrane towards the soma causes an abrupt change in the configuration of these proteins, they will probably gradually relax back towards their original disposition. Further stimulation should be able to prevent this from happening, but there could be no such possibility during non-dreaming sleep. Whence the need for refreshment.

Given sufficient time, the otherwise innocuous changes in individual synapses would begin to link up into patterns that would pose a serious signal-to-noise threat to recently acquired memories. It seems likely that such modifications, as long as they were still only local at least, would be nullified by coherently established memory patterns, because the latter are distributed over many synapses. In coherent excitation, the phase of a wave is of paramount importance, and the refreshing wave would force out-of-phase synaptic strengths to get into step, as it were. The different memories stored in a given cortical region would be excited at mutually random phases and should therefore not interfere.

Nothing has been mentioned, as yet, about long-term memory, although it has been tacitly assumed that the refreshing process would not have to be administered indefinitely. It is possible that the alterations to a synapse provoked by the changes in the configuration of the actin–myosin complex are gradually consolidated and made permanent by the fabrication of other protein structures, such as microtubules and microfilaments, and that this is the way in which short-term memory becomes long-term memory. The latter would not be vulnerable to the constant turnover of protein material which is known to occur, because the superstructure of tubules and filaments would be unaffected by such local changes. The same is true of any historic building, which retains its shape despite periodic renovation.

Although we have probably already strayed beyond our brief, it is tempting to close with a remark on one of the ultimate mysteries of the brain, namely the nature of consciousness. Gregory (1977) has suggested that the brain is conscious because it is able to 'read' itself. If the main thrust of this article is correct, such self-reading would be predicated on coherent firing of certain neurons in order to obviate pinch-out. An interesting example of consciousness, because it appears to be pared down to the bare essentials, occurs when one's full bladder provokes a nocturnal visit to the bathroom. Signals are passed up to the brain, and consciousness is produced, presumably because the organism realises that coordination between sensory inputs and muscular responses are going to be necessary. As further investigations of the type reported here are undertaken, it will be of interest to check whether coordination is contingent on coherence.

Acknowledgements

It is a pleasure to acknowledge stimulating discussions with John Clark, and with the members of the Lundtofte Brain Study Group: Øyvind Aabling, Stig Benthin, Ulla Binau, Steen Sloth Christensen, Eva Gamwell Davids, Uffe Hansen, Kenneth Hebel, Michael Hebel, Malene Dal Jensen, Allan Krebs, Carlo Lund, Stephan Mannestædt, Kaare Olsen, Lars Petersen, Tonny Haldorf Petersen, Henrik Kaare Poulson, Carsten Rogaard, Nils Svendsen and Jørgen Villadsen.

References

Barlow, H. B. & Levick, W. R. (1965). 'The mechanism of directional selective units in rabbits' retina.' *J. Physiol. (Lond.)*, **178**, 477–504.

Bastian, J. & Heiligenberg, W. (1980). 'Phase-sensitive midbrain neurons in *Eigermannia*: neural correlates of the jamming avoidance response.' *Science*, **209**, 828–31.

Bradley, P. & Horn, G. (1979). 'Neuronal plasticity in the chick brain: morphological effects of visual experience on neurones in hyperstriatum accessorium.' *Brain Res.*, **162**, 148–53.

Brandon, J. G. & Coss, R. G. (1982). 'Rapid dendritic spine stem shortening during one-trial learning: the honeybee's first orientation flight.' *Brain Res.*, **252**, 51–61.

Clark, J. W., Rafelski, J. & Winston, J. V. (1985). 'Brain without mind: computer simulation of neuronal networks with modifiable neuronal interactions.' *Physics Reports*, **123**, 215–73.

Cotterill, R. M. J. (1985). 'Fever in autistics.' *Nature*, **313**, 426.

Cotterill, R. M. J. (1986). 'The brain: an intriguing piece of condensed matter.' *Physics Scripta*, **T13**, 161–8.

Crick, F. (1982). 'Do dendritic spines twitch?' *Trends Neuroscience*, **5**, 44–6.

Crick, F. & Mitchison, G. (1983). 'The function of dream sleep.' *Nature*, **304**, 111–14.

Da Masio, A. R. (1978). 'A neurological model for childhood autism.' *Arch. Neurol.*, **35**, 777–86.

Fifkova, E. & Daley, R. J. (1982). 'Cytoplasmic actin in neuronal processes as a possible mediator of synaptic plasticity.' *J. Cell. Biol.*, **95**, 345–50.

Fifkova, E. (1985). 'A possible mechanism of morphometric changes in dendritic spines induced by stimulation.' *Cellular and Molecular Neurobiology*, **5**, 47–63.

Folstein, S. & Rutter, M. (1977). 'Genetic influences and infantile autism.' *Nature*, **265**, 726–8.

Gabor, D. (1968a). 'Holographic Model of Temporal Recall.' *Nature*, **217**, 584.

Gabor, D. (1968b). 'Improved holographic model of temporal recall.' *Nature*, **217**, 1288.

Gerstein, G. L., Bloom, M. J., Espinosa, I. E., Evanczuk, S. & Turner, M. R. (1983). 'Design of a laboratory for multineuron studies.' *IEEE Trans. on Systems, Man and Cybernetics*, **13**, 668–76.

Gerstein, G. L., Perkel, D. H. & Dayhoff, J. E. (1985). 'Cooperative firing activity in simultaneously recorded populations of neurons: detection and measurement.' *J. Neuroscience*, **5**, 881–9.

Gevins, A. S., Doyle, J. C., Cutillo, B. A., Schaffer, R. E., Tannehill, R. S., Ghannam, J. H., Gilcrease, V. A. & Yeager, C. L. (1981). 'Electrical potentials in human brain during cognition: new method reveals dynamic patterns of correlation.' *Science*, **213**, 918–22.

Gregory, R. L. (1977). 'Consciousness.' In *The Encylopaedia of Ignorance*, edited by R. Duncan and M. Weston-Smith. Pergamon Press, Oxford.

Hebb, D. O. (1949). *The Organization of Behaviour*. Wiley, New York.

Hodgkin, A. L. & Huxley, A. F. (1952). 'A quantitative description of membrane current and its application to conduction and excitation in nerve.' *J. Physiol.*, **117**, 500–44.

Hopfield, J. J. (1982). 'Neural networks and physical systems with emergent collective computational abilities.' *Proc. U.S. Nat. Acad. Sci.*, **79**, 2554–8.

Hopfield, J. J., Feinstein, D. I. & Palmer, R. G. (1983). 'Unlearning' has a stabilizing effect in collective memories.' *Nature*, **304**, 158–9.

188   *Rodney M. J. Cotterill*

Hubel, D. H. & Wiesel, T. N. (1962). 'Receptive fields, binocular interaction and functional architecture in the cat's visual cortex.' *J. Physiol.*, **160**, 106–54.

Kawato, M., Hamaguchi, T., Murakami, F. & Tsukahara, N. (1984). 'Quantitative analysis of electrical properties of dendritic spines.' *Biol. Cybernetics*, **50**, 447–54.

Knox, C, K. & Poppele, R. E. (1977). 'Correlation analysis of stimulus-evoked changes in excitability of spontaneously firing neurons. *J. Neurophysiology*, **40**, 616–25.

Kohonen, T. (1984). *Self-Organization and Associative Memory*, 2nd edn. Springer-Verlag, Berlin.

Kuffler, S. W. & Nicholls, J. G. (1976). *From Neuron to Brain*. Sinauer Associates, Sunderland, Massachusetts, p. 179 *et seq.*

Kuperstein, M. & Eichenbaum, H. (1985). 'Unit activity, evoked potentials and slow waves in the rat hippocampus and olfactory bulb recorded with a 24-channel microelectrode.' *Neuroscience*, **15**, 703–12.

Lashley, K. S. (1963). *Brain Mechanism and Intelligence*. Dover, New York.

Longuet-Higgins, H. C. (1968). 'Holographic model of temporal recall.' *Nature*, **217**, 104.

Mackey, M. C. & an der Heiden, U. (1984). 'The dynamics of recurrent inhibition.' *J. Math. Biol.*, **19**, 211–25.

Nobili, R. (1985). 'Schrödinger wave holography in brain cortex.' *Phys. Rev.*, **A 32**, 3618–26.

Pellionisz, A. & Llinas, R. (1982). 'Space–time representation in the brain. The cerebellum as a predictive space–time metric tensor.' *Neuroscience*, **7**, 2949–70.

Piggott, L. R. (1979). 'Overview of selected basic research in autism.' *J. Autism Dev. Disorders*, **9**, 199–218.

Reitboek, H. J. P. (1983). 'A 19-channel matrix drive with individually controllable fiber microelectrodes for neurophysiological applications.' *IEEE Trans. on Systems, Man and Cybernetics*, **13**, 676–83.

Russell, D. F. & Hartline, D. K. (1978). 'Bursting neural networks: a re-examination.' *Science*, **200**, 453–6.

Sachs, M. B., Voigt, H. F. & Young, E. D. (1983). 'Auditory nerve representation of vowels in background noise.' *J. Neurophysiol.*, **50**, 27–45.

Shepherd, G. M. (1979). *The Synaptic Organization of the Brain*. Oxford University Press, Oxford.

Soroko, L. (1980). *Holography and Coherent Optics*. Plenum, New York.

Sullivan, R. C. (1980). 'Why do autistic children . . .?' *J. Autism Dev. Disorders*, **10**, 231–41.

Sutton, R. S. & Barto, A. G. (1981). 'Toward a modern theory of adaptive networks: expectation and prediction.' *Psychological Review*, **88**, 135–71.

Träuble, H., Tuebner, M., Wooley, P. & Eibl, H. (1976). 'Electrostatic interactions at charged lipid membranes. I. Effects of pH and univalent cations on membrane structure.' *Biophys. Chem.*, **4**, 319–37.

Traub, R. D. & Wong, R. K. S. (1982). 'Cellular mechanism of neuronal synchronization in epilepsy'. *Science*, **216**, 745–7.

Westlake, P. R. (1970). 'The possibilities of neural holographic processes within the brain.' *Kybernetik*, **7**, 129–53.

Zemon, V. & Ratliff, R. (1984). 'Intermodulation components of the visual evoked potential: responses to lateral superimposed stimuli.' *Biol. Cybern.*, **50**, 401–8.

11

Simulations of the trion model and the search for the code of higher cortical processing

GORDON L. SHAW and DENNIS J. SILVERMAN

11.1 Introduction

The quest or search for the 'code' or 'codes' involved in short-term memory and information processing in higher mammalian cortex is one of the most exciting and challenging problems in all of science. The recent experimental progress and results from recording in cortex using large arrays of microelectrodes (Krüger & Bach, 1981; Bach & Krüger, 1986) and using optical dye techniques (Blasdel & Salama, 1986; Grinvald *et al.*, 1981) offer great opportunities in the search for the code. The cross-correlation analyses of these type of data are enormously difficult (Gerstein, Perkel & Dayhoff, 1985; Aertsen, Gerstein & Johannesma, 1986). Thus the close interplay of new theoretical models and experiment will be crucial.

The basis for the tremendous magnitudes of the processing capabilities and the memory storage capacities remain mysteries despite the substantial efforts and results in modeling neural networks; see, e.g., references in Amari & Arbib (1982), Ballard (1986) and Pisco (1984). We believe the Mountcastle (1978) columnar organizing principle for the functioning of neocortex will help provide a basis for these phenomena and we constructed the trion model (Shaw, Silverman & Pearson, 1985; Shaw, Silverman & Pearson, 1986; Silverman, Shaw & Pearson, 1986). Mountcastle proposed that the well-established cortical column (Goldmann–Rakic, 1984), roughly 500 μm in diameter, is the basic network in the cortex and is comprised of small irreducible processing sub-units. The sub-units are connected into the columns or networks having the capability of complex spatial–temporal firing patterns. We strongly believe that *higher, complex* mammalian processes involve the creation and transformation of *complex* spatial–temporal network neuronal firing patterns. This is in contrast to the 'usual' assumption that neurons fire asynchronously and that the 'code' for information processing only involves sets of neurons firing with high frequency. It is very likely that there are several codes in the central nervous system for communication among various regions, depending on the sophistication of the information processing involved *and* the urgency of the information. For example, the sensing of perilous information *must* be responded to immediately and thus the alerting code presumably would be a neuronal population firing at a high rate leading to a fast motor response. In the opposite extreme, the playing of chess at the grand master level or the composing or recall of a Mozart opera must involve incredibly precise, sophisticated spatial–temporal neuronal processes. We believe that the key to finding the code for higher brain function involves presenting the appropriately simple, yet sophisticated stimuli, *and* looking *simultaneously* at the appropriate spatial and temporal separations: we suggest scales of ~100 μm and 50 ms, respectively. Clearly if one looks at too large a scale, everything will be washed out; whereas at too fine a scale, one will be lost in a morass of detail and fluctuations.

The spatial scale of a minicolumn of ~100 μm in diameter was suggested by Mountcastle (1978). We presented (Shaw, Harth & Scheibel, 1982; Shaw & Pearson, 1985) an additional number of anatomical, physiological and theoretical arguments for this spatial scale (or roughly 30–100 neurons). For further recent evidence see: Fig. 12*a* of Gilbert & Wiesel (1983) which shows a clustering of axonal boutons at spacings of 90 μm; Fig. 2 of Wiesendanger (1986) which shows the sophisticated, fine organization pattern of microzones (Asanuma, 1975) in motor cortex; and the voltage-sensitive dye optical recording in monkey primary visual cortex which shows a beautiful modular organization at this spatial scale (Blasdel & Salama, 1986). An elegant *anatomical* demonstration of a spatial structure of ~100 μm in rat somatosensory cortex was reported by Killackey (1983). In Fig. 11.1 we present some results from his laboratory. Furthermore, these structures are highly reproducible from one rat preparation to another! Similarly, a number of arguments (Merzenich & Shaw, unpublished) suggest the temporal scale for groups of neurons to burst is ~50 ms. For example, see (Morrell, 1967; Morrell, Hoeppner & de Toledo-Morrell, 1983; Shaw, Rinaldi & Pearson, 1983; Pearson *et al.*, 1983; von Seelen *et al.*, 1986). We conclude that there is *increasing* evidence in cortex for both an organized spatial structure of scale ~100 μm and a temporal scale ~50 ms; much more work needs to be done, *especially* on the temporal aspect of neuronal firing.

The question we addressed theoretically in the trion model is what qualitatively new phenomena can occur as a result of having such a spatial substructure ~100 μm and a temporal scale ~50 ms. Our early theoretical studies (Little & Shaw, 1975) were based on an Ising-spin system analogy (Little, 1974) which explicitly included known statistical fluctuations (Shaw & Vasudevan, 1974). Examination of the solutions of the large fluctuation limit (Little & Shaw, 1978) revealed a sub-unit organization (Shaw, 1978; Shaw & Roney, 1979; Roney & Shaw, 1980) in which only a few levels of firing of these sub-units was important. Then Fisher & Selke (1980) and Fisher (1981) showed that a precise, yet simple extension of the Ising-spin system model led to an *enormous* increase in the number of

Fig. 11.1. Photomicrograph from the laboratory of H. Killackey (prepared by D. Dawson) of a flattened section of layer IV of rat somatosensory cortex as shown by succinic dehydrogenase staining. The dark patches of staining are related to areas of dense thalamic projections, while the interdigitating lightly stained areas have dense callosal projections. This is an entire body representation where, e.g., the lower three large segments, reading from left to right, are the cortical representations of the rat lower lip, forepaw and hindpaw, respectively. The scale bar represents 500 μm so that many of the dark patches have a spatial scale ~ 100 μm. Furthermore, these structures are *highly reproducible* from rat to rat!

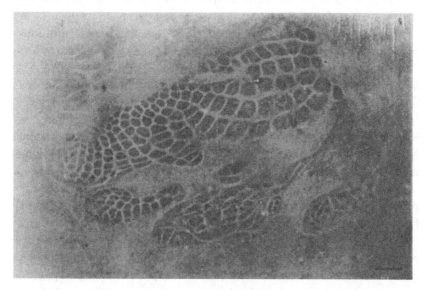

solutions. We incorporated Fisher's precise relationship between inhibitory and excitatory interactions among our idealized sub-units of neurons, trions having *three* levels of bursting. Further, we wanted a network of trions to have a *large* repertoire of sophisticated spatial–temporal patterns (in particular, long time sequences, since we believe this is one of the key features of higher cortical processing). Thus we update the state of the network at discrete time steps τ in a probabilistic way related to the states at the *two* previous time steps. The resulting trion model combines the computational power of cellular automata (Wolfram, 1983, 1984a, 1984b) with the highly adaptive and associative recall features of neural network models (Amari & Arbib, 1982; Ballard, 1986; Pisco, 1984). Table 11.1 contrasts the trion model with the 'usual' cellular automata and with the 'usual' neuronal network model.

The probability $P_i(S)$ of the ith trion attaining state S at time $n\tau$ is given by

$$P_i(S) = \frac{g(S)\cdot \exp\,[B\cdot M_i\cdot S]}{\Sigma_s\, g(s)\, \exp\,[B\cdot M_i\cdot s]},$$

$$M_i = \Sigma_j\,(V_{ij}S'_j + W_{ij}S''_j) - V_i^{\mathrm{T}},$$

$$(1)$$

where S'_j and S''_j are the state of the jth trion at times $(n-1)\tau$ and $(n-2)\tau$ respectively; V_{ij} and W_{ij} are the interactions between trions i and j between time $n\tau$ and times $(n-1)\tau$ and $(n-2)\tau$ respectively; V_i^{T} is an effective firing threshold. The three possible firing states S (of each trion) $= +1, 0, -1$ are, respectively, a large 'burst', an average burst and a below average firing. The statistical weighting term $g(S)$ with $g(0) \geqslant g(\pm 1)$ takes into account the number of equivalent firing configurations of the trion's internal neuronal constituents. (For example in a group of 75 neurons, firing levels of $+1$, 0 and -1 could correspond to 75–51, 50–26, and 25–0 neurons firing. There are many more combinatorial ways of generating the 50–26 level so that $g(0) \geqslant (g \pm 1)$, which is crucial in giving the firing patterns stability.) The fluctuation parameter B is inversely proportional to the level of noise, 'temperature', or random fluctuations in the network. The deterministic limit is B approaching infinity (or the noise going to zero).

Eqn (1) completely describes the trion model. We have analyzed the properties of a number of networks consisting of a small number of trions ($\leqslant 8$) connected in a ring (as would correspond to the Braitenberg & Braitenberg (1979) picture of the cortical column in primary visual cortex with a trion representing an orientation minicolumn). For example, consider a six-trion network. For a given set of parameters $V_{ij}, W_{ij}, g(S)$

Table 11.1. *Comparison of some features of the trion model versus the 'usual' cellular automata (Wolfram, 1983, 1984a,b) and the 'usual' neural model (see references in Amari & Arbib, 1982; Ballard, 1986; Pisco, 1984).*

Features of model	Trion model	'Usual' cellular automata	'Usual' neuronal network model
Spatial scale of basic elements	group of ~100 neurons	precise structure	single neuron
Temporal updating	synchronous (~50 ms) for 2 time steps	synchronous for 1 time step	asynchronous (~few ms)
Statistical fluctuations or noise	explicitly present	deterministic	sometimes added
Firing levels of basic elements	3 (with larger degeneracy of middle level)	2 (or more)	2
Firing patterns of network	complex spatial–temporal	complex spatial–temporal	mainly spatial
Connectivity	precise with symmetry to start	precise with symmetry	random to start
Adaptive	Hebb-modification of connections	none	Hebb-modification of connections
Associative memory recall	rapid recall by many stimuli	none	rapid recall by many stimuli
Storage capacity	*large*	none	moderate

and B, we examine all $3^{6+6} = 531,441$ possible firing configurations of the first two time steps. The computer is instructed to search for all the quasi-stable (high probability of cycling), periodic firing patterns, defined as MPs. The MPs are found by computing the most probable temporal evolution of the trion states from *each* of the 3^{6+6} initial conditions using (1) and determining if that evolution leads to a pattern that repeats within some (up to 24) time steps with a high probability (an MP). These full analyses require a substantial length of time (~50 hours of VAX 780 time for a seven-trion network). However, given the MPs from a full analysis, other calculations are *readily* performed. For example, we calculate the selective learning of an MP through 'experience' by using the Hebb (1949)-type algorithm

$$\Delta V_{ij} = \varepsilon \, \Sigma_{\text{cycle}} \, S_i(\tau)S_j(\tau - 1), \left.\right\}$$
$$\Delta W_{ij} = \varepsilon \, \Sigma_{\text{cycle}} \, S_i(\tau)S_j(\tau - 2), \; \varepsilon > 0. \quad (2)$$

We assume that the cycling of the trion network through a firing pattern will produce small changes in the coupling strengths V_{ij} and W_{ij} given by eqn (2). We also *readily* calculate the time evolution of the firing activity in a network using a standard Monte Carlo simulation. Some of the *striking* results of these calculations are: networks composed of a small number of trions with highly symmetric interactions (see, e.g. Table 1 in Shaw *et al.*, 1985; and Tables 1–6 in Silverman *et al.*, 1986) supported hundreds to thousands of MPs which can *evolve* from one to another (see Fig. 1 of Shaw *et al.*, 1985). Experience or learning would then modify the interactions (away from the symmetric values) using the Hebb algorithm (2) and select out or enhance the firing probability of the MP that had been cycled through as in the selection principle of Changeaux & Danchin (1976) or Edelman (1978). Remarkably, we found that (for a range in the fluctuation parameter B) *any* MP (that we have found in our studies) could be enhanced with only a small value of ε in (2), *even* the 18 cycle MPs in Tables 1, 2 and 5 of Silverman *et al.* (1986). In studying the associative recall properties of these networks, we found that, on the average, any of the initial firing configurations rapidly (in two to four time steps) projects onto an MP, and that many of the MPs can be individually accessed by thousands of different initial patterns (see Table 11.1).

Having summarized, above, the rich, general nature of the model from our one-dimensional ring-like network of trions we now turn to the present work: in section 11.2, we report some examples of Monte Carlo simulations of a 7×7 *two*-dimensional network of trions. These early investigations again give results similar to those found in our much more extensive one-dimensional studies. The crucial ideas on how to look for such complex spatial–temporal patterning (suggested by the trion model) in cortex are given in Section 11.3. In particular, we suggest a very specific type of analysis of multi-microelectrode data in sensory cortex along with suggested presentation of stimuli to test our ideas.

11.2 Monte-Carlo simulation of a two-dimensional network of trions

We present some Monte Carlo simulations using eqn (1) of a specific 7×7 network of trions for several initial firing configurations (see Tables 11.2–11.6). Clearly, we are unable to perform the full analysis described in Section 11.1 for the six or seven trion ring-like networks in which the computer follows the most probable firing behavior for each of the possible firing configurations: the 7×7 network has 3^{49+49} initial firing configurations for the first two time steps. The examples in Tables 11.2–11.6 are illustrative of our *preliminary* investigations.

The network connections extend to nearest neighbors, and are excitatory for the first time step and inhibitory for the second time step. Two types of boundary conditions were separately used, periodic and fixed average level (see Table captions for definition). Each 7×7 block shows the firing pattern of the network of trions at that discrete time step. The symbols #, 0 and = represent firing levels $S = 1, 0$ and -1, respectively, which correspond to firing above, at and below background respectively. Time increases from left to right for each row of blocks and from top row down. The first two (top left) blocks of firing levels are the initial firing configurations.

We note the following interesting features:

(1) A number of initial firing configurations lead to the same quasistable periodic firing pattern, MP.

(2) It usually takes only two time steps for the MP to be excited.

(3) Most of the MPs found have cycle lengths 6 (all of those in Tables 11.2–11.6).

(4) Some of the six time frames of these MPs appear to be closely related to the initial firing configurations, whereas others bear *no* obvious relation.

(5) As we see from comparing Tables 11.2 and 11.3 that although fixed average and periodic boundary conditions give different MPs, the patterns near the center of the trion array are very similar. (Of course, larger arrays should be used to investigate this.)

(6) For low fluctuations, an MP will run through many cycles, and will 'repair' an error, see, e.g., Table 11.2. At larger fluctuations, smaller B, an MP can quickly make transitions to a sequence of other MPs, as in Table 11.4.

Note to Tables 11.2–11.6: The symbols #, 0, = represent firing levels $S = 1, 0, -1$ respectively which correspond to firing levels above, at and below background respectively for each trion in the 7×7 block. Time increases from left to right for each row of blocks and from top row down. The first two (top left) blocks of firing levels are the initial firing configuration which evolve using eqn (1) via a Monte Carlo simulation. The network parameters are $V_i^T = 0, g(0) = 500, g(\pm 1) = 1, B = 15$. The synaptic connections into each trion are from itself and its nearest eight spatial neighbors with strengths $V = \begin{smallmatrix} 1\,1\,1 \\ 1\,2\,1 \\ 1\,1\,1 \end{smallmatrix}$ from the previous time step, and $W = -V$ for the second previous time step. The boundary conditions are fixed at an average level $S = 0$ by enlarging the array (to a 9×9 size) with the additional trions always firing at $S = 0$.

Gordon L. Shaw & Dennis J. Silverman

Table 11.2. *Simulation of a two-dimensional* 7 × 7 *array of trions.*

```
0 0 0 0 0 0 0   0 0 0 0 0 0 0   0 0 0 0 0 0 0   0 # # # # # #   # # # # # # #
0 0 0 0 0 0 0   0 0 0 0 0 0 0   0 0 # # # # 0   0 # # # # # #   # # # # # # #
0 0 0 0 0 0 0   0 0 0 # # 0 0   0 0 # # # # 0   # # # # # # #   # # # 0 0 # #
0 0 0 0 0 0 0   0 0 0 0 0 0 0   0 # # # # # 0   # # # # # # #   # # # 0 0 # #
0 0 0 0 0 0 0   0 0 # 0 # 0 0   0 # # # # # 0   # # # # # # #   # # 0 0 0 # #
0 0 0 0 0 0 0   0 0 0 0 0 0 0   0 # # # # # 0   # # # # # # #   # # # # # # #
0 0 0 0 0 0 0   0 0 0 0 0 0 0   0 0 0 0 0 0 0   # # # # # # #   # # # # # # #

# # 0 0 0 0 0   0 = = = = = =   = = = = = = =   = = 0 0 0 0 0   0 # # # # # #
# # = = = = 0   0 = = = = = =   = = = = = = =   = = # # # # 0   0 # # # # # #
# # = = = = 0   = = = = = = =   = = = 0 0 = =   = = # # # # 0   # # # # # # #
0 = = = = = 0   = = = = = = =   = = = 0 0 = =   0 # # # # # 0   # # # # # # #
0 = = = = = 0   = = = = = = =   = = 0 0 0 = =   0 # # # # # 0   # # # # # # #
0 = = = = = =   = = = = = = =   = = = = = = =   0 # # # # # 0   # # # # # # #
0 0 0 0 0 0 0   = = = = = = =   = = = = = = =   0 0 0 0 0 0 0   # # # # # # #

# # # # # # #   # # 0 0 0 0 0   0 = = = = = =   = = = = = = =   = = 0 0 0 0 0
# # # # # # #   # # = = = = 0   0 = = = = = =   = = = = = = =   = = # # # # 0
# # # 0 0 # #   # # = = = = 0   = = = = = = =   = = = 0 0 = =   = = # # # # 0
# # # 0 0 # #   0 = = = = = 0   = = = = = = =   = = = 0 0 = =   0 # # # # # 0
# # 0 0 0 # #   0 = = = = = 0   = = = = = = =   = = 0 0 0 = =   0 # # # # # 0
# # # # # # #   0 = = = = = 0   = = = = = = =   = = = = = = =   0 # # # # # 0
# # # # # # #   0 0 0 0 0 # 0   = = = = = = =   = = = = = = =   0 0 0 0 0 0 0

0 # # # # # #   # # # # # # #   # # 0 0 0 0 0   0 = = = = = =   = = = = = = =
0 # # # # # #   # # # # # # #   # # = = = = 0   0 = = = = = =   = = = = = = =
# # # # # # #   # # # 0 0 # #   # # = = = = 0   = = = = = = =   = = = 0 0 = =
# # # # # # #   # # # 0 0 # #   0 = = = = = 0   = = = = = = =   = = = 0 0 = =
# # # # # # #   # # 0 0 0 # #   0 = = = = = 0   = = = = = = =   = = 0 0 0 = =
# # # # # # #   # # # # # # #   0 = = = = = 0   = = = = = = =   = = = = = = =
# # # # # # #   # # # # # # #   0 0 0 0 0 0 0   = = = = = = =   = = = = = = =

= = 0 0 0 0 0   0 # # # # # #   # # # # # # #   # # 0 0 0 0 0   0 = = = = = =
= = # # # # 0   0 # # # # # #   # # # # # # #   # # = = = = 0   0 = = = = = =
= = # # # # 0   # # # # # # #   # # # 0 0 # #   # # = = = = 0   = = = = = = =
0 # # # # # 0   # # # # # # #   # # # 0 0 # #   0 = = = = = 0   = = = = = = =
0 # # # # # 0   # # # # # # #   # # 0 0 0 # #   0 = = = = = 0   = = = = = = =
0 # # # # # 0   # # # # # # #   # # # # # # #   0 = = = = = 0   = = = = = = =
0 = 0 0 0 0 0   # # # # # # #   # # # # # # #   0 0 0 0 0 0 0   = = = = = = =

= = = = = = =   = = 0 0 0 0 0   0 # # # # # #   # # # # # # #   # # 0 0 0 0 0
= = = = = = =   = = # # # # 0   0 # # # # # #   # # # # # # #   # # = = = = 0
= = = 0 0 = =   = = # # # # 0   # # # # # # #   # # # 0 0 # #   # # = = = = 0
= = = 0 0 = =   0 # # # # # 0   # # # # # # #   # # # 0 0 # #   0 = = = = = 0
= = 0 0 0 = =   0 # # # # # 0   # # # # # # #   # # 0 0 0 # #   0 = = = = = 0
= = = = = = =   0 # # # # # 0   # # # # # # #   # # # # # # #   0 = = = = = 0
= = = = = = =   0 0 0 0 0 0 0   # # # # # # #   # # # # # # #   0 0 0 0 0 0 0
```

Table 11.3. *Simulation of a two-dimensional 7 × 7 array of trions, as in Table 11.2, except that we use periodic boundary conditions (ring-like along horizontal, vertical and main diagonal directions).*

```
0 0 0 0 0 0 0   0 0 0 0 0 0 0   0 0 0 0 0 0 0   0 # # # # # #   # # # # # # #
0 0 0 0 0 0 0   0 0 0 0 0 0 0   0 0 # # # # 0   0 # # # # # #   # # # # # # #
0 0 0 0 0 0 0   0 0 0 # # 0 0   0 0 # # # # 0   # # # # # # #   # # # 0 0 # #
0 0 0 0 0 0 0   0 0 0 0 0 0 0   0 # # # # # 0   # # # # # # #   # # # 0 0 # #
0 0 0 0 0 0 0   0 0 # 0 # 0 0   0 # # # # # 0   # # # # # # #   # # 0 0 0 # #
0 0 0 0 0 0 0   0 0 0 0 0 0 0   0 # # # # # 0   # # # # # # #   # # # # # # #
0 0 0 0 0 0 0   0 0 0 0 0 0 0   0 0 0 0 0 0 0   # # # # # # #   # # # # # # #

# # 0 0 0 0 #   0 = = = = = =   = = = = = = =   = = 0 0 0 0 =   0 # # # # # #
# # = = = = #   0 = = = = = =   = = = = = = =   = = # # # # =   0 # # # # # #
# # = = = = #   = = = = = = =   = = = 0 0 = =   = = # # # # =   # # # # # # #
0 = = = = = 0   = = = = = = =   = = = 0 0 = =   0 # # # # # 0   # # # # # # #
0 = = = = = 0   = = = = = = =   = = 0 0 0 = =   0 # # # # # 0   # # # # # # #
0 = = = = = 0   = = = = = = =   = = = = = = =   0 # # # # # 0   # # # # # # #
# # 0 0 0 0 #   = = = = = = =   = = = = = = =   = = 0 0 0 0 =   # # # # # # #

# # # # # # #   # # 0 0 0 0 #   = = = = = = =   = = = = = = =   = = 0 0 0 0 =
# # # # # # #   # # = = = = #   0 = = = = = =   = = = = = = =   = = # # # # =
# # # 0 0 # #   # # = = = = #   = = = = = = =   = = = 0 0 = =   = = # # # # =
# # # 0 0 # #   0 = = = = = 0   = = = = = = =   = = = 0 0 = =   0 # # # # # 0
# # 0 0 0 # #   0 = = = = = 0   = = = = = = =   = = 0 0 0 = =   0 # # # # # 0
# # # # # # #   0 = = = = = 0   = = = = = = =   = = = = = = =   0 # # # # # 0
# # # # # # #   # # 0 0 0 0 #   = = = = = = =   = = = = = = =   0 0 0 0 0 0 0

# # # # # # #   # # # # # # #   # # 0 0 0 0 #   = = = = = = =   = = = = = = =
0 # # # # # #   # # # # # # #   # # = = = = #   0 = = = = = =   = = = = = = =
# # # # # # #   # # # 0 0 # #   # # = = = = #   = = = = = = =   = = = 0 0 = =
# # # # # # #   # # # 0 0 # #   0 = = = = = 0   = = = = = = =   = = = 0 0 = =
# # # # # # #   # # 0 0 0 # #   0 = = = = = 0   = = = = = = =   = = 0 0 0 = =
# # # # # # #   # # # # # # #   0 = = = = = 0   = = = = = = =   = = = = = = =
# # # # # # #   # # # # # # #   0 0 0 0 0 0 0   = = = = = = =   = = = = = = =

= = 0 0 0 0 =   # # # # # # #   # # # # # # #   # # 0 0 0 0 #   = = = = = = =
= = # # # # =   0 # # # # # #   # # # # # # #   # # = = = = #   0 = = = = = =
= = # # # # =   # # # # # # #   # # # 0 0 # #   # # = = = = #   = = = = = = =
0 # # # # # 0   # # # # # # #   # # # 0 0 # #   0 = = = = = 0   = = = = = = =
0 # # # # # 0   # # # # # # #   # # 0 0 0 # #   0 = = = = = 0   = = = = = = =
0 # # # # # 0   # # # # # # #   # # # # # # #   0 = = = = = 0   = = = = = = =
0 0 0 0 0 0 0   # # # # # # #   # # # # # # #   0 0 0 0 0 0 0   = = = = = = =

= = = = = = =   = = 0 0 0 0 =   # # # # # # #   # # # # # # #   # # 0 0 0 0 #
= = = = = = =   = = # # # # =   0 # # # # # #   # # # # # # #   # # = = = = #
= = = 0 0 = =   = = # # # # =   # # # # # # #   # # # 0 0 # #   # # = = = = #
= = = 0 0 = =   0 # # # # # 0   # # # # # # #   # # # 0 0 # #   0 = = = = = 0
= = 0 0 0 = =   0 # # # # # 0   # # # # # # #   # # 0 0 0 # #   0 = = = = = 0
= = = = = = =   0 # # # # # 0   # # # # # # #   # # # # # # #   0 = = = = = 0
= = = = = = =   0 0 0 0 0 0 0   # # # # # # #   # # # # # # #   0 0 0 0 0 0 0
```

Table 11.4. *Simulation of a two-dimensional 7 × 7 array of trions, as in Table 11.2, except that we use B = 10 instead of 15.*

```
0 0 0 0 0 0 0    0 0 0 0 0 0 0    0 0 0 0 0 0 0    0 0 # # # # #    0 # # # # # #
0 0 0 0 0 0 0    0 0 0 0 0 0 0    0 0 0 # # # 0    0 0 # # # # #    # # # # # # #
0 0 0 0 0 0 0    0 0 0 0 # 0 0    0 0 0 # # # 0    # # # # # # #    # # # # 0 # #
0 0 0 0 0 0 0    0 0 0 0 0 0 0    0 # # # # # 0    # # # # # # #    # # # # 0 # #
0 0 0 0 0 0 0    0 0 # 0 # 0 0    0 # # # # # 0    # # # # # # #    # # 0 0 0 # #
0 0 0 0 0 0 0    0 0 0 0 0 0 0    0 # # # # # 0    # # # # # # #    # # # # # # #
0 0 0 0 0 0 0    0 0 0 0 0 0 0    0 0 0 0 0 0 0    # # # # # # #    # # # # # # #

# # # 0 0 0 0    # # = = = = =    0 = = = = = =    = = = 0 0 0 0    = = # # # # #
# # # = = = 0    # # = = = = =    = = = = = = =    = = = # # # 0    = = # # # # #
# # # = = = 0    = = = = = = =    = = = = 0 = =    = = = # # # 0    # # # # # # #
0 = = = = = 0    = = = = = = =    = = = = 0 = =    0 # # # # # 0    # # # # # # #
0 = = = = = 0    = = = = = = =    = = 0 0 0 = =    0 # # # # # 0    # # # # # # #
0 = = = = = 0    = = = = = = =    = = = = = = =    0 # # # # # 0    # # # # # # #
0 0 0 0 0 0 0    = = = = = = =    = = = = = = =    0 0 0 0 0 0 0    # # # # # # #

0 # # # # # #    # # # 0 0 0 0    # # = = = = =    0 = = = = = =    = = = 0 0 0 0
# # # # # # #    # # # = = = 0    # # = = = = =    = = = = = = =    = = = # # # 0
# # # # 0 # #    # # # = = = 0    = = = = = = =    = = = = 0 = =    = = = # # # 0
# # # # 0 # #    0 = = = = = 0    = = = = = = =    = = = = 0 = =    0 # # # # # 0
# # 0 0 0 # #    0 = = = = = 0    = = = = = = =    = = 0 0 0 = =    0 # # # # # 0
# # # # # # #    0 = = = = = 0    = = = = = = =    = = = = = = =    0 # # # # # 0
# # # # # # #    0 0 0 0 0 0 0    = = = = = = =    = = = = = = =    0 0 0 0 0 0 0

= = # # # # #    0 # # # # # #    # # # 0 0 0 0    # # = = = = =    0 = = = = = =
= = # # # # #    # # # # # # #    # # # = = = 0    # # = = = = =    = = = = = = =
# # # # # # #    # # # # 0 # #    # # # = = = 0    = = = = = = =    = = = = 0 = =
# # # # # # #    # # # # 0 # #    0 = = = = = 0    = = = = = = =    = = = = 0 = =
# # # # # # #    # # 0 0 0 # #    0 = = = = = 0    = = = = = = =    = = 0 0 0 = =
# # # # # # #    # # # # # # #    0 = = = = = 0    = = = = = = =    = = = = = = =
# # # # # # #    # # # # # # #    0 0 0 0 0 0 0    = = = = = = =    = = = = = = =

= = = 0 0 0 0    = = # # # # #    0 # # # # # #    # # # 0 0 0 0    # # = = = = =
= = = 0 # # 0    = = # # # # #    # # # # # # #    # # # 0 0 0 0    # # = = = = =
= = = # # # 0    # # # # # # #    # # # # # # #    # # # = = = 0    = = = = = = =
0 # # # # # 0    # # # # # # #    # # # # 0 # #    0 = = = = = 0    = = = = = = =
0 # # # # # 0    # # # # # # #    # # 0 0 0 # #    0 = = = = = 0    = = = = = = =
0 # # # # # 0    # # # # # # #    # # # # # # #    0 = = = = = 0    = = = = = = =
0 0 0 0 0 0 0    # # # # # # #    # # # # # # #    0 0 0 0 0 0 0    = = = = = = =

0 = = = = = =    = = = 0 0 0 0    = = # # # # #    0 # # # # # #    # # # 0 0 0 0
= = = = = = =    = = = 0 0 0 0    = = # # # # #    # # # # # # #    # # # 0 0 0 0
= = = = = = =    = = = # # # 0    # # # # # # #    # # # # # # #    # # # = = = 0
= = = = 0 = =    0 # # # # # 0    # # # # # # #    # # # # 0 # #    0 = = = = = 0
= = 0 0 0 = =    0 # # # # # 0    # # # # # # #    # # 0 0 0 # #    0 = = = = = 0
= = = = = = =    0 # # # # # 0    # # # # # # #    # # # # # # #    0 = = = = = 0
= = = = = = =    0 0 0 0 0 0 0    # # # # # # #    # # # # # # #    0 0 0 0 0 0 0
```

Table 11.5. *Simulation of a two-dimensional 7 × 7 array of trions, as in Table 11.2, except the lower left V is 0.7 instead of 1 (no change in W).*

```
0 0 0 0 0 0 0   0 0 0 0 0 0 0   0 0 0 0 0 0 0   0 0 # # # # #   0 # # # # # #
0 0 0 0 0 0 0   0 0 0 0 0 0 0   0 0 0 # # # 0   0 0 # # # # #   # # # # # # #
0 0 0 0 0 0 0   0 0 0 0 # 0 0   0 0 0 # # # 0   # # # # # # #   # # # # 0 # #
0 0 0 0 0 0 0   0 0 0 0 0 0 0   0 # # # # # 0   # # # # # # #   # # # # 0 # #
0 0 0 0 0 0 0   0 0 # 0 # 0 0   0 # # # # # 0   # # # # # # #   # # 0 0 0 # #
0 0 0 0 0 0 0   0 0 0 0 0 0 0   0 # # # # # 0   # # # # # # #   # # # # # # #
0 0 0 0 0 0 0   0 0 0 0 0 0 0   0 0 0 0 0 0 0   # # # # # # #   # # # # # # #

# # # 0 0 = 0   # # = = = = =   0 = = = = = =   = = = 0 0 0 0   = = # # # # #
# # # = = = =   # # = = = = =   = = = = = = =   = = = # # # 0   = = # # # # #
# # # = = = 0   = = = = = = =   = = = = 0 = =   = = = # # # 0   # # # # # # #
0 = = = = = 0   = = = = = = =   = = = = 0 = =   0 # # # # # 0   # # # # # # #
0 = = = = = 0   = = = = = = =   = = 0 0 0 = =   0 # # # # # 0   # # # # # # #
0 = = = = = 0   = = = = = = =   = = = = = = =   0 # # # # # 0   # # # # # # #
0 0 0 0 0 0 0   = = = = = = =   = = = = = = =   0 0 0 0 0 0 0   # # # # # # #

0 # # # # # #   # # # 0 0 = =   # # = = = = =   0 = = = = = =   = = = 0 0 0 0
# # # # # # #   # # # = = = 0   # # = = = = =   = = = = = = =   = = = # # # 0
# # # # 0 # #   # # # = = = =   = = = = = = =   = = = = 0 = =   = = = # # # 0
# # # # 0 # #   0 = = = = = 0   = = = = = = =   = = = = 0 = =   0 # # # # # 0
# # 0 0 0 # #   0 = = = = = 0   = = = = = = =   = = 0 0 0 = =   0 # # # # # 0
# # # # # # #   0 = = = = = 0   = = = = = = =   = = = = = = =   0 # # # # # 0
# # # # # # #   0 0 0 0 0 0 0   = = = = = = =   = = = = = = =   0 0 0 0 0 0 0

= = # # # # #   0 # # # # # #   # # # 0 0 0 =   # # = = = = =   0 = = = = = =
= = # # # # #   # # # # # # #   # # # = = = 0   # # = = = = =   = = = = = = =
# # # # # # #   # # # # = # #   # # # = = = 0   = = = = = = =   = = = = 0 = =
# # # # # # #   # # # # 0 # #   0 = = = = = 0   = = = = = = =   = = = = 0 = =
# # # # # # #   # # 0 = 0 # #   0 = = = = = 0   = = = = = = =   = = 0 0 0 = =
# # # # # # #   # # # # # # #   0 = = = = = 0   = = = = = = =   = = = = = = =
# # # # # # #   # # # # # # #   0 0 0 0 0 0 0   = = = = = = =   = = = = = = =

= = = 0 0 0 #   = = # # # # #   0 # # # # # #   # # # 0 0 0 0   # # = = = = =
= = = # # # 0   = = # # # # #   # # # # # # #   # # # = = = 0   # # = = = = =
= = = # # # 0   # # # # # # #   # # # # = # #   # # # = = = 0   = = = = = = =
0 # # # # # 0   # # # # # # #   # # # # 0 # #   0 = = = = = =   = = = = = = =
0 # # # # # 0   # # # # # # #   # # = 0 0 # #   0 = = = = = 0   = = = = = = =
0 # # # # # #   # # # # # # #   # # # # # # #   0 = = = = = 0   = = = = = = =
0 0 0 0 0 0 0   # # # # # # #   # # # # # # #   0 0 0 0 0 0 0   = = = = = = =

0 = = = = = =   = = = 0 0 0 0   = = # # # # #   0 # # # # # #   # # # = 0 0 0
= = = = = = =   = = = # # # 0   = = # # # # #   # # # # # # #   # # # = = = 0
= = = = 0 = =   = = = # # # 0   # # # # # # #   # # # # 0 # #   # # # = = = 0
= = = = 0 = =   0 # # # # # 0   # # # # # # #   # # # # 0 # #   0 = = = = = 0
= = 0 0 0 = =   0 # # # # # 0   # # # # # # #   # # 0 = = # #   0 = = = = = 0
= = = = = = =   0 # # # # # #   # # # # # # #   # # # # # # #   0 = = = = = 0
= = = = = = =   0 0 0 0 0 0 0   # # # # # # #   # # # # # # #   0 0 0 0 0 0 0
```

Table 11.6. *Simulation of a two-dimensional* 7 × 7 *array of trions.*

```
0 0 0 0 0 0 0   0 0 0 0 0 0 0   0 0 0 0 0 0 0   0 0 # # # # #   0 # # # # # #
0 0 0 0 0 0 0   0 0 0 0 0 0 0   0 0 0 # # # 0   0 0 # # # # #   = # # # # # #
0 0 0 0 0 0 0   0 0 0 0 # 0 0   0 0 0 # # # 0   0 = # # # # #   = = 0 # = # #
0 0 0 0 0 0 0   0 0 0 0 0 0 0   0 0 = 0 0 # 0   0 = = = 0 # #   = = = = = # #
0 0 # # # 0 0   0 0 # 0 # 0 0   0 0 = = = 0 0   0 = = = = = #   = = = = = = #
0 0 0 0 0 0 0   0 0 0 0 0 0 0   0 0 = = = 0 0   0 = = = = = 0   = = = = = = =
0 0 0 0 0 0 0   0 0 0 0 0 0 0   0 0 0 0 0 0 0   0 = = = = = 0   = = = = = = =

# # # 0 0 0 0   # 0 = = = = =   = = = = = = =   = = = 0 0 0 0   # # # # # # #
= 0 # = = = 0   0 = = = = = =   0 = = = = = =   0 0 0 # # # 0   # # # # # # #
= = = = = = 0   = = = = = = =   # 0 = = 0 = =   # # # # # # 0   # # # # # # #
= = = = = = 0   0 0 = = = = =   # # # # # = =   # # # # # # #   # # # # # # #
= = 0 = = = =   0 # # # 0 = =   # # # # # # 0   # # # # # # #   0 = = = # # #
= = 0 0 0 = =   0 # # # # 0 =   # # # # # # #   # # 0 # # # #   0 = = = = # #
= = 0 0 0 = =   0 # # # # # 0   # # # # # # #   # # 0 0 # # #   0 = = = = 0 0

# # # # # # #   0 0 0 0 0 0 0   = = = = = = =   = = = = = = =   0 0 0 0 0 0 0
# # # # # # #   0 0 0 = = = 0   = = = = = = =   = = = = = = =   0 0 0 # # # =
# # # # 0 # #   = = = = = = 0   = = = = = = =   = = = = 0 = =   # # # # # # 0
= = = = = # #   = = = = = = =   = = = = = = =   # # # # = = =   # # # # # # #
= = = = = = 0   = = = = = = =   0 # # # = = =   # # # # # # 0   # # # # # # #
= = = = = = =   = = 0 = = = =   0 # # # # = =   # # # # # # #   # # 0 # # # #
= = = = = = =   = = 0 0 = = =   0 # # # # 0 0   # # # # # # #   # # 0 0 # # #

# # # # # # #   # # # # # # #   0 0 0 0 0 0 0   = = = = = = =   = = = = = = =
# # # # # # #   # # # # # # #   0 0 0 = = = 0   = = = = = = =   = = = = = = =
# # # # # # #   # # # # 0 # #   = = = = = = 0   = = = = = = =   = = = = 0 = =
# # # # # # #   = = = = = # #   = = = = = = =   = = = = = = =   # # # # # = =
0 = = = # # #   = = = = = = 0   = = = = = = =   0 # # # = = =   # # # # # # 0
0 = = = = # #   = = = = = = =   = = 0 = = = =   0 # # # # = =   # # # # # # #
0 = = = = 0 0   = = = = = = =   = = 0 0 = = =   0 # # # # 0 0   # # # # # # #

0 0 0 0 0 0 0   # # # # # # #   # # # # # # #   0 0 0 0 0 0 0   = = = = = = =
0 0 0 # # # 0   # # # # # # #   # # # # # # #   0 0 0 = = = 0   = = = = = = =
# # # # # # 0   # # # # # # #   # # # # 0 # #   = = = = = = 0   = = = = = = =
# # # # # # #   # # # # # # #   = = = = = # #   = = = = = = =   = = = = = = =
# # # # # # #   0 = = = # # #   = = = = = = 0   = = = = = = =   0 # # # = = =
# # 0 # # # #   0 = = = = # #   = = = = = = =   = = 0 = = = =   0 # # # = = =
# # 0 0 # # #   0 = = = = 0 0   = = = = = = =   = = 0 0 = = =   0 # # # 0 0

= = = = = = =   0 0 0 0 0 0 0   # # # # # # #   # # # # # # #   0 0 0 0 0 0 0
= = = = = = =   0 0 0 # # # 0   # # # # # # #   # # # # # # #   0 0 0 = = = 0
= = = = 0 = =   # # # # # # 0   # # # # # # #   # # # 0 # #     = = = = = = 0
# # # # = = =   # # # # # # #   # # # # # # #   = = = = = # #   = = = = = = =
# # # # # # 0   # # # # # # #   0 = = = # # #   = = = = = = 0   = = = = = = =
# # # # # # #   # # 0 # # # #   0 = = = = # #   = = = = = = =   = = 0 = = = =
# # # # # # #   # # 0 0 # # #   0 = = = = 0 0   = = = = = = =   = = 0 0 = = =
```

(7) More complicated initial firing configurations, as in Table 11.6, may take longer to lead to an MP.

(8) Moderate perturbations in the connections among the trions will not affect the MPs. See Table 11.5 in which one of the Vs is changed from 1 to 0.7.

As stressed in the next section, our main use for *future* Monte-Carlo calculations of two-dimensional arrays of trions will be in support of analysis of multiple-microelectrode experiments in sensory cortex. In addition to simply specifying the initial two firing configurations, we would add inputs corresponding to the cortical inputs from the applied sensory stimuli.

11.3 The quest for the code of higher cortical processing and the analysis of multi-microelectrode data

As we have stressed earlier, the key to decoding higher cortical processing activity is to examine neuronal firing data at the appropriate spatial and temporal scales. The single neuron is *not* the appropriate unit: the output of one cortical neuron cannot fire another. We have presented arguments that minicolumns (Shaw *et al.*, 1982; Shaw & Pearson, 1985; Mountcastle, 1978) ~100 μm in diameter are the units that one wishes to monitor (also see Fig. 11.1). Similarly, the appropriate temporal scale is *not* the recovery time of a few ms of the single neuron, but the much longer time scale of ~50 ms. (Morrell, 1967; Morrell *et al.*, 1983; Shaw *et al.*, 1983; Pearson *et al.*, 1983; von Seelen *et al.*, 1986; Krone *et al.*, 1986). Undoubtedly, *much* local processing takes place among the roughly 100 (pyramidal and stellate) neurons within the minicolumn through the six layers of cortex. In the computer simulations of Krone *et al.* (1986), circulation of neural activity through the cortical layers yields (see their Fig. 9) bursting activity with a 50-ms period! They find a layer dependent pattern of activity in nice agreement with the data of Best & Dinse (1984) from primary visual cortex of cat. An important message is that the neural activity has both strong spatial and temporal dependence and *cannot* be factorized.

Having established the plausibility of the appropriate spatial scale of ~100 μm and temporal scale of ~50 ms for cortical processing, we stress their significance in the theoretical setting of the trion model. The trion combines (see Table 11.1) the computational power of cellular automata (Wolfram, 1983, 1984*a,b*) with the highly adaptive and associative recall features of neural network (Amari & Arbib, 1982; Pisco, 1984; Ballard, 1986) models of memory. In particular, networks composed of a small number of trions support up to *thousands* of quasi-stable, periodic firing patterns (MPs). Clearly, this is just a highly idealized model. However, we believe it offers much insight in how to analyze multielectrode data from cortex to search for the code of information processing.

Consider an array of closely spaced ($\sim$100–200 μm) microelectrodes placed in sensory cortex of an animal which is being presented an appropriate variety of sensory stimuli each with many trials (for example, the very impressive primary, visual cortex experiments done in the laboratory by Krüger (Krüger & Bach, 1981; Bach & Krüger, 1986) using a 5 × 6 rectangular array spaced at 160 μm). Each electrode records one neuron or a small number of neurons. The number of cross-correlation calculations of pairs of spike trains are *enormous*, and methods have been devised recently (Gerstein *et al.*, 1985; Aertsen *et al.*, 1986) to analyze such large arrays. While these difficult analyses lead to interesting results, we believe that they are really suited for *local* circuits, and not for the more *global* picture we have in mind for decoding the communication among larger groups of neurons. Here a *key* element to the global analysis is the *assembly hypothesis* (Shaw, 1978; Shaw & Roney, 1979; Shaw *et al.*, 1982) which is imbedded in the trion model and tells us that we *necessarily* want to deal directly with the PSHs or poststimulus histograms rather than the individual trial spike trains. Consider the presentation of a 'meaningful' stimulus to an animal that has some 'repeatable' behavioral response. It is well known (Burns, 1968; Dill, Vallecalle & Verzeano, 1968; John, 1972) that although the spike train response of a single cortical neuron is not reproducible, the PSH (see Fig. 11.2) or *experiment* or *trial* summed response of a single neuron to many presentations (*roughly* 20–50) of the stimulus to the animal is 'reproducible' (clearly, the criteria are somewhat subjective). Furthermore, it is significant that neurons have been found (see Fig. 3 of Thompson, 1976) for which the PSH changes as a result of classical conditioning. Now consider the physiological significance of this widely used quantity, the PSH, determined from the sum over trials: we expect the firing response of a 'network' containing the individual neuron to be repeatable because the behavioral correlates to a single stimulus presentation are repeatable (as in the eye-blink paradigm described by Thompson, 1976). Assume that the network is divided into assemblies of neurons *defined* so that the 'output' firing response (to a single stimulus presentation) of the assembly summed over the localized group of 'output' pyramidal neurons in it would be the same as the PSH of a single pyramidal neuron in the assembly. (Clearly, there are also local circuit stellate neurons in the assembly which would also have PSHs equivalent to their assembly sums.) It is the output of the assembly that is meaningful for cortical–cortical processing. Our definition for the assembly *directly* relates the number of constituent neurons to the number of presentations necessary to achieve a 'reliable' PSH, i.e., *roughly* 20–50 pyramidal cells (plus an equivalent number of stellate cells). This translates to a minicolumn (Mountcastle, 1978; Shaw *et al.*, 1982) of ~100 μm diameter. We *identify* the *assembly* or minicolumn with our idealized *trion*.

Fig. 11.2. Schematic drawing illustrating our definition of an assembly of neurons. The spatial sum of firings across neurons in the assembly for one trial is assumed equal to (denoted by question marks) the sum for different experimental trials or the poststimulus histogram (PSH) for each individual neuron in the assembly. The upper left part of the drawing represents the spike train responses of a typical cortical neuron to a repeated brief 'meaningful' stimulus to the animal. They vary from experimental (numbered) trial to trial. However, the sum over trials or PSH (~20–50 trials) in the lower center is 'reproducible'. The dashed line represents the background activity of this cell. The 'size' of the time bins and the relevant 'levels' of firing will probably vary from region to region in the cortex. The upper right part of the drawing illustrates the spike train responses of the individual (numbered) neurons in the assembly to one stimulus presentation. This drawing refers to the 'output' pyramidal neurons. Presumably there are an equivalent number of stellate cells in the assembly.

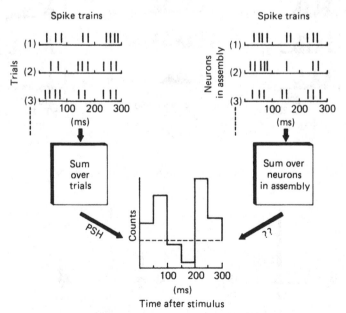

Fig. 11.3. Single-unit data from visual area III of cat from the published work of Morrell. A1, A2, and A3 are derived from Figs. 11, 14 and 12, respectively, of Morrell (1967). B1 and B2 are derived from Fig. 2 of Morrell *et al.* (1983). (*a*) All stimuli were presented during the 0 to 50 ms interval. In A1 and A2, (L) denotes a light line, (C) denotes an auditory click, and (L + C) denotes simultaneous presentation of the light line and the click. In A3, the same light line was presented to the left eye (L), the right eye (R), and to both eyes (R + L). In A2, spont. denotes the spontaneous or background level of discharge. The data displayed in each histogram were acquired in consecutive sets of 20 trials, as indicated. The calibration bar at time 0 equals 20 spikes. (*b*) The visual stimulus was a light line presented during the time marked below the axis. The calibration bar indicates 20 spikes, and about 150 trials were given. In B1 the light line was vertical while in B2 it was horizontal. These data demonstrate *possible* complex coding occurring at burst intervals of roughly 50 ms with burst levels of large, small or no peaks.

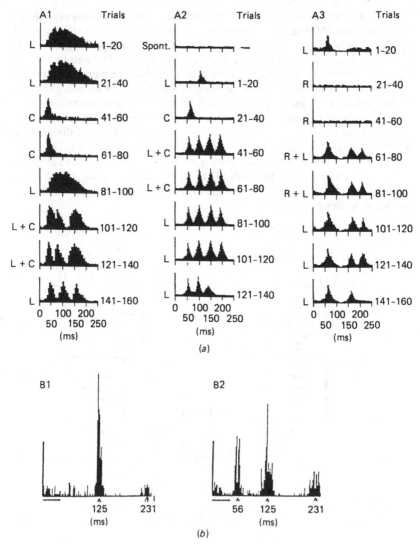

Two important features of the trion model are the assumptions of *three* firing levels ($S = 1, 0, -1$) and *periodic* bursting in cortex; both are necessary for the *many* MPs in a given network. An illustration of these features can also be seen in PSH data. In particular, Morrell (1967) and Morrell *et al.*, (1983) found multipeak responses in cat visual cortex with peak separation of approximately 50 ms. In addition, Morrell observed dramatic changes in these bursting patterns when he paired stimuli in conditioning experiments. Some of these PSH data are shown in Fig. 11.3. We suggest that these burst pattern data might be consistent with exciting and enhancing different MPs in our three-level trion model. We stress, however, that three levels are only a *minimum* requirement for the richness of our model. Thus we suggest that a *five*-level firing analysis of actual data be performed. The number of levels and the criteria for setting them along with the optimum value for the time bin (~50 ms) *must be* determined from the analysis of the data. *Two* obvious, but *crucial* features must be kept in mind during the search for complex spatial–temporal patterning; it *must* be reproducible and it *must* be specific to the stimulus (the patterning could, of course, depend on other 'variables' such as context (Fuster & Jervey, 1981)).

Our suggested analysis to search for the code of higher cortical processing from a multi (horizontal) microelectrode array (spaced $\geq 100\,\mu m$) in sensory cortex consists of:

(1) For an 'appropriate' stimulus (see below) perform a series of trials (at least 20); each trial some few seconds long.
(2) For *each* electrode perform the trial summed PSH.
(3) Bin the PSH data in ~50 ms time bins τ.
(4) Choose (after rough examination of the data) an 'appropriate' number of firing levels; at least three, probably five. The ranges of these levels should be set from the *average number* of *counts* per time bin τ for *each electrode*, with perhaps three (or more) standard deviations (from the average) for the width of each level. Note that the statistics are then built into the analysis.
(5) *Color* code the levels in (4). The human visual system is incredibly good for finding patterns in color.
(6) Display the data as in Tables 11.2–11.6, but with color codes rather than symbols to search for spatial–temporal patterns (which are reproducible and stimulus specific).
(7) Repeat (1)–(6) for a number of stimulus parameters. In *particular*, from our experience from using a dynamic time sequence of light bar stimuli at different orientations and recording from cat visual cortex (Shaw *et al.*, 1983; Pearson *et al.*, 1983) we suggest varying

the interstimulus interval around multiples of τ to *resonantly* enhance the network response of the cortex.

(8) We suggest that the most interesting stimuli to present to animals in order to find a complex spatial–temporal coding are dynamic time sequences (Shaw *et al.*, 1983; Pearson *et al.*, 1983) involving human psychophysics type illusions (Shaw & Ramachandran, 1982) or conditioning type pairing of stimuli (Morrell, 1967; Morrell *et al.*, 1983). Presumably, one would find as a result of carrying out the suggested experiments and analysis a *large* repertoire of complex spatial–temporal patterning.

(9) Finally, a *crucial* part of the program is the computer simulation of these experiments with a two-dimensional network of trions as described in Section 11.2 (along with the relevant stimuli) looking for MPs matching those found in the experimental analysis. Thus with relatively *few* parameters, one would hope to understand the sophisticated coding of this region of cortex. The test of course would be then to suggest additional stimuli to use *and* the predicted MP response. Such a close continuing interplay of experiment and theory is, we believe, absolutely necessary.

It is important to emphasize that this program *must* be done with *simultaneous* recording from an array of microelectrodes, rather than moving a single electrode to various sites: the relative timing among recording sites is *crucial*; there are *other* inputs (cortical and subcortical) to a network in addition to that directly related to the stimuli (Bach & Krüger, 1986), so that it is important to get the global picture as time evolves; it is imperative to re-do selected series of stimuli to test reproducibility of the spatial–temporal responses. In fact, our suggested analysis of the data is such that it can be done *on line*! Thus interesting results can be further explored *during* the experiment.

The goals of such a program are quite *ambitious*: to discover and decipher a code for higher cortical processing within a small region ($\sim 1000\ \mu$m diameter) or column of sensory cortex. Even if this (combined experimental and theoretical) program were successful, it would represent just the beginning of the quest for the understanding of higher information processing in the cortex.

Acknowledgements

We thank A. Aersten, T. Allard, M. Arbib, T. Bullock, D. Dawson, E. Harth, W. Jenkins, J. Krüger, M. Merzenich, J. Patera, J. Pearson, C. Schreiner and J. Ward for helpful discussions. GS would like to thank

M. Merzenich and members of his laboratory for the very kind hospitality shown him during his visit, and the Aspen Center for Physics where part of this work was done.

References

Aertsen, A., Gerstein, G. & Johannesma, P. (1986). 'From neuron to assembly: neuronal organization and stimulus representation.' In *Brain Theory*, eds. G. Palm & A. Aertsen, pp. 7–24. Berlin: Springer-Verlag.

Amari, S. & Arbib, M. A., ed. (1982). *Competition and Cooperation in Neural Nets*. Berlin: Springer-Verlag.

Andersen, P. & Andersson, S. A. (1968). *Physiological Basis of the Alpha Rhythm*. New York: Appleton-Century-Crofts.

Asanuma, H. (1975). 'Recent developments in the study of the columnar arrangement of neurons within the motor cortex.' *Physiological Review*, **55**, 143–56.

Bach, M. & Krüger, J. (1986). 'Correlated neuronal variability in monkey visual cortex revealed by a multi-microelectrode.' *Experimental Brain Research*, **61**, 451–6.

Ballard, D. (1986). 'Cortical connections and parallel processing: structure and function.' *The Behavioral and Brain Sciences*, **9**, 67–120.

Best, J. & Dinse, H. R. O. (1984). 'Laminar dependent visual information processing in the cat's area 17.' *Neuroscience Letter Supplement*, **18**, S76.

Blasdel, G. C. & Salama, G. (1986). 'Voltage-sensitive dyes reveal a modular organization in monkey striate cortex.' *Nature*, **321**, 579–85.

Braitenberg, V. & Braitenberg, C. (1979). 'Geometry of orientation columns in the visual cortex.' *Biological Cybernetics*, **33**, 179–87.

Burns, B. D. (1968). *The Uncertain Nervous System*. London: Arnold.

Changeaux, J.-P. & Danchin, A. (1976). 'Selective stabilization of developing synapses as a mechanism for the specification of neuronal networks.' *Nature*, **264**, 705–12.

Dill, R. C., Vallecalle, E. & Verzeano, M. (1968). 'Evoked potentials, neuronal activity and stimulus intensity in the visual system.' *Physiological Behavior*, **3**, 797–801.

Edelman, G. M. (1978). 'Group selection and phasic reentrant signaling: a theory of higher brain function.' In *The Mindful Brain*, eds. G. M. Edelman & V. B. Mountcastle, pp. 51–100. Cambridge: MIT.

Fisher, M. E. & Selke, W. (1980). 'Infinitely many commensurate phases in a simple Ising model.' *Physical Review Letters*, **44**, 1502–5.

Fisher, M. E. (1981). 'Low temperature analysis of the axial next-nearest neighbour Ising model near its multiphase point.' *Philosophical Transactions of the Royal Society of London, Serial A*, **302**, 1–44.

Fuster, J. M. & Jervey, J. P. (1981). 'Inferotemporal neurons distinguish and retain behaviorally relevant features of visual stimuli.' *Science*, **212**, 952–5.

Gerstein, G. L., Perkel, D. H. & Dayhoff, J. E. (1985). 'Cooperative firing activity in simultaneously recorded populations of neurons: detection and measurement.' *Journal of Neuroscience*, **5**, 881–9.

Gilbert, C. D. & Wiesel, T. N. (1983). 'Clustered intrinsic connections in cat visual cortex.' *Journal of Neuroscience*, **3**, 1116–33.

Goldmann-Rakic, P. S. (1984). 'Modular organization of prefrontal cortex.' *Trends in Neuroscience*, **7**, 419–24.

Grinvald, A., Cohen, L. B., Lesher, S. & Boyle, M. B. (1981). 'Simultaneous optical monitoring of activity of many neurons in invertebrate ganglia using a 124-element photodiode array.' *Journal of Neurophysiology*, **45**, 829–40.

Hebb, D. O. (1949). *The Organization of Behavior*. New York: Wiley.

John, E. R. (1972). 'Switchboard versus statistical theories of learning and memory.' *Science*, **177**, 85–864.

Killackey, H. P. (1983). 'The somatosensory cortex of the rodent.' *Trends in Neuroscience*, **6**, 25–429.

Krone, G., Mallot, H., Palm, G. & Schüz, A. (1986). 'Spatiotemporal receptive fields: a dynamical model derived from cortical architectonics.' *Proceedings of the Royal Society of London*, **B226**, 421–44.

Krüger, J. & Bach, M. (1981). 'Simultaneous recording with 30 microelectrodes in monkey visual cortex.' *Experimental Brain Research*, **41**, 191–4.

Little, W. A. (1974). 'Existence of persistent states in the brain.' *Mathematical Biosciences*, **19**, 101–20.

Little, W. A. & Shaw, G. L. (1975). 'A statistical theory of short and long term memory.' *Behavioral Biology*, **14**, 115–33.

Little, W. A. & Shaw, G. L. (1978). 'Analytic study of the storage capacity of a neural network.' *Mathematical Biosciences*, **39**, 281–90.

Morrell, F. (1967). 'Electrical signs of sensory coding.' In *The Neurosciences: A Study Program*, eds. G. C. Quarton, T. Melnechuk & F. O. Schmitt, pp. 452–69. New York: Rockefeller University.

Morrell, F., Hoeppner, T. J. & Toledo-Morrell, L. de (1983). 'Conditioning of single units in visual association cortex: cell-specific behavior within a small population.' *Experimental Neurology*, **80**, 111–46.

Mountcastle, V. B. (1978). 'An organizing principle for cerebral function: the unit module and the distributed system.' In *The Mindful Brain*, eds. G. M. Edelman & V. B. Mountcastle, pp. 1–50. Cambridge: MIT.

Pearson, J. C., Diamond, D. M., McKennan, T. M., Rinaldi, P. C., Shaw, G. L. & Weinberger, N. M. (1983). 'The neuronal coding of rotating bar stimuli in primary visual cortex of cat.' *13th Annual Meeting of the Society for Neuroscience, abstr. 238.9.*

Pisco, G. V. D. (1984). 'Hebb synaptic plasticity.' *Progress in Neurobiology*, **22**, 89–102.

Roney, K. J. & Shaw, G. L. (1980). 'Analytic study of assemblies of neurons in memory storage.' *Mathematical Biosciences*, **51**, 25–41.

Seelen, W. von, Mallot, H. A., Krone, G. T., Dinse, H. (1986). 'On information processing in the cat's visual cortex.' In *Brain Theory*, eds. G. Palm & A. Aertsen, pp. 49–77. Berlin: Springer-Verlag.

Shaw, G. L. (1978). 'Space-time correlations of neuronal firing related to memory storage capacity.' *Brain Research Bulletin*, **3**, 107–113.

Shaw, G. L., Harth, E. & Scheibel, A. B. (1982). 'Cooperativity in brain function: assemblies of approximately 30 neurons.' *Experimental Neurology*, **77**, 324–58.

Shaw, G. L. & Pearson, J. C. (1985). 'Information processing in the cortex: the role of small assemblies of neurons.' In *Information Processing in Biological Systems*, eds. S. L. Mintz & A. Perlmutter, pp. 1–31. New York: Plenum.

Shaw, G. L., Rinaldi, P. C. & Pearson, J. C. (1983). 'Processing capability of the primary visual cortex and possible physiological basis for an apparent motion illusion.' *Experimental Neurology*, **79**, 293–8.

Shaw, G. L. & Ramachandran (1982). 'Interpolation during apparent motion.' *Perception*, 11, 491–4.

Shaw, G. L. & Roney, K. J. (1979). 'Analytic solutions of a neural network theory based on an Ising spin system analogy.' *Physics Letters*, 74A, 146–9.

Shaw, G. L., Silverman, D. J. & Pearson, J. C. (1985). 'Model of cortical organization embodying a basis for a theory of information processing and memory recall.' *Proceedings of the National Academy of Science, USA*, 82, 2364–8.

Shaw, G. L., Silverman, D. J. & Pearson, J. C. (1986). 'Trion model of cortical organization: toward a theory of information processing and memory.' In *Brain Theory*, eds. G. Palm & A. Aertsen, pp. 177–91.

Shaw, G. L. & Vasudevan, R. (1974). 'Persistent states of neural networks and the random nature of synaptic transmission.' *Mathematical Biosciences*, 21, 207–18.

Silverman, D. J., Shaw, G. L. & Pearson, J. C. (1986). 'Associative recall properties of the trion model of cortical organization.' *Biological Cybernetics*, 53, 259–71.

Wiesendanger, M. (1986). 'Redistributive function of the motor cortex.' *Trends in Neuroscience*, 9, 120–4.

Wolfram, S. (1983). 'Statistical mechanics of cellular automata.' *Reviews of Modern Physics*, 55, 601–44.

Wolfram, S. (1984a). 'Cellular automata as models of complexity.' *Nature*, 311, 419–24.

Wolfram, S. (1984b). 'Twenty problems in the theory of cellular automata.' *Physica Scripta*, T9, 170–83.

12

And–or logic analogue of neuron networks

Y. OKABE, M. FUKAYA and M. KITAGAWA

12.1 Introduction

The function of the brain is a far cry from that of existing computer systems. Our knowledge of the information processing mechanism of the brain is rather limited, but we know that the brain consists of a large number of neurons and that the individual neuron can be regarded as a sort of threshold element. So, we can find some similarities between the neuron systems and the existing computer systems.

The similarity we are especially interested in is that both of them can be considered as aggregates of digital circuits. Any function of the digitial circuit which is independent of the previous state can be easily implemented by a two-level AND-to-OR gate network. In addition the threshold element which substitutes for a neuron performs the function of an AND gate or an OR gate according to its threshold value. Those facts inspired us with some ideas about our AND–OR analog of neuron networks. Our neuron network also has two levels. The first level of the network acts as an analyzer of the input patterns, and the second level acts as a generator of the output patterns. The operations assigned to the two levels correspond to those of the AND plane and the OR plane, respectively.

The function of a standard AND-to-OR gate network is determined by its inherent wiring. However, that of our neuron network is to be formed by the interaction with the given environment. The learning process of the network we assume is based on the biological hypothesis that the creatures which have neuron systems tend to avoid continuous and invariable stimuli, in other words, they are fond of moderate changes of the environment. For instance, the reflex including the avoidant behavior from danger should be explained by this hypothesis. We interpret the constant inputs to the reflex systems as a kind of demand on them. The environment keeps requiring the systems to change their outputs until the outputs are satisfactory for the environment. If the output patterns are appropriate for the input patterns, the demands to change their outputs will vanish. Then the different input patterns are to be given, for the neuron systems tend to like some moderate stimuli. Giving the same inputs continuously to the system is equivalent to teaching them that their outputs are inappropriate for the environment. As we adopt this learning principle, special teacher's signals for the individual neurons are unnecessary.

Considering the circumstances mentioned above, we simulate the neuron network which consists of six elements. Four of the elements are for the first level of the network and the rest are for the second level. Each element has qualitatively the same characteristic irrespective of its position. The output of the element takes two possible states: 0 and 1, according to the relation between its threshold and the summation of its weighted inputs.

Our purpose in this paper is to show how the circuits are built by the interaction with the environment and that our hypothesis is reasonable in several situations.

12.2 The structure of the model

We describe here the structure of our neuron network model. The functions of the elements which are the components of the network and the wiring of the elements are mentioned in detail.

Symbolic notation

f_1, f_2: assigned function.

i, j, m, n: integer.

m_1, m_2, m_3, m_4: intermediate state.

t: time.

T_{ai}: active time.

T_{ri}: resting time.

u, u_a: post-synaptic potential.

w_i, w_m, w_n, w_1, w_2: weighting factor.

w_{min}, w_{max}: range of weighting factor.

w_θ: critical weighting factor.

$x_i, x_m, x_n, x_1, x_2, x_{ai}, x_{am}, x_{an}, x_{a1}, x_{a2}$: input signal.

x_a: vector of input pattern.

y, y_1, y_2: output signal.

z: variable.
1: quantizing function.
$\Delta w_i^+, \Delta w_i^-$: change of weighting factor.
$\theta, \theta_\mathrm{p}, \theta_\mathrm{n}$: threshold value.

12.2.1 The functions of the elements

We should imitate the actual neurons when we design the functions of the elements. However, those of actual neurons are not yet clearly elucidated. So, we take this hypothetical neural element. For the characteristics we give to it, the element is expected to fire selectively to the particular input patterns which are generated in the preceding level or the environment.

The block diagram symbol for the neural element is shown in Fig. 12.1. The specification of the element is described in the following four points:

(1) The element has a single output and several inputs that take two possible states: 0 and 1. The output is a function of its post synaptic potential u and its threshold value θ. The potential u is a weighted sum of the input signals $x_1, x_2, \ldots, x_n$ with the weighting factors denoted by $w_1, w_2, \ldots, w_n$, where n is the number of the input nodes or the synapses. The value of u is defined as

$$u = \sum_{i=1}^{n} w_i \cdot x_i \tag{1}$$

We use the quantizing function **1** defined as

$$\mathbf{1}(z) = \begin{cases} 0 & \text{when } z \leq 0 \quad \text{and} \\ 1 & \text{when } z > 0. \end{cases} \tag{2}$$

Then, the output y is described as

$$y = \mathbf{1}(u - \theta). \tag{3}$$

Fig. 12.1. Block diagram symbol for neural element.

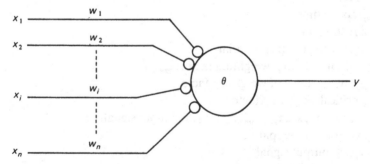

This rule is well-known as the McCulloch–Pitts model proposed in 1943 (McCulloch & Pitts, 1943).

(2) We now describe the dynamics of the weighting factor w_i. As we have already stated, the input patterns should be analyzed in the first level of the network on the analogy of the operation of the AND plane. If we impose the operation of the AND plane on the first level exactly, each element should be characterized to fire selectively to a specific input pattern. The necessary and sufficient condition for the element to fire only to the specific input signals which consist of a pattern $x_a = (x_{a1}, x_{a2}, \ldots, x_{an})$ is as follows:

$$u_a - \theta > 0, \tag{4}$$

$$u_a - w_m - \theta \leqq 0 \quad \text{for any } m \text{ satisfying } x_{am} = 1, \tag{5}$$

$$u_a + w_m - \theta \leqq 0 \quad \text{for any } m \text{ satisfying } x_{am} = 0, \tag{6}$$

$$\text{where } u_a = \sum_{i=1}^{n} w_i \cdot x_{ai}.$$

Considering these conditions, we can find some algorithms which provide the growth of the weighting factors of the element that fires only to a certain pattern x_a. One of the examples is as follows:

(1) In the first place, fix the threshold value at a certain positive number, and reset all of the weighting factors to 0.

(2) Then, give the input pattern x_a to the synapses of the element.

(3) Increase the weighting factor w_i if the input signal arriving at i's synapse x_{ai} is the 1 state.

(4) Decrease the weighting factor w_i, if the input signal x_{ai} is the 0 state.

(5) Stop increasing the weighting factor when the output of the element is in the 1 state.

(6) This algorithm is valid for any input pattern except the zero vector.

We adopt two items described in this algorithm, (3) and (4), when we design the dynamics of the weighting factors. It is inappropriate to accept the whole algorithm because we don't intend to design an element which has a perfect selectivity. Our aim is to get an element which is available for both the first and the second levels of the network. So, we adopt the only two items which are the indispensable extractions of selectivity from the algorithm. The element with such characteristics should have a tendency, in some degree, to fire selectively to a certain pattern.

Considering the circumstances mentioned above, we design the dynamics of the weighting factors. The weighting factor of the i's synapse w_i changes according to the relationship with the input signal x_i arriving at the i's synapse. The weighting factor w_i at time t is given as follows:

Y. Okabe, M. Fukaya & M. Kitagawa

$$w_i(t + 1) = \begin{cases} \begin{rcases} w_i(t) + \Delta w_i^+ & \text{for } x_i = 1 \\ w_i(t) - \Delta w_i^- & \text{for } x_i = 0 \end{rcases} \text{ when } w_i \geqq 0, \text{ and} \\[2ex] \begin{rcases} w_i(t) + \Delta w_i^- & \text{for } x_i = 1 \\ w_i(t) - \Delta w_i^+ & \text{for } x_i = 0 \end{rcases} \text{ when } w_i < 0, \end{cases} \tag{7}$$

where Δw_i^+ and Δw_i^- are the changes of the weighting factor w_i. They are positive constants attributing to the i's synapse and we set conditions on them as

$$\Delta w_i^+ > \Delta w_i^- > 0. \tag{8}$$

This condition contributes toward reducing the disturbance of the weighting factors when some input patterns different from x_a are given to the element. For the sake of preventing divergence of weighting factors, we set them a range given by

$$w_{\min} \leqq w_i \leqq w_{\max}, \tag{9}$$

where $w_{\min}$ is a negative and $w_{\max}$ is a positive constant attributing to the element.

(3) The weighting factor w_i has two kinds of time constants. They are an active time T_{ai} and a resting time T_{ri}. If the state of the input x_i keeps on the same value during T_{ai}, w_i is reset to 0 forcibly. Then the value of w_i is fixed at 0 independent of the input signals during T_{ri}. After that, the weighting factor changes to eqn (7).

By giving such conditions on the element, it should have the nature we proposed in the introduction. That is, the nature of the creatures to tend to avoid constant stimuli.

Fig. 12.2 shows how the weighting factor w_i changes with the input signal x_i.

(4) This element has two possible threshold values: the positive threshold value θ_p is required if the element fires to a pattern including non-zero components on account of the condition (5). On the other hand, the negative threshold value θ_n is required if it fires to the pattern of zero vector on account of the condition (4). So, the mechanism to change the threshold value is necessary for the element. The element changes its threshold value when all of the weighting factors turn to negative, for the state that all of the weighting factors are negative occurs when the zero vector continues to be given to the element. The element chooses its threshold value θ as follows:

$$\theta = \begin{cases} \theta_p & \text{when max } (w_m) > w_\theta, \text{ and} \\ \theta_n & \text{when max } (w_m) \leqq w_\theta \end{cases} \tag{10}$$
$$(m = 1, 2, \ldots, n),$$

where w_θ is a negative constant and is greater than $w_{\min}$.

12.2.2 *The connection between the elements*

Our model is a two-level neuron network, the first level roughly corresponds to the AND plane and the second to the OR plane. Let us consider the network which has k inputs and j outputs. If the first level of the network forms the perfect AND plane, there are 2^k different minterms, so, 2^k neural elements with k inputs are necessary for the first level at least. The number of the elements in the second level is equal to j, whether it forms perfect OR plane or not, and each of them has 2^k inputs.

The wiring diagram of the network is shown in Fig. 12.3. There is no connection between the elements which belong to the same level.

12.2.2 *The learning principle*

The function of this network should be formed by the interaction with the environment, so there is no special teacher which gives the individual elements the information whether the behavior of each element is correct or incorrect. The learning principle is as follows:

(1) The environment keeps on giving the network a certain pattern until it outputs the pattern required by the environment.

(2) The moment that the outputs of the network are satisfactory for the environment, the input pattern given by the environment changes to a different pattern than before.

(3) The weighting factors of the elements change according to eqn (7) while the frequency of the change of the input pattern generated by the environment is low.

Fig. 12.2. Temporal variation of variables. (*a*) An example of variation of input signal x_i, and (*b*) corresponding variation of weighting factor w_i.

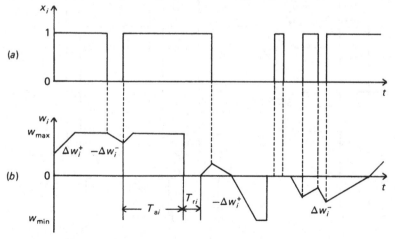

(4) If the input pattern changes frequently, the weighting factors are fixed during that time.

12.2.3 Individuality of the elements

Each element has qualitatively the same characteristic irrespective of its position. However, each has quantitatively a different characteristic from the other, in other words, the constants such as w_{min}, T_{ai}, . . ., etc., vary with the element. If each element has quantitatively the same characteristic, all of the elements which belong to the same level should behave exactly the same.

In order to specialize the operation of each level of the network, we assign different constants to the respective levels. The second level of the network is expected to generate the output pattern, therefore the characteristic time constants T_{ai} and T_{ri} of the elements which consist of the second level are set up rather smaller than those of the first level.

12.3 Computer simulation

Our neuron network model was simulated by a digital computer. There were two inputs and two outputs in the model we simulated, therefore six neural elements were used: four of them were for the first level and the rest were for the second, as shown in Fig. 12.4.

Fig. 12.3. Wiring of model.

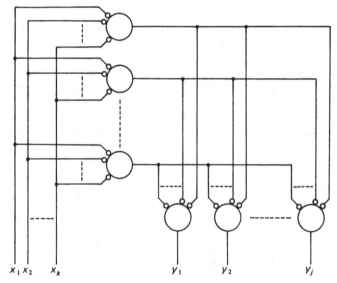

$x_1 x_2 \quad x_k$ $\qquad\qquad y_1 \qquad y_2 \qquad\qquad y_j$

First of all, the environment assigns the network a couple of functions $f_1(x_1, x_2)$ and $f_2(x_1, x_2)$, where x_1 and x_2 are the input signals given by the random-number generator in the computer. The output signals of the network y_1 and y_2 are generated simultaneously with the input signals. The environment requests the state as follows:

$$y_1 = f_1(x_1, x_2) \quad \text{and} \quad y_2 = f_2(x_1, x_2). \tag{11}$$

If the pair of outputs are content with the condition described in eqn (11) for a certain pattern, the environment changes the input patterns. The procedure mentioned above should be repeated until all weighting factors are fixed. The results of this simulation are summarized in Table 12.1.

In order to simplify the simulation program, we added some conditions to the model specifications mentioned in the preceding chapter, those are as follows:

(1) Every variable used in the simulation was quantized because an integer is easy to treat in a digital computer.

(2) If the input pattern of the network changes at time t, the weighting factors do not change at that time step. This is an abbreviation for the condition given in (3) and (4) in Section 12.2.3.

Fig. 12.4. Simulated model: x_1, x_2 – inputs of network; m_1, m_2, m_3, m_4 – intermediate states; y_1, y_2 – outputs of network.

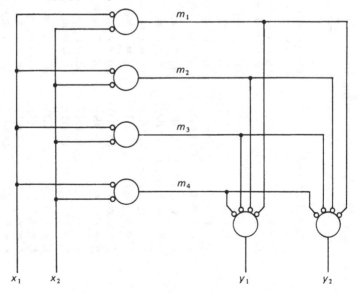

Table 12.1. *Results of simulation*

Assigned functions		Completed functions of each element 1st level/2nd level	Time steps for completion
$f_1 = x_1$		$m_1 = \bar{x}_1 x_2,\ m_2 = x_2,\ m_3 = x_1 + x_2,\ m_4 = \bar{x}_1 x_2$	645
$f_2 = x_2$		$y_1 = \bar{m}_1 m_3 + m_3 \bar{m}_4,\ y_2 = m_1 m_2 + m_2 m_3 + m_2 \bar{m}_4 + m_1 m_3 \bar{m}_4$	
$f_1 = x_1 \bar{x}_2 + \bar{x}_1 x_2$	(EOR)	$m_1 = 0,\ m_2 = x_1 x_2,\ m_3 = x_1 + x_2,\ m_4 = 0$	486
$f_2 = x_1 x_2$	(AND)	$y_1 = \bar{m}_2 m_3 + m_1 m_3 \bar{m}_4,\ y_2 = m_2 + m_4$	
$f_1 = \bar{x}_1$	(NOT)	$m_1 = 0,\ m_2 = \bar{x}_1 \bar{x}_2,\ m_3 = x_1 \bar{x}_2,\ m_4 = \bar{x}_1 + \bar{x}_2$	893
$f_2 = \bar{x}_1 + \bar{x}_2$	(NAND)	$y_1 = \bar{m}_1 m_2 m_4 + \bar{m}_1 \bar{m}_3 m_4 + m_2 \bar{m}_3 m_4,\ y_2 = m_4 + m_2 \bar{m}_3$	
$f_1 = x_1 \bar{x}_2 + \bar{x}_1 x_2$	(EOR)	$m_1 = 0,\ m_2 = \bar{x}_1 x_2,\ m_3 = x_1 \bar{x}_2,\ m_4 = 0$	4538
$f_2 = x_1 x_2 + \bar{x}_1 \bar{x}_2$	(EQU)	$y_1 = m_2 m_3 + m_2 \bar{m}_4 + m_3 \bar{m}_4,\ y_2 = \bar{m}_1 \bar{m}_2 \bar{m}_3 \bar{m}_4$	
$f_1 = x_1 x_2 + \bar{x}_1 \bar{x}_2$	(EQU)	$m_1 = \bar{x}_1 x_2,\ m_2 = x_1 \bar{x}_2,\ m_3 = \bar{x}_1 \bar{x}_2,\ m_4 = 0$	2230
$f_2 = x_1 \bar{x}_2 + \bar{x}_1 x_2$	(EOR)	$y_1 = \bar{m}_1 \bar{m}_2 \bar{m}_3 \bar{m}_4,\ y_2 = m_2 + m_3$	
$f_1 = x_1 x_2$	(AND)	$m_1 = \bar{x}_1 x_2,\ m_2 = x_2,\ m_3 = x_1 + x_2,\ m_4 = 0$	174
$f_2 = x_1 + x_2$	(OR)	$y_1 = \bar{m}_1 m_2 m_3 + \bar{m}_1 m_3 \bar{m}_4 + m_2 m_3 \bar{m}_4$	
$f_1 = \bar{x}_2$	(NOT)	$m_1 = 0,\ m_2 = x_1 \bar{x}_2,\ m_3 = \bar{x}_1 x_2,\ m_4 = \bar{x}_1 + \bar{x}_2$	1880
$f_2 = \bar{x}_1$	(NOT)	$y_1 = \bar{m}_3 m_4,\ y_2 = \bar{m}_1 \bar{m}_2 m_4$	
$f_1 = \bar{x}_1 + \bar{x}_2$	(NAND)	$m_1 = 0,\ m_2 = 0,\ m_3 = \bar{x}_1 \bar{x}_2,\ m_4 = \bar{x}_1 + \bar{x}_2$	440
$f_2 = \bar{x}_1 \bar{x}_2$	(NOR)	$y_1 = \bar{m}_2 m_3 + \bar{m}_2 m_4 + m_3 m_4,\ y_2 = \bar{m}_1 m_3$	
$f_1 = x_1 x_2$	(AND)	$m_1 = \bar{x}_1 + \bar{x}_2,\ m_2 = \bar{x}_1 \bar{x}_2,\ m_3 = \bar{x}_1 x_2,\ m_4 = 0$	1461
$f_2 = \bar{x}_1 + \bar{x}_2$	(NAND)	$y_1 = \bar{m}_1 \bar{m}_2 \bar{m}_3 \bar{m}_4,\ y_2 = m_1 + m_2 + m_4$	
$f_1 = x_2$		$m_1 = x_1 + x_2,\ m_2 = x_1,\ m_3 = x_2,\ m_4 = 0$	122
$f_2 = x_1 + x_2$	(OR)	$y_1 = m_3,\ y_2 = m_1 + \bar{m}_2 m_4$	

12.4 Discussion

The purpose of the paper is to show that some neuron systems are formed by interaction with the environment according to the learning principle we proposed before.

As is shown in Table 12.1, the network could learn the function assigned to it after several thousands of time steps, at most. There were a few functions that took comparatively large time steps to learn. It is hard to specify such functions. However, it seems to be a trend that the functions which need rather more independent minterms, such as the combination of EOR and EQU, take larger time steps. The number of the minterms appearing in the simulated model was less than or equal to four, whereas that of a standard AND–OR network with k inputs is usually equal to 2^k irrespective of the function. For the operation of the first level of the network was different from that of the AND plane. That is to say, the inner operation of the network was not separated completely into the AND plane and the OR plane. The neural element has more functions than a mere AND or OR gate, so it is possible to design a digital circuit elegantly by using the neural elements.

We have shown that our neuron network has the ability to learn some functions assigned by the environment in the case of 2-input, 2-output system. The system we simulated was too small, but our network is allowed to have only a few outputs because the increase of the number of the outputs reduces the chance of completion of the network. That is the nature of a system with a trial–error process. However, we think that this fault is essentially unimportant because the condition that all of the outputs should satisfy the request of the environment simultaneously seems to be too severe, even in the actual neuron systems.

This model leaves other problems to be solved; one of them concerns the learning process of the network. In the model we simulated, every element had the ability to get the information on the environment directly. It might be more natural that each element is influenced only by its own input signals. In this case, the weighting factors of the element should be fixed while the frequency of the change of the input signals arriving at its own synapses or that of its post synaptic potential is high.

12.5 Conclusion

We proposed the learning principle based on the biological hypothesis that creatures tend to avoid constant stimuli, and gave the model for such neuron systems which learn by the interaction with the environment. We adopted the two-level neuron network into our model on the analogy of the AND–OR logic circuits, and designed the hypothetical neural element which is suitable for the component of the network.

Our neuron network model, which consists of six elements, was simulated by a digital computer. As a result, we have shown that our neuron network has the ability to learn any function assigned by the environment in the case of a 2-input, 2-output system. The behavior of creatures observed in the several biological situations has something in common with that of our model. In this simulation, we might show the possibility that there are some natural neuron systems which are similar to our model.

Acknowledgement

The authors wish to thank Prof. T. Sugano for providing excellent working conditions and encouragement.

References

McCulloch, W. S. & Pitts, W. H. (1943). 'A logical calculus of the ideas immanent in nervous activity.' *Bulletin of Mathmatical Biophysics*, 5 (4), pp. 115.

13

Neural networks: learning and forgetting

J. P. NADAL, G. TOULOUSE, M. MÉZARD,
J. P. CHANGEUX and S. DEHAENE

13.1 Introduction

Networks of formal neurons provide simple models for distributed, content addressable, fault-tolerant memory. Many numerical and analytical results have been obtained recently, especially on the Hopfield model (Hopfield, 1982). In this model, a network of a large number of fully connected neurons, with symmetric interactions, has a memory capacity which increases linearly with the size of the network – that is, in fact, with the connectivity. When the total number of stored patterns exceeds this capacity, a catastrophic deterioration occurs, as total confusion sets in. Alternative schemes have been proposed (Hopfield, 1982; Nadal *et al.*, 1986; Parisi, 1986) that avoid overloading: new patterns can always be learned, at the expense of more anciently stored ones which get erased – for this reason, these schemes have been called palimpsest. Numerical and analytical results (Nadal *et al.*, 1986; Mézard *et al.*, 1986) detail the behavior of these models, which show striking analogies with the behavior of human short-term memory. We will review the main results, and point out the possible relevance for human working memory.

In Section 13.2 the origin of the catastrophic deterioration in the standard scheme (Hopfield model) is simply explained. In Section 13.3 simple modifications are shown to lead to short-term memory effects. In Section 13.4 properties of these networks are exposed in close analogy with known data of experimental psychology.

13.2 Basic formulation and memorization threshold

All the models we will consider share the same basic ingredients. The network is made of N fully connected formal neurons S_i, $i = 1, N$. A formal neuron (MacCulloch & Pitts, 1943) is represented by a spin-like

Nadal et al.

variable S_i, which can take two values: $S_i = +1$ (neuron firing), and $S_i = -1$ (neuron quiescent). The synaptic efficacies, which can be either excitatory (positive) or inhibitory (negative), are taken to be symmetric. Hence an energy function can be defined

$$E = -(1/2) \sum_{i \neq j} T_{ij} S_i S_j, \qquad (2.1)$$

and the neuron dynamic is a downhill motion on the energy landscape. (In numerical simulations the Monte-Carlo algorithm is used). The memory is defined by the set of attractors of this relaxational dynamic. Learning of a given pattern $S^\mu = (S_i^\mu)_{i=1,N}$ is obtained by storing some relevant information in the synaptic efficacies. The network should work as an associative memory: setting the network in an initial state identical or close to a stored pattern S^μ, it relaxes toward an attractor S^*; S^μ is said to be recognized if the retrieval quality m, defined by the overlap

$$m = (1/N) \left\langle \sum_i S_i^\mu S_i^* \right\rangle \qquad (2.2)$$

is close to one. In eqn (2.2) the bracket means an average over stochastic noise, whose level is defined by a temperature parameter T.

Each model we will consider is characterized by its learning scheme, that is to say the rules which fix the synaptic efficacies for any given set of patterns to be learned. The standard scheme (Hopfield, 1982) follows a generalized Hebbian rule:

$$T_{ij} = (1/N) \sum_{\mu=1,p} S_i^\mu S_j^\mu. \qquad (2.3)$$

The thermodynamic of this model has been solved (Amit *et al.*, 1985*a,b* and 1986; Crisanti *et al.*, 1986). From all the results obtained on the Hopfield model, we retain here only one of the main features. At any temperature T (below some critical value), there is a maximal capacity $\alpha_c(T)$: for $\alpha = p/N < \alpha_c$, the network works as an associative memory. For $\alpha > \alpha_c$, the system enters a spin-glass phase, and all retrieval properties are lost. Within the memory phase ($\alpha < \alpha_c$) retrieval quality is very good. At, say, zero temperature, it decreases slightly from $m = 1$ at $\alpha = 0$, to $m = 0.97$ at $\alpha = \alpha_c \simeq 0.14$.

Constructive criticisms of this model have been made, bearing on its biological relevance. Among other works, it has been shown (Hopfield, 1984) that networks of neurons described by continuous spin variables have the same qualitative recognition properties as networks of formal neurons. Similarly, dissymmetrisation of the synapses does not significantly impair the general picture (Hopfield, 1982) – although this can induce new features also (Parisi, 1986*b*; Hertz *et al.*, 1986). Analysis of partially connected networks (Sompolinsky, 1986) has clarified how connectivity governs the memory capacity. The dynamics of learning, the problem of time delays, have been tackled by Peretto (1986). One fundamental issue, the problem of instructive versus selective learning, has been addressed recently (Toulouse *et al.*, 1986). Here we will be concerned only with the afore-mentioned deterioration of the memory, as related to a lack of constraints on the plasticity of the synapses.

So let us consider the acquisition of a new pattern S^p, after $(p-1)$ have been stored. This is achieved through the rule:

$$T_{ij}(p) = T_{ij}(p-1) + \Delta T_{ij}(p), \tag{2.4}$$

with

$$\Delta T_{ij}(p) = \sigma(p)S_i^p S_j^p; \tag{2.5}$$

$\sigma(p)$ is the acquisition amplitude (which is kept constant in the Hopfield scheme). Now this pth pattern is effectively memorized if, for each neuron i (for simplicity we consider the zero temperature limit):

$$\sum_{i=j} T_{ij}(p)S_i^p S_j^p > 0. \tag{2.6}$$

The quantity on the left-hand side can be decomposed in two terms:

$$\sum_{i=j} T_{ij}(p-1)S_i^p S_j^p + \sum_{ij} \Delta T_{ij}(p)S_i^p S_j^p.$$

For patterns chosen independently at random, the first term is a sum of N independent random variables, of zero mean, and thus for large N behaves like $[NK(p-1)]^{1/2}$, where K is the cumulant

$$K(p) = \overline{T_{ij}^2} - \overline{T_{ij}}^2. \tag{2.7}$$

Here the bar means averaging over the distribution of patterns. The second term is simply equal to $(N-1)\sigma(p)$. Hence, the pth pattern is safely stored if $\sigma(p)$ is greater than some threshold value $\sigma^*(p)$:

$$\sigma(p) > \sigma^*(p) = \varepsilon[K(p-1)/N]^{1/2}, \tag{2.8}$$

where ε is some numerical parameter. Since the stored patterns are independent, the cumulant is simply the sum of the acquisition intensities:

$$K(p) = K(0) + \sum_{\mu=1,p} \sigma^2(\mu), \tag{2.9}$$

$K(O)$ being its value before learning.

Within the Hopfield scheme, the acquisition amplitude is uniform

$$\sigma(p) = \sigma. \tag{2.10}$$

Hence, starting from *tabula rasa* $(K(0) = 0)$,

$$K(p) = p\sigma^2 \tag{2.11}$$

and the pth pattern is memorized if the condition (2.8) is fulfilled, which gives

$$p/N < \alpha_c = 1/\varepsilon^2. \qquad (2.12)$$

Clearly, the threshold condition applies also at any time for any previously stored pattern. Since here all the amplitudes are equal, this means that as soon as p/N becomes greater than α_c, all the patterns are simultaneously forgotten.

From the estimate $\alpha_c = 0.14$, one finds $\varepsilon \simeq 2.6$. This value is in striking accord with the spin glass estimate (Toulouse *et al.*, 1986): starting with random initial interactions $T_{ij}(0) = \pm 1/\sqrt{N}$, and storing one pattern ξ by $T_{ij} = T_{ij}(0) + (\varepsilon/N)\xi_i\xi_j$, one finds that the retrieval quality is almost perfect for $\varepsilon \simeq 2.5 - 2.7$ (Fig. 13.1).

It is now clear that to avoid overloading effect, one has to control the amplitude acquisitions compared to the actual noise level K. The simplest way to achieve it is to increase, at each new learning event, the amplitude acquisition, in such a way that (at least) the newly stored pattern is safely memorized (Nadal *et al.*, 1986). This however leads to an exponential growth of this amplitude, and of the cumulant K, with the number of stored patterns. A more realistic method is to control the level K. This leads mainly to two models, which we discuss now.

Fig. 13.1. Retrieval quality of the first stored pattern, as a function of the acquisition amplitude ε. Before learning, the synaptic efficacies have random values, $\pm 1/\sqrt{N}$. The calculation is made at zero temperature, for $N = 100$ and $N = 200$.

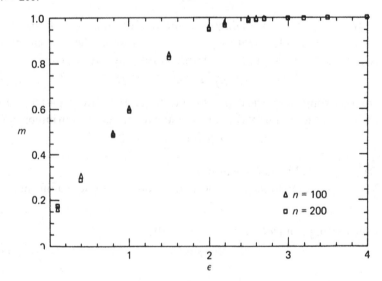

13.3 Palimpsest schemes

13.3.1 *Learning with bounded synaptic efficacies*

We make the assumption that the synaptic efficacies are bounded above and below (Nadal *et al.*, 1986; see also Hopfield, 1982; Vedenov & Levchenko, 1985; Parisi, 1986*a*):

$$0 \leq T_{ij} \leq A \quad \text{or} \quad -A \leq T_{ij} \leq 0. \tag{3.1}$$

The acquisition amplitude is kept constant. From the thermodynamic point of view the proper scaling is

$$A = 1/\sqrt{N}, \tag{3.2}$$

$$\Delta T_{ij}(\mu) = (\varepsilon/N) S_i^\mu S_j^\mu. \tag{3.3}$$

The learning protocol is now (see Fig. 13.2):

$$T_{ij}(p) = \begin{cases} T_{ij}(p-1) + \Delta T_{ij}(p), & \text{if no bound is reached,} \\ \text{value of the reached bound otherwise.} \end{cases} \tag{3.4}$$

For very small ε, the bounds will have no effect, and the catastrophic deterioration still occurs. For very large $\varepsilon(\varepsilon \geq \sqrt{N})$, the last pattern is optimally memorized. This suggests that a transition occurs as a function of ε. Indeed, numerical simulations show that for ε greater than some threshold ε_c, after a great number of patterns has been stored, the network has a stationary capacity: a well-defined number of the most recently stored patterns are memorized, and the older ones are forgotten. This stationary capacity goes through a maximum value $\alpha_{opt} \simeq 0.015\,N$ at $\varepsilon_{opt} \simeq 3$. Retrieval quality is about 0.93 at ε_c, and increases rapidly with ε, being 0.97 around ε_{opt}.

Fig. 13.2. Typical evolution (with the number of stored patterns) of an excitatory synaptic efficacy, in the model of learning within bounds.

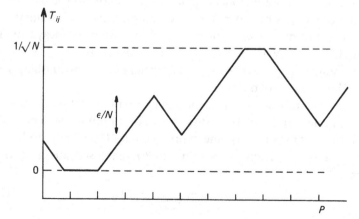

13.3.2 Marginalist scheme

In this scheme, it is the averaged cumulant of the synaptic efficacies which is kept fixed. This is done via the following learning rule:

$$T_{ij}(p) = \lambda[T_{ij}(p - 1) + (\varepsilon/N)S_i^p S_j^p]. \qquad (3.5)$$

That is, λ is chosen such that, after each new learning with amplitude acquisition ε/N, the cumulant K is brought back to its previous level. Hence, for a proper choice of ε (and λ), the threshold condition (2.8) can be valid for each new learning event – this is why this scheme has been called marginalist. For independent random patterns, after a great number of them have been learned, one can take

$$\lambda = \exp(-\varepsilon^2/2N). \qquad (3.6)$$

In this asymptotic regime, if we number the patterns according to remote ancestry, i.e., ξ^1 is the most recently stored pattern, ξ^2 the previously stored, and so on, one has

$$T_{ij} = (\varepsilon/N) \sum_{\mu \geq 1} \lambda^\mu \xi_i^\mu \xi_j^\mu \qquad (3.7)$$

and

$$K = 1/N. \qquad (3.8)$$

The thermodynamic of this model can be solved (Mézard *et al.*, 1986) in the very same way as for the Hopfield model. One finds that the qualitative properties of this scheme are very much the same as those of the previous scheme (of learning within bounds). In particular, there is a threshold value ε_c such that, for $\varepsilon > \varepsilon_c$, the network has a stationary capacity. This capacity goes through a maximum at some value ε_{opt}, and this optimal capacity is proportional to N (see Fig. 13.3). Note that the scaling is such that ε_c and ε_{opt} are independent of the size of the network – but, of course, they are model dependent. For both models one can see why the capacity is of order N: in the first one, the typical number of learning events during which a synaptic efficacy remains away from the bounds is of order N; in the second one, from the expression of λ one sees that the number of patterns whose actual weight λ^μ is non-vanishing in the large N limit, is also of order N.

In these palimpsestic schemes the serial order of the stored patterns is obviously relevant. It is here worth stressing the difference with models of non-linear synapses as, say, the clipping model (Hopfield, 1982; Sompolinsky, 1986; van Hemmen & Kühn, 1986): in this scheme the learning rule is

$$T_{ij}(p) = \text{sign} \left(\sum_{\mu=1, p} S_i^\mu S_j^\mu \right). \qquad (11.9)$$

Although the absolute value of the synaptic efficacies is kept constant, all the patterns are equivalent, as in the Hopfield scheme. Note also that the learning of a new pattern requires the knowledge of the complete sum $\Sigma\, S_i^\mu S_j^\mu$, an information which is not stored in the synapses.

We now come back to the main properties of the short-term memory models, in close relationship with known properties of the human working memory.

13.4 Neural networks and experimental psychology

Let us first recall some features of these neural networks models. The 'psychological tasks' that are performed are *recognition* tasks, as opposed to free recall tasks. Also, in most computations, independent random patterns are learned. Conversely, it is well known in experimental psychology that human memory performances can be qualitatively very different whether memory is tested by recognition or free recall, and whether the learned items are uncorrelated, nonsense material (digits, nonsense syllables . . .), or correlated, meaningful material (sentences . . .). Hence it is with recognition tasks, using nonsense material, that the analogies with human short-term memory are more likely to be relevant.

Fig. 13.3. Stationary capacity α_c in the marginalist scheme as a function of ε, at zero temperature.

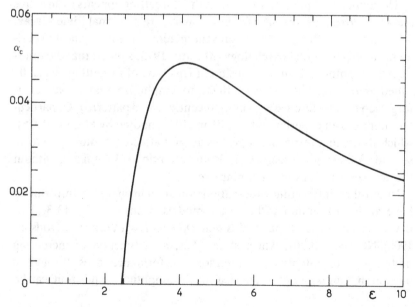

One remark – what is measured by psychologists is a *probability* of recall or recognition. In the analysis of the models, the decision of recognition was assumed to rely on the value of the retrieval quality, eqn (1.2). The unambiguity of such a decision is possible since, in the infinite N limit, the retrieval quality has with probability one a well-defined value, which is close to one for some patterns (the 'memorized' ones), and very small for all the other patterns ('forgotten' ones). However, for finite N, there are huge finite size effects. In particular distribution of the retrieval quality has two peaks, one at a value close to one, and one at a value close to zero, whose relative weight increases while the pattern is progressively erased. Hence the retrieval quality still provides a criterion for the decision, and the statistical fluctuations provide its probabilistic aspect.

The basic phenomenon is the *recency* effect. It implies the notions of serial position effect (Murdock, 1962), and of memory span. Human memory span is well known to be 'seven plus or minus two' (Ebbinghaus, 1885; Miller, 1956), largely independent of modality and material (digits, words, drawings, . . .). In our models, say in the scheme with bounded synaptic efficacies, such a capacity is reached for a connectivity of about 500 (we remark that the stronger the constraints, the lower the capacity). This suggests that the short-term memory span might essentially be determined by the cortex connectivity – which is known to be quite uniform.

The main consequence, however, is that forgetting appears as an active *masking effect*, as distinct from a passive relaxational time decay. Although both effects might be present in human memory, most experiments in experimental psychology (Masaro, 1975) suggest that the interference hypothesis is more plausible. (This type of forgetting is usually called *retroactive interference* effect, to emphasise that a pattern is forgotten by interference with more recently stored patterns). Of particular interest is an experiment by Shiffrin (1973, quoted by Masaro, 1975), which shows that retrieval properties are not affected if, during up to 40 seconds following the learning task, the attention is kept fixed, without the occurrence of any new learning event.

Now other interesting observations on human memory turn out to have an interpretation within these models. Consider Fig. 13.3. This is very reminiscent of the *Yerkes and Dodson law* (Yerkes & Dodson, 1908; Norman, 1976), which states that, as a function of increasing motivation, or intensity of attention, performance goes through a maximum. Our parameter ε, measuring the amplitude acquisition, can be thought of reflecting directly the intensity of attention during the learning process.

This interpretation of the amplitude acquisition leads immediately to an appealing explanation of the *primacy* effect. This is the fact that after learning a list of items, the probability of recall or recognition of the first stored item remains relatively high (Murdock, 1962; Masaro, 1975). It is quite natural to assume that, just before the learning task begins, the attention – hence ε – is held very high. Thus the first item is perfectly memorized. However, in order to memorize more than one item, the attention has to be lowered – so that ε is shifted toward the optimal value. We have simulated this effect for the scheme with bounded T_{ij}. The first pattern is stored with maximal acquisition amplitude, each synaptic efficacy reaching its lower or upper bound. Subsequent patterns are stored with a uniform value of ε, $\varepsilon = 4$. For 100 neurons, the 'time' during which the first pattern can still be recognized is about twice the normal capacity at this value of ε.

Finally, we mention two effects, one expected and one unexpected, but of similar basis. Learning by reinforcement is a well-known and used effect ('to teach is to repeat'). It is interesting that, for the marginalist scheme, an analytical study can be made, quantifying the increase of the capacity due to repetitive learning (see Mézard *et al.*, 1986). Numerical simulations give very similar results for the other scheme. A limitation to the capacity is the noise due to anciently stored patterns, uncorrelated to the actual ones, as explained in Section 13.2. Clearly, repetitive learning will diminish this noise.

Obviously, the lowest noise level is obtained at the beginning of learning, when starting with *tabula rasa*. Indeed, when storing random patterns with uniform amplitude ε, all of them are memorized, until some critical number $p^* = \alpha^* N$. Although smaller than the optimal value in the Hopfield model, α^* can be much larger than α_c – especially for small ε. If more and more patterns are stored, the capacity decreases, eventually reaching its stationary value α_c. (Note that this effect subsists when starting with non-zero synaptic efficacies, provided the cumulant $K(0)$ is significantly smaller than its asymptotic value). Surprisingly, this is in striking analogy with the so-called *proactive interference* effect (Keppel & Underwood, 1962; Postman, 1976): at the beginning of a learning session, the memory span is typically much higher than its final asymptotic value. Although psychologists admit that this loss of capacity comes from interference with the previously stored items, its basis is not at all understood.

13.5 Conclusion

We have shown that, within the framework of formal networks, the introduction of a natural constraint leads to improved performances of the system: the network becomes robust to new learning events. Different models, taking into account in different manners the same type of constraint, have been introduced and shown to lead to the same qualitative behavior. Their properties have been studied by numerical and analytical means. The analogies with human short-term memory are very suggestive: the main effects observed in experimental psychology have a simple explanation within the context of these neural network models.

Let us conclude with a word on long-term memory. From the above discussion, one may wonder how these neural networks can be used for long-term memory modeling. Within the Hopfield scheme, obviously one can avoid the deterioration if the plasticity of the synapses is limited to a short enough time duration. This is not unrealistic for some early learnings. Another way to obtain the same result is, again, to assume that each synaptic efficacy is bounded, but this time that it is fixed once it reaches a bound. This mechanism is used, for example, by Linsker (1986), in modeling some early learning in the visual cortex, and by Peretto (1986), in a general model of long- and short-term memory. We note that, in similarity with the effect of proactive interference described in Section 13.4, the capacity of such an everlasting memory, still linear in the connectivity, can however be significantly higher than the short-term capacity.

Acknowledgements

We acknowledge K. O'Regan for providing us with some useful references of experimental psychology.

References

Amit, D. J., Gutfreund, H. & Sompolinsky, H. (1985a). *Physical Review*, **A32**, 1007.
Amit, D. J., Gutfreund, H. & Sompolinsky, H. (1985b). *Physical Review Letter*, **55**, 1530–3.
Amit, D. J., Gutfreund, H. & Sompolinsky, H. (1986). *Ann. Phys.*, **173**, 30.
Crisanti, A., Amit, D. J. & Gutfreund, H. (1986). *Europhysics Letters*, **2**, 337–41.
Ebbinghaus, H. (1885). *Uber das Gedachtnis*. Leipzig: Duncker und Humblot.
Hertz, J. A., Grinstein, G. & Solla, S. A. (1987). In *Heidelberg Colloquium on Glassy Dynamics*, edited by van Hemmen, J. L. and Morgenstern, I. (Springer, Berlin), p. 538.
Hopfield, J. J. (1982). *Proc. Natl. Acad. Sci. USA*, **79**, 2554–8.
Hopfield, J. J. (1984). *Proc. Natl. Acad. Sci. USA*, **81**, 3088–92.
Keppel, G., Underwood, J. (1962). *Journal of Verbal Learning and Verbal Behavior*, **1**, 153–61.

Linsker, R. (1986). *Proc. Natl. Acad. Sci. USA*, **83**, 7508, 8390, 8779.

MacCulloch, W. W. & Pitts, W. (1943). *Bull. Math. Biophys.*, **5**, 115–33.

Masaro, D. W. (1975). *Experimental Psychology and Information Processing*. Chicago: Rand McNally College Publishing Co.

Mézard, M., Nadal, J. P. & Toulouse, G. (1986). *Journal de Physique (Paris)*, **47**, 1457–62.

Miller, G. A. (1956). *Psychological Review*, **63**, 81–97.

Murdock Jr, B. B. (1962). *Journal of Experimental Psychology*, **64**, 482–8.

Nadal, J. P., Toulouse, G., Changeux, J. P. & Dehaene, S. (1986). *Europhysics Letters*, **1**, 535–42.

Norman, D. A. (1976). *Memory and Attention*, 2nd edn. J. Wiley and Sons.

Parisi, G. (1986a). *Journal of Physics A: Math. Gen.*, **19**, L617–20.

Parisi, G. (1986b). *Journal of Physics A: Math. Gen.*, **19**, L675–80.

Peretto, P. (1986). (This volume).

Postman, L. (1976). In *Recall and Recognition*, ed. J. Brown, p. 157. J. Wiley and Sons.

Shiffrin, R. M. (1973). *Journal of Experimental Psychology*, **100**, 39–49.

Sompolinsky, H. (1986), in press.

Toulouse, G., Dehaene, S. & Changeux, J. P. (1986). *Proc. Natl. Acad. Sci. USA*, **83**, 1695–8.

van Hemmen, J. L. & Kühn, R. (1986). *Physical Review Letter*, **57**, 913–16.

Vedenov, A. A., Levchenko, E. B. (1985). *JETP Letters*, **41**, 402–6.

Yerkes, R. M. & Dodson, J. D. (1908). *Journal of Comparative Neurology and Psychology*, **18**, 459–82.

14

Learning by error corrections in spin glass models of neural networks

S. DIEDERICH, M. OPPER, R. D. HENKEL
and W. KINZEL

14.1 Introduction

Neural networks of spin glass type reveal remarkable properties of a content-addressable memory (Hopfield, 1982; Amit *et al.*, 1985; Kinzel, 1985*a*). They are able to retrieve the full information of a learned pattern from an initial state which contains only partial information. Recently much effort has been devoted to the modeling of networks based on Hebb's learning rule (Cooper *et al.*, 1979). These networks are the Hopfield model and its modifications. All have in common a local learning rule which allows the storage of orthogonal patterns without errors. The learning rule is local if the change of the synaptic coefficient depends only on the states of the two interconnected neurons and possibly on the local field of the postsynaptic one. This property seems to be essential from a biological point of view. However, the storing capability of these networks is strongly limited by the fact that they are not able to store correlated patterns without errors (Kinzel, 1985*b*).

On the other hand a storing procedure for correlated patterns is available (Personnaz *et al.*, 1985; Kanter & Sompolinsky, 1986). But it involves matrix inversions which are not equivalent to a local learning mechanism. It is the purpose of this paper to present a new local learning rule for neural networks which are able to store both correlated and uncorrelated patterns. Moreover, this learning rule enables the network to fulfil two further important properties of natural networks: the learning process does not reverse the signs of the synaptic coefficients and leads to a network with unsymmetric bonds even if it starts from a symmetric one. Of course we do not claim to represent all features of a natural network. But we think that our model does bring a network of two-state neurons substantially closer to physiological evidence.

The paper is organized as follows. In Section 14.2 we define and explain the learning rule. The learning behaviour for random patterns is investigated in Section 14.3. Section 14.4 presents some results for the retrieval of noisy patterns. Concluding remarks follow in Section 14.5.

14.2 The learning rule

The neural network is modeled analogous to a spin glass, i.e., as a system of N interconnected two-state neurons S_i, $S_i = 1$ (firing) or $S_i = -1$ (inactive), $i = 1 \ldots N$. Neuron i receives a local field E_i from the other neurons j given by

$$E_i = \sum_{j=1}^{N} J_{ij} S_j .$$

The bond strength J_{ij} characterizes the synaptic efficacy from neuron j to neuron i. Self-coupling terms J_{ii} are excluded ($J_{ii} = 0$).

The dynamics of this model are assumed to be sequential single spin-flip dynamics used in $T = 0$ Monte Carlo calculations. That means, a spin-flip occurs if $S_i E_i < 0$. All the local fields are updated before the next spin is tested.

Dynamically stable states $S = (S_1, \ldots, S_N)$ of the system are characterized by

$$S_i E_i = \sum_{j=1}^{N} S_i J_{ij} S_j > 0 \qquad (1)$$

for $i = 1, \ldots, N$, i.e., all spins are aligned with their local fields.

We initiate our learning procedure with a random network which is fully connected. We start with a spin-glass (Sherrington & Kirkpatrick, 1975), i.e., the synaptic couplings J_{ij}^o are assumed to be independent random variables. They are symmetric, $J_{ij}^o = J_{ji}^o$, and Gaussian distributed with mean zero and variance $1/N$.

The prescribed patterns $S^\nu = (S_1^\nu, \ldots, S_N^\nu)$ $\nu = 1, \ldots, p$ – they may be correlated or not – are to be embedded in this network. To guarantee the local stability of an embedded pattern with respect to the dynamics of the system it is not sufficient to satisfy eqn (1). Indeed, this system of equations merely characterizes time independent states. For a state to act as a local attractor it is important to replace the threshold on the right-hand side of eqn (1) by a positive number T of O(1). This can be proven easily for a large network with $J_{ij} = O(1/\sqrt{N})$. For simplicity's sake we choose $T = 1$ and characterize the embedding of a pattern ν by the following modification of eqn (1):

$$S_i^\nu E_i^\nu = \sum_{j=1}^{N} S_i^\nu J_{ij} E_j^\nu > 1 \qquad (2)$$

for $i = 1, \ldots, N$. Note that the corresponding equation in the case of Hebb's learning rule with orthogonal patterns is given by

$$S_i^\nu \sum_{j=1}^{N} J_{ij} S_j^\nu = 1$$

for $i = 1, \ldots, N$.

The purpose of the learning procedure is to establish the embedding condition (2) for every pattern $S^\nu = (S_1^\nu, \ldots, S_N^\nu)$ $\nu = 1, \ldots, p$ to be stored. To achieve this goal we start from the random network $\{J_{ij}^0\}$ defined above. Then the system is led to memorize the set of patterns $\{S^\nu\}$ via a sequence of modifications of the synaptic strengths J_{ij}.

To define and to explain the learning rule, we start with pattern $\nu = 1$ and check if this pattern is already embedded in the network, i.e., the system of eqn (2) is obeyed for $\nu = 1$. In case, for example, eqn (2) is not satisfied for neuron i, we change the synaptic strengths $J_{ij} = J_{ij}^0$ according to the rule

$$J_{ij} \rightarrow J_{ij}(1 + S_i^\nu S_j^\nu \operatorname{sgn} (J_{ij})\Delta) \tag{3}$$

for $j = 1, \ldots, N$. Here we have introduced a parameter $\Delta > 0$. This simultaneous updating of the bonds J_{ij} occurs only if the embedding condition is not satisfied for i. In case it is satisfied we leave the bonds J_{ij} unchanged for $j = 1, \ldots, N$. The updating leads to a change of the local field at site i by

$$S_i^\nu \delta E_i^\nu = \sum_{j=1}^{N} S_i^\nu J_{ij} S_i^\nu S_j^\nu \operatorname{sgn} (J_{ij}) \cdot \Delta \cdot S_j^\nu = \sum_{j=1}^{N} |J_{ij}| \cdot \Delta,$$

which is of $O(\sqrt{N}) \cdot \Delta$. Together with the embedding condition this result suggests the scaling $\Delta = \lambda/\sqrt{N}$, thus introducing a free parameter λ.

The essential point of this storage mechanism is based on a coherent modification of the magnitudes of the synaptic connections. Frustrated bonds ($S_i^\nu S_j^\nu \operatorname{sgn} (J_{ij}) < 0$) become reduced in absolute magnitude ($|J_{ij}| \rightarrow |J_{ij}|(1 - \Delta)$), whereas unfrustrated bonds ($S_i^\nu S_j^\nu \operatorname{sgn} (J_{ij}) > 0$) become enhanced ($|J_{ij}| \rightarrow |J_{ij}|(1 + \Delta)$). In contrast to the individual changes $\delta J_{ij} = \pm J_{ij} \cdot \Delta$, which are of $O(1/N)$, the sums $S_i^\nu \delta E_i^\nu = \Sigma_j^N S_i^\nu S_j^\nu \delta J_{ij}$ are positive and of $O(1)$.

To proceed with the learning process we pass to pattern $\nu = 2$ and update the synaptic strengths J_{ij} in the same way, and so on. This leads to a sequence of modifications of the synaptic coefficients from $\nu = 1$ up to $\nu = p$, which altogether constitute one step of the learning procedure. These steps have to be performed again and again up to that point where the embedding conditions become satisfied simultaneously for every pattern ν and every site i. This completes the learning process.

We summarize the main issues of our learning rule.

(1) Proceeding from a random network the learning mechanism generates an unsymmetric synaptic matrix.

(2) According to the local learning rule

$$\delta J_{ij} = |J_{ij}|S_i^\nu S_j^\nu \cdot \theta(1 - S_i^\nu E_i^\nu) \cdot \Delta. \tag{4}$$

($\theta(x)$ is the step function: $\theta(x < 0) = 0$, $\theta(x > 0) = 1$), the synaptic couplings become gradually modified. The individual changes of each coupling depend only on the actual states of the presynaptic S_j^ν and postsynaptic S_i^ν neurons and of the local field E_i^ν.

(3) The synaptic coefficients preserve their signs throughout the learning procedure.

(4) Correlated patterns can be memorized without producing errors.

One may doubt the necessity of point (3), arguing that J_{ij} represents only the net effect of many synaptic couplings between the two neurons. Therefore, it could well change sign. In this case eqn (4) could be replaced by the additive learning rule

$$J_{ij} \rightarrow J_{ij} + (\lambda/N)S_i^\nu S_j^\nu \cdot \theta(1 - S_i^\nu E_i^\nu), \tag{5}$$

allowing for sign reversals. The simulation of this learning rule also leads to a convergent procedure.

A few remarks may be added. In the course of the learning process the patterns are presented sequentially $\nu = 1, \ldots, p$ to the network following one and the same order. We may equally well select the patterns randomly. By this way a procedure is obtained which does not single out one order.

Another point worth mentioning, concerns the parameter $\Delta = \lambda/\sqrt{N}$, which may be chosen dependent on the local field E_i^ν, for example $\lambda = f(1 - E_i^\nu S_i^\nu)$. By a suitable choice of the function $f()$ this may provide a fine tuning of the variations of the local fields with respect to the threshold T in eqn (2).

14.3 Learning of random patterns

The storage properties of the network with respect to $p = \alpha N$ random patterns $S^\nu = (S_1^\nu, \ldots, S_N^\nu)$ $\nu = 1, \ldots, p$ have been investigated numerically. The S_i^ν are independent random variables which take the values $+1$ and -1 with equal probability. Fig. 14.1 shows that our learning procedure indeed converges for the range of α values investigated. Remarkably, the average number of steps $\langle l \rangle$ needed to memorize a set of $p = \alpha N$ patterns depends on λ and $\alpha = p/N$, not on the systems size N, i.e., $\langle l \rangle =$ function (α, λ). This is a good approximation at least for small values of α. At larger values of α there seems to be an additional dependence on the system size N, i.e., the number of steps needed to store a set of $p = \alpha N$ patterns decreases slightly with increasing N (α remains fixed).

Of course, we expect that the system cannot store any arbitrary large number of patterns. But a huge amount of CPU time would be needed to carry out the calculation up to higher values of α and to determine, for example, the storage capacity of the network. An analytic approximate analysis of the learning process will be presented in a subsequent paper.

14.4 Retrieval of noisy patterns

In this section we demonstrate that a network equipped with this learning rule will act as a content-addressable memory. For this purpose we present a pattern to the network which differs slightly from a memorized one $S^\beta = (S_1^\beta, \ldots, S_N^\beta)$. It is easily obtained from the memorized pattern

Fig. 14.1. Average number of steps $\langle l \rangle$ needed to embed $p = \alpha N$ patterns as a function of α, $\langle l \rangle$ is calculated as an average over 40 different samples (sets of $p = \alpha N$ random patterns to be embedded in a random network). The simulations have been carried out for three different system sizes N: $N = 144$ (squares); $N = 256$ (triangles); $N = 400$ (circles), a solid line is drawn to join these circles. All these calculations have been performed with the parameter choice $\lambda = 1$. The corresponding results for parameter choice $\lambda = 3.2$ and system size $N = 400$ are indicated by the broken line.

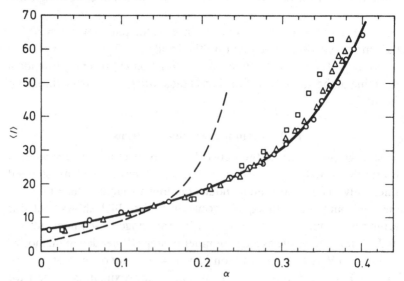

by reversing $p_n \cdot N$ randomly selected neurons. Serving as initial state S(o) for the retrieval process, this noisy pattern evolves into a final state S(t → ∞). The overlap $q = (1/N) \Sigma_{i=1}^{N} S_i(t \to \infty)$. S_i^β measures the extent to which the retrieved pattern coincides with the memorized pattern S^β.

We consider first the case of random patterns ($S_i^\nu = \pm 1$ with equal probability). The average overlap $\langle q \rangle$ is depicted in Fig. 14.2 as a function of noise level p_n. We find that a pattern with up to 20% neurons flipped is recognized with only minor retrieval errors.

To give an example of the performance in the case of highly correlated patterns the network is led to store the six capital letters A → F drawn in Fig. 14.3 (lines I). The retrieval process is carried out with 30% errors (lines II). The recovered states are depicted in Fig. 14.3 (lines III). One pattern (A) was not recognized at all. In fact, by visual inspection we observe that a lot of information has been destroyed by the noise.

14.5 Concluding remarks

In a previous approach the storing of the patterns was achieved by replacing all frustrated bonds by zero (Kinzel, 1985; van Hemmen & van

Fig. 14.2. Average retrieval overlap $\langle q \rangle$ versus noise level p_n for $N = 256$ neurons, $p = 26$ patterns ($\alpha = 0.1$). The parameter λ is chosen as $\lambda = 3.2$.

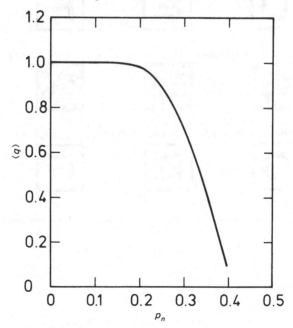

Fig. 14.3. The six patterns of A → F (lines I) are stored in a network with $N = 16 \times 16$ neurons. The patterns in lines II are provided with $p_n = 30\%$ errors.

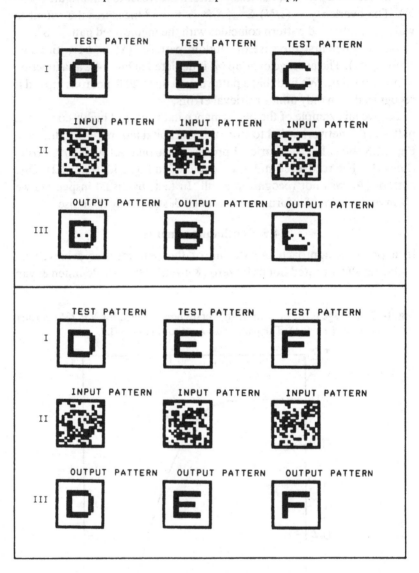

Enter, 1986). In the course of our learning process the synaptic coefficients become gradually modified. But they only change if required, that is if a presented pattern does not yet fulfil the embedding condition. The change of the bonds is controlled by the outcome, i.e., the local potential. This seems reasonable from a biological point of view. The same is true for the additive learning rule (5). Results for this modified learning rule will be published elsewhere.

We would like to point out that the retrieval process (Section 14.4) has never run into cycles, i.e., periodic sequences of states. These are generally expected to be present in unsymmetric neural networks. We explain this phenomena by the 'weak' asymmetry of our network, which was completely symmetric before we initiated our learning procedure. Moderate asymmetry has little effect on dynamic stability (Hopfield & Tank, 1986).

Acknowledgement

One of the authors (S.D.) thanks Eberhard Fetz, Seattle for the inspiring talks which turned out to be germinal for the present work.

References

Amit, D. J., Gutfreund, H. & Sompolinsky, H. (1985). 'Storing infinite numbers of patterns in a spin-glass model of neural networks.' *Physical Review Letters*, **55**, 1530–3.

Cooper, L. N., Liberman, F. & Oja, E. (1979). *'Biological Cybernetics'*, **33**, 9–28.

Hopfield, J. J. (1982). 'Neural networks and physical systems with emergent collective computational abilities.' *Proceedings of the National Academy of Sciences of the USA*, **79**, 2554–8.

Hopfield, J. J. & Tank, D. W. (1986). 'Computing with neural circuits: a model.' *Science*, **233**, 625–33.

Kanter, I. & Sompolinsky, H. (1986). 'Associative recall of memory without errors.' *Physical Review A*, **35**, 380–92.

Kinzel, W. (1985a). 'Spin glasses as model systems for neural networks.' In *Complex Systems – Operational Approaches in Neurobiology, Physics and Computers*, ed. H. Haken, pp. 107–15. Berlin: Springer Verlag.

Kinzel, W. (1985b). 'Learning and pattern recognition in spin glass models.' *Zeitschrift für Physik B*, **60**, 205–13.

Personnaz, L., Guyon, I. & Dreyfus, G. (1985). 'Information storage and retrieval in spin-glass like neural networks.' *Journal de Physique Lettres*, **46**, L359–L365.

Sherrington, D. & Kirkpatrick, S. (1975). 'Solvable model of a spin-glass.' *Physical Review Letters*, **35**, 1792–6.

Van Hemmen, J. L. & van Enter, A. C. D. (1986). 'Chopper model of pattern recognition.' *Physical Review A*, **34**, 2509–12.

15

Random complex automata: analogy with spin glasses

H. FLYVBJERG

15.1 Introduction

We have seen several approaches to randomly connected neural networks in this book. This chapter is about the properties such networks have *before* you teach them anything. Whenever one has a large system with some degree of homogeneity to it *self-averaging* may occur. So, it makes sense to ask: if something is 'big and dumb', will it demonstrate some 'character' anyway, if only it is big enough? We shall also look at large ensembles, or populations, if you wish, of random networks, and see some statistical properties of an apparently universal nature emerge.

Fig. 15.1. (*a*) Example of wiring pattern for $N = 5$ formal neurons with connectivity $K = 2$. (*b*) Same as (*a*) in a representation showing each neuron twice: as source of output and as receiver of input.

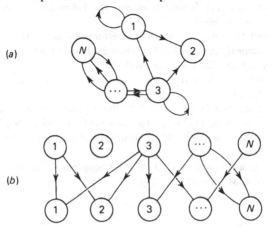

15.2 Kauffman's model

Random boolean networks were introduced by S. Kauffman as models for cell differentiation in embryonic development (Kauffman, 1969, 1970*a*,*b*, 1971, 1972, 1974, 1979, 1984). They have been studied for their applications (Kauffman, 1969, 1970*a*,*b*, 1971, 1972, 1974, 1979, 1984; Gelfand & Walker, 1977; Walker & Gelfand, 1979; Gelfand & Walker, 1980; Thomas, 1979; Fogelman-Soulié, Goles-Chacc & Weisbuch, 1982; Fogelman-Soulié, 1985) and in their own right, as examples of deterministic, disordered systems (Derrida & Pomeau, 1986; Derrida & Stauffer, 1986; Derrida & Weisbuch, 1986; Weisbuch & Stauffer, 1986; Hilhorst & Nijmijer, 1986; Derrida & Flyvbjerg, 1986*a*,*b*; Derrida, 1986). One has N boolean variables, or formal neurons, or Ising spins, depending on one's field, at any rate N variables σ_i that can equal 0 or 1. Time is discrete, and these N variables evolve in time in a synchronous way.† The value of σ_i at time $t + 1$ depends on the value of K of the N variables $\sigma_{j_1(i)}, \sigma_{j_2(i)}, \ldots,$ $\sigma_{j_K(i)}$ at time t through a boolean function f_i:

$$\sigma_i(t + 1) = f_i(\sigma_{j_1(i)}(t), \ldots, \sigma_{j_K(i)}(t)). \qquad (1)$$

Like N, the *connectivity* K is a parameter of Kauffman's model. For given parameter values a *sample* of such a network is defined by giving the *wiring pattern* $(j_1(i), \ldots, j_K(i))_{i=1, \ldots, K}$ (see Fig. 15.1) and the boolean functions $(f_i)_{i=1, \ldots, K}$. For each value of i we choose $j_1(i), \ldots, j_K(i)$ at random between 1 and N, and f_i at random amongst the 2^{2^K} possible boolean functions of K variables. These functions and the wiring pattern are held fixed as time evolves.‡ Notice that since the wiring pattern was

---

† A few words about synchronous vs. asynchronous time. We had a long discussion of the artificiality of synchronous time based upon Littleworth's article. I would like to draw to your attention a small work by Ingerson & Buvel (1984). These authors have taken S. Wolfram's 32 one-dimensional cellular automata with legal, totalistic rules and rerun them both with random updating and with individual, asynchronous clocks with a 20% standard deviation in relative periods. They found that much of the apparent self-organization of synchronous automata disappears, and conclude that it is an artifact of the synchronous time development. But lots of non-trivial behavior survives. The work is very unconclusive. It consists mainly of pictures, so you will have to look for yourself.

   I will be using synchronous time. The quantities I will be showing can, however, also be generalized to asynchronous and random updating. But now I am getting ahead of myself!

‡ This may be called the quenched model. It is the one introduced by Kauffman. Derrida & Pomeau (1986) have introduced an annealed model: $(f_i)_{i=1, \ldots, N}$ are rechosen at each timestep. This makes some quantities analytically calculable. More surprising, in the thermodynamic limit $N = \infty$, these analytic results hardly differ from simulation results for the quenched model (Derrida & Weisbuch, 1986).

randomly chosen there is no such thing as 'neighbours' or any kind of 'geometry' in this model. Its finite dimensional versions, to which such concepts do apply (Fogelman-Soulié, Goles-Chacc & Weisbuch, 1982; Fogelman-Soulié, 1985; Derrida & Stauffer, 1986; Weisbuch & Stauffer, 1986), we shall not consider here.

15.3 Dynamical partitioning of configuration space

A sequence $\sigma_1, \sigma_2, \ldots, \sigma_N$ of zeros and ones we may call a *firing pattern* or a *configuration*, or a *point* in *configuration space*. Configuration space is finite and consists of 2^N points for N finite. So after at most 2^N timesteps the trajectory of any initial configuration will have passed twice through one point in configuration space. Since the time evolution is deterministic, it is cyclic, starting its second cycle the moment a configuration is visited the second time. Thus every configuration after, at most, 2^N timesteps evolves onto a cycle. Every cycle is an *attractor* with a certain *basin of attraction*, and configuration space is partitioned into basins of attraction. See Fig. 15.2. With Ω_s being the number of points in the sth basin of attraction, we introduce its relative size, or weight:

$$W_s = \Omega_s/2^N, \tag{2}$$

$$\sum_s W_s = 1. \tag{3}$$

Fig. 15.2. Highly symbolic representation of configuration space as a rectangle with area 1 broken into basins of attraction with areas $W_s, s = 1, 2, \ldots$, each basin containing a limit cycle as attractor.

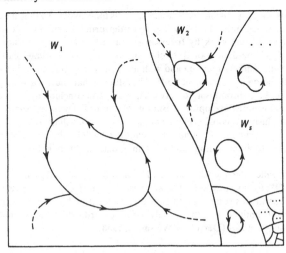

Now we may ask about the properties of large networks for N going to infinity:

Does the *number* of basins of attraction grow with N while Ω_s remains finite, and W_s therefore goes to zero?

Or do at least *some* of the weights W_s remain finite, because the absolute basin size Ω_s grows with N?

If the latter is the case, do only definite values of W_s occur, due to self-averaging in the individual network, or do the values of W_s occurring fluctuate from sample to sample even when N is infinite?

With an eye on spin glasses we consider the quantities

$$Y_P = \sum_s W_s^P \qquad (4)$$

in particular $Y = Y_2$, for each sample network, and the averages over samples $\bar{Y}_P$. Since a point chosen randomly in configuration space belongs to the sth basin of attraction with probability W_s, Y_P is the probability that P randomly chosen points belong to the same basin of attraction. Y_P remains finite for $N \to \infty$ if and only if some weights W_s remain finite. And if this is the case, Y_P remains constant from sample to sample if and only if all W_s self-average. In the mean field theory for spin glasses one finds $\bar{Y}_P$ finite for N infinite, and sample-to-sample fluctuations survive in the N-infinite limit, since $\sigma^2(Y) = \bar{Y^2} - \bar{Y}^2$ remains finite in that limit.

15.4 Results

Fig. 15.3 shows results for $\bar{Y}$ as a function of N and K. Results for $K = 1$, 2, 3, 4 are numerical, $\bar{Y}$ is averaged over 10^4 samples. Results for $K = \infty$ are analytical: for $K = \infty$ every variable $\sigma_i(t + 1)$ depends on *all* N variables $\sigma_1(t), \ldots, \sigma_N(t)$. Thus time-evolution is just the random map of configuration space into itself, and a number of quantities can be obtained analytically (Derrida & Flyvbjerg, 1986*b*). For $N \leqq 14$ the numerical results were obtained by going through the entire configuration space of each sample, and following the time evolution of each configuration up to the point where it either coincided with a point already encountered in a previous evolution, or until a new cycle was formed. For $N > 14$ this method proved too time consuming, and $\bar{Y}$ was measured as the probability that two points chosen at random fall in the same basin of attraction. $\bar{Y}_3$, $\bar{Y}_4$, and $\bar{Y^2}$ were measured in similar ways (Derrida & Flyvbjerg, 1986*a*).

Fig. 15.3 shows for $K = 1, 2, 3, 4$, and ∞ that as N goes to infinity, some basins of attraction keep a finite weight. For $K = 2$ it is not clear whether or not $\bar{Y}$ goes to zero for N going to infinity. However, since $\bar{Y}$ and $\bar{Y}^2$ are moments of a probability distribution $\pi(Y)$ with support in $[0, 1]$, $\sigma(\bar{Y})$ must vanish if $\bar{Y}$ does. Fig. 15.4 shows $\sigma(\bar{Y})$ as a function of K and N. Within the errorbar there is no indication that $\sigma(\bar{Y})$ vanishes as N goes to infinity for $K = 2$. The results shown for $K = 2$ in Figs. 15.3 and 15.4 differ nevertheless somewhat from those of other K-values. This is not so surprising, since in the annealed model $K = 2$ has been shown to be a critical value (Derrida & Pomeau, 1986).

The finite values for $\bar{Y}$ are similar to what one gets for infinite range spin glasses for N infinite. Quantitative tests of this similarity are shown in Figs. 15.5, 15.6, and 15.7. The various points are numerical results for Kauffman's model (Derrida & Flyvbjerg, 1986a) with values of K and N as in Figs. 15.3 and 15.4. The one cross in each figure is the exact, analytical result for $K = \infty$ (Derrida & Flyvbjerg, 1986b). The full line in each diagram is the analytical result from the mean field theory for infinite range spin glasses (Mézard, Parisi, Sourlas, Toulouse & Virasoro, 1984). The dashed lines outline the area in which the data point *must* fall, because $\bar{Y}_3$, $\bar{Y}_4$, and $\bar{Y}^2$ are moments of probability distributions with support in $[0, 1]$.

Fig. 15.3. $\bar{Y}$ versus number N of formal neurons for connectivities $K = 1, 2, 3, 4$, and ∞. Each point represents an average over 10 000 samples, except the crosses ($K = \infty$) which are exact, analytic results.

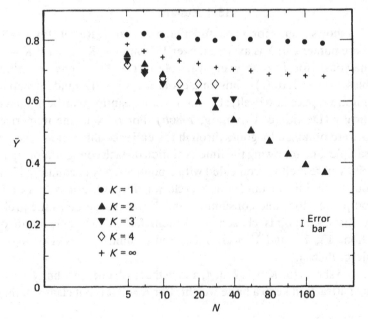

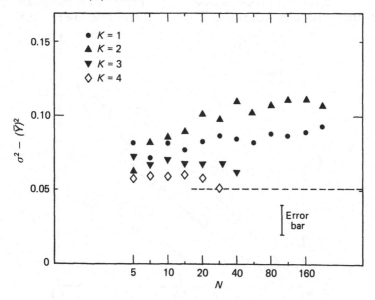

Fig. 15.4. $\sigma^2(\bar{Y})$ versus N for $K = 1, 2, 3$, and 4. Each point represents an average over $10\,000$ samples. The dashed line represents the value $\lim_{N\to\infty}\lim_{K\to\infty}\sigma^2(\bar{Y}) = \frac{16}{315}$.

Fig. 15.5. $\bar{Y}_3$ versus $\bar{Y}$. Each point represents an average over $10\,000$ samples, except the cross, which is the exact, analytic result for $K = \infty$ and $N = \infty$. Results for $K = \infty$, N finite, interpolate between this cross and $(1, 1)$, and fall only slightly below the full curve. The full curve represents the mean field result for spin glasses (Mézard *et al.*, 1984), $\bar{Y}_3 = \bar{Y}(1 + \bar{Y})/2$. The dashed curves are bounds $\bar{Y}^2 \leqq \bar{Y}_3 < \bar{Y}$ that $\bar{Y}_3$ must satisfy.

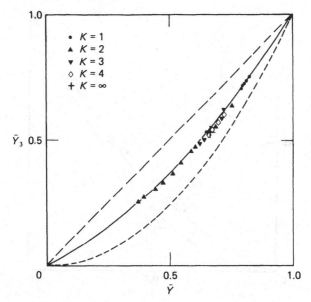

Fig. 15.6. $\bar{Y}_4$ versus $\bar{Y}$. Full curve represents $\bar{Y}_4 = \bar{Y}(1 + \bar{Y})(2 + \bar{Y})/6$ (Mézard *et al.*, 1984). Dashed curves are bounds $\bar{Y}^3 \leqq \bar{Y}_4 \leqq \bar{Y}$. Otherwise like Fig. 15.5.

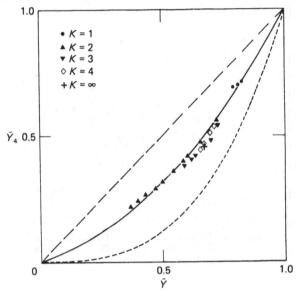

Fig. 15.7. $\overline{Y^2}$ versus $\bar{Y}$. Full curve represents $\overline{Y^2} = \bar{Y}(1 + 2\bar{Y})/3$ (Mézard *et al.*, 1984). Dashed curves are bounds $\bar{Y}^2 \leqq \overline{Y^2} \leqq \bar{Y}$. Otherwise like Fig. 15.5.

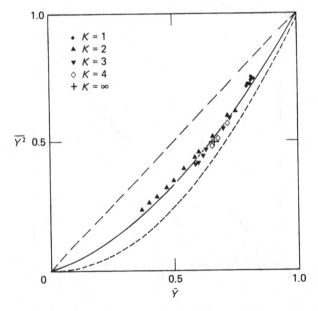

Table 15.1. *The agreement between Kauffman's model and spin glasses.*

	Kauffman's model for $K = \infty$	Spin glasses (MFT)	Kauffman's model / Spin glasses
$\bar{Y}$	$\frac{2}{3}$	$\frac{2}{3}$	1
$\bar{Y}_3$	$\frac{8}{15} = 0.533$	$\frac{5}{9} = 0.556$	0.96
$\bar{Y}_4$	$\frac{16}{35} = 0.457$	$\frac{40}{81} = 0.494$	0.93
$\overline{Y^2}$	$\frac{52}{105} = 0.495$	$\frac{14}{27} = 0.519$	0.96

Note: (*a*) The mean field result for spin glasses contains a free parameter, which is fixed by choosing $\bar{Y} = \frac{2}{3}$ (see eqn (6)). The other values in this column then follow from this choice.

The quantitative agreement between Kauffman's model and spin glasses is surprisingly close, since the errors on the data points are approximately the size of the points. The agreement is not *exact*, however, since the crosses do not fall exactly on the full lines, see Table 15.1. More specifically, for Kauffman's model with $K = \infty$ the average number of attractors with weight between W and $W + \mathrm{d}W$ is $f(W)\mathrm{d}W$, where (Derrida & Flyvbjerg, 1986*b*):

$$f(W) = \tfrac{1}{2}W^{-1}(1 - W)^{-1/2}. \tag{5}$$

For spin glasses, on the other hand, the average number of states with weight W is given by (Mézard, Parisi, Sourlas, Toulouse & Virasoro, 1984)

$$f_{\mathrm{sg}} = \frac{W^{y-2}(1 - W)^{-y}}{\Gamma(y)\Gamma(1 - y)}; \quad y \text{ parameter}. \tag{6}$$

The form of f is strikingly similar to that of f_{sg}, but for no value of the parameter y in f_{sg} are the two functions identical.

15.5 Conclusion

We have seen that the individual random network in Kauffman's model does not selfaverage the weights of its attractors. They fluctuate from sample to sample.

On the other hand, when we consider ensembles, or populations, of such random networks, they show a rather universal kind of behavior: populations differing w.r.t. *two* parameters, K and N, are characterized by probabilities $\bar{Y}_3$, $\bar{Y}_4$ and $\overline{Y^2}$ that depend essentially only on one parameter, $\bar{Y}$. Moreover, this dependence is strikingly similar, though not identical to what is found in the mean field theory of spin glasses.

This book is on brain science, so it would have been appropriate if we had also tried to *teach* these automata a trick or two, and studied their ability to memorize, associate, and recall. We have not, but maybe we will, now that we know their 'prerequisites'.

References

Derrida, B., 'Phase transitions in random networks of automata.' Proc. of Summer School: Les Houches, July, 1986, 'Chance and matter'.
Derrida, B. & Flyvbjerg, H., *J. Phys. A: Math. Gen.*, **19**, L1003 (1986a).
Derrida, B. & Flyvbjerg, H., 'The random map model: A disordered model with deterministic dynamics' (1986b). *J. Physique*, **48**, 971 (1987).
Derrida, B. & Pomeau, Y., *Europhys. Letters*, **1**, 45 (1986).
Derrida, B. & Stauffer, D., *Europhys. Letters*, **2** (1986).
Derrida, B. & Weisbuch, G., *J. Physique*, **47**, 1297 (1986).
Fogelman-Soulié, S., Goles-Chacc, E. & Weisbuch, G., *Bull. Math. Biol.*, **44**, 715–730 (1982).
Fogelman-Soulié, F., *Theor. Comp. Sci.*, **40**, 275–300 (1985).
Gelfand, A. E. & Walker, C. C., *Int. J. Gen. Systems*, **4**, 39–45 (1977).
Gelfand, A. E. & Walker, C. C., *Behavioral Sci.*, **25**, 250–60 (1980).
Hilhorst, H. J. & Nijmijer, M., *J. Physique*, **48**, 85 (1987).
Ingerson T. E. & Buvel R. L., *Physica*, **10D**, 59 (1984).
Kauffman, S. A., *J. Theor. Biol.*, **22**, 437 (1969).
Kauffman, S., 'Behavior of randomly constructed genetic nets.' In *Towards a Theoretical Biology*, vol. 3, pp. 18–37. C. H. Waddington (ed.) (Edinburgh Univ. Press, 1970a).
Kauffman, S., *Math. Life Sci.*, **3**, 63–116 (1970b).
Kauffman, S., 'Gene regulation networks: a theory for their global structure and behaviors.' In *Current Topics in Developmental Biology*, vol. 6, pp. 145–82. A. A. Moscona & A. Monroy, eds. (Academic Press, New York, 1971).
Kauffman, S. A., 'The organization of cellular genetic control system.' In *Lectures on Mathematics in the Life Sciences*, vol. 3, pp. 63–116. J. D. Cowan (ed.) (Amer. Math. Soc., Providence, RI, 1972).
Kauffman, S. A., *J. Theor. Biol.*, **44**, 167 (1974).
Kauffman, S. In *Lecture Notes in Biomathematics*, vol. 29, pp. 30–61. R. Thomas, ed. (Springer Verlag, Berlin, 1979).
Kauffman, S. A., *Physica*, **D10**, 145 (1984).
Mézard, M., Parisi, G., Sourlas, N., Toulouse, G. and Virasoro, M., *J. Physique*, **45**, 843 (1984).
Thomas, R., 'Kinetic logic: a Boolean approach to the analysis of complex regulatory systems.' In *Lecture Notes in Biomathematics*, vol. 29. R. Thomas, ed. (Springer Verlag, Berlin, 1979).
Walker, C. C. & Gelfand, A. E., *Behav. Sci.*, **24**, 112–20 (1979).
Weisbuch, G. & Stauffer, D., *J. Physique*, **48**, 11 (1987).

16

The evolution of data processing abilities
in competing automata

MICHEL KERSZBERG and AVIV BERGMAN

16.1 Introduction

It is probably fair to say that we have not, to this day, formed a clear picture of the learning process; neither have we been able to elicit from artificial intelligence machines a sort of behavior which could possibly compare in flexibility and performance with that exhibited by human or even animal subjects.

Leaving aside the issue of what actually happens in a learning brain, research on the question of how to generate 'intelligent' behavior has oscillated between two poles. The first, which today predominates in artificial intelligence circles (Nilsson, 1980), takes it for granted that solving a particular problem entails repeated application, to a data set representing the starting condition, of some operations chosen in a *predefined* set; the order of application may be either arbitrary or determined heuristically. The task is completed when the data set is found to be in a 'goal' state. This approach can be said to ascribe to the system, 'from birth', the capabilities required for a successful solution. The second approach, quite popular in its early version (Samuel, 1959), has been favored recently by physicists (Hopfield, 1982; Hogg & Huberman, 1985), and rests on the idea that 'learning machines' should be endowed, not with specific capabilities, but with some *general architecture*, and a set of *rules*, which are used to modify the machines' internal states in such a way that progressively better performance is obtained upon presentation of successive sample tasks. The rules themselves may be of two types: either 'free', i.e., not built in reference to any particular problem (D'Humières & Huberman, 1984), or 'task-bound', i.e., adapted narrowly to the task at hand (Hopfield, 1982; Hogg & Huberman, 1985; Personnaz, Guyon & Dreyfus, 1985). In both cases, the systems are initially 'ignorant', i.e. they are started from some 'null' situation where all parameters to be modified by the rules are either set to zero or to some random values (Toulouse, Dehaene & Changeux, 1986).

Recent consideration of human or animal intelligence, however, has revealed that biological reality seems actually to be located somewhere between these two extremes. We are neither perfect *tabulae rasae*, nor totally preprogrammed robots. For instance, the acquisition of linguistic competence (the ability to form or understand correct sentences in one's native language) seems to rest (Chomsky, 1968) on the existence of high-level capabilities present at birth. Thus we all learn some natural language as a mothertongue, but we are able to do so only because the structure of natural languages is not arbitrary: instead, it obeys some deep universal laws, to which we are 'tuned' from the outset. It is interesting to note that some of the best candidates for such universal features are *hierarchical* in nature, e.g. the so-called *A-over-A* rule which is respon-sible for the fact that, when converting 'The man who is on the chair is tall' to interrogative form, a native speaker will say 'Is the man who is on the chair tall?', and not 'Is the man who on the chair is tall?', because there is a clear separation of levels between 'The man . . . is tall' and '. . . who is on the chair . . .'. This translates technically, that the best 'learning machines' presumably have an ultrametric structure (Rammal, Toulouse & Virasoro, 1986; Huberman & Kerszberg, 1985) and the one we shall use here satisfies such a condition (Kerszberg, 1986).

The question whether 'intelligent' behavior can be generated more efficiently by using a proper balance of 'nature' versus 'nurture' in the learning process thus remains open. Given that the information encoded into the brain at birth must mainly be of genetic origin, and that such information is conceived today as having emerged through a process of evolution, we are led naturally to think in terms of populations of individuals (see, e.g. Mayr, 1982), each endowed with a structure it has inherited (for the most part) from its 'parent(s)', and learning as a result of adaptation to its environment. Learning better, some machines leave more descendents than the others; and, statistically, the population cannot fail to improve its performance. However simple the idea (Hol-land, 1975; Braitenberg, 1984), its implementation can be very tricky, as we shall see below.

In what follows, we describe the structure of the machines we are considering; the basic scheme is general enough that a large class of tasks is in principle executable; however, we do *not* attempt in any way to 'program' at the outset a particular task into the system. We give an outline of the way populations of machines were simulated, discuss the results and under which conditions they could be efficiently obtained. We also stress the limitations of the current approach and briefly sketch the ways in which we plan to overcome them in future work.

16.2 A general machine architecture

Holland has introduced, in his 'genetic algorithms', the notion of genetically adaptable programs. These programs consist of modules which can be combined in various ways, and contain a variety of parameters which have specified values in each individual program (Holland, 1975; Grefenstette, 1985). The design of such modular programs calls for knowledge about the task to be executed; here, we would like to avoid having to provide such advance knowledge, and propose to start from an architecture sufficiently general that a wide variety of tasks can in principle be performed. We expect the population of machines to adapt progressively, in such a way that one or several machines will ultimately meet our requirements: examining their structure should then inform us about how they are actually producing a solution. Presumably, since the procedure 'found' by the successful machines is of evolutionary origin, it will exhibit various redundancies and useless complications: this has been referred to by Jacob as 'evolutionary tinkering' (Jacob, 1982). However, it should be possible to iron out these accidental features, leaving us with an efficient structure which can then be used in practical design: thus, we hope the evolutionary approach will eventually be of help in the conception of artificial intelligence systems.

The architecture we use is cellular, and consists of successive layers. Such a structure insures that data processing will be hierarchical in nature (Kerszberg, 1986). The layers are one-dimensional in the current implementation; connections to and from cellular elements ('neurons') run exclusively between nearest and next-nearest neighbors on the square lattice (see Fig. 16.1). All links have the same strength but may be excitatory ($+$) or inhibitory ($-$), and two elements may be connected by more than one link. Each neuron is a simple processor: it sums its inputs (with their sign) and sets its output at a value equal to that sum S, provided S lies between zero and some saturation value M; if S is negative, output is zero; while if $S > M$, output is M. This operation is carried out in parallel at each layer, at discrete time intervals: time will, in the following, always be measured in units of this basic updating process. The top elements are fed, at their 'downcoming' inputs, a set of integers $\{I_i\}$ all lying between 0 and M: this set constitutes the *input string* of the system.

The neurons at the bottom of the array then generate a new set of integers $\{O_i\}$, the *output string*. Changes in input propagate to the output in a time equal to the number of layers. Note that if M is large enough, the limitation to integers becomes irrelevant.

The network just defined is certainly equipped with a vast potential for complex computational tasks. This is particularly true, considering the possibility of lateral and backward connections, which allow for feedback control; this feature, together with the strong non-linearity of the neurons, sets our model clearly apart from perceptron-like architectures (Minsky & Papert, 1969). Carrying out a particular goal, i.e., obtaining a given (possibly time dependent), input–output relationship, requires, however, setting up a very precise set of connections. We avoid having to specify this ourselves by running a population–dynamical simulation as described in Sections 16.3 and 16.4. There, we consider in more detail three sorts of automata, namely totally periodic (P-arrays), i.e., the pattern of links to and from each neuron is the same for all neurons; layer-wise periodic, i.e., all neurons in a given layer are identically connected (LP-arrays); and non-periodic (NP-arrays).

16.3 Population dynamics

The basic idea is to *select*, as contributors to a new generation of automata, those machines which are performing best. This requires that we set up a *test* indicative of performance. Several tasks have been

Fig. 16.1. A three-layer, four-neuron-wide automaton. The links indicate which elements may be joined by one or more connections going either way. The state of each of the top elements is *forced* by an input integer I_j. The outputs are collected as the integers O_j delivered by the neurons in the last layer.

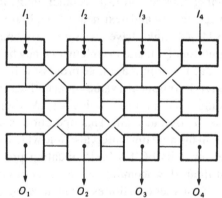

implemented (Bergman & Kerszberg, 1986); here we choose, as an illustration, the following problem: three strings, comprising ten integers each, are presented successively to our machines for a certain time ('persistence time'); two of these can be matched by translation invariance, e.g. $S_1 = \{0, 0, 0, a, b, c, d, 0, 0, 0\}$ and $S_2 = \{0, a, b, c, d, 0, 0, 0, 0, 0\}$; while the third is unrelated to these, e.g. $S_3 = \{0, 0, 0, 0, f, g, h, i, 0, 0\}$. To a population of N ten-neuron wide arrays, each of which typically contains five layers, we now present these strings, with a persistence time of at least five units, and in random order; N is usually on the order of ten. We require that, upon successive presentation of $S_1 S_2$ (case TR1) or $S_2 S_1$ (case TR2), some output cell will assume a large activity, while after $S_1 S_3$ (i.e., NTR1), $S_3 S_1$ (NTR2), $S_2 S_3$ (NTR3), or $S_3 S_2$ (NTR4), that same neuron will be as close to 0 activity as possible. In a sense, we are thus asking for a 'grandmother neuron' which fires specifically when detecting translation invariance (TR). We believe programming the array *a priori* to perform this exercise is not easy. In practice, all we have to do here is assign to each machine, upon completion of the test, a *grade*; the closer the machine comes to achieving the goal, the higher its grade: this can be, for instance, the sum of output values delivered by a certain output cell after TR minus the sum of output values at the same cell after NTR, properly normalized. In practice, the output cell which is selected for grading is the one which, at 'birth', already produces the sharpest contrast. After testing, we set up a new population, to which each machine contributes in rough proportion to its grade. Each newborn automaton inherits the connectivity pattern of its ancestor, but a small number of connections are either added or deleted randomly (Bergman & Kerszberg, 1986). The new population again consists of N machines, and is submitted to another test, and so on, until satisfactory performance is obtained. Certainly, provided the task we have chosen can be carried out at all using the architecture we use, a solution will ultimately be found. However, the question remains as to whether this can be achieved in reasonable computer time, and as to how efficient and elegant the solution will be. Here, the answers are quite subtle.

16.4 Results

The problem described above, among others, has been successfully solved; the quality of the results, however, depends strongly on how gradually we present problems to our machines, and on how constrained (P, LP or NP) their architecture is. Ideally, we should like not to supply the automata with any sort of initial information. Therefore, the populations we begin with may typically consist of ten machines with *random* connections. Not surprisingly, random machines do not perform well; neither do they improve rapidly. Thus, we encounter the nature versus nurture problem: a stupid start leads you nowhere.

Interestingly, much better results are obtained when rather unspecific bits of information are supplied. One is that a successful machine probably possesses more forward than backward or lateral connections; another concerns the likely predominance of inhibition, that is, negative connections. If we build our random initial population such that these conditions are statistically satisfied, the first useful machines emerge. It is remarkable that populations where no biases of this type were imposed seemed to evolve them, but very slowly; and that so little information makes such a difference. Even then, however, before it can be learned in a reasonable amount of time (say, 30 minutes CPU, or roughly 100 generations), the task must be presented in a rather restricted form. A 'startup' procedure, where the strings are not modified at all, but only the order of presentation is changed, is necessary; thereafter, the integers a, b, c, . . . , i (or *alphabet*) used in the definition of S_1, S_2 and S_3 are not varied, but only the position of the non-zero range in the strings (or *translation amount*) is modified from one test (used to grade generation j) to the next (used with $j + 1$). A striking difference appears at this stage between P, LP and NP machines.

P-machines never manage. Their architecture is apparently too limited. On the other hand, NP-machines have an *embarras de richesses*: they do succeed in learning, but the connectivity space they are searching might be so wide that they never quite hit the perfect solution. This is illustrated in Fig. 16.2(a), where a portion of a relatively good machine is shown. This machine could detect translation invariance for fixed alphabet but varying translation amounts with a success rate of about 80%; no obvious pattern can be discerned in its connections.

The LP-machines are by far the best. Not only do they perform the limited test just described, the better ones among them are able to go on to the harder feat of performing well no matter what the alphabet. After they have learned with their first alphabet, they learn the second one much faster, and the learning time drops even further with the third. Note that with each new alphabet learned, there is a slight loss in performance using the *previous* alphabets. This can be alleviated with a measure of 'reinforcement', that is, by presenting instances of all alphabets previously learned even while teaching the new one; at any rate, machines which have gone through some ten alphabets seem to recognize translation invariance no matter what the alphabet or the translation amount; they still do very well, even when persistence times are changed randomly: it would seem that they have learned the TR *concept*.

Before we ask ourselves in what sense this last sentence should be understood, it is worth reflecting that, once more, we have come across complex nature/nurture interactions: LP-automata are the better learners because they had the structural features adapted to the problem to begin with: not too complicated, like the NP-machines, but not too simple, like the P's. Furthermore, the LP-arrays whose structure embodied their experience of learning with previous alphabets, did better on the next alphabets, demonstrating that an evolutionary process can by itself endow its products with a better adapted 'nature'.

Fig. 16.2. Parts of three different 10 by 5 automata which are proficient in detecting translation invariance. The neurons are symbolized by asterisks. The figures around them denote the number of connections (with their sign) going *from* a neuron to its neighbors in the corresponding directions. The neurons at the top (layer zero) have their output *forced* by the input integers and are used only to feed the first layer; the neurons at the bottom have of course no elements to feed in the downward directions. (*a*) Two columns from a non-periodic (NP) machine. The other layers of the automaton bear no evident resemblance to those displayed here. The machine has a success rate of about 80% in detecting translation invariance (TR) with one alphabet and varying translation amount (see text). (*b*) A layer-wise periodic (LP) machine. All elements in a given layer are identically connected. The machine knows TR perfectly with one alphabet and any translation amount. (*c*) An LP machine which has learned TR with any alphabet or translation amount.

```
    *        *                  *         *                   *            *
1  3 -2  -1 -2  9        0-35  7    0-35  7          14-86 54    14-86 54

 1 -1  0   0 -1  0        0  7 -2    0  7 -2          -2  1  1    -2  1  1
 5  *  2   0  * -1        3  *  1    3  *  1         -15  *-14   -15  *-14
-10-10 0  -7  6  0        2 -3  3    2 -3  3         -21-11 24   -21-11 24

 0 -4 -1   0  0  0       -1  5  0   -1  5  0          -6-16 -9    -6-16 -9
 0  *  0  -3  * -6       -1  * -6   -1  * -6          -3  *-12    -3  *-12
-4  0  6   2 11  2       16-12  4   16-12  4        -120-22 84  -120-22 84

 0 -1  0   0  1 -1       -2  2  1   -2  2  1           1-70 -5     1-70 -5
 0  *  1  -1  *  3       -2  * -3   -2  * -3         -20  *  9   -20  *  9
-9 -4  2  -2  0 -3      -15  5  4  -15  5  4          12 88 -1    12 88 -1

 0 -2  0   0 -1  0        1 -1  0    1 -1  0          -3  1  3    -3  1  3
-4  * -2  -3  *  2        1  *  3    1  *  3          -4  *  4    -4  *  4
-3 -4  4  -6 -7  2       3-10 10    3-10 10           58 -4 38    58 -4 38

 0 -2  0   0  0  0        0 -4  0    0 -4  0          -2-38 -1    -2-38 -1
-1  * -3   1  *  0        3  * -6    3  * -6          -37  *-35   -37  *-35

       (a)                      (b)                        (c)
```

When we say that our machines have learned the concept of translation invariance, we mean that, embedded implicitly in their connectivity pattern, is an *algorithm* which embodies this concept. A sample of the connectivity associated with TR is displayed in Figs. 16.2(*b*) and (*c*). Before analyzing these patterns, let us first inquire what an explicit algorithm for translation invariance would be. This is not difficult to imagine: one would have to store the first pattern presented, say S_1, then the second one, say S_3; then either would be subjected to all possible translations, and subtracted from the other: if and only if one of the differences would consist only of zeros, would TR be detected. Note that, for strings ten integers long, with four non-zero members, this process would imply storage of both strings, performing between zero and seven subtractions, and detecting a row of zeros in one of the results: it can be said in this respect that our arrays, invariably performing an equivalent set of operations in ten ticks of their internal clock (i.e., two persistence times), appear to be fairly efficient!

Furthermore, their algorithm is naturally parallel, which allows us to implement it on modern processors built with this sort of application in mind. In addition, simulations of population dynamics, used to discover the procedure, are themselves genuinely parallel, in the sense that, at a given generation, each machine can be tested independently of the others: this is the time-consuming part of the calculation. Only when the tests have been completed, do we need to compare all the members of the group; suppressing the inefficient automata, while preserving and repro- ducing the successful ones can again be performed simultaneously over the whole population.

Thus, with no design effort beyond that of setting up the initial architecture, and designing a testing routine which progressively and faithfully represents the task we actually desire our automata to learn, we can claim to have reached a stage where success, and efficient success at that, became possible. The general procedure illustrated above with translation invariance, has proved its flexibility by being used just as successfully to solve a variety of other computational problems, with virtually no additional conceptual effort (Bergman & Kerszberg, 1986).

We now take a closer look at the structure of our automata. It should be stressed at the outset that the machines we have chosen for display are not the only ones of their kind: many other machines, with rather different 'innards', seem to behave just as satisfactorily. Thus, on Fig. 16.2(*b*), we have displayed a portion of an LP-machine which has successfully learned TR with one alphabet. The figure is not easy to decipher, but certain regularities are apparent. Thus, in the last layer, excitatory and inhibitory connections alternate in a way very suggestive of multistable electronic circuits; this part of the automaton seems to be in charge of *short-term memory*, temporarily storing the results of some computation on a first string. Another readily visible feature is the presence of strong lateral inhibition. This is in accord with what we know about perception in biological systems. The same trends seem to subsist in the machine partially displayed in Fig. 16.2(*c*), which recognizes TR with any alphabet. As learning proceeds, the predominance of inhibition over excitation becomes more and more noticeable. We see also that this machine has been undergoing many learning cycles, and that some of the connection strengths have grown quite large: we have not checked as yet whether limiting the explosion of connection strengths leads to a difference in performance.

It seems clear to us that, by developing further the analysis of such circuitry, one should be able to abstract, from the 'raw' structures obtained through evolution, the essential elements of the algorithm involved, thus paving the way for the design of actual VLSI chips. These chips would come in various 'strains', each capable of certain predefined operations (*nature*), and presumably able to learn a slightly more difficult set of tasks (*nurture*). The non-uniqueness of structure among the 'learned' automata certainly suggests that it must be worthwhile maintaining a whole population of chips: while all automata may do certain things, they are probably not equivalent in terms of their future learning potential.

It may well be that the major weakness of the present approach is the current impossibility to predict whether a given problem can be solved using some predefined set of architectural constraints. We cannot even say what depth is needed in general to solve problems like TR. Perhaps one should let the automata themselves adjust some of the variables involved, such as the number of layers; but we have seen that increasing the dimensions of the space being searched is not always a good idea.

On the other hand, instead of analyzing the contents and mode of operation of our machines, we may just want to enjoy the pleasure of seeing them work without having had to bother to program them!

16.5 Perspectives

In the present work, we have tried to tread an intermediate path between the extremes of, on the one hand, a fixed operations repertoire acquired at birth, and on the other, that of random but adaptive architectures. We have discovered that the automata we start with, which in general do already possess computational capabilities, can refine them in many interesting ways in the process of competing among themselves. In a limited sense, we have thus demonstrated the complex interactions between nature and nurture in learning. We found that, from generation to generation, specific connectivity patterns develop; concomitantly, one can observe that certain groups of cells become active, while others lapse into disuse. This brings us in close contact with the group-selection theory of the brain (Edelman & Mountcastle, 1978). In this respect, one should remark that our singling out of 'grandmother neurons' for the completion of various tasks is not really at variance with group-selection theory, if only because our 'neurons', with their small number of connected neighbors, need not consist of single physical neurons, but may instead by representative of larger assemblies.

It is difficult to say *a priori* whether the introduction of recombination – i.e., sexual relationships among our automata – is warranted (Holland, 1975). The reason is that the tasks we are attempting to teach them are *epistatic*: we need a whole set of connections to be established, and there are strong correlations between them; therefore, it is not likely that combining some of the synapses of one machine with part of another's will lead to much improvement, quite the contrary. The choice of the *units* which undergo recombination is crucial and, most probably, recombination will, if ever, be of advantage only at a higher level of combining the capabilities of large assemblies of cells.

A clear shortcoming of the approach presented here is that adaptation is entirely *Mendelian*, i.e., properties inherited from the ancestor are immediately translated into fixed properties of the descendant; the next natural step would consist in introducing a new level of adaptation, that of the child learning to behave in its environment (Bergman & Kerszberg, 1986). These later adaptations would *not* be transferred to the following generations, but would presumably interact profoundly with the heritable properties and possibly lead to a measure of (indirect) *Lamarckism*.

Acknowledgments

This work was begun while one of us (MK) was a visitor at the Xerox Palo Alto Research Center. We should like to thank PARC and its staff for their hospitality; we are particularly grateful to B. A. Huberman for stimulating ideas and criticism.

References

Bergman, A. & M. Kerszberg (1986). In preparation.

Braitenberg, V. (1984). *Vehicles, Experiments in Synthetic Psychology*. Cambridge: The MIT Press.

Chomsky, N. (1968). *Language and Mind*. New York: Harcourt, Brace & World.

Edelman, G. M. & V. B. Mountcastle (1978). *The Mindful Brain*. Cambridge: The MIT Press.

Grefenstette, J. (1985), ed., *Proceedings of a Conference on Genetic Algorithms*. The Robotics Institute, Carnegie-Mellon University.

Hogg, T. & B. A. Huberman (1985). 'Parallel computing structures capable of flexible associations and recognition of fuzzy inputs.' *J. Stat. Phys.*, **41**, 115–23.

Holland, J. (1975). *Adaptation in Natural and Artificial Systems*. Ann Arbor: The University of Michigan Press.

Hopfield, J. J. (1982). 'Neural networks and physical systems with emergent collective computational abilities.' *Proc. Nat. Acad. Sci. (USA)*, **79**, 2554–8.

Huberman, B. A. & M. Kerszberg (1985). 'Ultradiffusion: the relaxation of hierarchical systems.' *J. Phys. A: Math. Gen.*, **18**, L331–6.

D'Humières, D. & B. A. Huberman (1984). 'Dynamics of self-organization in complex adaptive networks.' *J. Stat. Phys.*, **34**, 361–79.

Jacob, F. (1982). *The Possible and the Actual*. New York: Pantheon Books.

Kerszberg, M. (1986). 'The emergence of hierarchical data structures in parallel computation.' In *Disordered Systems and Biological Organization*, E. Bienenstock et al., eds., Berlin, Heidelberg: Springer Verlag.

Mayr, E. (1982). *The Growth of Biological Thought*. Cambridge: The Bellknap Press of Harvard University Press.

Minsky, M. & S. Papert (1969). *Perceptrons*. Cambridge: The MIT Press.

Nilsson, N. J. (1980). *Principles of Artificial Intelligence*, Palo Alto: Tioga Publishing Company.

Personnaz, L., I. Guyon & G. Dreyfus (1985). 'Information storage and retrieval in spin-glass-like neural networks.' *J. Phys. Lett. (Paris)*, **46**, L359–65.

Rammal, R., G. Toulouse & M. A. Virasoro (1986). 'Ultrametricity for physicists.' *Rev. Mod. Phys.*, **58**, 765–88.

Samuel, A. L. (1959). 'Some studies in machine learning using the game of checkers.' *IBM J. Res. and Dev.*, **3**, 211–29.

Toulouse, G., S. Dehaene & J. P. Changeux (1986). 'Spin-glass model of learning by selection.' *Proc. Nat. Acad. Sci. (USA)*, **83**, 1695–8.

17

The inverse problem for neural nets and cellular automata

EDUARDO R. CAIANIELLO and MARIA MARINARO

17.1 Introduction

The belief that complex macroscopic phenomena of everyday experience are consequences of cooperative effects and large-scale correlations among enormous numbers of primitive microscopic objects subject to short-range interactions, is the starting point of all mathematical models on which our interpretation of nature is based. The models used are basically of two types: continuous and discrete models.

The first have been until now the most current models of natural systems; their mathematical formulation in terms of differential equations allows analytic approaches that permit exact or approximate solutions. The power of these models can be appreciated if one thinks that complex macroscopic phenomena, such as phase transitions, approach to equilibrium and so on, can be explained in terms of them when infinite (thermodynamic) limits are taken.

More recently, the great development of numeric computation has shown that discrete models can also be good candidates to explain complex phenomena, especially those connected with irreversibility, such as chaos, evolution of macroscopic systems from disordered to more ordered states and, in general, self-organizing systems. As a consequence, the interest in discrete models has vastly increased. Among these, cellular automata,† C.A. for short, have received particular attention; we recapitulate their definition:

> A discrete lattice of sites, the situation of which is described at time t by integers whose values depend on those of the sites at the previous time $t - \tau$ (τ is a fixed finite time delay).

† A collection of several papers on cellular automata can be found in *Physica*, **100** (1984), pp. 1–248.

Such integers are assumed to belong to a ring r_h;

The value assumed by each site at each time step depends only on a local neighborhood of sites around it; it can be obtained (in any case, but most immediately by taking $h = 2$, as we assume from now on) by means of the same equations (neuronic equations, NE) that were introduced by one of us to model neural activity (Caianiello, 1961, 1984).

Thus, the evolution of a cellular automaton can be studied with the same formalism developed for NE. The key idea is to describe the evolution of the system in the functional space of system states. We shall thus use results obtained for NE to study here the behaviour of a cellular automaton of N sites which assumes values belonging to the ring R_2 in the 2^N functional space of all possible states or configurations of the C.A. This leads to the linearization of the dynamics: the evolution of the automaton is described by a $2^N \times 2^N$ permutation matrix, possibly degenerate, which we denote by P_N.

The existence of transient states (configurations that die out after a finite number of steps) and of cycles (self-repeating sequences of states) is simply expressed in terms of the eigenvalues of P_N.

In fact, since P_N is a permutation matrix, its eigenvalues are zero or roots of the unit. The eigenvalues zero denotes degeneration and correspond to transient states, the roots of the unit to the cycles of the automaton. These features appear in the characteristic equation of the permutation matrix P_N which is

$$\lambda^{n_0} \sum_i (\lambda^{l_i} - 1)^{n_i} = 0,$$

where n_0 gives the total number of transient states (the fraction of the 2^N possible states of the automaton which die in the evolution); n_i is the number of cycles of length l_i. The sum is over all the possible cycles. The integer parameters n_0, l_i and n_i depend on N and on the evolution rule; they are connected by the relation

$$n_0 + \sum_i n_i l_i = 2^N.$$

The above equation establishes, in a completely general way, that all possible states of a finite automaton of N sites are either transient states or enter into a cycle. Relevant information on the global behaviour of C.A. for $t \to \infty$ obtains from the computation of the parameters n_0, l_i, and n_i.

In previous papers N.E. were studied with greater detail in the case in which the evolution law is a binary function of linear arguments, i.e., in the language of boolean functions, a boolean separable function. This paper is dedicated to the study of additive (Martin, Odlyzko & Wolfram, 1984) cellular automata: we show that their evolution laws are monomials, i.e., the most simple non-separable boolean functions, C.A. are treated in the literature by studying their evolution once the dynamic laws connecting their sites are preassigned; this is the direct problem. Our formalism also explicitely solves the inverse problem, that of determining, given any arbitrary sequence of 2^N states, the dynamic law that realizes it.

17.2 Notation

The symbol $\vec{\xi}$ will be used to denote the state of a cellular automaton of N sites

$$\vec{\xi} \equiv (\xi^1, \xi^2, \ldots, \xi^N) \quad (\xi^i = \pm 1). \tag{2.1}$$

On the ensemble of the 2^N automaton states we define the following combination rule (component-wise product): Given m automaton states

$$\vec{\xi}_{l_i} = (\xi^1_{l_i}, \ldots, \xi^N_{l_i}) \quad (i = 1, \ldots, m).$$

their 'combination' is the state defined by

$$\vec{\xi}_{l_1} \times \vec{\xi}_{l_2} \times \ldots \times \vec{\xi}_{l_m} \equiv ((-1)^{m+1}\xi^1_{l_1}, \ldots, \xi^1_{l_m}, (-1)^{m+1}\xi^2_{l_1}, \ldots, \xi^2_{l_m}, \ldots) \tag{2.2}$$

It is easy to see that, taken N distinct states, all 2^N states can be obtained by using the combination rule (2.2) with $m = 0, i, \ldots, N$, where we define, for convenience, the ground state $\vec{\xi}_0 \equiv (-1, -1, \ldots, -1)$ in correspondence of $m = 0$. A possible complete set of distinct states is obtained taking the states with all their site values but one equal to -1:

$$\vec{\xi}_{l_i} = \underbrace{(-1, -1, \ldots,}_{i-1} \underbrace{1,}_{i} \underbrace{-1, \ldots, -1)}_{N-i} \quad (i = 1, 2, \ldots, N). \tag{2.3}$$

In R_2 the evolution of the cellular automaton is determined by the N boolean functions:

$$\xi^i_{t+\tau} = \sigma[\mathcal{F}_i(\xi^1_t, \ldots, \xi^N_t)] \quad (i = 1, 2, \ldots, N) \tag{2.4}$$

where σ is the signum function:

$$\sigma[\mathcal{F}_i] = \begin{cases} 1 & \text{if } \mathcal{F}_i > 0, \\ -1 & \text{if } \mathcal{F}_i < 0, \end{cases}$$

with the assumption $\mathcal{F}_i \neq 0$ always.

By using the properties of boolean functions it is easy to show (Caianiello, 1961) that

$$\xi^i_{t+\tau} = \sum_\alpha f^i_\alpha \eta^\alpha_t \tag{2.5}$$

where η_t^α is the αth component of the 2^N vector:

$$\vec{\eta}_t = \begin{pmatrix} 1 \\ \xi_t^N \end{pmatrix} \otimes \begin{pmatrix} 1 \\ \xi_t^{N-1} \end{pmatrix} \cdots \begin{pmatrix} 1 \\ \xi_t^1 \end{pmatrix}; \qquad (2.6)$$

$$f_\alpha^i = \langle \eta^\alpha \sigma(\mathcal{F}_i) \rangle = \langle \sigma[\eta^\alpha \mathcal{F}_i] \rangle;$$

$$\langle \rangle \equiv 1/2^N \sum_{\xi_1 = \pm 1 \ldots \xi_N = \pm 1};$$

and $\otimes$ denotes direct product. From (2.5) and (2.6) it follows that the 2^N 'vector' η evolves *linearly*:

$$\vec{\eta}_{t+\tau} = F_N \vec{\eta}_t. \qquad (2.7)$$

In eqn (2.7) F_N is the $2^N \times 2^N$ matrix determined by eqns (2.5). A well-defined vector $\vec{\eta}$ is thus associated to each state; the N *linear* components of $\vec{\eta}$, $\eta^\alpha = \xi^i$, take the site values of that state. This allows us to introduce the $2^N \times 2^N$ matrix ϕ_0 whose columns are the 2^N vectors obtained by giving all the possible values ± 1 to each ξ_t^i in (2.6). A convenient representation of the ϕ_0 matrix is the following:

$$\phi_0 = C_N \begin{pmatrix} 1 & 1 \\ 1 & -1 \end{pmatrix} \otimes \begin{pmatrix} 1 & 1 \\ 1 & -1 \end{pmatrix} \otimes \cdots \begin{pmatrix} 1 & 1 \\ 1 & -1 \end{pmatrix}; \quad C_N = 2^{-N/2}. \qquad (2.8)$$

It is easy to see that:

$$\phi_0 = \phi_0^T \qquad (2.9)$$

and from (2.7) that:

$$\phi_\tau = F_N \phi_0. \qquad (2.10)$$

The evolution law (2.10) is relevant for us because the matrix ϕ_τ is a (possibly degenerate) permutation of the matrix ϕ_0, effected on its column symbols

$$\phi_\tau = \phi_0 P_n, \qquad (2.11)$$

where

$$P_N = \phi_0 F_N \phi_0 \qquad (2.12)$$

is a (possibly degenerate) permutation matrix. In conclusion, the study of the time evolution of a C.A. is reduced to that of the corresponding permutation matrix P_N. The problem is thus *completely linearized*.

17.3 The P_N matrix for additive cellular automata

In this section we construct the P_N matrix for the special class of cellular automata referred to as 'additive' in the literature (Martin, Odlyzko & Wolfram, 1984). A cellular automaton is additive when the evolution rule (2.5) does not change the combination relations (2.2) among the states.

In formulae, if

$$\vec{\xi}_t = \vec{\xi}_{l_1,t} \times \vec{\xi}_{l_2,t} \times \ldots \times \vec{\xi}_{l_m,t}$$

then

$$\vec{\xi}_{t+\tau} = \vec{\xi}_{l_1,t+\tau} \times \vec{\xi}_{l_2,t+\tau} \times \ldots \times \vec{\xi}_{l_m,t+\tau}$$

where $\vec{\xi}_{l+\tau}$ and $\vec{\xi}_{l_{i,t+\tau}}$ are obtained after one time step from $\vec{\xi}_t$ and $\vec{\xi}_{l_i,t}$ respectively.

From eqns (2.5) and eqn (2.2) it is evident that C.A. are additive if their evolution laws are expressed by monomials, i.e. all the f_α^i but one in (2.5) vanish. In the language of boolean functions, such monomials are typical examples of 'non-separable functions'.

Symmetric nearest-neighbors one-dimensional additive C.A. of N sites have evolution laws expressed by one of the following equations:

$$\xi_{t+\tau}^K = \xi_t^{K-n} \ldots \xi_t^{K-1} \xi_t^K \xi_t^{K+1} \xi_t^{K+n}, \tag{3.1a}$$

$$\xi_{t+\tau}^K = -\xi_t^{K-n} \ldots \xi^{K-1} \xi_t^{K+1} \xi_t^{K+n}. \tag{3.1b}$$

Periodic boundary conditions are assumed. The construction of the matrix P_N for the automaton under consideration is obtained in the following way: eliminate all rows of ϕ_0 except those whose elements coincide with the site values of the automaton (the linear components of η). Denote the rectangular matrix $N \times 2^N$ so obtained with φ_0. The generic elements of φ_0 are $a_{kh} = 2^{-N/2}(-1)^{[h/2^{k-1}]}$, where φ_0 is the collection of the distinct 2^N states of the automaton; each column of φ_0 corresponds to a state, each row to a site. By applying to the first, second, and so on, columns of φ_0 the evolution rule (3.1) we generate a new $N \times 2^N$ matrix whose columns coincide with the columns of φ_0 modulo a permutation (repetitions are not excluded). We call the new matrix φ_0'. It corresponds to the one-time step evolution of all the 2^N states. The matrix P_N is thus immediately determined by the equation

$$\varphi_0' = \varphi_0 P_N. \tag{3.2}$$

It is convenient to number the 2^N columns of φ_0 in binary base; the mth column of φ_0 is thus individuated by the sequence: $(m_1, \ldots, m_N)$ with

$$m_i = \begin{cases} 0 \\ 1 \end{cases} \tag{3.3}$$

The sequence $(0, 0, \ldots, 0)$ corresponds to the first column of φ_0, the sequence $(1, 1, \ldots, 1)$ to the last. The application of the rule (3.1) to a column of φ is expressed by an operation acting on the sequence $(m_1, \ldots, m_N)$, which changes thereby into a sequence $(r_1, \ldots, r_n)$. In correspondence of equation (3.1a), one has

$$r_k \approx m_{k-n} + \ldots + m_{k-1} + m_k + m_{k+1} + \ldots + m_{k+n}, \quad (3.4a)$$

and in correspondence of equation (3.1b):

$$r_{k+1} \approx m_{k-n} + \ldots + m_{k-1} + m_{k+1} + \ldots + m_{k+n} \quad (3.4b)$$

or respectively with

$$\vec{S} \equiv (S_1, \ldots, S_N) \quad \text{and} \quad \vec{1} = (1, \ldots, 1),$$
$$\vec{r} \approx \tilde{T}_N \vec{m},$$
$$\vec{r} + \vec{1} \approx T_N \vec{m},$$

The symbol $\approx$ means that summations are modulo 2. $\tilde{T}_N$ and T_N are $N \times N$ matrices determined by (3.4a) and (3.4b) respectively.† In a previous (Caianiello & Marinaro, 1986) work the evolution of C.A. described by (3.1b) for $k = 2$ was analyzed in detail.

From eqn (3.2) numbering the rows and columns of P_N in binary base the elements of P_N can be easily determined; we have

$$\text{(case a)} \quad (P_N)_{r,m} = \begin{cases} 1 & \text{if} \quad \vec{r} \approx \tilde{T}_N \vec{m} \\ 0 & \text{otherwise} \end{cases},$$

$$\text{(case b)} \quad (P_N)_{r,m} = \begin{cases} 1 & \text{if} \quad \vec{r} \approx \tilde{1}_N \vec{m} + T \\ 0 & \text{otherwise} \end{cases}.$$

It can also immediately be seen that the Kth power of P_N is a matrix with elements:

$$\text{(case a)} \quad (P_N^K)_{r,m} = \begin{cases} 1 & \text{if} \quad \vec{r} = \tilde{T}_N^K + \vec{1} \\ 0 & \text{otherwise} \end{cases},$$

$$\text{(case b)} \quad (P_N^K)_{r,m} = \begin{cases} 1 & \text{if} \quad \vec{r} = T_N^K + \vec{1} \\ 0 & \text{otherwise} \end{cases},$$

The equations above imply that
(1) On each column of P_N there is only one non-vanishing element.
(2) The presence of all zero elements on the Kth row denotes the disappearance in one time step of the automaton state corresponding to the Kth column of φ_0.
(3) The presence of two or more elements different from zero in the Kth row, for example the elements $(K, S^1) \ldots (KS^n)$, denote that the state corresponding to the Kth column of φ_0 can be generated in one time step by *any* of the states corresponding to the columns $S^1, \ldots, S^n$ of the φ_0 matrix: the state corresponding to the Kth column of φ_0 has n predecessors.

---

† The linearity of eqn (3.4) is peculiar to additive C.A.; in general $\vec{r} = f(\vec{m})$ where f is not necessarily a linear function.

(4) The presence of a diagonal element (k, k) different from zero denotes that the state k is left invariant by the evolution. Thus the trace of P_N gives the number of cycles of length one; the number of cycles of length l_i is given by

$$n_i = (\text{Tr}(P_N)^{l_i} - \sum_j \text{Tr}(P_N)^{l_j})/l_i,$$

where l_j are divisors of l_i and Tr indicates the trace operation.

17.4 The inverse problem

Our attention has thus far concentrated on the *direct problem* and on *additive* C.A. Of far greater interest, at least in principle, is the *inverse problem*, i.e., the determination of the dynamic law that secures that a C.A. will evolve according to an arbitrarily preassigned sequence of 2^N states.

The solution in terms of the P_N matrix formalism is immediate; only exceptionally, of course, the corresponding automaton will be found to be additive. It suffices to notice that, since

$$P_N = \Phi_0 F_N \Phi_0, \tag{2.12}$$

F_N is given by

$$F_N = \Phi_0 P_N \Phi_0. \tag{4.1}$$

Each column of Φ_0 denotes one of the possible 2^N states of the automaton, in 'standard' order; we number them, as $0, 1, 2, \ldots, 2^N - 1$. If $S^0, S^1, \ldots, S^{2^N} - 1$ is the wanted sequence of states (with repetitions and omissions, if so desired, from the standard sequence) the permutation P_N is the matrix of elements

$$(P_N)_{h,k} = \delta_{h,s}k \tag{4.2}$$

$(h,k = 0, 1, 2, \ldots, 2^N - 1)$. Insertion into (4.1) gives the wanted dynamical law. As a trivial example, if $N = 3$ and

$$S^0 = 7, \quad S^1 = 0, \quad S^2 = 1, \quad S^3 = 2, \quad S^4 = 3, \quad S^5 = 4, \quad S^6 = 5, \quad S^7 = 6,$$

one finds

$$\begin{aligned}
\xi^1_{t+\tau} &= \xi^1_t, \\
\xi^2_{t+\tau} &= \xi^1_t \xi^2_t, \\
\xi^3_{t+\tau} &= 1/2(\xi^3_t - \xi^1_t \xi^3_t - \xi^2_t \xi^3_t - \xi^1_t \xi^2_t \xi^3_t).
\end{aligned}$$

References

Caianiello, E. R., *J. Theor. Biol.*, **2**, 204 (1961); with W. E. L. Grimson: *Biol. Kybernetik*, **18**, 111 (1975); *Kybernetik*, **12**, 90 (1973).

Caianiello, E. R., *in Brain Theory*, eds. G. Palm & A. Aertsen, Springer, Berlin, 1984 and references therein.
Caianiello, E. R. & M. Marinaro, *Physico Scrip.*, **4** (1986).
O. Martin, A. M. Odlyzko & S. Wolfram, *Com. Math. Phys.*, **93** (1984), 219.

18

A new synaptic modification algorithm and rhythmic oscillation

KAZUYOSHI TSUTSUMI and HARUYA MATSUMOTO

18.1 Introduction

Rhythmic oscillation is a fundamental component which can be found in the various kinds of nervous systems (Friesen & Stent, 1977; Thompson, 1982). In a neural network with a ring-structured set of synaptic connections, a set of oscillations with different phases can be generated (Morishita & Yajima, 1972; Stein *et al.*, 1974), and the occurrence of such rhythmic oscillation is also confirmed in different types of neural networks (Matsuoka, 1985). Since, however, various additional connections can cause a disturbance which easily extinguishes the rhythmic oscillation in the neural network, some function for maintaining the rhythmic oscillation should be expected to exist in the synapses if such signals play an important role in the nervous system.

A new synaptic modification algorithm is proposed which employs the average impulse density (AID) and the average membrane potential (AMP); examination of the effect of synaptic modification on rhythmic oscillation has been attempted (Tsutsumi & Matsumoto, 1984*a*). Simulation demonstrated some cases in which rhythmic oscillation reappears, by applying the algorithm to the disturbed ring neural network where the rhythmic oscillation was previously extinguished.

If that is the case, how can such oscillation derived from the neural network with feedback inhibition be processed in the following neural network with, for example, the feedforward system? Here we take, as an instance, the cerebellar circuitry including both feedback and feedforward systems, and discuss the relationship between synaptic modification and rhythmic oscillation in the neural network.

The cerebellum has a homogeneous arrangement of cells and it has in recent years attracted the attention of neural modelers. The perceptron was compared in detail with the cerebellar cortex (Marr, 1969; Eccles, 1973), and this collation is still often quoted. A template matching model, functioning under a certain improved synaptic modification algorithm, has been proposed and is also collated with the cerebellum (Hirai, 1980*a,b*). Even though many models for explaining the cerebellum's mechanism of information processing have been constructed, the principal discussions by modellers have concentrated on spatial pattern processing.

Since, however, the cerebellum is involved in the control of the actuator, both spatially and temporally, its mechanism should be explained using a model which illustrates both the spatial and temporal surfaces of control simultaneously. Recently the temporal control surface has come under investigation and the time delay of the signals passing through the cells and traveling on the fibres has been researched. An adaptive linear filter model of the cerebellum has been proposed on the basis of a hypothesis that the granule–Golgi (GR–GO) network works as a phase lead/lag compensator (Hassul & Daniels, 1977; Fujita, 1982*a,b*).

The impulse sequence for controlling the muscles is not of a constant interval; it is in the form of bursts of nerve impulses. Therefore any model of the cerebellum must show how that organ is able to learn this type of signal, and draw it out as a final output. In this paper, developing on the interpretation of the GR–GO network described in a previous paper (Tsutsumi & Matsumoto, 1984*b*), a model of the cerebellar circuitry employing rhythmic oscillation is advanced. In Section 18.2, the synaptic modification algorithm employed here is described, and an account is given of how the five kinds of cells in the cerebellum are modelled and classified. Then dividing the cerebellar circuitry into the two stages, that is the GR–GO network and the basket–stellate–Purkinje (BA–ST–PU) network, the functions of each stage are described separately in Sections 18.3 and 18.4. In Section 18.5, the two stages are connected and the total model of the cerebellar circuitry is detailed. Simulation shows that the output from the PU cells after learning has the inverse phase of the signals from the climbing (CL) fibres. In Section 18.6, the results are summarized and the course of future research is discussed.

18.2 Modifiable synapses and neural cells

In current research on the neural network, one of the most important themes is the way in which synaptic strength changes according to the number of nerve impulses passing through the synapse, the membrane potential of the post-synaptic cell, etc. Although various synaptic modification algorithms have been proposed, the algorithm put forward by Tsutsumi & Matsumoto (1984*a*) is employed here. According to this algorithm, synaptic strength $w_{ji}(t)$ from cell i in layer q to cell j in layer r at time t will be modified after a unit of time Δt as follows:

$$w_{ji}(t + \Delta t) = w_{ji}(t) + \Delta w_{ji}(t), \tag{2.1}$$

$$\Delta w_{ji}(t) = -\delta^{(rq)}[av[[x_i^{(q)}(t)]^+] - \theta^{(rq)}]^+ \times [av[x_j^{(r)}(t)] - \eta^{(r)}]^+, \tag{2.2}$$

where $x_i^{(q)}(t)$ and $x_j^{(r)}(t)$ represent the membrane potentials of the corresponding cells and

$$[\xi]^+ = \begin{cases} \xi & \xi > 0 \\ 0 & \xi \leq 0. \end{cases} \tag{2.3}$$

Here $av[\cdot]$ is defined by

$$av[\zeta(t)] = \int_{-\infty}^{t} \psi(t', \sigma)\zeta(t') \, dt', \tag{2.4}$$

and the following rectangular window function $\psi(t', \sigma)$ is employed:

$$\psi(t', \sigma) = \begin{cases} 1/\sigma & t - \sigma \leq t' \leq t, \\ 0 & \text{otherwise.} \end{cases} \tag{2.5}$$

Introducing (2.4) and (2.5), the average impulse density (AID) and the average membrane potential (AMP) of $\zeta(t)$ are represented as follows:

$$\text{AID: } av[[\zeta(t)]^+], \tag{2.6}$$

$$\text{AMP: } av[\zeta(t)]. \tag{2.7}$$

In (2.2), $\theta^{(rq)}$ and $\eta^{(r)}$ indicate, respectively, the pre-synaptic and post-synaptic thresholds and $\delta^{(rq)}$ represents the proportional constant. Therefore $w_{ji}(t)$ decreases in proportion to the differences between the pre-synaptic AID and $\theta^{(rq)}$ and the post-synaptic AMP and $\eta^{(r)}$.

In the cerebellar cortex, there are five kinds of neural cells. In this paper, the ordinary analog neuron models with integral time constants shown in Fig. 18.1 (Type A cell) are employed as the excitatory GR,

Fig. 18.1. A model of a neural cell with integral time constant and analog threshold (Type A cell). Here this model is employed as the granule, Golgi, basket, or stellate cell. (*a*) Schematic diagram. (*b*) Symbolic expression.

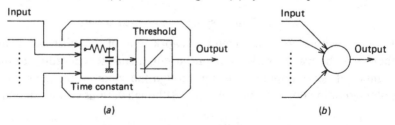

inhibitory GO, inhibitory BA, and inhibitory ST cells. In the modifiable synapses connected to the Type A cell, the synaptic modification is carried out according to the algorithm described by (2.1) and (2.2).

The inhibitory PU cells have synaptic connections from the BA and ST cells and the CL and parallel (PA) fibres. The synapses from the BA cells exist on the cell bodies, while those from the ST cells and the CL and PA fibres connect to the dendritic trees (Szentagothai, 1968). It has been reported recently that there exist considerable non-linear interactions between the adjacent inputs on the dendritic trees. Basing our arguments on this structural difference, we assume here that every part of the well-grown dendrite has a threshold effect. Hence the PU cells are modeled as shown in Fig. 18.2 (Type B cell), which can be represented equivalently using Type A cells. In the modifiable synapses connected to the Type B cell, the synaptic modification progresses in a similar way to that of the Type A cell, except that the post-synaptic AMP is not that of any particular part of the dendrite but is that of the cell body.

18.3 Feedback system (Granule–Golgi network)

18.3.1 Learning process

The GR–GO network, the first stage of the cerebellar circuitry, forms feedback inhibition composed of the GR and GO cells. The network is

Fig. 18.2. A model of a neural cell with a well-grown dendrite (Type B cell). Here this model is employed as the Purkinje cell. A Type B cell can be equivalently represented using Type A cells.

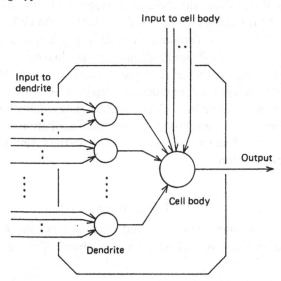

assumed to have two input channels from the outside: the GR cells receive the input from the mossy (MO) fibres and the GO cells do so from the CL fibres. Ignoring for the moment the input channel from the CL fibres to the GO cells, the network behaviour is examined here. The equations for the network employing Type A cells are as follows:

$$\left. \begin{aligned} \tau_g \frac{d}{dt} x_i^{(g)}(t) + x_i^{(g)}(t) &= u_i^{(g)}(t) - \sum_{j=1}^{N_G} d_{ij}^* \left[x_j^{(G)}(t) \right]^+ \\ & \qquad\qquad (i = 1, 2,\ldots, N_g), \\ \tau_G \frac{d}{dt} x_j^{(G)}(t) + x_j^{(G)}(t) &= \sum_{i=1}^{N_g} c_{ji}^* \left[x_i^{(g)}(t) \right]^+ \\ & \qquad\qquad (j = 1, 2,\ldots, N_G). \end{aligned} \right\} \quad (3.1)$$

Here $x_i^{(g)}(t)$ and $x_j^{(G)}(t)$ are the membrane potentials of the GR and GO cells, and τ_g and τ_G are their integral time constants; c_{ji}^* and d_{ij}^* indicate the modifiable synaptic strengths between the GR and GO cells.

The synaptic modification algorithm is applied to the network with a disturbed ring structure as illustrated in Fig. 18.3(*a*) (the network constants, etc., are listed in Appendix 1). Fig. 18.3(*b–d*) shows the output in impulse density of the GR cells before modification (Network 1), after 2760 modification steps, and after 6000 modification steps (Network 2), respectively. Each GR cell initially outputs a non-oscillatory signal, and with the progress of the synaptic modification, rhythmic oscillation appears, as happened in the networks described and discussed in the previous papers. The period of the rhythmic oscillation has a tendency to converge rapidly on a certain value.

Fig. 18.4(*a–c*) shows the changes in, respectively, the AIDs of the GR cells, the AMPs of the GR cells, and the AIDs of the GO cells during the synaptic modification. The parameters all vary greatly until the oscillation appears at around 2700 modification steps and then the AIDs of both the GR and GO cells gather around the threshold $\theta^{(Gg)}$ or $\theta^{(gG)}$. Since the progress of the synaptic modification depends on the difference of the AID and θ as is evident from (2.1) and (2.2), the modification speed drops to an extremely low level once the rhythmic oscillation is restored. The GR–GO network should be considered to have the function of generating rhythmic oscillation.

18.3.2 *Period locking process*

Taking into account now the input channel from the CL fibres, the behaviour of the GR–GO network is analysed. The equations of the

Fig. 18.3. Learning process as a result of the synaptic modification of c_{ji}^* and d_{ij}^* in the granule–Golgi network. (*a*) The schematic diagram of the simulated network (see Appendix 1). (*b*) The output $[x_i^{(g)}(t)]^+$ of the granule cells before modification (Network 1). (*c*) After 2760 modification steps. (*d*) After 6000 modification steps (Network 2).

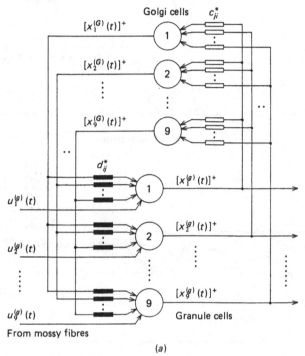

(a)

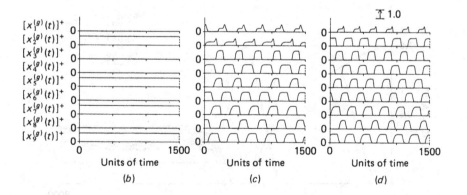

(b)   (c)   (d)

Fig. 18.4. The changes in the AIDs and the AMPs during the synaptic modification. (a) AID of the granule cells. (b) AMP of the granule cells. (c) AID of the Golgi cells.

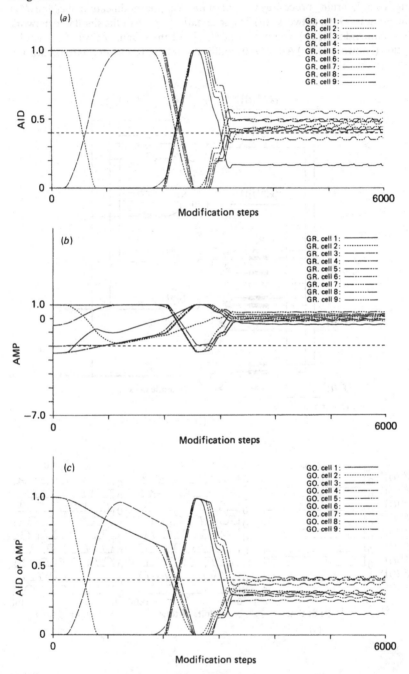

Fig. 18.5. Period locking process due to the square input $u_1^{(G)}(t)$ from the climbing fibre to the Golgi cell in the granule–Golgi network. Here the peak value of $u_1^{(G)}(t)$ is 0.2 and the set of synaptic strengths is fixed as in Network 2. (a) The schematic diagram of the simulated network. (b) The output $[x_i^{(g)}(t)]^+$ of the granule cells when $u_i^{(g)}(t) = 1.0$. (c) When $u_i^{(g)}(t) = 0.5$.

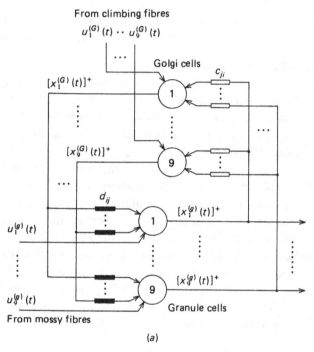

(a)

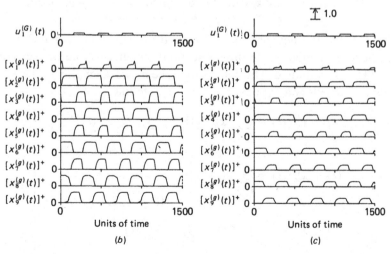

(b)   (c)

network can be given as follows:

$$
\left.
\begin{aligned}
\tau_g \frac{d}{dt} x_i^{(g)}(t) + x_i^{(g)}(t) &= u_i^{(g)}(t) - \sum_{j=1}^{N_G} d_{ij}[x_j^{(G)}(t)]^+ \\
&\qquad\qquad (i = 1, 2, \ldots, N_g), \\
\tau_G \frac{d}{dt} x_j^{(G)}(t) + x_j^{(G)}(t) &= u_j^{(G)}(t) + \sum_{i=1}^{N_g} c_{ji}[x_i^{(g)}(t)]^+ \\
&\qquad\qquad (j = 1, 2, \ldots, N_G),
\end{aligned}
\right\} \quad (3.2)
$$

where c_{ji} and d_{ij} are taken to be fixed.

Fig. 18.5(*a*) illustrates schematically the simulated network with the same set of synaptic strengths as Network 2 and Fig. 18.5(*b*) and (*c*) shows the result when the oscillatory and excitatory signal $u_1^{(G)}(t)$ is applied from the CL fibre. The period of the oscillatory signal $u_1^{(G)}(t)$ is set differently from that of the already generated rhythmic oscillation. If the level of $u_1^{(G)}(t)$ with an adequate period is high enough, the period of the output $[x^{(g)}(t)]^+$ of the GR cells coincides with that of $u_1^{(G)}(t)$ (see Fig. 18.5(*b*)). If c_{ji} and d_{ij} are modifiable, the dispersion of the AIDs caused by the application of $u_1^{(G)}(t)$ often restarts the synaptic modification and obstructs the period locking. As detailed in the previous paper (Tsutsumi & Matsumoto, 1984*b*), the two-mode selection mechanism solves this obstruction: even if the level of $u_1^{(g)}(t)$ is reduced to half, a locked output can be obtained (see Fig. 18.5(*c*)). Hence the input channel from the CL fibres to the GO cells should be considered to control the period of the rhythmic oscillation in the GR–GO network.

18.4 Feedforward system (Basket–Stellate–Purkinje network)
18.4.1 Suppression of large input

The BA–ST–PU network located behind the GR–GO network forms feedforward inhibition. In this subsection, the effect of the BA cells on the PU cells is studied. The equations of the network employing Type A cells as BA cells and Type B cells as PU cells follow:

$$
\left.
\begin{aligned}
\tau_P \frac{d}{dt} x_l^{(P)}(t) + x_l^{(P)}(t) &= \sum_{q=1}^{N_d} [x_{lq}^{(d)}(t)]^+ - \sum_{n=1}^{N_b} o_{ln}[x_n^{(b)}(t)]^+ \\
&\qquad\qquad (l = 1, 2, \ldots, N_P), \\
\tau_d \frac{d}{dt} x_{lq}^{(d)}(t) + x_{lq}^{(d)}(t) &= \sum_{p=1}^{N_F} e_{lqp} v_p^{(F)}(t) \\
&\qquad\qquad (q = 1, 2, \ldots, N_d), \\
\tau_b \frac{d}{dt} x_n^{(b)}(t) + x_n^{(b)}(t) &= u_n^{(b)}(t) + \sum_{p=1}^{N_F} h_{np} v_p^{(F)}(t) \\
&\qquad\qquad (n = 1, 2, \ldots, N_b).
\end{aligned}
\right\} \quad (4.1)
$$

Here $x_l^{(P)}(t)$ and $x_n^{(b)}(t)$ represent the membrane potentials of the PU cell bodies and the BA cells, and $x_{lq}^{(d)}(t)$ represent the local membrane potentials of the PU dendrites. τ_P, τ_d, and τ_b are the corresponding integral time constants and e_{lqp}, h_{np}, and o_{ln} are the synaptic strengths between cells or from fibres to cells, which are fixed in this case. The thresholds of the BA cells are assumed to be higher than those of the other cells. The input $u_n^{(b)}(t)$ from the outside to the BA cells is taken into account in order to control the thresholds equivalently, since Type A cells are employed as the BA cells.

The simulation is carried out in the network illustrated in Fig. 18.6(a) (the network constants etc. are listed in Appendix 2), and the result is shown in Fig. 18.6(b) and (c). When rhythmic oscillation is applied from the PA fibres, the oscillation is combined in the BA cell via homogeneous $h_{n'p}$ and non-oscillatory inhibition is provided to the PU cell body. Since $u_{n'}^{(b)}(t)$ is set negative, the threshold of the BA cell increases correspondingly. Therefore the inhibition starts to work only when the amount of the input from the PA fibres exceeds $u_{n'}^{(b)}(t)$. With the application of a large input, the membrane potential $x_l^{(P)}(t)$ of the PU cell body is suppressed within a certain value (see Fig. 18.6(b)). In other words, even if the peak level of rhythmic oscillation is reduced in order to obtain a locked output without synaptic modification in the GR–GO network, the membrane potential of the PU cell body can be kept almost constant (see Fig. 18.6(c)). Choosing the level of $u_{n'}^{(b)}(t)$ and $h_{n'p}$ adequately, one also obtains a case in which the positive membrane potential of the PU cell body can be attained only if the peak level of rhythmic oscillation is reduced.

Although various sets of synaptic strengths are conceivable, those used in this section enable the BA cells to work most effectively as the suppressor of a large input to the PU cells. It is evident that this effect can be obtained in a similar way when a Type A cell, instead of a Type B cell, is employed as a PU cell.

18.4.2 *Filtering of rhythmic oscillation*

Since the synapses from the ST cells are connected to the PU dendrites, the inhibitory effect of the ST cells must differ from that of the BA cells. The non-linear interaction on the PU dendrites as stated in Section 18.2 may give rise to the functional difference. The equations of the ST–PU network are as follows:

Fig. 18.6. Suppression of the large input in the basket-Purkinje network. (*a*) The schematic diagram of the simulated network (see Appendix 2). (*b*) The output $[x_{l'}^{(P)}(t)]^+$ of the Purkinje cell when the peak value of the input $v_p^{(F)}(t)$ is equal to 1.0. (*c*) When the peak value of $v_p^{(F)}(t)$ is equal to 0.5.

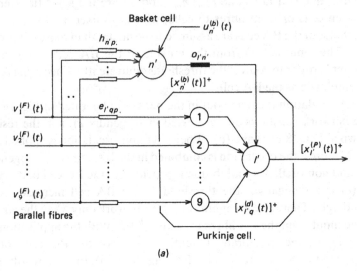

(a)

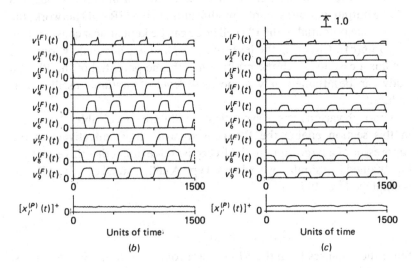

Units of time

(b)

Units of time

(c)

$$\left.\begin{array}{l} \tau_P \dfrac{\mathrm{d}}{\mathrm{d}t} x_l^{(P)}(t) + x_l^{(P)}(t) = \sum_{q=1}^{N_d} [x_{lq}^{(d)}(t)]^+ \quad (l = 1, 2, \ldots, N_P), \\[3mm] \tau_d \dfrac{\mathrm{d}}{\mathrm{d}t} x_{lq}^{(d)}(t) + x_{lq}^{(d)}(t) = \sum_{p=1}^{N_F} e_{lqp} v_p^{(F)}(t) - \sum_{m=1}^{N_s} g_{lqm} [x_m^{(s)}(t)]^+ \\[3mm] \hspace{5cm} (q = 1, 2, \ldots, N_d), \\[3mm] \tau_s \dfrac{\mathrm{d}}{\mathrm{d}t} x_m^{(s)}(t) + x_m^{(s)}(t) = \sum_{p=1}^{N_F} f_{mp} v_p^{(F)}(t) \quad (m = 1, 2, \ldots, N_s). \end{array}\right\} \quad (4.2)$$

Here $x_m^{(s)}(t)$ and τ_s represent the membrane potentials and the integral time constant of the ST cells; f_{mp} and g_{lqm} indicate, respectively, the synaptic strengths from the PA fibres to the ST cells and from the ST cells to the PU dendrites.

The simulated network is illustrated in Fig. 18.7(*a*) (the network constants etc. are listed in Appendix 3) and the result is shown in Fig. 18.7(*b*) and (*c*). When the non-oscillatory signals generated in Network 1 are applied to the network, the membrane potential $x_l^{(P)}(t)$ of the PU cell body is inhibited below zero shortly after the time delay (see Fig. 18.7(*b*)). When, on the other hand, the oscillatory signals generated in Network 2 are applied, the phases of the direct signals and the inhibition via the ST cells are shifted in the PU dendrite. In this case, the negative membrane potentials caused by the inhibition of the ST cells do not interfere with each other, because of the threshold effect in every part of the PU dendrite. Therefore rhythmic oscillation passes through the PU dendrite and reaches the cell body, where the non-oscillatory membrane potential is created by combining the signals (see Fig. 18.7(*c*)).

As mentioned above, the ST–PU network employing a Type B cell as a PU cell may function as a filter through which only rhythmic oscillation can pass. Although we have considered only the case in which $g_{l'qm}$ are diagonal, it is clear that the same effect can be obtained even if the $g_{l'qm}$ are fairly disturbed.

18.4.3 Learning process on Purkinje cell

In this subsection, the synaptic modification algorithm is applied to the synapses from the PA fibres to the PU cells and the second stage of the learning mechanism is examined. This algorithm which effectively generates rhythmic oscillation in the GR–GO network acts on the PU cells in a notable manner. The network including the PA and CL fibres and the PU cells are as follows:

Fig. 18.7. Filtering of rhythmic oscillation in the stellate–Purkinje network. (*a*) The schematic diagram of the simulated network (see Appendix 3). (*b*) The output $[x_{l'}^{(P)}(t)]^+$ of the Purkinje cell when the input $v_p^{(F)}(t)$ is non-oscillatory (the output of Network 1). (*c*) When the input $v_p^{(F)}(t)$ is oscillatory (the output of Network 2).

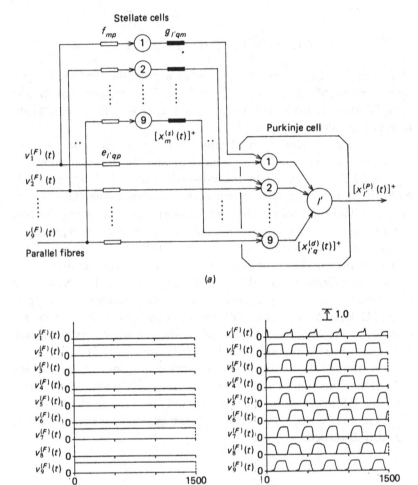

$$
\left.\begin{aligned}
\tau_P \frac{d}{dt} x_l^{(P)}(t) + x_l^{(P)}(t) &= \sum_{q=1}^{N_d} [x_{lq}^{(d)}(t)]^+ + [x_l^{(c)}(t)]^+ \\
&\qquad\qquad (l = 1, 2, \ldots, N_P), \\
\tau_d \frac{d}{dt} x_{lq}^{(d)}(t) + x_{lq}^{(d)}(t) &= \sum_{p=1}^{N_F} e_{lqp}^* v_p^{(F)}(t) \quad (q = 1, 2, \ldots, N_d), \\
\tau_c \frac{d}{dt} x_l^{(c)}(t) + x_l^{(c)}(t) &= u_l^{(M)}(t).
\end{aligned}\right\} \quad (4.3)
$$

Here $x_l^{(c)}(t)$ represent the local membrane potentials of the PU dendrites which are produced by the input $u_l^{(M)}(t)$ from the CL fibres; τ_c is the corresponding integral time constant.

Fig. 18.8(a) shows the simulated network (the network constants etc. are listed in Appendix 4) and Fig. 18.8(b–f) shows the result. In this case, σ in the window function is set up at 20 units of time, while σ was equal to 500 units of time in the first stage. This means that the changes in the synaptic strengths $e_{l'qp}^*$ are assumed to have less hysteresis than those in c_{ji}^* and d_{ij}^*.

With the application of rhythmic oscillation from the PA fibres (see Fig. 18.8(b)), the non-oscillatory membrane potential appears in the PU cell body by way of homogeneous $e_{l'qp}^*$ (see Fig. 18.8(c)). Synaptic modification does not start yet since the threshold $\eta^{(P)}$ in the algorithm is set up at 0.4.

At this point, the square input $u_l^{(M)}(t)$ with the same period as that of the rhythmic oscillation from the PA fibres is applied via the CL fibre to the PU cell. The two inputs, from the PA fibres and the CL fibre, are combined in the PU cell body. As a result, $x_l^{(P)}(t)$ exceeds $\eta^{(P)}$ in the interval during which $u_l^{(M)}(t)$ is positive (see Fig. 18.8(d)).

Although the wave shape of $[x_l^{(P)}(t)]^+$ shown in Fig. 18.8(d) is caused by $u_l^{(M)}(t)$, the synaptic modification algorithm with a small σ attenuates $e_{l'qp}^*$ so as to reduce the projection. That is, when both $v_p^{(F)}(t) - \theta^{(PF)}$ and $x_l^{(P)}(t) - \eta^{(P)}$ are positive at the same time, the corresponding $e_{l'qp'}^*$ are reduced. The periods of $u_l^{(M)}(t)$ and $v_p^{(F)}(t)$ are equal and therefore the $e_{l'qp}^*$ to be modified are always the same. Within a short time, the membrane potential $x_l^{(P)}(t)$ of the PU cell body drops below the threshold $\eta^{(P)}$ in spite of the application of $u_l^{(M)}(t)$ (see Fig. 18.8(e)). Then the synaptic modification stops.

When the application of $u_l^{(M)}(t)$ is ceased, a signal with the inverse phase of $u_l^{(M)}(t)$ appears in the membrane potential of the PU cell body (see Fig. 18.8(f)).

As a consequence of the above-mentioned mechanism, the network can synthesize the signals from the PA fibres, producing an output which has the inverse phase of the signal from the CL fibre. The learning is accomplished by the network's copying of the signal from the CL fibre, the timing of which is constant. This enables it to control the actuator directly, so the process differs from error–correction learning such as is employed in the perceptron. In this sense, the signal from the CL fibre should be referred to as 'master' rather than 'teacher'.

Fig. 18.8. Learning process on the Purkinje cell as a result of the synaptic modification of e_{lqp}^*. (*a*) The schematic diagram of the simulated network (see Appendix 4). (*b*) The input $v_p^{(F)}(t)$ from the parallel fibres. (*c*) The output $[x_{l'}^{(P)}(t)]^+$ of the Purkinje cell without the input $u_{l'}^{(M)}(t)$ from the climbing fibre. (*d*) $[x_{l'}^{(P)}(t)]^+$ immediately after the application of $u_{l'}^{(M)}(t)$. (*e*) $[x_{l'}^{(P)}(t)]^+$ after 6000 modification steps. (*f*) $[x_{l'}^{(P)}(t)]^+$ without $u_{l'}^{(M)}(t)$.

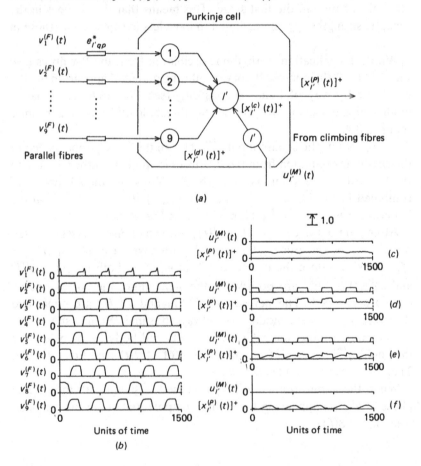

18.5 Total behaviour of the cerebellar circuitry

Total behaviour of the cerebellar circuitry is now illustrated, incorporating all the preceding functions of the cells and the fibres. Putting

$$
\left.\begin{aligned}
[x_i^{(g)}(t)]^+ &= v_p^{(F)}(t) \quad (i = p, \ N_g = N_F), \\
u_i^{(g)}(t) &= \sum_{k=1}^{N_B} a_{ik} v_k^{(B)}(t), \\
u_j^{(G)}(t) &= \sum_{l=1}^{N_P} s_{jl} v_l^{(M)}(t), \\
u_l^{(M)}(t) &= r_l v_l^{(M)}(t),
\end{aligned}\right\}
\tag{5.1}
$$

in order to connect (3.1), (3.2), (4.1), (4.2), and (4.3), the equations of the model of the cerebellar circuitry can be represented as follows:

$$
\left.\begin{aligned}
\tau_g \frac{\mathrm{d}}{\mathrm{d}t} x_i^{(g)} + x_i^{(g)}(t) &= \sum_{k=1}^{N_B} a_{ik} v_k^{(B)}(t) - \sum_{j=1}^{N_G} d_{ij}^* [x_j^{(G)}(t)]^+ \\
&\qquad (i = 1, 2, \ldots, N_g), \\
\tau_G \frac{\mathrm{d}}{\mathrm{d}t} x_j^{(G)}(t) + x_j^{(G)}(t) &= \sum_{l=1}^{N_P} s_{jl} v_l^{(M)}(t) + \sum_{i=1}^{N_g} c_{ji}^* [x_i^{(g)}(t)]^+ \\
&\qquad (j = 1, 2, \ldots, N_G), \\
\tau_P \frac{\mathrm{d}}{\mathrm{d}t} x_l^{(P)}(t) + x_l^{(P)}(t) &= \sum_{q=1}^{N_d} [x_{lq}^{(d)}(t)]^+ + [x_l^{(c)}(t)]^+ \\
&\qquad - \sum_{n=1}^{N_b} o_{ln} [x_n^{(b)}(t)]^+ \\
&\qquad (l = 1, 2, \ldots, N_P), \\
\tau_d \frac{\mathrm{d}}{\mathrm{d}t} x_{lq}^{(d)}(t) + x_{lq}^{(d)}(t) &= \sum_{i=1}^{N_g} e_{lqi}^* [x_i^{(g)}(t)]^+ \\
&\qquad - \sum_{m=1}^{N_s} g_{lqm} [x_m^{(s)}(t)]^+ \quad (q = 1, 2, \ldots, N_d), \\
\tau_c \frac{\mathrm{d}}{\mathrm{d}t} x_l^{(c)}(t) + x_l^{(c)}(t) &= r_l v_l^{(M)}(t), \\
\tau_b \frac{\mathrm{d}}{\mathrm{d}t} x_n^{(b)}(t) + x_n^{(b)}(t) &= u_n^{(b)}(t) + \sum_{i=1}^{N_g} h_{ni} [x_i^{(g)}(t)]^+ \\
&\qquad (n = 1, 2, \ldots, N_b), \\
\tau_s \frac{\mathrm{d}}{\mathrm{d}t} x_m^{(s)}(t) + x_m^{(s)}(t) &= \sum_{i=1}^{N_g} f_{mi} [x_i^{(g)}(t)]^+ \\
&\qquad (m = 1, 2, \ldots, N_s),
\end{aligned}\right\}
\tag{5.2}
$$

Fig. 18.9 gives the block diagram of the simulated model with parameters corresponding to those in (5.2). Fig. 18.10(*a–e*) shows a typical operation of the model, where the synaptic strengths (the initial values in the case of c_{ji}^*, d_{ij}^*, and e_{lqi}^*), the constants in the algorithm, etc., are listed in Appendix 5. The sequences of its behavior are:

Sequence 1. Rhythmic oscillation is applied as the input $v_k^{(B)}(t)$ from the MO fibres. The master signals $v_l^{(M)}(t)$ are not applied. This is equivalent to applying the non-oscillatory input uniformly to the GR cells, because of the homogeneous a_{ik}. In the GR–GO network with a disturbed ring structure, the imbalance of the inhibition produces the non-oscillatory outputs $[x_i^{(g)}(t)]^+$ and $[x_j^{(G)}(t)]^+$ from the GR and GO cells. If the level of $v_k^{(B)}(t)$ is high enough, some values of $[x_i^{(g)}(t)]^+$ or $[x_j^{(G)}(t)]^+$ exceed the threshold $\theta^{(Gg)}$ or $\theta^{(gG)}$ and the synaptic modification of c_{ji}^* and d_{ij}^* starts. At this point, the membrane potentials of the PU cell bodies are inhibited below zero by the ST cells (see Section 18.4.2). Therefore the e_{lqi}^* are not modified (see Fig. 18.10(a)).

Sequence 2. With the progress of the synaptic modification of c_{ji}^* and d_{ij}^*, rhythmic oscillation appears in the GR–GO network. Once it appears, the AIDs of the GR or GO cells gather around $\theta^{(Gg)}$ or $\theta^{(gG)}$, after which the speed of the modification becomes very low and the rhythmic oscillation is caught and held (see Section 18.3.1). The filtering effect of the ST cells may produce the non-oscillatory membrane potentials of the PU cell bodies. However the inhibition by the BA cells suppresses the

Fig. 18.9. The block diagram of the simulated model of the cerebellar circuitry (see Appendix 5).

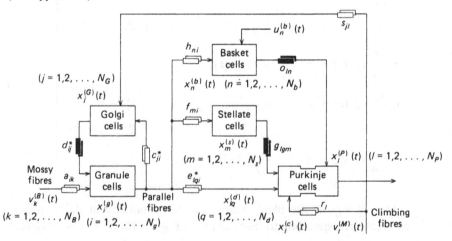

potentials below zero (see Section 18.4.1). Therefore the e_{lqi}^* are not yet modified (see Fig. 18.10(b)).

Sequence 3. After 6000 modification steps, the level of $v_k^{(B)}(t)$ is reduced and a certain level of the oscillatory master signals $v_l^{(M)}(t)$ is applied simultaneously. This procedure helps the period of rhythmic oscillation in the GR–GO network coincide with that of the master signals, as well as avoiding the restarting of the synaptic modification of c_{ji}^* and d_{ij}^* (see Section 18.3.2). As a result of the application of the master signals, the PU cells output signals with square wave shapes. Since the inhibition by the BA cells is still in effect, the non-oscillatory bias components of the membrane potentials $x_j^{(P)}(t)$ of the PU cell bodies due to $v_k^{(B)}(t)$ are held below $\eta^{(P)}$ (see Fig. 18.10(c)).

Sequence 4. The projection of $[x_j^{(P)}(t)]^+$ exceeds $\eta^{(P)}$ and therefore the synaptic modification of e_{lqi}^* starts. Since the periods of $[x_i^{(g)}(t)]^+$ and $v_l^{(M)}(t)$ are equal, the synaptic modification algorithm selectively attenuates the e_{lqi}^* which contribute to the projection of $x_j^{(P)}(t)$. After a short time, this modification suppresses $x_j^{(P)}(t)$ below $\eta^{(P)}$ again in spite of the application of $v_l^{(M)}(t)$, after which the e_{lqi}^* are no longer modified (see Fig. 18.10(d)).

Sequence 5. Ceasing the application of the master signals $v_l^{(M)}(t)$ after a further 6000 modification steps, the PU cells output signals which have the inverse phase of $v_l^{(M)}(t)$. When this occurs, the period of the rhythmic oscillation in the GR–GO network returns to its original length and therefore the period of the output $[x_j^{(P)}(t)]^+$ of the PU cells also changes. However this model can learn the relative timing of the master signals (see Fig. 18.10(e)).

Thus, the model of the cerebellar circuitry has finished learning. This state is maintained without any synaptic modification, since $[x_i^{(g)}(t)]^+$, $[x_j^{(G)}(t)]^+$, or $x_j^{(P)}(t)$ are less than $\theta^{(Gg)}$, $\theta^{(gG)}$, or $\eta^{(P)}$ respectively.

18.6 Discussion

In this paper, we have discussed the relationship between synaptic modification and rhythmic oscillation, constructing a model of the cerebellar circuitry which includes both feedback and feedforward systems. The synaptic modification algorithm was applied to all of the modifiable synapses in the model. Simulation shows that the algorithm is effective for the generation of rhythmic oscillation in the GR–GO network, while working to synthesize the output in the BA–ST–PU network. This

Fig. 18.10. A typical operation of the model. (*a*) Sequence 1: the application of $v_k^{(B)}(t)$. (*b*) Sequence 2: the synaptic modification in the granule–Golgi network (after 6000 modification steps). (*c*) Sequence 3: the reduction of the level

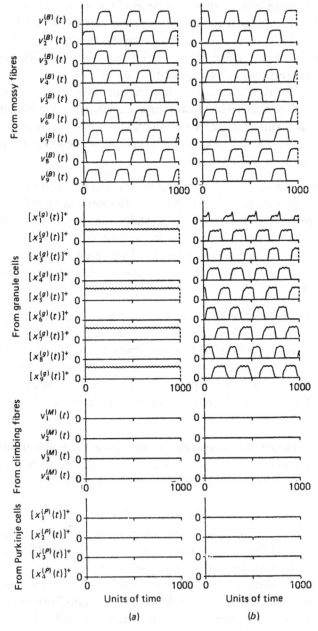

of $v_k^{(B)}(t)$ and the application of $v_l^{(M)}(t)$. (d) Sequence 4: the synaptic modification in the basket–stellate–Purkinje network (after a further 6000 modification steps). (e) Sequence 5: The stoppage of $v_l^{(M)}(t)$.

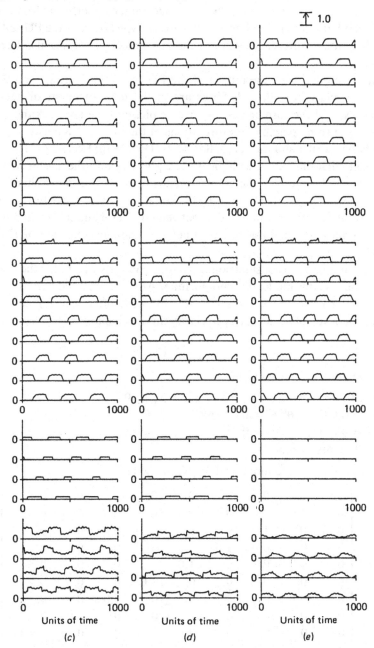

behaviour agrees with the technological principle that the superposition of periodic components is effective in order to create arbitrary patterns, and it is also analogous to the process of mathematical interpolation. In this sense, it should be noted that one algorithm can perform these two different but related functions. By the use of Type B cells as the PU cells, the functional difference between the BA and ST cells has also been clarified.

In the model, both the output of the PU cells after learning and the master signals from the CL fibres are in the form of bursts of nerve impulses, and the former has the inverse phase of the latter. Although there exist some possible interpretations of the interaction between the cerebellar cortex and the cerebellar nuclei (Ito, 1970; Eccles, 1973), it is probable that the output with the inverse phase against the master signal from the PU cell craves the uniform mainstream into the wave shape of the original master signal, since the PU cell is inhibitory. It will further be important to detail the interaction between the cerebellum itself and the related nuclei on the basis of recent neurophysiological knowledge (Ito, 1982).

It is important to consider some synaptic channels which, for the sake of simplicity, this model does not include. Also not analysed here is how the period of the final output of the PU cells after learning can be controlled. It will be necessary to clarify this mechanism.

Appendix 1

(1) The network constants, etc.

$\tau_g = 2.0$, $\tau_G = 10.0$, $N_g = 9$,   and $N_G = 9$.
$\delta^{(Gg)} = 0.0004$, $\theta^{(Gg)} = 0.4$, $\eta^{(g)} = -2.0$,
$\delta^{(gG)} = 0.0012$, $\theta^{(gG)} = 0.4$,   and $\eta^{(G)} = 0.0$.
$\sigma = 500$ units of time.

(2) c_{ji}^* and d_{ij}^* before modification (Network 1):

$$c_{ji}^* = \begin{bmatrix} 1.0 & 0. & 0. & 0. & 0. & 0. & 0. & 0. & 0. \\ 0. & 1.0 & 0. & 0. & 0. & 0. & 0. & 0. & 0. \\ 0. & 0. & 1.0 & 0. & 0. & 0. & 0. & 0. & 0. \\ 0. & 0. & 0. & 1.0 & 0. & 0. & 0. & 0. & 0. \\ 0. & 0. & 0. & 0. & 1.0 & 0. & 0. & 0. & 0. \\ 0. & 0. & 0. & 0. & 0. & 1.0 & 0. & 0. & 0. \\ 0. & 0. & 0. & 0. & 0. & 0. & 1.0 & 0. & 0. \\ 0. & 0. & 0. & 0. & 0. & 0. & 0. & 1.0 & 0. \\ 0. & 0. & 0. & 0. & 0. & 0. & 0. & 0. & 1.0 \end{bmatrix}$$

$$d_{ij}^* = \begin{bmatrix} 0. & 3.0 & 2.0 & 0. & 0. & 0. & 0. & 0. & 0.5 \\ 0.5 & 0. & 3.0 & 1.0 & 0. & 0. & 0. & 0. & 0. \\ 0. & 0.5 & 0. & 3.0 & 0. & 0. & 1.0 & 0. & 0. \\ 0. & 0. & 0.5 & 0. & 3.0 & 0. & 0. & 0. & 0. \\ 0. & 0. & 0. & 0.5 & 0. & 3.0 & 0. & 0. & 0. \\ 0. & 0. & 0. & 0. & 0.5 & 0. & 3.0 & 0. & 0. \\ 0. & 0. & 0. & 0. & 0. & 0.5 & 0. & 3.0 & 0. \\ 0. & 0. & 0. & 0. & 0. & 0. & 0.5 & 0. & 3.0 \\ 3.0 & 0. & 0. & 0. & 0. & 0. & 0. & 0.5 & 0. \end{bmatrix}$$

(3) c_{ji}^* and d_{ij}^* after 2760 modification steps:

$$c_{ji}^* = \begin{bmatrix} 0.924 & 0. & 0. & 0. & 0. & 0. & 0. & 0. & 0. \\ 0. & 0.908 & 0. & 0. & 0. & 0. & 0. & 0. & 0. \\ 0. & 0. & 0.719 & 0. & 0. & 0. & 0. & 0. & 0. \\ 0. & 0. & 0. & 0.926 & 0. & 0. & 0. & 0. & 0. \\ 0. & 0. & 0. & 0. & 0.575 & 0. & 0. & 0. & 0. \\ 0. & 0. & 0. & 0. & 0. & 0.921 & 0. & 0. & 0. \\ 0. & 0. & 0. & 0. & 0. & 0. & 0.579 & 0. & 0. \\ 0. & 0. & 0. & 0. & 0. & 0. & 0. & 0.918 & 0. \\ 0. & 0. & 0. & 0. & 0. & 0. & 0. & 0. & 0.592 \end{bmatrix}$$

$$d_{ij}^* = \begin{bmatrix} 0. & 2.989 & 0.851 & 0. & 0. & 0. & 0. & 0. & 0. \\ 0.119 & 0. & 2.586 & 0.630 & 0. & 0. & 0. & 0. & 0. \\ 0. & 0.003 & 0. & 2.923 & 0. & 0. & 0. & 0. & 0. \\ 0. & 0. & 0.135 & 0. & 2.769 & 0. & 0. & 0. & 0. \\ 0. & 0. & 0. & 0.472 & 0. & 2.964 & 0. & 0. & 0. \\ 0. & 0. & 0. & 0. & 0.271 & 0. & 2.779 & 0. & 0. \\ 0. & 0. & 0. & 0. & 0. & 0.470 & 0. & 2.964 & 0. \\ 0. & 0. & 0. & 0. & 0. & 0. & 0.267 & 0. & 2.798 \\ 2.963 & 0. & 0. & 0. & 0. & 0. & 0. & 0.462 & 0. \end{bmatrix}$$

(4) c_{ji}^* and d_{ij}^* after 6000 modification steps (Network 2):

$$c_{ji}^* = \begin{bmatrix} 0.906 & 0. & 0. & 0. & 0. & 0. & 0. & 0. & 0. \\ 0. & 0.886 & 0. & 0. & 0. & 0. & 0. & 0. & 0. \\ 0. & 0. & 0.714 & 0. & 0. & 0. & 0. & 0. & 0. \\ 0. & 0. & 0. & 0.824 & 0. & 0. & 0. & 0. & 0. \\ 0. & 0. & 0. & 0. & 0.565 & 0. & 0. & 0. & 0. \\ 0. & 0. & 0. & 0. & 0. & 0.863 & 0. & 0. & 0. \\ 0. & 0. & 0. & 0. & 0. & 0. & 0.549 & 0. & 0. \\ 0. & 0. & 0. & 0. & 0. & 0. & 0. & 0.883 & 0. \\ 0. & 0. & 0. & 0. & 0. & 0. & 0. & 0. & 0.537 \end{bmatrix}$$

$$
d^*_{ij} = \begin{bmatrix}
0. & 2.946 & 0.851 & 0. & 0. & 0. & 0. & 0. & 0.5 \\
0. & 0. & 2.586 & 0.103 & 0. & 0. & 0. & 0. & 0. \\
0. & 0. & 0. & 2.704 & 0. & 0. & 0. & 0. & 0. \\
0. & 0. & 0.135 & 0. & 2.769 & 0. & 0. & 0. & 0. \\
0. & 0. & 0. & 0.288 & 0. & 2.908 & 0. & 0. & 0. \\
0. & 0. & 0. & 0. & 0.271 & 0. & 2.779 & 0. & 0. \\
0. & 0. & 0. & 0. & 0. & 0.388 & 0. & 2.912 & 0. \\
0. & 0. & 0. & 0. & 0. & 0. & 0.267 & 0. & 2.798 \\
2.924 & 0. & 0. & 0. & 0. & 0. & 0. & 0.364 & 0.
\end{bmatrix}
$$

Appendix 2

$\tau_P = 2.0, \quad \tau_d = 2.0, \quad \tau_b = 10.0,$

$N_P = 1, \quad N_d = 9, \quad N_b = 1, \quad \text{and} \quad N_F = 9.$

$e_{l'qp} = \begin{cases} 0.25 & \text{if } p = q, \quad h_{n'p} = 0.25, \quad \text{and} \quad o_{l'n'} = 1.0. \\ 0. & \text{otherwise} \end{cases}$

$u_n^{(b)}(t) = -0.5.$

Appendix 3

$\tau_P = 2.0, \quad \tau_d = 2.0, \quad \tau_s = 200.0,$

$N_P = 1, \quad N_d = 9, \quad N_s = 9, \quad \text{and} \quad N_F = 9.$

$e_{l'qp} = \begin{cases} 0.25 & \text{if } p = q, \\ 0. & \text{otherwise} \end{cases} \quad f_{mp} = \begin{cases} 0.25 & \text{if } p = m, \\ 0. & \text{otherwise} \end{cases}$

$\text{and} \quad g_{l'qm} = \begin{cases} 1.00 & \text{if } m = q \\ 0. & \text{otherwise.} \end{cases}$

Appendix 4

$\tau_P = 2.0, \quad \tau_d = 2.0, \quad \tau_c = 2.0, \quad N_P = 1, \quad N_d = 9, \quad \text{and} \quad N_F = 9.$

$e^*_{l'qp} = \begin{cases} 0.15, & \text{if } p = q \\ 0. & \text{otherwise.} \end{cases}$

$\delta^{(PF)} = 0.0012, \quad \theta^{(PF)} = 0.4, \quad \text{and} \quad \eta^{(P)} = 0.4.$

$\sigma = 20 \text{ units of time.}$

Appendix 5

(1) The granule–Golgi network

$\tau_g = 2.0 \quad \text{and} \quad \tau_G = 10.0.$

$N_g = 9 \quad \text{and} \quad N_G = 9.$

$a_{ik} = 0.25.$

c_{ji}^* and d_{ij}^* are the same as those in Network 1:

$$s_{jl} = \begin{cases} 1.00 & \text{if} \quad l = j = 1 \\ 0. & \text{otherwise.} \end{cases}$$

$\delta^{(Gg)} = 0.0004$, $\theta^{(Gg)} = 0.4$, $\eta^{(g)} = -2.0$,

$\delta^{(gG)} = 0.0012$, $\theta^{(gG)} = 0.4$, and $\eta^{(G)} = 0.0$.

$\sigma = 500$ units of time.

(2) The basket–stellate–Purkinje network

$\tau_P = 2.0$, $\tau_d = 2.0$, $\tau_c = 2.0$, $\tau_s = 200.0$, and $\tau_b = 10.0$.

$N_P = 4$, $N_d = 9$, $N_s = 9$, and $N_b = 4$.

$$e_{1qi}^* = e_{2qi}^* = e_{3qi}^* = e_{4qi}^* = \begin{cases} 0.60 & \text{if} \quad i = q \\ 0. & \text{otherwise.} \end{cases}$$

$$f_{mi} = \begin{cases} 0.60 & \text{if} \quad i = m \\ 0. & \text{otherwise.} \end{cases}$$

$$g_{1qm} = g_{2qm} = g_{3qm} = g_{4qm} = \begin{cases} 1.00 & \text{if} \quad m = q \\ 0. & \text{otherwise.} \end{cases}$$

$h_{ni} = 0.25$.

$$o_{ln} = \begin{cases} 5.00 & \text{if} \quad n = l \\ 0. & \text{otherwise} \end{cases}$$

$r_l = 2.00$.

$u_n^{(b)}(t) = -0.5$.

$\delta^{(Pg)} = 0.003$, $\theta^{(Pg)} = 0.2$, and $\eta^{(P)} = 0.4$.

$\sigma = 20$ units of time.

References

Eccles, J. C. (1973). 'The cerebellum as a computer: patterns in space and time.' *Journal of Physiology*, **229**, 1–32.

Friesen, W. O. & Stent, G. S. (1977). 'Generation of a locomotory rhythm by a neural network with recurrent cyclic inhibition.' *Biological Cybernetics*, **28**, 27–40.

Fujita, M. (1982a). 'Adaptive filter model of the cerebellum.' *Biological Cybernetics*, **45**, 195–206.

Fujita, M. (1982b). 'Simulation of adaptive modification of the vestibulo–ocular reflex with an adaptive filter model of the cerebellum.' *Biological Cybernetics*, **45**, 207–14.

Hassul, M. & Daniels, P. D. (1977). 'Cerebellar dynamics: the mossy fiber input.' *IEEE Transactions on BME*, **24**, 449–56.

Hirai, Y. (1980a). 'A new hypothesis for synaptic modification: an interactive process between postsynaptic competition and presynaptic regulation.' *Biological Cybernetics*, **36**, 41–50.

Hirai, Y. (1980b). 'A template matching model for pattern recognition: self-organization of templates and template matching by a disinhibitory neural network. *Biological Cybernetics*, **38**, 91–101.

Ito, M. (1970). 'Neurophysiological aspects of the cerebellar motor control system.' *International Journal of Neurology*, 7, 162–76.

Ito, M. (1982). 'Cerebellar control of the vestibulo–ocular reflex around the flocculus hypothesis.' *Annual Review of Neuroscience*, 5, 275–96.

Marr, D. (1969). 'A theory of cerebellar cortex.' *Journal of Physiology*, 202, 437–70.

Matsuoka, K. (1985). 'Sustained oscillation generated by mutually inhibiting neurons with adaptation.' *Biological Cybernetics*, 52, 367–76.

Morishita, I. & Yajima, A. (1972). 'Analysis and simulation of networks of mutually inhibiting neurons.' *Kybernetik*, 11, 154–65.

Stein, R. B., Leung, K. V., Mangeron, D. & Oguztöreli, M. N. (1974). 'Improved neuronal models for studying neural networks.' *Kybernetik*, 15, 1–9.

Szentagothai, J. (1968). 'Structuro–functional considerations of the cerebellar neuron network.' *Proceedings of IEEE*, 56, 960–8.

Thompson, R. S. (1982). 'A model for basic pattern generating mechanisms in the lobster stomatogastric ganglian.' *Biological Cybernetics*, 43, 71–8.

Tsutsumi, K. & Matsumoto, H. (1984a). 'A synaptic modification algorithm in consideration of the generation of rhythmic oscillation in a ring neural network.' *Biological Cybernetics*, 50, 419–30.

Tsutsumi, K. & Matsumoto, H. (1984b). 'Ring neural network and a generator of rhythmic oscillation with period control mechanism.' *Biological Cybernetics*, 51, 181–94.

19

'Normal' and 'abnormal' dynamic behaviour during synaptic transmission

G. BARNA and P. ÉRDI

19.1 Introduction

Rhythmic behaviour is characteristic for the nervous system at different hierarchical levels. Periodic temporal patterns can be generated both by endogenous pacemaker neurons and by multicellular neural networks. At single-cell level it was demonstrated, both experimentally and theoretically, that periodic membrane potentials could bifurcate to more complex oscillatory behaviour (ultimately identified by chaos) in response to drug treatment (Holden, Winlow & Haydon, 1982; Chay, 1984). Even the alteration of periodically synchronized oscillation and chaotic behaviour has been found in periodically forced oscillators of squid giant axons (Aihara, Matsumoto & Ichikawa, 1985).

The appearance of quasi-periodicity and chaos has been associated with abnormal neural phenomena not only at single neural level but as well at macroscopic scale connecting chaotic EEG dynamics to epileptic seizure (Babloyantz, Salazar & Nicholis, 1985). At intermediate level, chaotic behaviour was found in a model of the central dopaminergic neuronal system, and was associated with schizophrenics (King, Barchas & Huberman, 1984).

'Normal' and 'abnormal' dynamic behaviour, also at intermediate, namely synaptic level, has recently been investigated (Érdi & Barna, 1986; Érdi & Barna, 1987). Preliminary numerical calculations suggested that the regular periodic operation of synaptic level rhythmic generator of cholinergic system requires a *fine-tuned neurochemical control system*. Even mild impairment of the metabolism might imply 'abnormal' dynamic synaptic activity.

Memory disorders associated with Alzheimer's disease, partially due to disturbance of the control system of acetylcholine (ACh) synthesis, can be accompanied by change of dynamic patterns of firing frequency (Wurtman, Hefti & Melamed, 1981). Newer results (see Price, 1986) reinforced the connection between lesions in cholinergic system and disorders in behaviour, cognition and memory, as syndromes of Alzheimer's disease.

The basis of the model investigated here is the transmitter-recycling (TRC) hypothesis (Érdi, 1983) adopted to explain the 'integrated' synaptic activity at cholinergic system. The model is supplemented by an independent, harmonic oscillator to take into consideration, at least approximately, the effect of other neural oscillators.

The neurochemical background is shortly analyzed (Section 19.2). The driven TRC model is presented (Section 19.3). Extensive numerical calculations demonstrate the transition from 'normal' to 'abnormal' (and what is clinically more important) from 'abnormal' to 'normal' dynamic behaviour. Further difficulties and problems are mentioned (Section 19.5).

19.2 Neurochemical background

Experimental evidence has accumulated to connect neural and mental disorders to disturbance of control of neurotransmitter synthesis. The hypoxia and hypoglycemia due to the failure of cholinergic metabolism leads to reduced ACh synthesis and neurological disorders (Gibson & Blass, 1976a,b). A precursor of ACh, namely choline (Ch) seemed to be useful in treating memory disorders associated with Alzheimer's disease and ageing (Wurtman et al., 1981), reinforcing the view that the understanding of the operation of the dynamic control system of ACh metabolism would conclude in suggestions for new clinical treatment of such diseases.

At least three different neurochemical and neurophysiological oscillatory phenomena appear at different hierarchical levels of cholinergic synaptic transmission (Érdi & Tóth, 1981; Érdi, 1983), see Table 19.1. The 'rapid' and 'slow' oscillations of free, presumably cytoplasmic ACh were presented (Dunant et al., 1977; Israel et al., 1977). Other oscillatory phenomena are the series of miniature – end-plate potential (Fatt & Katz, 1952).

The skeleton model of slow oscillation due to the 'integrated synaptic activity' (Fig. 19.1) suggests that the state of the system can be characterized by four variables, and five subprocesses can be defined. The state variables of the system:

cytoplasmic ACh concentration: X;

Table 19.1. *Hierarchical chemical oscillators*

Oscillators	Cellular localization presumed	Primary effects	
		Neurochemical	Neurophysio-logical
I	Bound partially to the mitochondria of nerve terminal	Rapid ACh and ATP oscillation	No electrophysio-logical correlate has been observed
II	Synaptic cleft	Supposed ACh oscillation in the cleft	MEPP
III	'Integrated' synaptic activity	Slow ACh oscillation	Conductance change

Fig. 19.1. Skeleton model of integrated synaptic activity associated with the transmitter-recycling hypothesis. The eight-compartments system has been lumped into a four-variables system.

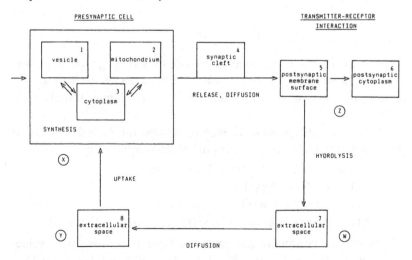

ACh concentration at the postsynaptic membrane surface: Z;
Ch concentration near postsynaptic cell: W;
Ch concentration near presynaptic cell: Y.
The subprocesses taken into account:
  transmitter release, cleft processes, transmitter–receptor interaction;
  ACh hydrolysis;
  metabolic products (mostly Ch) diffuse to the vicinity of the presynaptic cell;
  (re)uptake of Ch;
  autocatalytic synthesis of Ch.

It might be plausible to assume that rhythmic integrated synaptic activity is perturbed at least by another oscillator coupled to the ACh synthesis. ACh synthesis is controlled by the sodium-dependent high-affinity choline uptake (Barker & Mittag, 1975) and by the transport of acetyl group (Jope, 1979; Tucek, 1983). Periodically added Ch might lead complex oscillatory behaviour of the state variables.

19.3 The driven transmitter-recycling model

The skeleton model of slow oscillation can be given in terms of formal chemical reactions as

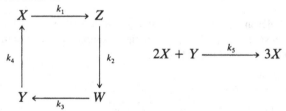

The mass action kinetic model of this mass-conserving model reaction, containing a single non-linearity, can exhibit sustained oscillation. The 'limit shell' character of the oscillation has been demonstrated (Tóth, 1985).

Assuming an independent choline oscillation the periodically driven system is described by the system of differential equations:

$$\dot{x}(t) = -k_1 x(t) + k_4 y(t) + k_5 x^2(t) y(t),$$
$$\dot{z}(t) = k_1 x(t) - k_2 z(t),$$
$$\dot{w}(t) = k_2 z(t) - k_3 w(t),$$
$$\dot{y}(t) = k_3 w(t) - k_4 y(t) - k_5 x^2(t) y(t), + a \cdot \cos(\omega t + \varphi).$$

Simulation experiments demonstrated here were done with values $k_1 = 10, k_2 = 100, k_3 = k_4 = 0.1, k_5 = 1$; the value of the total mass was 110.

Earlier simulation experiments (Érdi & Barna, 1986; Érdi & Barna, 1987) gave some information about the behaviour of the system for different parameter values of the perturbation. Phase locking has been demonstrated in the neighbourhood of the main entrainment band. The existence of rather long-lived transient arrhythmicities and their abrupt decay to simple periodicity seemed to be in accordance with the view, according to which the normal rhythmic dynamics is the result of the operation of a fine-tuned control system.

19.4 Results

The system of differential equations mentioned above was solved numerically (Gottwald & Wanner, 1981) for different parameter values of the perturbation. For the visual illustration of the dynamic behaviour the Poincaré and Lorenz plots are added to the time evolution curve. The Poincaré plot is the x_n versus x_{n+1} mapping, where x_n is the value of the perturbed variable at the moment t_n. t_0 is an arbitrarily chosen initial point, $t_{n+1} - t_n = 2\pi/\omega$ (ω is the period of the impressed oscillation). The Lorenz plot is obtained by plotting successive maxima.

In our notation a limit cycle is denoted with a pair of numbers: (m, n) where m and n are natural numbers. Let this mean that the frequency of the m-fold limit cycle is the $1/n$ part of the perturbed frequency. In the observed region it was found that $|n/m - \omega/\omega_0| < 1$ where ω_0 denotes the inherent frequency of the undriven system ($\omega_0 = 2.343\,977\ldots$). (In an arbitrary perturbed system in case of limit cycle the above absolute value tends to zero if α tends to zero.) In the case of an (m, n) limit cycle the number of fixed points on the Lorenz plot is m at least, while on the Poincaré plot it is exactly n.

On the α–ω phase plane in cases of minor amplitudes ($\alpha < \sim3$) around ω_0, $2\omega_0$, $3\omega_0$, . . ., were found limit cycles $(1, 1)$, $(1, 2)$, $(1, 3)$ . . . respectively (Fig. 19.2), with quasi-periodic area among them (Fig. 19.3).

Fig. 19.2. Single limit cycles at $\alpha = 5.0$, the figures show the α–w phase plane: (*a*) (1,1) $\omega = 2.3$; (*b*) (1,2) $\omega = 5.6$; (*c*) (1,3) $\omega = 8.0$.

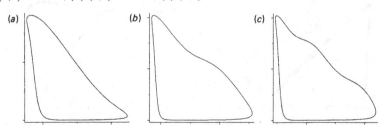

The borders of the quasi-periodic and $(1, i)$ areas are almost straight, the borders of the $(1, i)$ area meet at $i\omega_0$ enclosing an acute angle.

In cases of major amplitudes the $(1, i)$, $(1, i + 1)$ regions may meet directly, intercepting a very thin $(2, i + i + 1)$ region (Fig. 19.4). The border between the areas $(1, 2)$ and $(1, 3)$ is almost entirely independent of α at $\omega = 6.2 \pm 0.02$. Along this border there is a characteristic $(3, 8)$ cycle (Fig. 19.5(a)). The trajectories along the imaginary elongation of this border into the quasi-periodic part intercepted by $(1, 2)$ and $(1, 3)$ are similar to the $(3, 8)$ limit cycle found at greater amplitudes (Fig. 19.3(a)). Naturally, these cannot be limit cycles but their orbits are enclosed in a narrow band around an imaginary $(3, 8)$ cycle.

Our investigation is limited by the chemically plausible constraint that

Fig. 19.3. Quasi-periodic cycles, the figures show the α–w phase plane, the Poincaré and the Lorenz plot respectively. The central part of the phase plane enlarged ten times as shown in the upper right quarter. (a) $\alpha = 1.0$, $\omega = 6.18$; (b) $\alpha = 1.0$, $\omega = 5.6$; (c) $\alpha = 7.0$, $\omega = 13.7$.

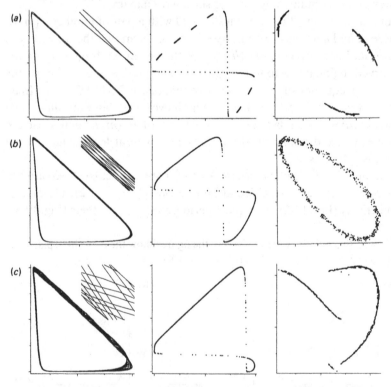

concentrations cannot be negative; therefore the value of a can only be inside a region $[0, g]$, where g is a function of ω (though it is not proved, that g is a function in mathematical meaning). It is continuous inside an area, but it leaps between them, e.g., on the border of (1, 2) and (1, 3) from ~11.5 onto ~8.

The quasi-periodic orbit on the Poincaré plot has a trace where the points form a closed curve, in the sense that they cover the curve totally as t tends to infinity (Fig. 19.3(b)). In some cases tearing occurs. The x_i, x_{i+k}, x_{i+2k} . . . elements of the x_n sequence of the stroboscopic mapping stay in a certain closed interval, where they cannot get out, and they fill it entirely when t tends to infinity. This is a kind of transition from the quasi-periodic to the limit cycle behaviour (Fig. 19.3(a)).

Fig. 19.4. (2,i) cycles, the figures show phase plane, Poincaré and Lorenz plot respectively: (a) (2,5) $\alpha = 3.0$, $\omega = 5.86$; (b) (2,7) $\alpha = 7.0$, $\omega = 8.6$; (c) (2,11) $\alpha = 7.0$, $\omega = 13.0$.

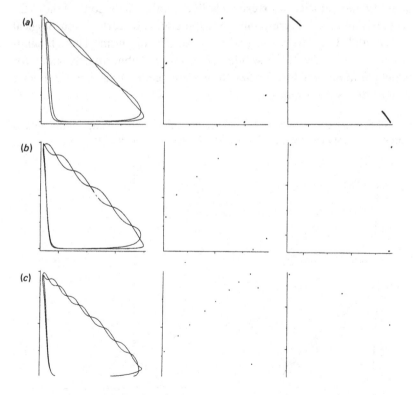

19.5 Conclusions

The driven TRC model investigated here is, technically, a periodically perturbed four-variables system of differential equations. Since the formal chemical model exhibits mass-conserving property, the total system is four-dimensional.

Response of a lower, namely two-dimensional non-linear, oscillator for perturbation by an independent harmonic oscillator was thoroughly examined by Tomita (1982). His studies resulted in the fine classification of the perturbing amplitude–frequency phase space in terms of the qualitative behaviour of the system: regions of entrainment, of period-doubling cascade and of chaos were demonstrated.

Extensive numerical calculations aided the discovery of many details of the fine-structure of the amplitude–frequency space in the driven TRC model. The occurrence of different types of complex oscillations and transitions to simple periodic behaviour was clearly obtained.

Simulation results in terms of neurochemistry and neurology suggest the existence of a fine-tuned control system of ACh metabolism. The quantity and velocity of external choline uptake might control the ACh synthesis and can severely influence the course of certain neurological and mental disorders associated with ACh metabolism. Though simulation results predict the possibility of the onset of abnormal dynamics for many parameter values, further studies are needed to give more precise quantitative suggestions.

Fig. 19.5. $(3,i)$ cycles at $\alpha = 7$, the diagram shows phase plane, Poincaré and Lorenz plot respectively: (a) $(3,8)$ $\omega = 6.16$; (b) $(3,19)$ $\omega = 14.0$.

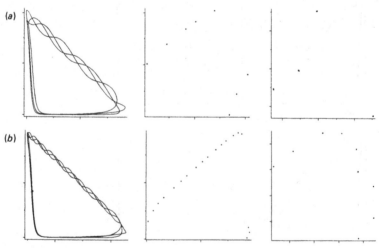

Acknowledgement

Special thanks are due to Prof. T. Kohonen since many simulation experiments were made in his laboratory at the Helsinki University of Technology, using a Data General Eclipse S/250 minicomputer when one of us (G.B.) spent two months there within the framework of the International Trainee Exchanges program between the Finnish Ministry of Labour and the Hungarian International Cultural Institute.

References

Aihara, K., Matsumoto, G. & Ichikawa, M. (1985). 'An alternating periodic–chaotic sequence observed in neural oscillators.' *Physics Letters*, **111A**, 251–5.

Babloyantz, A., Salazar, J. M. & Nicholis, C. (1985). 'Evidence of chaotic dynamics of brain activity during the sleep cycle.' *Physics Letters*, **111A**, 152–6.

Barker, L. A. & Mittag, T. W. (1975). 'Comparative studies of substrates and inhibitors of choline transport and choline acetyltransferase.' *Journal of Pharmacology and Experimental Therapeutics*, **192**, 86–94.

Chay, T. R. (1984). 'Abnormal discharges and chaos in a neuronal model system.' *Biological Cybernetics*, **50**, 301–11.

Dunant, Y., Israel, M., Lesbats, B. & Manaranche, R. (1977). 'Oscillation of acetylcholine during nerve activity in the Torpedo electric organ.' *Brain Research*, **125**, 123–40.

Érdi, P. (1983). 'Hierarchical thermodynamic approach to the brain.' *International Journal of Neuroscience*, **20**, 193–216.

Érdi, P. & Barna, G. (1986). 'Pattern formation in neural systems I. In *Cybernetics and Systems* (1986), ed. R. Trappl, pp. 335–42. D. Reidel Publishing Company.

Érdi, P. & Barna, G. (1987) 'Self-organization in the nervous system: some illustrations.' In *Lecture Notes in Biomathematics*, vol. 71. Berlin–Heidelberg–New York–Tokyo: Springer-Verlag, pp. 301–12.

Érdi, P. & Tóth, J. (1981). 'Oscillatory phenomena at the synapse.' *Advances in Physiological Sciences*, **34**, 113–21.

Fatt, P. & Katz, B. (1952). 'Spontaneous subthreshold activity at motor nerve endings.' *Journal of Physiology*, **117**, 109–28.

Gibson, G. E. & Blass, J. (1976a). 'Inhibition of acetylcholine synthesis and of carbohydrate utilization by maple-syrupurine disease metabolites.' *Journal of Neurochemistry*, **26**, 1073–8.

Gibson, G. E. & Blass, J. (1976b). 'Impaired synthesis of acetylcholine in the brain accompanying mild hypoxia and hypoglycemia.' *Journal of Neurochemistry*, **27**, 37–42.

Gottwald, B. A. & Wanner, G. A. (1981). 'A reliable Rosenbrock Integrator for stiff differential equations.' *Computing*, **26**, 355–60.

Holden, A. V., Winlow, W. & Haydon, P. G. (1982). 'The induction of periodic and chaotic activity in a molluscan neuron.' *Biological Cybernetics*, **43**, 169–73.

Israel, M., Lesbats, B., Manaranche, R., Marsal, J. & Mastour-Frachon, P. (1977). 'Related changes in amounts of ACh and ATP in resting and active torpedo nerve electroplaque synapse.' *Journal of Neurochemistry*, **28**, 1259–67.

Jope, R. S. (1979). 'High affinity choline transport and acetyl CoA production in brain and their roles in the regulation of acetylcholine synthesis.' *Brain Research Review*, **1**, 313–44.

King, R., Barchas, J. D. & Huberman, B. A. (1984). 'Chaotic behaviour in dopamine neurodynamics.' *Proceedings of the National Academy of Sciences of the USA*, **81**, 1244–7.

Price, O. L. (1986). 'New perspectives on Alzheimer's disease.' *Annual Review of Neuroscience*, **9**, 489–518.

Tomita, K. (1982). 'Chaotic response of nonlinear oscillators.' *Physics Reports*, **86**, 113–67.

Tóth, J. (1985). 'A mass action kinetic model of neurochemical transmission.' In *Dynamic Phenomena in Neurochemistry and Neurophysics: Theoretical Aspects*, ed. P. Érdi, pp. 522–55. Budapest.

Tucek, S. (1983). 'Acetylcoenzyme A and the synthesis of acetylcholine in neurons. Review of recent progress.' *General Physiology and Biophysics*, **2**, 313–24.

Wurtman, R. J., Hefti, F. & Melamed, E. (1981). 'Precursor control of neurotransmitter synthesis.' *Pharmacological Reviews*, **32**, 315–35.

20

Computer simulation studies to deduce the structure
and function of the human brain

P. A. ANNINOS and G. ANOGIANAKIS

20.1 Introduction

A prominent feature of the brain is the apparent diversity of its structure: the distribution of neurons and the way in which their dendrites and axon fibers differ in various brain centers. The pattern of inputs and outputs of each neuron in the brain most probably differs from that of any other neuron in the system, and this possibility clearly imposes constraints on any attempts at generalization. Yet, since its inception, microscopy of the central nervous system (CNS) has involved a sustained effort to define the laws of spatial arrangement and of connectivity distinguishing specific structures. However, the question which naturally arises from the above is whether these structural features may reflect, and perhaps determine, fundamental differences in the mode of operation of distinct brain structures. Alternatively, the possibility may exist that such structural specializations merely represent anatomical 'accidents of development', perhaps reflecting phylogenic origin, but playing a functional role which is no more significant than, for example, that of the appendix or the coccygeal vertebrae in man.

It is difficult to provide an answer to this question from the presently available anatomical and physiological data. Although substantial neurohistological data, on one hand, and neurophysiological information, on the other, are available, meaningful correlation of these two sets of data can only be accomplished in very isolated instances. In general, unlike recording from invertebrates, where the simplicity and viability of the nervous system makes it feasible to observe the elements recorded, physiological studies of the mammalian CNS are performed in a 'blind' fashion and it is exceedingly difficult to correlate these studies with the microscopical anatomy of the tissue.

While the ultimate answer to the question of the functional meaning of anatomical structure eventually must come from increased sophistication in experimental design and methodology, some insight also may be obtained through the use of computer simulation models. It is, of course, impractical to create a model which is a perfect replica of the system under study; to do so would presuppose perfect knowledge of the system and thus would obviate the need for the model. Rather, one may choose a certain smaller subset of properties and employ the model to study the effect of these properties on operation of the model.

Thus, in this paper we present the investigation of the relationship between structure, as expressed in the pattern of interneuronal connectivity, and the 'spontaneous' neuronal activity in neural nets, which is in the form of cyclic or self-maintaining activity (Anninos, 1972) and which is required for the simulation of the human electroencephalogram (EEG). After we succeed in obtaining the simulated EEG then we will try to correlate the EEG with the experimental measured Magnetoencephalogram (MEG) which is obtained from human subjects several cm away from their skull, using the new sophisticated device known as SQUID (Superconducting Quantum Interference Device). With such correlation it was possible to deduce certain microstructures which might be responsible for the normal or abnormal behavior observed in the MEG data.

20.2 Theoretical methods

20.2.1 Unit properties

The model employed for analysis of the EEG activity of small neuronal populations is based on earlier work (Anninos *et al.*, 1970; Anninos, 1972, 1973). A family of nerve nets was constructed in those studies, which allowed study of firing patterns, and of the conditions necessary for sustained activity. To preserve generality, connections between individual 'neurons' were made following a random pattern, but once established, such connections were kept fixed for the duration of the experiment. A certain percentage of the neurons was defined as inhibitory. These elements were allowed to deliver over their connections to other neurons only, hyperpolarizing potentials. The remainder of the neuronal population was excitatory. Firing would be triggered in each 'nerve' cell whenever the combination of excitatory and inhibitory potentials reached or exceeded an arbitary threshold. In previous work (Anninos *et al.*, 1970; Anninos, 1972, 1973) it had been considered that when a neuron fires, its threshold is raised to a maximum value and stays there for the duration of the specified absolute refractory period, throughout which the neuron cannot receive excitation. After the absolute period, the neuron is returned to its normal state and is ready to fire again whenever the summed excitatory and inhibitory input exceeds the specified threshold. To achieve greater realism, in the present work we modified the above assumption so that although the threshold of a generator which has been fired previously is high for the duration of the refractory period, it nevertheless continues to receive excitatory and inhibitory inputs throughout the period.

20.2.2 Parameters of the neural net model

The synaptic delay is represented by τ; A is the total number of neurons in the netlet; h is the fraction of inhibitory neurons in the netlet; μ^+ is the average number of axon branches emanating from an excitatory neuron; μ^- is the average number of axon branches emanating from an inhibitory neuron; K^+ is the average EPSP produced by an excitatory neuron in arbitrary units; K^- is the average IPSP produced by an inhibitory neuron in arbitrary units, and ϑ is the firing threshold of the neurons in the netlet.

20.2.3 The EEG model

In the research reported here, the model was further modified to generate EEG activity (i.e. spontaneous wave-like activity), so as to allow investigation of the questions raised above. EEG activity was defined simply as the sum at any instant of all potentials, depolarizing and hyperpolarizing, in the entire cell population. This is in keeping with the experimental evidence from intracellular recordings on generation of the EEG which indicates that the EEG is produced by summation of transmembrane currents in cortical nerve cells (Elul, 1962, 1964; Creutzfeldt, Watanabe & Lux, 1966; Jasper & Stefanis, 1965). Spontaneous and continued 'EEG activity' was assured through use of nerve nets, which, in preceding analyses have been shown to maintain spontaneous activity (Anninos, 1969; Anninos *et al.*, 1970; Anninos, 1972, 1973). In the present study all netlets are class A netlets, according to our classification (Anninos *et al.*, 1970). These are netlets in which any initial activity, however small, will initiate sustained activity. These nets are also classifiable as monostable according to the classification by Amari (1974); that is, nets with one stable equilibrium level to which the activity of the net eventually converges.

After a connectivity pattern was established by fixing the parameters: A, $\mu^\pm$, K, h, an initial state of activity was generated by triggering spikes in a number of neurons according to a random pattern. In networks which are capable of sustained activity, this 'priming' results in the next iteration, in excitation sufficient to induce firing in a number of other neurons, which in turn cause firing in the third iteration, etc. In this way spontaneous activity is maintained, usually on a stable level, although in some cases activity is oscillatory. Samples of the activity generated by this procedure are shown in Fig. 20.1. The activity along time of a typical 'neuron' is shown (Fig. 20.1(a)) in comparison with actual intracellular activity (Fig. 20.1(b) registered with a digital recorder (Varian Statos I). It can be seen that the activity produced by the model is reasonably close to the experimental data. The summed activity of the entire net is shown in Fig. 20.1(c)–(e) for three different model nets. The spontaneous fluctuations in the summed activity – 'gross EEG' may be compared with typical EEG activity (Fig. 20.1(f)). An interesting point in Fig. 20.1 is

Fig. 20.1. Activity of an artificial nerve net (a), (c)–(e), and brain activity recorded in animal experiments (b). (f) The activity of a single generator in the artificial net (a) is compared with the activity of a nerve cell in cat's cerebral cortex obtained in intracellular recording (b)–(e), some of which resemble quite closely the electroencephalogram recorded from the surface of the cat's brain (f).

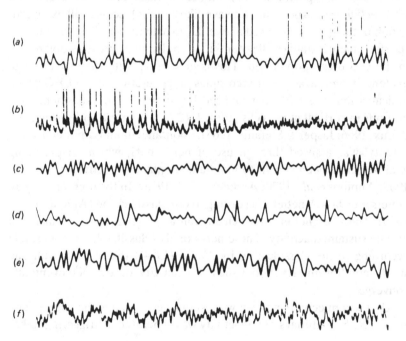

that, depending on the parameters of the nerve net model, the summed activity (Figs. 20.1(c)–(e)) may vary quite markedly in appearance, but with each set of parameters produces a characteristic 'spindling EEG' which exhibits bursts of high amplitude, interspersed with periods of low-voltage activity (Fig. 20.1(c)). Utilizing a different set of parameters, the activity resembles high-voltage sleep (Fig. 20.1(e)).

As we stated in our introduction we are interested in the correlation of the computer simulated EEG with experimental MEG data recorded from the human brain. The justification for this comes from the fact that since we cannot penetrate the human brain with electrodes in order to study its microstructure, the proposed simulated model and the experiment should give quantities which can be measured macroscopically in both systems. In the computer simulated model this quantity is the EEG, which is easy to obtain, as we described above; but for the experiments such quantity should give the real state of neural activity which takes place in the human brain at every moment. One of the most important contributions for such experimental study, and for the relation between structure and function of the human brain, was the development of the SQUIDs. These systems are the most refined tools for this technique. The SQUID operates on the basis of the Josephson effect of superconductivity (Josephson, 1962). With this instrument, which can be used as sensitive magnetometer, we can measure magnetic fields of the order 2×10^{-8} G from the brain which corresponds to brain activities for α-frequencies (8–13 cm s^{-1}) or 5×10^{-9} G for evoked potentials from optical stimulations (Brenner *et al.*, 1975) a few cm away from the scalp. The critical problem, largely solved with this device, is not the amplification of such small signals, but the amplification of the signal (S) to noise (N) ratio (S/N). In this device we have practically eliminated the problem of intrinsic instrumentation noise, while the major problem of ambient noise associated with extraneous sources is eliminated with a proper arrangement of the superconducting coils. Thus with the proper coil arrangement we can eliminate the necessity for costly and elaborate magnetic shielding (Cohen, 1972). Furthermore, with the use of SQUID the inherent noise, due to the use of electrodes as in the case of EEG technique, is eliminated. The fact that the detector is not in contact with the scalp offers the best technique for eliminating the dc potentials appearing at the surface between skin and electrode which are typically larger than any dc potential of neuronal origin. So the SQUID is capable of measuring the dc and the lowest frequency components of electromagnetic radiation from the brain, the result being known as the magnetoencephalogram (MEG). Therefore, from what we have stated so far we can see that the MEG is the only macroscopic quantity which can be correlated to the simulated EEG in order to study the normal and abnormal behaviour observed in the human MEG data.

Thus, the methodology which we considered in this work consists of the following stages:

(1) Using the SQUID gradiometer in an acoustically and electrically shielded room (Anninos *et al.*, 1986) we measured the MEG from different individuals. The noise level in the SQUID environment was of the order of 50 fT/(Hz) (Fig. 20.2). Using the 10–20 International point system (IPS), as in the case of placing EEG electrodes, for recording MEG data from the subjects after positioning the SQUID at each particular point, we asked the subjects to relax and close their eyes. This was done for two reasons: (i) to avoid any artifact from eye flickering, and (ii) to record α-waves (8–13 cm s^{-1}), since we were interested in getting the MEG from the occipital area of the cortex. Furthermore, we introduced acoustically a tone of 12 Hz in order to enhance the α-state of the individual for better MEG recording in the magnetically unshielded room. In these experiments for each measured point and for each individual we took 32 records for a total duration time of 1 s for each record. Thus, using the above experimental set up we detected in several of our patients that their MEG spectra showed definite peaks of 3–4 Hz which is an indication of *petit mal* epilepsy (Brazier, 1968). One such patient is shown in Fig. 20.3.

Fig. 20.2. The noise spectrum of the SQUID which is of the order of 50 fT/(HZ).

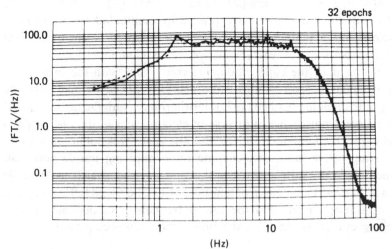

(2) The second stage of our methodology was to analyze the MEG data of our patient (Fig. 20.3) by Fourier series ($\phi = a_0 + \Sigma_{f=1}^{\infty} a_f \cos 2\pi ft + b_f \sin 2\pi ft$) (Anninos & Raman, 1975) the coefficient (a_f, b_f) of which we fit with our MEG data (Fig. 20.4).

(3) Finally, the third stage was to construct a neural net model of the human brain with such parameters as to exhibit similar behaviour as that of Fig. 20.3, and find the specific microstructure which was responsible for such abnormal behaviour. In order to do that we chose the following neural parameters for the connectivity: $A = 1000$, $h = 45\%$, $\mu^+ = 3$, $\mu^- = 3$, $K^\pm = 10$, and $\theta = 10$. On starting our simulation program (Anninos, 1972) we found that such neural network exhibits sustained EEG activity in the form of cyclic activity (Anninos, 1972, 1973) of 3 cm s^{-1} which is indeed similar to the frequency observed in the MEG spectrum of our patient (Fig. 20.3). Analyzing again the simulated EEG data in Fourier series we tried to fit the previously found MEG Fourier coefficients (a_f, b_f) with those obtained from the EEG. Such a fit is shown in (Fig. 20.5). After succeeding in fitting the set of coefficients (a_f, b_f) from both MEG and EEG data we searched to find the microstructure of the theoretical EEG which might be related for such observed MEG abnormal behaviour. Thus, by examining such microscopic structure, as we can see from the following diagrams, we can get some information regarding the arrangement of inhibitory versus excitatory neurons (Fig. 20.6), the distribution of the total number of incoming connections/

Fig. 20.3. Average magnetic field spectrum of 32 records, over a period of 1 s for each record, from a patient with epileptic focus near the P3 of the 10–20 IPS, showing a peak of 3 Hz and another peak of 10 Hz (α-frequency).

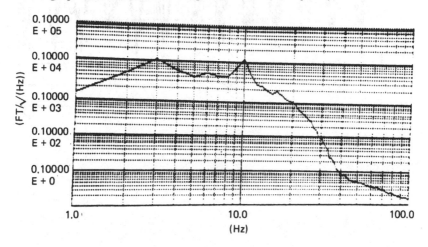

P. A. Anninos & G. Anogianakis

Fig. 20.4. The fit of MEG data recorded from the scalp of the patient shown in Fig. 20.3 with a Fourier series.

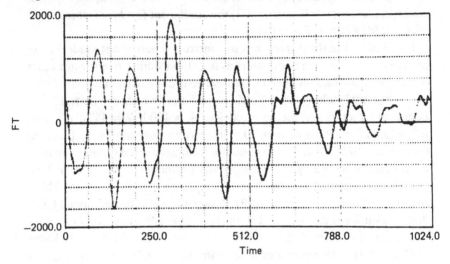

Fig. 20.5. The combined fit of MEG and EEG data to the same Fourier series.

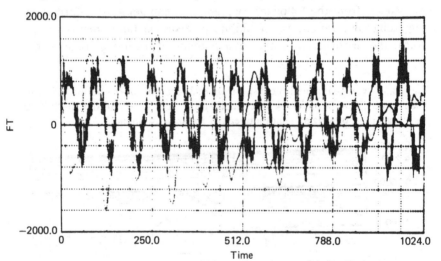

Fig. 20.6. The arrangement of inhibitory and excitatory neurons in the simulated brain. Open and closed circles represent the excitatory and inhibitory neurons respectively.

```
O●O●C●O●O●  OOOOO●O●OO  O●●●●OOOOO  ●OOO●O●O●O  OOO●O●●OOO
OOOOO●●OOO  ●OOO●O●OOO  OO●OOCO●OO  ●OO●OO●●C●  ●●●OO●●●OO
OO●●●●OOO●  OO●OOO●O●●  O●O●OOOOOO  OO●OOO●OOO  OOO●OO●●O●
O●O●OC●O●●  OOO●OO●OO●  ●OOOOOO●OO  O●OO●O●OOO  OO●●●OC●O●
●OOOCO●OO●  ●O●●●●OO●O  OOOO●OOO●●  OO●O●●●●C●  O●OOOOOO●O
O●●●●●C●OO  OOOO●●O●OO  OOOOO●●OOO  OOO●OO●O●O  OOOO●OOOOO
O●OOO●OO●●  OOOOO●OO●●  O●OOOO●O●●  OO●O●●●●O●  ●OOOO●●OO●O
OO●●OOO●OO  OO●O●●●●●O  ●●O●●OOOO●  ●OOOOO●OOO  ●OOOOOO●O●
OO●OO●●●●O  O●OOOOOOO●●  OOO●●OOOOO  O●OOOOOO●O  OO●●●●OO●O
OOOO●●●●●O  O●OOOOOO●O  ●OOOOOOOO●  ●●●OOO●●OO  OO●O●OO●O●O
●OOOOOOOOO  ●OOO●OOOOO  O●OO●●OO●O  OOOO●OOOOO  OOOOCO●O●O
OO●O●●●OOO  OOO●OOOO●O  O●OOO●O●●O  ●OO●OOOO●●  O●OOO●OOOO●
●O●●OOO●O●  OOOO●OOOOO  ●OOOOO●OOO  OOO●●●●●O●  ●OO●OO●●O●
O●●OOOOOOO  O●O●OOOO●O●  O●O●OOOO●O●  OOOO●OOO●●  ●●OOO●OOOO
O●●OO●OOOO  ●O●●●O●OOO  O●OOOO●O●O  ●●OOOOOOOO  OO●●OOO●●O
O●●OO●OOOO  ●O●●●●OOOO  OOO●OOOO●●  O●OOOO●O●O  ●O●OOO●OO●
●OOO●OOOOO  O●OOO●●●●O  OOO●●O●OOO  OOOOOOOOOO  OOO●●OO●O●
●OOO●O●OOO  O●●OOOO●O●  ●OOOOOOOOO  O●O●OO●●●O  OO●OOO●●OO
●O●OOO●O●●  O●OO●OOO●●  O●●C●OOOO●  ●O●●OOO●O●  OOOOOOOOOO
OO●OOOOOOO  OOOOO●O●●●  OO●OOOOOOO  ●●OOOOOOO●  ●●●●●OOOOO
```

neuron (Fig. 20.7), the total number of excitatory incoming connections/ neuron (Fig. 20.8) and the total number of inhibitory incoming connec- tions/neuron (Fig. 20.9). Therefore the above obtained information with the use of simulation studies indeed offer a useful technique for investigat- ing the relationship between mode of operation and CNS structure.

20.3 Discussion

The principal question posed in this study is whether differences in structure in the nervous system reflect, or perhaps even determine, distinct modes of function. There are various aspects of function which might differ from one CNS structure to another. Physiologists would be inclined to accept bioelectric activity in general and spike discharges in particular as a valid, if limited, estimator of nervous function. Therefore, we have to investigate the structure of the CNS for this purpose. Thus the present study up to this point was concentrated on the analysis in terms of

Fig. 20.7. The distribution of the total number of incoming connections per neuron.

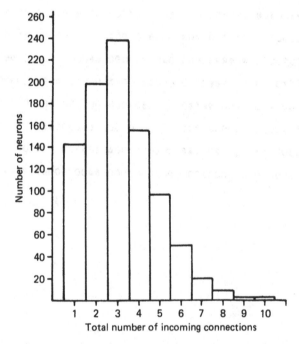

computer simulation of the EEG and its correlation with a measured MEG from human subjects showing abnormal behaviour. Our results indicate that the statistical parameters of our computer simulated brain determine the actual connections reaching any given neuron (Anninos, 1972). In order to determine the actual connections reaching any given neuron in the simulated brain we have to look into the microscopic structure, as we indicated in the previous section (Figs. 20.6–20.8).

Thus by inspecting the microscopic structure of the simulated brain, which exhibits a particular mode of function, we can obtain information, for instance, on how the specified percentage of inhibitory elements are distributed in the network; it is clear that these elements may be arranged within the net in many different ways, according to the choice of the initial random number which is used for establishing the connectivity matrix (Anninos, 1972). Therefore the question which naturally arises is whether these 'microscopic' permutations, as long as they do not violate the 'law' of structure, have any effect on the functioning of the net. This possibility

Fig. 20.8. The distribution of the total excitatory incoming connections per neuron.

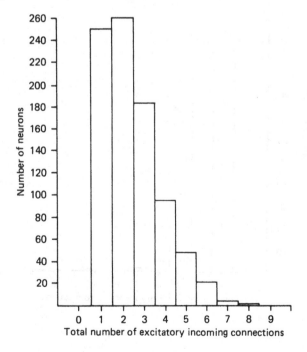

314   *P. A. Anninos & G. Anogianakis*

is also of great interest in relation to the question of variation among nervous systems in similar organisms. Therefore modelling approach provides an attractive method for answering such questions. If the importance of 'microscopic' variations can be demonstrated, which have any effect on the mode of operation in models containing only relatively few elements, these variations are certain to become important in larger systems, such as the human brain. Thus by using the above adopted simulation technique it was possible to explore the effect of structural changes, in microscopic structure, on the mode of operation in terms of the rhythmic activity (Anninos, 1972). Our results indeed indicated that there is a definite relationship between microstructure and function and the 'law' of structure responsible for the abnormal behaviour observed in MEG data (Fig. 20.3), as is given by Figs. 20.6–20.9.

Fig. 20.9. The distribution of the total inhibitory incoming connections per neuron.

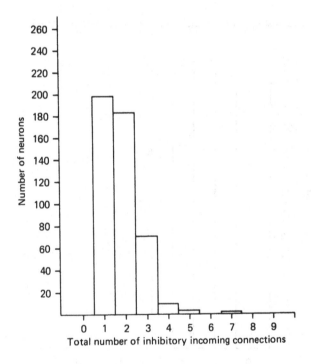

Acknowledgement

This work has been supported by the Ministries of Research and Technology of Greece and of the Federal Republic of Germany. The authors are very indebted to Prof. Hoke and his colleagues from Münster University in the laboratory of which we performed our experimental work.

References

Amari, S. (1974). *Kybernetik*, **14**, 201.

Anninos, P. A. (1969). *Dynamics and Function of Neural Structures*. Doctoral dissertation, Syracuse University, Syracuse, N.Y. Ann Arbor: University Microfilm.

Anninos, P. A., Beek, B., Csermely, T. J., Harth, E. M. & Pertile, G. (1970). *J. Theoret. Biol.*, **26**, 121–48.

Anninos, P. A. (1972). *Kybernetik*, **11**, 5–14.

Anninos, P. A. (1973). *Kybernetik*, **13**, 24–9.

Anninos, P. A. & Raman, S. (1975). *Intern. J. of Theoret. Phys.*, **12**, 9.

Anninos, P. A., Kokkinidis, M., Hoke, M., Pantev, Ch., Lehnertz, K. & Lütkenhöner, B. (1986). *Brain Research Bulletin*, **16**(4), 549.

Brazier, M. A. (1968). *The Electrical Activity of the Nervous System*. Baltimore: The Williams and Wilkins Company, p. 293.

Brenner, D. S., Williamson, J. & Kaufman, L. (1975). *Science*, **190**, 480.

Cohen, D. (1972). *Science*, **175**, 664.

Creutzfeldt, O. D., Watanabe, S. & Lux, H. D. (1966). *Electroenceph. Clin. Neurophys.*, **20**, 19.

Elul, R. (1962). *Expl. Neurol.*, **6**, 285.

Elul, R. (1964). *The Physiologist*, **7**, 125.

Jasper, H. & Stefanis, S. (1965). *Nature*, **238**, 413.

Josephson, B. D. (1962). *Physics Letters*, **1**, 251.

21

Access stability of cyclic modes in quasirandom networks of threshold neurons obeying a deterministic synchronous dynamics

J. W. CLARK, K. E. KÜRTEN and J. RAFELSKI

21.1 Introduction

Computer simulation has become a valuable – even indispensable – tool in the search for viable models of the self-organizing and self-replicating systems of the biological world as well as the inanimate systems of conventional physics. In this paper we shall present selected results from a large number of computer experiments on model neural networks of a very simple type. In the spirit of McCulloch & Pitts (1943) and Caianiello (1961), the model involves binary threshold elements (which may crudely represent neurons); these elements operate synchronously in discrete time. The synaptic interactions between neurons are represented by a non-symmetric coupling matrix which determines the strength of the stimulus which an arbitrary neuronal element, in the 'on' configuration, can exert on a second neuron to which it sends an input connection line. Within this model, the classes of networks singled out for study are defined by one or another prescription for random connection of the nodal units, implying that the entries in the coupling matrix are chosen randomly subject to certain overall constraints governing the number of inputs per 'neuron', the fraction of inhibitory 'neurons' and the magnitudes of the non-zero couplings.

We are primarily concerned with the statistics of cycling activity in such model networks, as gleaned from computer runs which follow the autonomous dynamical evolution of sample nets. An aspect of considerable interest is the stability of cyclic modes under disturbance of a single neuron in a single state of the cycle. Thus our study is intended – in several respects – to parallel that of Kauffman (1969) (see also Kauffman, 1984) for randomly constructed genetic nets.

In Section 21.2 we spell out the assumptions of the model, listing the aspects of neuronal and synaptic structure and function which it is intended to embody. We present a critical discussion of the limitations of the model, with a view to clarifying the conditions under which its behavior may be of neurobiological relevance, and especially the circumstances under which cyclic modes might be involved in sequential content-addressable memory phenomena. Two elementary classes of quasi-random nets are specified in Section 21.3. 'Representative' (or else particularly interesting) results from simulation runs for sample nets from these classes are examined, and trends (or peculiarities) are sought with respect to numbers of accessible cycles, periods of cyclic modes, distances between accessible cyclic modes, average activity levels, relative accessibilities, and relative stabilities of cycles. Ideally, we would like to understand the dependence of these properties on overall network parameters, such as number of neurons, number of inputs per neuron, inhibitory fraction and threshold. However, the set of experiments which have been analyzed so far is not large enough to allow meaningful inferences to the drawn, except in the simplest cases. As stressed in Section 21.4, the most conspicuous feature of our empirical results is the wide variation in the properties of individual nets, which hampers the induction of useful general rules of behavior.

21.2 A synchronous finite-state model and its cyclic modes

21.2.1 Specifications of the model

In order that it might bear some useful resemblance to actual biological systems, the neural network model should incorporate at least the following empirical properties of individual neurons and neuronal interactions:

(1) all-or-none character of the action potential;
(2) spatio-temporal summation of postsynaptic potentials;
(3) such synaptic properties as connectivity, strength or efficiency, excitatory versus inhibitory nature, and delay time;
(4) absolute refractory period.

The model to be specified below has roots in the seminal (if streamlined) construct of McCulloch & Pitts (1943) and is basically identical to that studied extensively in the early 70s by Harth and coworkers (Harth *et al.*, 1970; Anninos *et al.*, 1970; Anninos, 1972). It may be regarded as a simplified or limiting version of the more realistic models proposed by Caianiello (1961) and by Little and Shaw (Little, 1974; Little & Shaw,

1975). For thorough discussion of models of this class, see Clark, Rafelski & Winston (1985).

1. Each model neuron (or formal neuron) of the N-body assembly is assigned a binary state variable π_i, which takes on the value $+1$ when neuron i is *on* (firing an action potential) and the value 0 when i is *off* (inactive or not firing). This reflects the all-or-none character of the action potential.

2. The stimulus at neuron i due to all connections from neuron j ($j \to i$) is expressed as V_{ij}/π_j. This assumption reflects (in part) the spatio-temporal summation of incoming signals. The synaptic organization and essential synaptic properties are summarized in the matrix (V_{ij}) of coupling strengths, also known as the connection matrix. If the net effect of synapses of j onto i is excitatory [inhibitory], then V_{ij} is taken positive [negative]; if j sends no connections to i, then of course $V_{ij} = 0$. It is to be stressed that, in general, $V_{ij} \neq V_{ji}$.

3. The delay τ for direct signal transmission from one neuron to another is taken the same for all neuron pairs (and implicitly for all synapses). Together with the other assumptions made here, the imposition of a universal delay implies that the collection of neurons will fire *synchronously* on a discrete-time grid with uniform spacing τ. Physiologically, τ would be about a millisecond or a few milliseconds, if we identify our model neurons with real neurons, and add the various delay times (including synaptic delay) associated with signal propagation from axon hillock to axon hillock. However, such a literal interpretation would limit the applicability of the model, which might be used to describe neural decision processes at larger or smaller scales of distance and time.

4. The firing of neuron j at time t is felt by i at time $t + \tau$ with strength V_{ij}, but *zero* strength thereafter. In other words, it is supposed that postsynaptic potentials have negligible decay times. This Markovian assumption can easily be relaxed, as in more refined modeling (Clark *et al.*, 1985) not described here.

5. If neuron i fires at time t, it is restrained from firing again until time $t + R\tau$, where R may be taken as any positive integer. This incorporates the absolute refractory property of neurons. If $R = 1$ is chosen (corresponding to a refractory period less than τ), there is no real effect of refractoriness, since a neuron active at t must anyway wait until $t + \tau$, the next time-step, before it can fire again. With $R = 2$ (chosen in much of the earlier work (Harth *et al.*, 1970; Anninos *et al.*, 1970; Anninos, 1972) and also commonly by Clark *et al.* (1985)) there is indeed a non-trivial constraint, since the neuron must skip a time-step before it is ready to fire again.

6. *Equations of motion* of the system are formulated in terms of the *firing function*

$$F_i(t + \tau) = \sum_j V_{ij}\pi_j(t) - V_{0i} + [U_i(t + \tau)], \tag{1}$$

where the first term is the net internal stimulus from neurons synapsing onto neuron i, V_{0i} is the threshold assigned to i and U_i is a possible external stimulus. When i is not in its absolute refractory condition, the rule for updating its state is simply deterministic threshold logic:

$$\pi_i(t + \tau) = \Theta(F_i(t + \tau)), \tag{2}$$

where $\Theta(x) = $ zero for $x < 0$ and unity for $x \geq 0$. Thus the neuron fires if and only if the threshold is exceeded (or equaled) by the signal.

7. The *state of the network* at a given time t is specified by the set of values of all the individual neuronal state variables π_i at that time, i.e., by the *firing pattern*

$$\nu = \{\pi_1(t), \pi_2(t), \dots \pi_N(t)\}. \tag{3}$$

There are exactly 2^N states for N neurons. With this definition of state and $R = 1$ or 2, the dynamics is Markovian in the sense that the state at time t suffices to determine the state at time $t + \tau$, through eqns (1) and (2). The *activity* of the network at time t is defined as $\alpha(t) = N^{-1} \sum_i \pi_i(t)$.

This model is extreme in several respects, notably (a) representation of the neuron in terms of a *nodal element* whose intrinsic structure is suppressed, (b) emphasis on the *non-linearity* of neuronal response, epitomized in the step function of eqn (2), which might more generally be replaced by a smooth sigmoid function, (c) strict *synchronicity* of network operation, with all N neurons updating their states simultaneously according to eqn (2) and (d) strict *deterministic evolution*. The work of Rall & Segev (1988) typifies the modern view transcending (a): there is abundant evidence of the importance of non-linear processing in dendritic trees. The work of Cooper's group (Scofield & Cooper, 1985; Cooper, 1988) is predicated on a view opposite to (b), placing the emphasis instead on linear aspects of neural information processing. As a counterpoint to aspect (c) of our model, Hopfield's (1982) threshold-logic model goes to the opposite extreme in the timing of individual neuronal updating events: only *one* neuron at a time is allowed to update its state, the other neuronal states being frozen. (The tested neuron is chosen randomly from the pool at each trial; or else each neuron makes an updating attempt at random times with mean waiting period W^{-1}.) The drastic nature of features (a)–(c) may be absolved somewhat, at least in certain contexts, if we are allowed to interpret the nodal elements of the model as more fundamental information-processing units present *within* neurons or, alternatively, as coherent modular assemblies of tens or hundreds of neurons. With regard to (d), it should be noted that Little (1974) and Little & Shaw (1975) have explored a generalization of the present model, which is supposed to incorporate, in a reasonable fashion, the effects of neuronal spontaneity and the stochastic nature of information transfer in neural systems (see also Clark *et al.*, 1985). In this stochastic synchronous model, the deterministic updating rule for receptive (non-refractory) neurons, eqn (2), is replaced by the ansatz

$$p_i(\pi_i(t + \tau)) = \frac{1}{\exp\left[-\beta F_i(t + \tau)\right] + 1} \tag{4}$$

for the *probability* that neuron i will assume state π_i at time $t + \tau$, where β^{-1} measures the amount of noise in the system. It is seen that eqn (2) is essentially the noiseless limit of this probabilistic rule.

Even for the primitive model embodied in specifications 1–7, it is not ordinarily possible to obtain the full set of explicit solutions for the time evolution of the network state. Nevertheless, we can easily reach some general conclusions about the dynamical behavior of the system. The progression of states according to eqn (2) is unambiguous: with $R = 1$ or 2. The state of the system at time t determines the successor state at time $t + \tau$ uniquely. Mathematically, we are dealing with a deterministic finite-state sequential machine. Let us focus on the autonomous behavior of this machine, which means that the network is not subjected to any external stimuli U_i after time 0, when the system is put in some arbitrarily chosen initial state (firing pattern). We shall also assume that the intrinsic network parameters (the individual neuronic thresholds V_{0i} and the asymmetric neuron–neuron couplings V_{ij}) are constant in time.

21.2.2 Autonomous motions of the model; cyclic modes as associative memories

After an initial transient period during which the detailed motion of the net may be quite sensitive to the starting state, the system will inevitably settle into an ordered condition – a terminal cycle or cyclic mode – which persists indefinitely. A cyclic mode is characterized (in strict terms) by the periodicity condition

$$\nu(t + k\tau) = \nu(t) \tag{5}$$

on the sequence of network states. The period K of the cyclic mode is the smallest integer k satisfying this condition. Thus in a cyclic mode the same set of firing patterns is repeated over and over, in the same order. That the autonomous system will sooner or later lock into such a mode is obvious:

with only a finite number of states available, and an infinite time to run, some state will eventually be repeated, establishing a terminal cycle. Steady states are of course just cyclic modes of period $K = 1$, among which 'death' (persistence of the dead state $\{\pi_i = 0, \text{ all } i\}$) and 'epilepsy' (persistence of the totally active state $\{\pi_i = 1, \text{ all } i\}$) are trivial special cases.

Aside from the intrinsic theoretical interest of dynamical systems of this type, what aspects of the motion of such a system might be of psychobiological relevance? More specifically, in what sense are cyclic modes of biological interest? The answer is that cyclic modes, or the reverberating excitations underlying them, have often been proposed (see, e.g., Caianiello, 1961; Anninos, 1972; Scott, 1977; Clark *et al.*, 1985) as model analogs of active short-term memory traces, or thoughts. With this proposal in mind, we make the following observations.

(1) Using simple combinatorics, the total number C of *distinct* cyclic modes, in the case $R = 1$, lies in the range $(2^N - 1)! < C < (2^N)!(1 + 2^{-N})$. For $N = 10^{10}$, we have a lower bound of 10^{10^9}, raised to the power of 10^{10^9}, an impressively huge number. However, such estimates are misleading:

(a) For one thing, the longer modes (with $K \sim 2^N$) predominate in the combinatoric accounting; even if τ were as short as a millisecond, it would take much longer than the age of the universe for such a mode to run through just one cycle. But if we restrict attention to modes of length K less than 1000, the number of distinguishable cyclic conditions is still quite staggering.

(b) A much more critical consideration is that the number of these distinct cyclic modes which are *actually accessible* to a given network, with frozen V_{ij} and V_{0i} and not subject to any external stimulus after $t = 0$, may be quite limited. For deterministic updating (eqn (2)), an upper bound on this measure is clearly just 2^N, since there can be no more distinct long-term behaviors than there are initial states. In the nets which are studied in practice, the number of accessible cyclic modes is found to be much smaller than this, usually some small fraction of N. With probabilistic updating (eqn (4)), at large enough β so that cyclic modes are not lost in the noise, a broader repertoire of modes of relevant length might be more readily elicited, since the system need no longer be trapped in a particular 'rut' – spontaneity allows escape to other cyclic pathways. (Of course, in the probabilistic network, any cyclic mode that surfaces is subject to eradication by spontaneous firings or misfirings. Hence the number of long-lived modes may well be reduced compared to the deterministic case, because of the relative instability of some deterministic 'ruts' compared to others. The phenomenon of drifting from one cycle to another is suggestive of 'trains of thought.')

(2) At any rate, we must expect that the number of memories which can be stored in a given network, counted as the number of cyclic modes which can be excited by arbitrary instantaneous stimuli U_i, is ordinarily only a modest fraction of N. This limitation is circumvented in an important sense if one invokes *plasticity*: allowing the intrinsic net parameters V_{ij} and V_{0i} (for all i, j) to be adjustable at will, the full assortment of cyclic modes becomes accessible. The modification of synaptic couplings (and/or thresholds) – particularly, such modification induced by internal neural activity associated with external stimuli – is commonly held to be the mechanism for engramming (or storing) memory traces. For completeness we remark that even for a frozen network, it is possible to realize an arbitrary cyclic mode by the imposition of a suitably chosen sequence of external stimuli.

To summarize: In this discussion we are entertaining a form of *distributed, superimposed, associative, sequential* memory. Cyclic modes correspond to the active (or short-term) phase of the memory process (i.e., to 'remembering', under an appropriate stimulus), while plasticity provides the means for laying down new memories, either permanent or semi-permanent.

21.2.3 Are cyclic modes relevant to neurobiology?

Severe reservations may be expressed as to the neurobiological relevance of the cyclic modes displayed by synchronous models of the kind studied here. Basically, it is objected that timing in the nervous system cannot be nearly so precise as would be required for cycles of appreciable length to be identifiable and reproducible. It is correctly pointed out that delay times show a wide dispersion because of the differences in communication pathways (axonal, synaptic, dendritic, somic) between different neurons, rendering quite unrealistic the assumption of a universal time-step τ and concomitant synchronous updating. Moreover, various stochastic effects endemic to neural processing would tend to destroy the coherence required for cycles involving cooperation of neural populations over large distances and long times. While these judgments are essentially valid, especially if the time-step τ is indeed interpreted as a 'typical' synaptic delay of a millisecond or so, there are several mitigating arguments which can be put forward.

(1) The first is based on the visualization of a cyclic mode in terms of an underlying system of *reverberations*. A reverberation is taken to mean a closed loop of successive neuronal firings, involving a definite subset of the N neurons. The individual firings repeat with some period $\varkappa$ equal to the number of neurons involved. A reverberation of period $\varkappa = 8(\tau)$ is represented diagrammatically in Fig. 21.1(*a*). In general, a cyclic mode corresponds to a *superposition* of several reverberations – which may intersect or be connected by extra neuron-neuron links, or may be disjoint – together with assorted 'dead-end' pathways or 'spurs'. Fig. 21.1(*b*) provides a simple illustration in which a cyclic mode of period $K = 6$, with 12 participating neurons, is built out of four reverberations (with no extra neuron-neuron links joining them, and no loose ends). We observe that the network can be partitioned into non-overlapping subsets of neurons in many ways. Irrespective of what is happening in the rest of the net, a cyclic mode may be established in any one of these subsets – and would constitute a 'subcycle', corresponding in an obvious manner to some reverberation or system of reverberations. A cyclic mode of the full net prevails if and only if a subcycle has been established in each and every subset of some partition. On the other hand, the transient phase of network activity is in general characterized by the coexistence of ordered and disordered behavior. Evidently, interesting questions can be raised

Fig. 21.1. (*a*) A reverberation of period $\varkappa = 8$. Triangles symbolize participating neurons, the lines joining triangles represent direct neuron–neuron links, and the arrows indicate the direction of propagation of the successive impulses, separated in time by τ. (*b*) Superposition of four reverberations yielding a cyclic mode or subcycle of period $K = 6$; the neuron triangles indicate the direction of propagation of the signal.

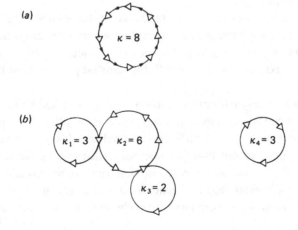

concerning the approach to complete order in a given (deterministic) network exposed to a given initial stimulus; in particular, how sudden is the 'phase transition' from an initial condition of disorder or partial order to the final 'crystalline' order of the terminal cyclic mode of the system? Such issues are taken up in another contribution to this book (Littlewort, Clark & Rafelski, 1988). Without much question, it makes better sense to describe active short-term memory in terms of reverberations (and extra links and loose ends) rather than in terms of cyclic modes of the full network: asking the *whole* net to participate rhythmically in a given 'thought', rather than some smaller subset of neurons, is extreme. Moreover, depicting specific, organized neural activity in terms of reverberations does not hinge on synchronicity in the strict sense. The time interval between successive network states need not be a global constant (τ) – it is sufficient that synchronism is adequately maintained *independently* in each of the prevailing disjoint loop systems, during the active course of the given 'memory impression'. In this sense, cyclic activity in neural-network models like that specified in 1–7 may be pertinent so long as none of the reverberatory loops is very large, i.e., so long as $\varkappa$ remains fairly small. Note that this *does not* imply that the period K of the full cyclic mode must be small, since it could arise from a large number of reverberations with relatively small $\varkappa$ values which do not have a small least common multiple. (See Clark *et al.*, 1985.) Still it would be best to concentrate on modes with periods not exceeding, say, $K \sim 100$, when attempting to attribute neurobiological significance to the behaviors of the model. The upshot of the argument, however, is that reverberatory activity will survive in some meaningful degree when the rigid synchronism of our model is relaxed, and may well be an important aspect of real neural systems.

(2) Within the model 1–7, as it stands, synchronous updating of all the neurons becomes a less harmful assumption when the average activity in the network is low, so that in fact not many neurons fire at any one time-step. Of course, the system will still manifest precise cyclic behavior at large times.

(3) Even with asynchronous updating, as in Hopfield's model, non-steady cyclic conditions can be reached if the assumption of symmetrical couplings, ordinarily made within that model, is relaxed. Grondin *et al.* (1983) have pointed out that the possibilities for cycling are *narrowed*, relative to the synchronous case, in that the undirectionality of the threshold test implies that no asynchronous map can have an inverse. Thus, the minimum (non-trivial) limit cycle must involve four states, and

only cycles of even length are allowed. On the other hand, these authors also point out that that the situation grows *more complicated* in that the stochastic nature of the asynchronous dynamics can give rise to *multifrequency* oscillations, which cannot occur in the model studied here. Another complication arising from the non-uniqueness of state → state transitions is the possibility of chaotic wandering among a set of states with small relative Hamming distances. The computer simulations of nonsymmetric asynchronous systems which have been discussed in the literature (Hopfield, 1982) suggest that (non-trivial) cycles are reached only occasionally when starting from randomly chosen initial states, that the structure of these cycles is quite simple (long complex cycles being apparently disfavored by the stochastic single-neuron updating rule), and that chaotic wandering is also the exception rather than the rule. By contrast, rather complex cycles of large period K are observed in some realizations of the synchronous, deterministic model specified in 1–7 above (e.g., see Section 21.3), and in some cases these modes collect the flow from a large fraction of the 2^N initial states. However, these more elaborate cycles tend to wash out in the probabilistic version of the model corresponding to eqn (4). In comparing the properties of Hopfield and McCulloch-Pitts type models, it is perhaps well to reiterate the comment of Grondin *et al.* that: 'synchronous and asynchronous systems with an identical interconnection matrix and identical thresholds will have identical stable (i.e., absorbing) states even though the dynamics of the two systems may be very different'.

(4) Shaw (1986) (see Shaw & Silverman, 1988; and Silverman, Shaw & Pearson, 1986) maintains that results from the synchronous model become relevant if the time τ is interpreted not as a transmission delay time for communication between single cells but, rather, as the observed bursting interval of roughly 50 ms manifested by small, localized groups of neurons (~30–100 in number). There is impressive evidence of such a clock-like timing unit in the visual area III of cat (Morrell, 1967; Morrell *et al.*, 1983).

(5) Going to the other extreme, the stigma of synchronicity can be removed (for all practical purposes) by a brute-force treatment in which the elemental time τ is made much smaller than any physiological time entering the problem. A real-time description can then be approached by allowing different delay times from signal transmission via different synaptic links and modeling more realistically the time course of accumulation and decay of PSP's and the time course of absolute and relative refractory periods, with all times quantized in units of the computational

grid time τ. For a discussion of this approach and a description of preliminary results indicating that the crude model 1–7 has essentially the correct features with regard to periodic behavior, see Clark *et al.* (1985); see also Cotterill (1986) for a discussion of much more elaborate real-time simulations in this vein.

Periodic or nearly periodic activity is clearly important in the functioning of natural neural systems. While it is unjustified to make a literal identification of the cyclic modes of our primitive model with memories in the brain, the above considerations indicate that some aspects of its cyclic solutions may nevertheless be relevant to sequential memory phenomena. In physics we have a long tradition of devoting serious study to simple model problems, e.g. the Ising model in solid-state physics, the Lipkin model in nuclear physics and the Gross–Neveu model in field theory. There are many good reasons to do the same in theoretical neurobiology, not least the fact that as yet there exists no comprehensive theoretical superstructure in brain science.

21.3 Empirics of cycling in quasirandom model nets

It is known that natural nerve nets tend to have rather specific connections. However, in many cases there appears to be a substantial degree of randomness of the detailed synaptic organization; in such cases one is hard put to decide whether the appearance of randomness is due to ignorance of the rules of connection or represents a genuine stochastic aspect of the formation of synapses. Exploring the outer bounds of the possible, it is of considerable interest – within the general spirit of the model studies pursued in physics – to collect information on the systematics of cyclic modes in *randomly assembled* nets of threshold elements obeying the synchronous deterministic dynamics of eqn (2). For each sample net, we shall be concerned with (a) the *number n* of accessible cyclic modes (as determined by starting the net with as many different initial conditions as practicable and looking for different terminal cycles), (b) the *distribution of periods* of the accessible cycles, (c) the *average activities* α_{av} of the observed cycles (i.e. $N^{-1} \Sigma_i \pi_i$, averaged over each cycle), (d) the *relative accessibilities* a_c of the observed cyclic modes *c* (measured by the fraction of initial conditions leading to each terminal cycle), (e) the *distances between cycles* (in terms of the minimum and maximum Hamming distances H_{min} and H_{max} between states of one cycle and states of the other) and (f) the *relative stabilities* of the cycles detected.

There are a number of serviceable definitions of stability (or relative stability), depending on the disturbance imposed on the system. In our case, the disturbance consists of flipping the state variable of a single neuron, arbitrarily selected, at some time step, arbitrarily selected, when the system is playing out a given cyclic mode. If the cycle is *absolutely stable*, the system always returns to it, regardless of which state of the cycle is disturbed and no matter which neuron is affected. Otherwise, the cycle will be absolutely unstable (if the system never returns to that cycle), or, more commonly, relatively stable (if the system only returns to the given cycle on a portion of the trials). In the case of relative stability or absolute instability, we would of course like to know the percentage of trials leading to the various cycles which are accessible to the network. This leads to the introduction of a transition matrix $S = (S_{cc'})$, where $S_{cc'}$ gives the probability (or, rather, the fraction of instances) of going from cycle c to cycle c' upon changing the value of the state variable of a single neuron is one of the states of c. Thus our study of stability parallels that of Kauffman (1969), who has performed systematic computer experiments on randomly assembled binary Boolean automata (Kauffman, 1969, 1984; Derrida & Flyvbjerg, 1986). One could, naturally, go on to investigate stability under simultaneous flips of the states of two or more neurons in an arbitrarily chosen state of a cycle. An alternative approach to the issue of stability, not pursued in the current experiments, is to impose a finite 'noise temperature' β^{-1} at some point in a given cycle. This approach involves switching on the probabilistic dynamics associated with eqn (4), with reasonably large β, and looking for transitions to other cycles. In this case, since no cycle can be expected to survive forever, the relevant measure of stability is the share of time spent in a given cycle.

In our study, the prescription adopted for random connection of the N neuronal elements is the following.

(1) Each neuron i is assigned exactly M non-zero c_{ij}s, where $0 \le M \le N$, the distinct neurons j feeding information to i being picked at random and democratically from the N neurons of the pool. Every neuron has the *same* number M of inputs.

(2) A fraction h of the set of non-zero couplings c_{ij} is taken inhibitory, the choice of the NMh inhibitory links being random and unbiased. Any *particular* neuron will generally *not* have exactly Nh inhibitory inputs.

The foregoing specifications are the same as those adopted by Kürten & Clark (1986, 1988) in their demonstrations of chaotic activity in a continuous-time neural network model. However, they differ from those implemented by Littlewort *et al.* (1988) in other discrete-time simulations described in this book. In a given net of the class studied by Littlewort *et al.*, individual neurons will have variable numbers of inputs clustered around M, and the neurons are divided into separate excitatory and inhibitory subsets.

We explore two options for the strengths of the non-zero couplings:

● $|V_{ij}| = 1$, if non-zero,

●● $|V_{ij}| \le 1$, if non-zero.

In the latter case the actual values of the non-zero couplings are fixed by random sampling of a uniform distribution on $(0, 1]$. In the former case one is dealing with a class of nets rather similar to the Type I nets investigated by Clark *et al.* (1985), the main qualification being that in a Type I net a given neuron has exclusively an excitatory or an inhibitory effect on its target cells.

We also explore two options for the neuronal thresholds:

● *Normal thresholds*

$$V_{0i} = V_{0i}^{\text{norm}} = \tfrac{1}{2} \sum_j V_{ij}. \tag{6}$$

●● *Adjustable thresholds*,

$$V_{0i} = \tfrac{1}{2}(\sum_j V_{ij} + V_0) = V_{0i}^{\text{norm}} + \tfrac{1}{2}V_0, \tag{7}$$

where V_0 is an arbitrary constant, independent of i, chosen for a particular trial net or collection of trial nets.

In the simulation runs, the options marked with a ● are paired up to make a more primitive, more restricted case, while the ●● options are joined to define a less restricted, 'more realistic' class of models. With normal thresholds (also with adjusted thresholds) some neurons may have negative V_{0i}. In selected runs of the ● variety, we removed this presumably unrealistic feature by using *corrected normal thresholds*, meaning that V_{0i} is set to zero if V_{0i}^{norm} turns out to be negative, but is otherwise left at V_{0i}^{norm}. In all cases, $R = 1$.

A range of experiments were performed with a view to comparing the cycling properties (a)–(f) of these two fundamental classes of model systems and, more broadly, to detecting any prominent trends in their behavior as the gross parameters N, h, and M are varied.

We adopt the following notation for three kinds of averages: an 'av' subscript on a quantity indentifies it as an average over a given cycle; a bar signifies an average over the observed cycles of a given specimen net; and angle brackets ⟨⟩ indicate an average over a collection or 'ensemble' of specimen nets.

21.3.1 Normal thresholds; unit non-zero coupling magnitudes

First, we studied the simpler class of systems (the ● case, specified by $V_{0i} = V_{0i}^{\mathrm{norm}}$ and $|V_{ij}| = 1$ if non-zero), for $N = 10$. Two choices of inhibitory fraction h were considered, namely 0.35 and 0.5, and the number of inputs M was stepped from 2 to 10, i.e., from 'sparse' to full connectivity. For each h and M, we examined 100 sample nets and tried $I = 200$ different randomly picked initial conditions (out of the total of $2^{10} = 1024$). Some ensemble-averaged data on the numbers of accessible cycles and the periods of these cycles is given in Table 21.1. The average number of cycles is $\langle n \rangle \sim 2$–3, depending only weakly on h and increasing slowly with M. Periods are longer for larger M and for larger h. The standard deviation associated with these results amounts to about 10%.

Next, a large number of specimen nets were examined for $N = 100$, with various M values but generally keeping h at 0.35. An exhaustive numerical study of nets of size 100 is not possible and, in particular, we have not made a systematic exploration of the dependence of cycling properties on M. In lieu of such systematics, we feel that it is useful to

Table 21.1. *Cycling data for nets of $N = 10$ model neurons, with normal thresholds and non-zero couplings of unit magnitude. Average number of observed cycles $\langle n \rangle$ and average cycle length $\langle \bar{K} \rangle$ for ensembles of 100 sample nets, all with specified inhibitory fraction, h, and number of inputs per neuron, M. Each net was run for 200 different randomly chosen initial states*

M	$\langle n \rangle$	$\langle \bar{K} \rangle$	
2	2.19	3.62	$h = 0.35$
4	2.55	5.23	
6	2.74	5.59	
8	3.17	6.17	
10	3.31	6.48	
2	2.64	6.02	$h = 0.50$
4	2.74	8.20	
6	2.97	11.11	
8	3.26	12.46	
10	3.25	11.55	

Table 21.2. *Cycling data for sample nets of* $N = 100$ *model neurons, with normal thresholds and non-zero couplings of unit magnitude. Both specimens have inhibitory fraction* $h = 0.35$ *and* $M = 6$ *inputs per neuron. (a) Results for first specimen, from* $I = 50$ *runs with different randomly chosen initial states. Fourteen cells have negative thresholds. (b) Results for second specimen, from* $I = 40$ *runs. Nine cells have negative thresholds*

n	Cycle lengths						
6	24	40	8	3	18	3	Average length: $\bar{K} = 16$
$\alpha_{av.}$	0.784	0.779	0.780	0.817	0.793	0.793	Average activity
a_c	0.24	0.50	0.12	0.10	0.02	0.02	Accessibility

	24	40	8	3	18	3	24	40	8	3	18	3
24	□	3	1	6	7	7	□	21	18	21	28	18
40		□	1	10	8	10		□	19	25	32	23
8			□	10	9	9			□	19	26	17
3				□	3	2				□	21	7
18					□	6					□	21
3						□						□

$\bar{H}_{min} = 6 \pm 3$ $\bar{H}_{max} = 21 \pm 5$

(a)

n	Cycle lengths									$\bar{K} = 6.2$
10	2	30	6	1	6	2	5	2	6	2
α_{av}	0.87	0.85	0.91	0.86	0.88	0.86	0.84	0.90	0.90	0.87
a_c	0.20	0.55	0.03	0.05	0.03	0.03	0.03	0.03	0.03	0.05

	2	30	6	1	6	2	5	2	6	2	2	30	6	1	6	2	5	2	6	2
2	□	8	10	9	10	1	12	13	12	10	□	22	16	9	17	15	17	19	16	16
30		□	8	9	4	9	10	9	4			□	22	20	25	23	21	23	22	25
6			□	13	3	11	14	3	1	9			□	18	18	17	22	14	13	14
1				□	10	10	5	14	13	13				□	14	10	8	20	19	13
6					□	11	11	4	3	6					□	18	18	18	18	19
2						□	13	14	13	9						□	18	20	17	17
5							□	14	14	13							□	22	21	15
2								□	1	11								□	14	15
6									□	10									□	14
2										□										□

H_{min} H_{max}

$\bar{H}_{min} = 9 \pm 4$ $\bar{H}_{max} = 18 \pm 4$

(b)

present specific results for a selection of sample nets. It is not claimed that these examples necessarily depict typical behavior; in some cases they were chosen because they seemed (to the experimenters) to exhibit especially interesting properties or phenomena, which indeed may not be at all typical. The same qualifications apply to the set of results presented in Subsection 21.3.2, which are selected from computer experiments on the more flexible ●● class of nets.

In Tables 21.2(a) and (b) we provide data on the cycles reached by two different nets with $M = 6$ inputs per neuron; Tables 21.3(a)–3(c) give

Table 21.3. *Cycling data for sample nets of M = 20 but otherwise specified as in Table 21.2. (a) Results for first specimen, from I = 50 initial conditions; 7 negative thresholds. (b) Results for second specimen, from I = 250 initial conditions; 5 negative thresholds. (C) Results for third specimen, from I = 250 initial conditions; 6 negative thresholds*

n	Cycle lengths			
4	23	54	33	2
$\alpha_{av.}$	0.872	0.861	0.860	0.890
a_c	0.22	0.72	0.04	0.02

Average length: $\bar{K} = 28$
Average activity
Accessibility

	23	54	33	2	23	54	33	2
23	□	2	3	7	□	25	27	20
54		□	2	4		□	24	19
33			□	3			□	19
2	$\bar{H}_{min} = 4 \pm 2$			□	$\bar{H}_{max} = 22 \pm 3$			□

(a)

n	Cycle lengths						
7	2	1	3	2	2	4	1
$\alpha_{av.}$	0.920	0.890	0.893	0.935	0.945	0.880	0.940
a_c	0.52	0.13	0.15	0.15	0.03	0.00	0.02

Average length: $\bar{K} = 2.1$
Average activity
Accessibility

	2	1	3	2	2	4	1	2	1	3	2	2	4	1
2	□	6	6	1	2	6	3	□	8	9	3	4	10	5
1		□	1	5	6	3	5		□	4	6	7	4	5
3			□	5	6	3	5			□	7	8	8	6
2				□	1	6	2				□	2	10	3
2					□	7	1					□	11	2
4	$\bar{H}_{min} = 4 \pm 2$					□	6	$\bar{H}_{max} = 6 \pm 3$					□	9
1							□							□

(b)

n	Cycle lengths										$\bar{K} = 1.8$
11	1	2	1	3	4	2	1	1	1	1	3
α_{av}	0.93	0.92	0.91	0.89	0.94	0.93	0.94	0.91	0.92	0.90	0.91
a_c	0.33	0.02	0.24	0.01	0.17	0.09	0.04	0.02	0.03	0.03	0.02

	1	2	1	3	4	2	1	1	1	1	3	1	2	1	3	4	2	1	1	1	1	3
1	□	1	8	9	4	3	5	10	7	9	6	□	1	8	10	4	3	5	10	7	9	8
2		□	9	10	5	4	6	11	8	10	7		□	9	11	5	4	6	11	8	10	9
1			□	7	4	5	3	2	5	1	3			□	8	4	5	3	2	5	1	6
3				□	5	6	4	9	2	6	5				□	8	9	7	10	5	7	12
4					□	1	1	6	3	5	2					□	3	1	6	3	5	6
2						□	2	7	4	6	3						□	2	7	4	6	7
1	H_{min}						□	5	2	4	3	H_{max}						□	5	2	4	5
1								□	7	3	5								□	7	3	8
1	$\bar{H}_{min} = 5 \pm 3$								□	4	3	$\bar{H}_{max} = 6 \pm 3$								□	4	7
1										□	4										□	7
3											□											□

(c)

corresponding results for three nets with $M = 20$. Obviously, these few examples can tell us nothing about the dependence on M of proper ensemble averages of the various quantities in our list (a)–(f) (particularly n and $\bar{K}$). (*Note added in proof:* Recently, important aspects of the general dependence of dynamical behavior on M and other gross network parameters have been clarified by analytical studies of Kürten (1988a,b), carried out in the thermodynamic limit.) We certainly expect that when the activity clings around 50%, cycles will tend to be longer. We observe that the five sample normal-threshold nets in question, all with $h = 0.35$, run at fairly *high* average activity $\bar{a}$, which might favor shorter cycles than otherwise. The Hamming distances between the states in pairs of accessible cyclic modes are generally rather short in these specimen nets. This is a typical feature of networks of the class under study, but exceptions are not uncommon (as witnessed by further examples discussed below). The relative accessibilities of the individual cyclic modes vary widely for each of the nets examined in Tables 21.2 and 21.3.

Fig. 21.2. Histogram of observed cycle lengths K in a mini-ensemble of nets with normal thresholds and unit non-zero couplings. This distribution represents an average over results for eight sample nets, all with $N = 100$ model neurons, fraction $h = 0.35$ of inhibitors and $M = 20$ inputs per neuron. Each specimen was tested with $I = 200$ initial conditions.

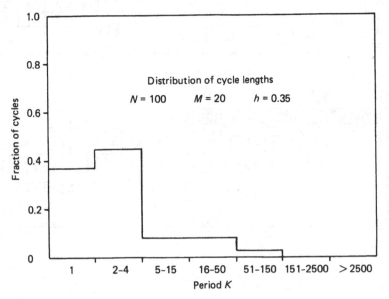

Table 21.4. *Cycling and stability data for sample net of* $N = 100$ *model neurons, with normal thresholds and non-zero couplings of unit magnitude, inhibitory fraction* $h = 0.35$ *and* $M = 30$ *inputs per neuron. The* 5×5 *array in the top display gives the transition matrix* $S = (S_{cc'})$, *where* $S_{cc'}$ *is the fraction of the single-neuron-flip trials* T *leading from cycle* c *to cycle* c'. *A dash indicates that the corresponding cycle* c' *is not reached in any trial*

n	Cycle lengths					$\bar{K} = 8.6$	
5	2	10	11	12	8	$\alpha_{av.}$	T
2	1	–	–	–	–	0.36	200
10	0.01	0.42	0.32	0.24	0.02	0.11	1000
11	0.01	0.13	0.47	0.35	0.04	0.09	1100
12	0.001	0.10	0.17	0.66	0.08	0.11	1200
8	0.006	0.172	0.318	0.274	0.23	0.08	800

Transition matrix S

	2	10	11	12	8
2	□	85	87	82	89
10		□	2	3	2
11			□	1	1
12	H_{min}			□	2
8					□

	2	10	11	12;	8
2	□	94	97	98	96
10		□	17	23	19
11			□	21	17
12	H_{max}			□	22
8					□

Averaging over the results obtained for eight sample nets all with $N = 100$, $M = 20$ and $h = 0.35$, each probed with $I = 200$ randomly selected initial conditions, we find $\langle n \rangle = 4.8$, $\langle \bar{K} \rangle = 6$. However, considerable deviations from these averages occur, as indicated by the distribution of cycle lengths in the eight net 'mini-ensemble' (Fig. 21.2). The accessibilities of the cycle modes detected in this set of nets span a broad range: $\frac{1}{200} - \frac{174}{200}$. The average activities α_{av} of these terminal cycles are uniformly high: 0.86–0.98. However, it is interesting to note that nets with the same gross specifications can be generated which display *low* $\bar{\alpha}$ values, indicating that the details of random assembly, and the concomitant formation of an individual topological loop structure, can have important dynamical consequences.

Tables 21.4 and 21.5 give two additional examples at $N = 100$, the former with the normal-threshold choice as above, but the latter with *corrected* normal thresholds. Besides the usual data on cycling, these

Table 21.5. *As in Table* 21.4, *except that sample net has* corrected *normal thresholds and M* = 19; *transition matrix is given by the upper* 6 × 6 *array*

n	Cycle lengths						$\bar{K}$ = 8.7	
6	1	5	27	1	7	11	α_{av}	T
1	0.42	0.27	0.07	0.23	–	0.01	0.0	100
5	–	0.36	0.11	0.49	–	0.04	0.1	500
27	0.00	0.11	0.39	0.49	–	0.03	0.1	2700
1	0.06	0.14	–	0.80	–	–	0.02	100
7	–	–	–	–	1	–	0.88	700
11	–	0.12	0.13	0.51	–	0.23	0.1	1100

Transition matrix *S*

	1	5	27	1	7	11
1	□	9	5	2	86	8
5		□	4	9	84	1
27			□	3	81	2
1				□	88	6
7		H_{min}			□	83
11						□

	1	5	27	1	7	11
1	□	12	13	2	91	14
5		□	15	10	90	13
27			□	13	94	16
1				□	93	14
7		H_{max}			□	92
11						□

tables provide information on stability as quantified by the respective transition matrices, in what may be regarded as 'representative' cases. In these examples, there is typically a chance of slightly better than 50% of returning to the same cycle, when only single neuron-state flips are imposed. In Table 21.4 we see that the cycle with period 2 is far away from the others (measured in terms of Hamming distances of its states from the states of the other cycles), and – thus not surprisingly – it is absolutely stable against decay into any of them. The cycles of periods 10, 11, 12 and 8 are all relatively close and communicate intimately. Table 21.5 also shows a cycle (of period 7) which is well separated from the others; it again turns out to be absolutely stable while the others decay into one another fairly readily.

As judged from a larger sample of experiments, there are no great changes in behavior when corrected normal thresholds are used instead of the original prescription allowing some negative V_{0i} values – provided of course that the inhibitory fraction does not grow too large. One naturally expects that with the elimination of negative thresholds, the characteristic level of activity in the net will be reduced. Indeed, low average activities are observed for most of the cycles found in the net of Table 21.5; on the other hand, the activities of most of the cycles recorded in Table 21.4 are also rather low. In both cases the absolutely stable cycle shows a quite distinct (and relatively high) level of activity.

One finding of our experiments on the ● class nets is particularly remarkable: in some cases cycles of great length (K up to ~6000) were authenticated, and certainly much longer cycles could be discovered, depending on the available computer space. To give a definite example, a cyclic mode with $K = 3175$ was established in a net of 100 neurons having $h = 0.35$ and $M = 19$. The firing function $F_i(t)$ for one of the neurons in this net is shown in Fig. 21.3. For the reasons discussed in Section 21.2, we should not attach biological significance to these modes in terms of detailed, temporally structured memories. Nevertheless they are of considerable interest in connection with the emergence of deterministic

Fig. 21.3. Firing function F_i of a particular neuron, during a cyclic mode of period $K = 3175$, occurring in a network of $N = 100$ neurons, with $h = 0.35$, $M = 19$, unit non-zero $|V_{ij}|$ and normal thresholds.

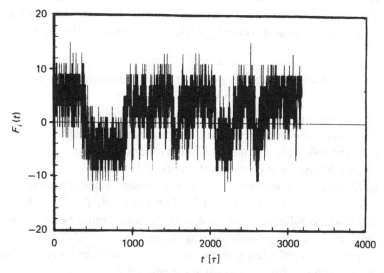

chaotic motion in neural systems (Choi & Huberman, 1983; Grondin *et al.*, 1983; Kürten & Clark, 1986, 1988). Strictly, such motion is not possible in the present model, which has only a finite number of states and, with deterministic synchronous updating, must eventually reach a fixed point or a cycle. However, the appearance and proliferation of long cycles, as one or another gross parameter (h, M, V_0 in the classes of nets studied here) moves through some critical region, is very suggestive of the bifurcation process leading to chaos in non-linear systems with continuous state variables. Indeed, it is common practice to simulate chaotic solutions using digital computers, operating discretely on a large but finite set of rational numbers. Although some state must sooner or later be repeated, implying a periodic solution, 'later' in the case of our neural nets can in principle be $\sim 2^N \tau$, a virtually infinite time if N is ~ 100 or greater. And although there is a limit on the separation, along an attractor, between two points tracing the evolution in state space from nearby initial conditions, this separation can still grow very large, in correspondence with the growing seed of uncertainty characteristic of deterministic chaos. Issues raised by the intimations of chaos in discrete neural-network models are discussed in some depth by Grondin *et al.* (1983). Also apropos is a recent explicit study by Binder & Jensen (1986), examining digital-computer simulations of chaotic behavior of iterates of the logistic map. These authors find that while relatively 'short' limit cycles are formed (with lengths $\sim \sqrt{N_s}$, where N_s is the number of discrete states), statistical properties of the original continuous-state problem are nevertheless preserved, including the invariant probability distribution and the Lyapunov exponent. Moreover, the transition between periodic and chaotic behavior is still clearly visible in the results for the discretized map.

21.3.2 Adjustable thresholds; non-zero coupling magnitudes bounded by unity

For illustrative purposes we shall focus on one of the many simulation studies which have been performed on quasirandomly assembled networks of the ●● class. The aim of this and other similar experiments was to gain insight into the influence of the adjustable threshold parameter V_0 of eqn (7) on cycling properties. The nets examined in the experiment all have $N = 100$, $M = 5$ and $h = 0.35$. For each net, $I = 50$ different random initial conditions were tried, and the autonomous behavior was followed until a cycling condition was attained or until 2500 time-steps had elapsed. Generally, ten specimen nets were considered for each value of the parameter V_0 from 1.0 to -0.7 in steps of 0.1.

(1) Perhaps the most noteworthy finding of this particular experiment concerns the distribution of cycling periods in the nets which were generated. In Fig. 21.4 we plot, for each mini-ensemble of (usually) ten nets, the fraction of periods lying in a specified period bin. Note that the bins marked off do not correspond to equal intervals in K; as in Fig. 21.2 we have chosen a subdivision of the K range in tune with the general behavior of the model, so that interesting variations are more readily

Fig. 21.4. Histograms of observed cycle lengths K in mini-ensembles of nets with adjusted thresholds and nonzero couplings bounded by unity. Each distribution represents an average over results for E sample nets with $N = 100$, $h = 0.35$ and $M = 5$ and with the specified threshold parameter V_o. $E = 9$ and 8 for $V_o = 1.0$ and -0.7 respectively, and $E = 10$ in all other cases. Each specimen was tested with $I = 50$ initial conditions.

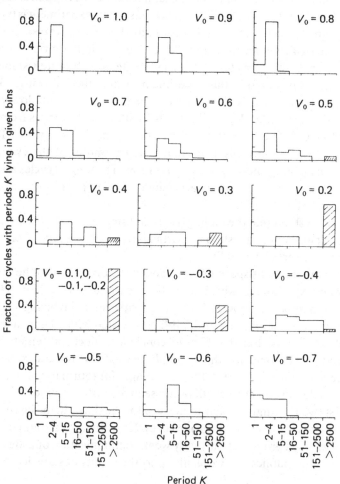

discernible. Runs which did not show any state repetitions over 2500 time-steps (and hence did not yield an identifiable cycle) are *arbitrarily* assigned to the highest period bin, $K > 2500$. One might well suspect that long cycles exist in at least some of these cases, since cycles of periods as long as $K = 1538$ and 1544 have been observed (in nets with $V_0 = -0.5$ and -0.4, respectively). However, in any given case we cannot rule out the possibility of a long transient followed by a short cycle. (Indeed, checks were made by allowing the net to run for 4000 time-steps from one or another of the initial conditions involved, and even then no state repetition was found, leaving the issue undecided.) With this reservation, it appears from inspection of Fig. 21.4 that the peak of the distribution of cycling periods moves to higher K as $|V_0| \to 0$. On the other hand, this behavior is *not* seen in many other examples which have been studied.

(2) The number of cycles found in the nets of this experiment is typically 2–4. Even so, 20 out of the total of 167 individual networks displayed only one cycle (which is accordingly called a *single*), and there were nets with as many as 16 and 18 cycles. Obviously, singles are absolutely stable.

Other trends noted in this experiment include the following. (3) The average activities α_{av} of the observed cycles run from quite low values, ~0.05–0.14, to rather high values, ~0.71−0.86, as V_0 ranges from $+1.0$ down to -0.7. There is not much variation in mean activity level for the cycles of a given net. (4) The relative accessibilities of the cycles of a specimen net are generally not very uniform. The longest cycles are often the most (or nearly the most) accessible. (5) The periods of singles are usually short.

We must stress that the findings ((1)–(5) listed above) apply specifically to the experiment in question; in particular, (5) and the second part of (4) cannot be asserted generally.

The limitations of space do not allow us to do justice to the 50 or so different experiments which have been carried out at $N = 100$ with different numbers of inputs M, etc., each experiment involving a substantial number of sample nets of the ●● class tested with a large number of initial conditions. Let it suffice to conclude explicit presentation with detailed cycling data for three sample nets of this more flexible class. Inspecting Tables 21.6–21.8, the percentages for return to the same cycle upon single-neuron perturbations are seen to cluster around 70–75% for the first two nets and average about 50% for the third. In the last example there are two well separated groups of cycles, with fairly strong communication within a group but only very weak communication outside.

In another publication we shall report the results of statistical analysis

Table 21.6. *Cycling and stability data for sample net of $N = 100$ model neurons, with threshold parameter $V_0 = 0.4$ and non-zero couplings bounded by unity, inhibitory fraction $h = 0.35$ and $M = 4$ inputs per neuron. Twenty cells have negative thresholds. Nine cycles, all of period 12, were observed, the first eight being found in runs from $I = 500$ initial conditions and the last being detected during the neuron-state-flip trials. The transition matrix $(S_{cc'})$ is given by the upper (left) array. A dash indicates that the corresponding cycle c' is never reached in any trial, while 0.00 indicates that c' is reached in less than 1% of the tries*

n	Cycle lengths																		
9	12	12	12	12	12	12	12	12	12	12	12	12	12	12	12	12	12	12	
12	0.77	0.08	0.12	0.02	0.00	–	–	–	0.00	0.28	0.28	0.27	0.29	0.28	0.29	0.29	0.28	0.28	α_{av}
12	0.18	0.73	0.04	0.00	0.02	0.02	–	–	0.00	0.41	0.21	0.19	0.02	0.12	0.01	0.02	0.01	0.00	a_c
12	0.19	0.01	0.73	0.00	0.04	–	–	–	0.02										
12	0.07	0.03	0.04	0.73	0.00	0.05	0.00	–	0.07										
12	0.16	0.03	0.15	0.00	0.63	–	0.02	–	0.00										
12	0.04	0.06	0.01	0.14	0.01	0.70	0.01	–	0.02	←——————— Transition matrix S									
12	0.09	0.00	0.03	0.02	0.05	0.03	0.68	–	0.09										
12	0.09	0.01	0.07	0.08	0.00	0.00	0.05	0.69	–										

n	Cycle lengths															
8	12	12	12	12	12	12	12	12	12	12	12	12	12	12	12
12	□	1	5	1	7	2	8	6	□	29	29	33	29	30	30	30
12		□	8	2	7	1	8	9		□	28	30	30	27	31	29
12			□	6	3	9	4	1			□	30	29	29	30	32
12				□	8	1	7	5				□	30	29	29	29
12					□	8	1	4					□	30	29	29
12	H_{min}					□	7	8	H_{max}					□	31	29	30
12							□	3							□	30	28
12								□								□	29
12																	□

of the accumulating data on nets with non-integer V_{ij} and adjusted thresholds. A finding which deserves special attention is that in a certain threshold regime the overall level of activity can be an extremely sensitive function of V_0.

21.4 Conclusions

We close with a summary of broad features of the simulation results discussed in Section 21.3, for net size $N = 100$.

(1) Typically, the *number of cyclic memories* built into a net upon random assembly might be around 3–5. However, this number is subject to wide variation, depending on the topology of the loops present in the net. Networks with only one or two cyclic modes are not uncommon, and as many as 16–18 cycles have been found in some of the sample nets considered in Section 21.3.

Table 21.7. *As in Table* 21.6, *except that sample net has* $M = 5$; *seventeen cells have negative thresholds. The last two cycles listed, of periods* 1 *and* 6, were not detected in the $I = 500$ *runs from random initial conditions.*

n	Cycle lengths																$\bar{K} = 8.9$
17	13	7	2	6	2	2	1	7	15	47	6	2	17	1	14	1	6
13	0.71	0.00	–	0.01	0.00	0.00	0.00	0.01	0.01	0.15	0.04	0.05	–	0.02	0.00	–	–
7	–	0.73	–	0.01	–	0.02	0.02	0.14	0.05	0.03	–	–	–	–	–	–	–
2	–	0.02	0.88	–	0.02	0.03	–	–	0.05	–	–	–	–	–	–	–	–
6	–	0.00	–	0.76	–	–	0.03	–	–	0.04	0.07	0.07	–	0.02	0.01	0.00	–
2	–	–	0.02	–	0.88	–	–	–	0.01	0.06	0.01	0.02	–	–	–	–	–
2	–	0.01	0.07	–	–	0.81	0.03	–	0.05	–	–	0.02	–	–	–	–	–
1	–	–	–	–	–	0.15	0.76	0.01	0.06	–	–	–	–	0.02	–	–	–
7	–	0.12	0.01	–	–	0.02	0.02	0.70	0.11	0.02	0.01	–	–	–	–	–	–
15	–	0.03	0.00	0.00	–	0.07	0.03	0.04	0.77	0.02	0.01	0.03	–	–	–	–	0.01
47	0.02	0.02	–	0.00	0.01	0.00	0.00	0.01	0.00	0.84	0.03	0.06	–	0.00	0.00	–	–
6	–	–	–	0.07	0.09	0.02	0.00	–	0.01	0.04	0.72	0.04	–	0.00	0.01	–	–
2	–	–	–	0.01	0.15	0.03	–	–	0.00	0.05	0.10	0.65	–	0.01	–	–	–
17	–	0.00	–	0.14	0.02	–	0.02	–	0.00	0.04	0.06	0.03	0.60	0.06	0.01	–	–
1	–	–	–	0.15	–	–	0.03	–	–	0.04	0.06	0.22	–	0.50	–	–	–
14	0.01	0.00	–	0.04	0.01	–	0.00	0.01	0.02	0.19	0.05	0.05	0.00	0.01	0.61	–	–
	Transition matrix S																
α_{av}	0.29	0.27	0.21	0.28	0.24	0.23	0.25	0.27	0.28	0.29	0.26	0.27	0.27	0.29	0.30	0.28	0.31
a_c	0.01	0.07	0.14	0.04	0.04	0.16	0.14	0.05	0.20	0.05	0.03	0.05	0.01	0.02	0.00	0.00	–

n	Cycle lengths														
15	13	7	2	6	2	2	1	7	15	47	6	2	17	1	14
13	□	8	19	9	18	18	14	9	9	4	17	17	9	13	5
7		□	21	14	22	20	16	1	4	3	23	21	12	18	9
2			□	12	3	3	5	23	21	20	9	7	12	9	21
6				□	9	11	7	13	14	10	6	8	3	4	9
2					□	6	8	24	23	18	6	4	9	6	19
2						□	4	22	20	19	5	3	11	8	20
1							□	18	17	15	9	7	7	4	16
7								□	2	3	21	23	11	20	6
15									□	4	24	22	14	19	7
47			Minimum Hamming distances							□	18	17	8	14	4
6											□	99	99	99	99
2												□	8	4	18
17													□	5	8
1														□	14
14															□

(2) *Cycle lengths* span a large range of values, again depending on the particular topology generated in random assembly of the network. Some very long cyclic modes, with periods K of several thousand, have been observed. On the other hand, K less than 50 appears to be more typical, and very short periods are not uncommon.

(3) *Distances between accessible cycles* are often short (cf. Harth *et al.*, 1970; Anninos *et al.*, 1970), as measured by the Hamming distances

Table 21.7 (continued)

n	Cycle lengths														
15	13	7	2	6	2	2	1	7	15	47	6	2	17	1	14
13	□	24	26	23	25	26	22	24	26	100	100	24	21	20	21
7		□	27	22	28	26	22	19	23	100	100	28	22	25	21
2			□	16	4	5	6	26	29	100	100	8	17	10	28
6				□	13	14	10	21	24	100	100	11	10	7	20
2					□	8	9	29	32	100	100	5	14	7	27
2						□	4	26	27	100	100	12	15	8	28
1							□	22	24	100	100	8	11	4	24
7								□	22	100	100	28	21	24	21
15									□	100	100	31	25	27	23
47										□	100	100	100	100	100
6			Maximum Hamming distances								□	100	100	100	100
2												□	13	5	26
17													□	9	21
1														□	22
14															□

Table 21.8. *As in Table* 21.6, *except that* $V_0 = 0.1$ *and* $M = 41$; *nine cells have negative thresholds.*

n	Cycle lengths								$\bar{R} = 3.4$								
8	7	2	2	4	2	2	4	4	7	2	2	4	2	2	4	4	
7	0.69	–	0.27	–	–	0.03	–	–	0.047	0.955	0.040	0.938	0.930	0.045	0.928	0.940	α_{av}
2	–	0.67	–	0.31	–	–	0.00	0.01	0.31	0.29	0.32	0.06	0.002	0.02	0.002	0.002	a_c
2	0.38	–	0.63	–	–	–	–	–									
4	–	0.22	–	0.68	–	–	0.04	0.06									
2	–	0.74	–	0.04	0.22	–	–	–									
2	0.53	–	0.16	–	–	0.31	–	–			Transition matrix S						
4	–	0.05	–	0.47	–	–	0.47	0.01									
4	–	0.20	–	0.46	–	–	0.09	0.26									

8	7	2	2	4	2	2	4	4	7	2	2	4	2	2	4	4
7	□	95	1	91	92	1	92	93	□	99	5	99	97	7	96	98
2		□	98	1	3	94	3	2		□	100	5	7	97	6	5
2			□	94	93	3	93	94			□	99	97	6	96	98
4				□	4	90	1	1				□	9	98	6	6
2					□	91	7	5					□	98	11	9
2						□	91	97						□	95	97
4			H_{min}				□	1			H_{max}				□	7
4								□								–

between states in one cycle and states in another. However, there are clear exceptions, as when conditions (gross parameters and detailed connectivity) are such that the activity level runs near 50%.

(4) *Relative accessibilities* of the cycles of a given net vary widely.

(5) We have not made a study of the *distribution of transient lengths.* Even so, it is clear that we are dealing with systems which are highly dissipative in the sense that the time required to enter a cycle is usually

quite short, far less than $2^N \tau$. For both $N = 10$ and $N = 100$, transients are ordinarily less than 500 time-steps, although some exceptions involving transient lengths greater than 4000 were noted in Section 21.3.

(6) Regarding the *stability of cycles under single-neuron state flips*, some interesting possibilities have been actualized. For· example, nets have been identified in which there are 'many' cycles ($\sim$10) and yet the chance of returning to a given cycle after perturbation is typically 50% or better. Some cyclic modes (*not* necessarily singles) are found to be *absolutely stable* under single-neuron flips. There are cases where the accessible cycles divide into groups, with strong transitions ('associations') within a group and weak transitions between groups. In other cases there is basically just one group, with relatively uniform communication between the member cycles. As yet, the collection of samples which has been analyzed is too small for any useful conclusions to be drawn about potential systematic dependences of stability measures on gross network parameters such as M, h and V_0. One expectation, yet to be verified, is that – other things being equal – stability might be better for smaller M (cf. Gardner & Ashby, 1970).

According to our experience, 'typical' behavior of these systems is very difficult to pin down; the more specimen nets one probes as one extends experiments over the ranges of adjustable parameters, the more one gets the impression that almost anything is possible. Exceptions in ample number can be produced to weaken practically any general rule.or general trend which seems to be emerging.

We are reminded of the following epigram due to Arbib (1972):

There are no universal statements about the nervous system except for the universal statement that there are no universal statements except for the universal statement that there are no universal statements except . . .

Thus, for better or worse, it can be justly claimed that the model nets simulated in our studies, consisting of randomly coupled threshold neurons operating deterministically and synchronously in discrete time, share at least this essential feature with living nerve networks.

In the above report, we have been concerned with the *direct* problem of neural nets (Caianiello & Marinaro, 1986, 1988): given the structure and dynamics, to find the evolution. More broadly, we have sought, with the aid of computer simulation, to discover and categorize the motions available to members of simple classes of models. If instead one has the more limited and more practical goal of constructing a specific network to carry out a specific task, through the realization of specific cyclic modes, one must instead solve the *inverse* problem. Important formal advances toward solution of this problem, involving linearization in functional space, are currently being made by Caianiello & Marinaro (1986, 1988). Another interesting approach to the inverse problem has been offered by Personnaz, Guyon & Dreyfus (1986).

Note added in proof

Recent analytic studies by one of us (Kürten, 1988*a*,*b*) indicate that the pessimistic view expressed in these concluding remarks is too extreme Certain universal dynamical properties of the models considered here are revealed by examination of the evolution of the normalized Hamming distance, in the thermodynamic limit. In particular, conditions on gross network parameters (e.g. M and V_o) for the existence of dynamical phase transitions can be established, thereby explaining – among other features – the glimpses of 'chaotic' activity seen in our experiments.

Acknowledgments

This work was supported in part by the Condensed Matter Theory Program of the Division of Materials Research of the U.S. National Science Foundation, under Grant No. DMR-8519077, and in part by the Foundation for Research Development, RSA. We thank E. Caianiello, R. M. J. Cotterill, R. Davé, H. Flyvbjerg and G. L. Shaw for useful remarks and illuminating discussions.

References

Anninos, P. A., Beck, B., Csermely, T. J., Harth, E. M. & Pertile, G. (1970). 'Dynamics of neural structures'. *J. Theoret. Biol.*, **26**, 121–48.

Anninos, P. A. (1972). 'Cyclic modes in artificial neural nets'. *Kybernetik*, **11**, 5–14.

Arbib, M. A. (1972). *The Metaphorical Brain: An Introduction to Cybernetics as Artificial Intelligence and Brain Theory*, p. 24. New York: Wiley.

Binder, P. M. & Jensen, R. V. (1986). 'Simulating chaotic behavior with finite-state machines'. *Phys. Rev. A*, **34**, 4460–3.

Caianiello, E. R. (1961). 'Outline of a theory of thought processes and thinking machines'. *J. Theoret. Biol.*, **2**, 204–35.

Caianiello, E. R. & Marinaro, M. (1986). 'Linearization and synthesis of cellular automata: the additive case'. *Physica Scripta*, **34**, 444–8.

Caianiello, E. R. & Marinaro, M. (1988). 'The inverse problem for neural nets and cellular automata'. These proceedings.

Choi, M. Y. & Huberman, B. A. (1983). 'Dynamic behavior of non-linear networks. *Phys. Rev. A*, **28**, 1204–6.

Clark, J. W., Rafelski, J. & Winston, J. V. (1985). 'Brain without mind: computer simulation of neural networks with modifiable neuronal interactions'. *Physics Reports*, **123**, 215–73.

344   *J. W. Clark, K. E. Kürten & J. Rafelski*

Cooper, L. N. (1988). 'Mean-field theory of a neural network'. These proceedings.
Cotterill, R. M. J. (1986). 'The brain: an intriguing piece of condensed matter'. *Physica Scripta*, **T13**, 161–8.
Derrida, B. & Flyvbjerg, H. (1986). 'Multivalley structure in Kauffman's model: Analogy with spin glasses'. *J. Phys. A*. **19**, L1003–8.
Gardner, M. R. & Ashby, W. R. (1970). 'Connectance of large dynamic (cybernetic) systems: critical values for stability'. *Nature*, **228**, 784.
Grondin, R. O., Porod, W., Loeffler, C. M. & Ferry, D. K. (1983). 'Synchronous and asynchronous systems of threshold elements'. *Biol. Cybern.*, **49**, 1–7.
Harth, E. M., Csermely, T. J., Beek, B. & Lindsay, R. D. (1970). 'Brain functions and neural dynamics'. *J. Theoret. Biol.*, **26**, 93–120.
Hopfield, J. J. (1982). 'Neural networks and physical systems with emergent collective computational abilities'. *Proc. U.S. Nat. Acad. Sci.*, **79**, 2554–8.
Kauffman, S. A. (1969). 'Metabolic stability and epigenesis in randomly constructed genetic nets'. *J. Theoret. Biol.*, **22**, 437–67.
Kauffman, S. A. (1984). 'Emergent properties in random complex automata'. *Physica*, **10D**, 145–56.
Kürten, K. E. & Clark, J. W. (1986). 'Chaos in neural systems'. *Phys. Lett.*, **114A**, 413–18.
Kürten, K. E. & Clark, J. W. (1988). 'Exemplification of chaotic activity in nonlinear neural networks obeying a deterministic dynamics in continuous time'. These proceedings.
Kürten K. E. (1988a). 'Transition to chaos in asymmetric neural networks'. In *Condensed Matter Theories*, eds. J. Arponen, E. Pananne & R. F. Bishop. New York: Plenum.
Kürten K. E. (1988b). 'Critical phenomena in model neural networks'. Submitted to *Physics Letters*.
Little, W. A. (1974). 'The existence of persistent states in the brain'. *Math. Biosci.*, **19**, 101–20.
Little, W. A. & Shaw, G. L. (1975). 'A statistical theory of short and long term memory'. *Behav. Biol.*, **14**, 115–33.
Littlewort, G. C., Clark, J. W. & Rafelski, J. (1988). 'Transition to cycling in neural networks'. These proceedings.
McCulloch, W. S. & Pitts, W. (1943). 'A logical calculus of the ideas immanent in nervous activity'. *Bull. Math. Biophys.*, **5**, 115–33.
Morrell, F. (1967). 'Electrical signs of sensory coding'. In *The Neurosciences: A Study Program*, eds. G. C. Quarton, T. Melnechuk & F. O. Schmitt, pp. 452–69. New York: Rockefeller University.
Morrell, F., Hoeppner, T. J. & de Toledo-Morrell, L. (1983). *Exp. Neurol.*, **80**, 111–46.
Personnaz, L., Guyon, I. & Dreyfus, G. (1986). 'Collective computational properties of neural networks: new learning mechanisms'. *Phys. Rev. A*, **34**, 4217–28.
Rall, W. & Segev, I. (1988). 'Excitable dendritic spine clusters: non-linear synaptic processing'. These proceedings.
Scofield, C. L. & Cooper, L. N. (1985). 'Development and properties of neural networks'. *Contemp. Phys.*, **26**, 125–45.
Scott, A. C. (1977). *Neurophysics*. New York: Wiley.
Shaw, G. L. (1986). Private communication.
Shaw, G. L. & Silverman, D. J. (1988). 'Large network simulations of the trion model of cortical organization'. These proceedings.
Silverman, D. J., Shaw, G. L. & Pearson, J. C. (1986). 'Associative recall properties of the trion model of cortical organization'. *Biol. Cybern.*, **53**, 259–71.

22

Transition to cycling in neural networks

G. C. LITTLEWORT, J. W. CLARK and J. RAFELSKI

22.1 Introduction

The mechanisms of the complex functions attributed mostly to the cerebral cortex are hidden in the collective behaviour of a vast neural network that cannot practically be described in detail or in general. Cyclic modes of activity which emerge spontaneously in the dynamics of neural networks may underly possible mechanisms of short-term memory and associative thinking. The transitions from seemingly random activity patterns to cyclic activity have been examined in isolated networks with pseudorandomly chosen synapses and in networks with very simple architectures.

The basic computer model (Clark, Rafelski & Winston, 1985) envisions a collection of neurons, linked by a network of axons and dendrites that synapse onto one another. The synaptic interactions are modeled by a connection matrix V. The net algebraic strength of the connections from neuron j to neuron i, represented by the matrix element V_{ij}, can be positive (excitatory), negative (inhibitory) or zero (no connection). In the present study, the V_{ij} were chosen randomly, but in accord with certain specified gross network parameters, viz.

N = net size = number of neurons in net,

m = connection density = probability that a given $j \rightarrow i$ link exists,

h = fraction of inhibitory neurons.

No more than one connection ('synapse') was allowed from any source neuron j to a given target neuron i.

The neurons update their states synchronously, corresponding to the assumption of a universal time delay τ for direct signal transmission. Each neuron i can be on ($\pi_i = 1$), off ($\pi_i = 0$) or recovering from its previous firing, the third (refractory) state not being considered in the present study. Neurons behave as threshold elements, turning on for one time step when there is sufficient integrated stimulation from incoming synapses. Thus

$$\pi_i(t + \tau) = \theta\left[\sum_j V_{ij}(t)\pi_j(t) - V_{0i} + \text{accumulated signal}\right.$$
$$\left. + \text{external input} + \text{noise}\right],$$

where $\theta[x]$ is the step function, V_{0i} is the threshold of neuron i and $\pi_i(t)$, $i = 1, \ldots, N$, forms the state vector. In the work reported here, there is no accumulation of signals, no noise and no external input, so the state of the net at time step $t + \tau$ depends only on the state vector at time t, the connection matrix and the threshold vector formed from V_{0i}, $i = , \ldots, N$. The two choices of V_{0i} are of particular interest as standards, namely

$$\text{normal threshold of neuron } i = \frac{1}{2}\sum_j V_{ij},$$

$$\text{uniform threshold for all neurons} = \frac{1}{2N}\sum_{ij} V_{ij}.$$

However, larger studies (Littlewort, 1986) were not restricted to these choices.

When the dynamics of the sample nets of the general type described above were followed by computer simulation, with the connection matrix held constant, the behaviour soon assumed a periodic character, i.e., the system was seen to enter a *cyclic mode*. In such deterministic nets, repetition of any state vector implies indefinite repetition of the sequence of states occurring from the first to the second appearance of the duplicated state. The period K of a cyclic mode is simply the number of time steps between any two identical states of the net, and the transition length is the time for the cycle to form, as described below.

Convenient choices for the ranges of the network parameters (net size, connection density and inhibitory fraction) were made. Uniform thresholds were adopted for the survey of transitions in unstructured nets, and normal thresholds were used in most studies of structured nets.

It was found that, ordinarily, a particular net generates only a small number of cyclic modes when plied with a variety of initial conditions. The time from initialisation of a net's activity to the entrance into a cycle (the *transient period*) was found to be short in most cases, that is, a cyclic mode was usually found within 500 time units, for the kinds and sizes of nets examined here. The *transition length*, measured from the time the first neuron starts to behave periodically (with the period of the eventual cycle) to the time the whole net is cycling, can naturally be quite protracted for very long cycles. However, the transition to ordered behaviour was generally found to be *relatively rapid*, in the sense that the transition length is shorter than the cycling period. This was in fact the case for 97% of the cycles with period $K \geq 12$ time steps. Long (or relatively long) transitions would be expected if the mechanism of transition involved one neuron or group of neurons steadily seeding the transition to cycling. This scenario may apply for modes of small K (cf. Clark *et al.*, 1985). However, our results for large K point to the existence of a more global condition which allows a sudden collective onset of cycling in the net.

22.2 Rapid transitions and network parameters

Ranges of gross network parameters explored include:

$N = 15$–100, limited by computer power,

$m = 0.08$–0.30, large enough to avoid disconnected neurons,

$h = 0.25$–0.45, to possibly include the physiological value.

Rapid transitions, in the relative sense, were found for all parameter sets, and particularly for small nets, small h or large m. The occurrence of relatively long transitions for long complicated cycles, although rare, placed some limits on the generality of the phenomenon of rapid transitions. Complexity of cycles, in terms of reverberatory composition (Clark *et al.*, 1985), was correlated with eligibility of neurons and the average distance between neurons. The simplest definition of the *distance* from one neuron to another is the shortest path length from one neuron to the other, in terms of number of synapses crossed (Clark, Littlewort & Refelski, 1987). *Eligible* neurons are defined here as those not locked into steady firing or silence, in the prevailing mode of operation of the network (cf. Clark *et al.*, 1985). By *eligibility* of a net we shall normally mean the fraction or percentage of neurons that qualify as eligible during some appropriately chosen time interval.

The influence of gross parameters on complexity may be summarised as follows. Raising the inhibitory fraction (e.g., to 0.45) enhanced complexity to the extent that it became inconvenient to search for the very long, less accessible cyclic modes. Larger nets (e.g., $N = 60$, 100) with lower connectivity (e.g., $m = 0.08$–0.15), that is, nets with say $M = 5$–10 inputs per neuron, were characterised by slightly longer distances and by long cycles and occasionally long transitions. It must be emphasized that individual nets with the same gross parameters displayed a wide variety of behaviour, but that general tendencies were visible. The effect of a blanket application of the 'brainwashing' plasticity algorithm was also varied, some nets being scarcely affected while others were over-brainwashed. (Brainwashing involves the selective punishment of active connections, i.e., reduction of $|V_{ij}|$ if the firing of neuron j is followed immediately by the firing of neuron i (Clark *et al.*, 1985).) Although cycling periods increased by an average factor of three after brainwashing, there were only slight increases in relative transition times and percentages of eligible neurons.

The longest transitions (measured relatively) were found for short cycles of up to twelve steps. However, unusually large eligibilities were associated with these cases (cf. the correlation between period of cycling and eligibility, to be documented below).

22.3 Effect of simple architecture on transitions to cycling

The above results lead one to ask whether some kind of structure was causing the nets to cycle easily with so few terminal cycles and to undergo relatively rapid transitions. A hidden accidental grouping could allow closely connected units to dominate activity, but the inherent structure of the nets considered to this point is rather intangible. Accordingly, a simple, controllable structure was imposed on the nets, with a concomitant increase in the average distance. Two main prescriptions were used for dividing the net into layers or netlets. The first, called *local emphasis*, is to vary the connection density by greatly enhancing the probability for two neurons in the same region or netlet to be connected, while reducing the probability of connection between neurons in different netlets (see Fig. 22.1).

The second prescription, called cutting, involves systematic disconnection of internetlet connections neuron by neuron (see Fig. 22.2). Changes

Fig. 22.1. Schematic connection matrices show simple architecture imposed by weighting the connection probability (shading density) in the block-diagonal region (left matrix) or near-diagonal region (right matrix). The corresponding grouping of neurons is into loosely cross-linked netlets (for the left matrix) or into a ring-like structure (for the other matrix).

Connection matrices with local emphasis

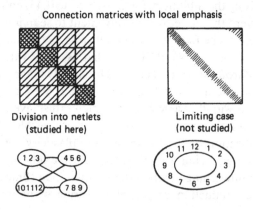

Division into netlets   Limiting case
(studied here)   (not studied)

in behaviour were observed as a function of cutting, until the netlets were completely separated.

There is obviously a problem dividing an already small net into netlets which are supposed to maintain some individual behaviour. The cases adopted most often in our experiments were 100 neurons divided into two netlets of 50, into four netlets of 25 and into ten netlets of 10 neurons each.

The purpose of monitoring subcycles or near subcycles in netlets of architectured nets was to gain a closer view of the process by which a cycle emerges from the 'wandering'. For example, in a long transition, one group of neurons may start cycling before the rest and the different netlets may display different periodicities until one eventually dominates the others. For this to happen, the number of connections between netlets must strike a balance between allowing sufficient communication for netlets to influence one another and eventually dominate or succumb, and yet allowing netlets enough independence to develop cycles individually without destructive interruption.

It was found that large local emphasis, a profusion of subcycles and long transients are correlated. Particular runs of nets which had transients longer than 500 steps, or runs which cycled trivially (period $k \leq 2$) showed little evidence of 'attempts' to subcycle. The former observation may indicate that nets operating with many eligible neurons, sample too many states for repetition to be likely. The latter may indicate that all the netlets need to cycle trivially, or else one longer subcycle would be a non-trivial common multiple of periods.

Applying local emphasis to the connection matrix did not substantially alter the influence of gross network parameters on average cyclic

Fig. 22.2. The connection matrix (with shaded regions set to zero as synaptic links are cut) and the effective grouping of neurons caused by this cutting process are shown. The diagonal blocks of the matrix (corresponding to internal connections, within netlets) are unaltered, while the off-diagonal regions (netlet–netlet connections) are encroached by shading (severed links) as the netlets become progressively more disconnected. Arrows indicate communication from set to set.

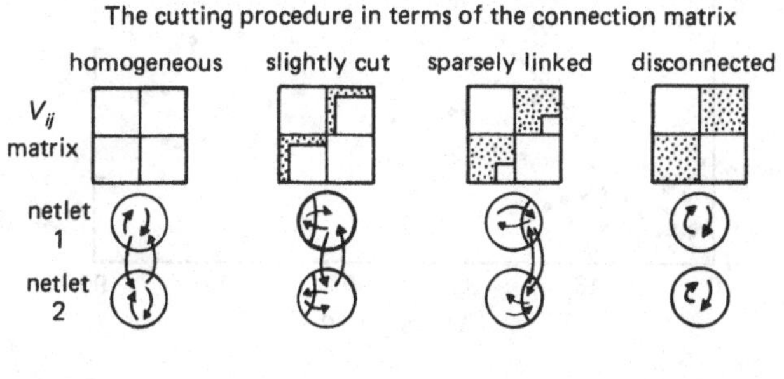

The cutting procedure in terms of the connection matrix

Fig. 22.3. (*a*) Transition time versus period, for local-emphasis nets. The maximum run time was 500 steps, and each dot represents one run. Thus the distributions of cycle lengths and transition times are also illustrated. Note that in this set of runs, T_t (transition time) is less than K for $K > 12$ and $T_t < K/2$ for $K > 160$, but the ratio T_t/K is extremely varied from case to case.

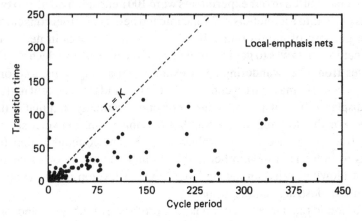

Fig. 22.3. (*b*) Magnified view of small-period region of Fig. 22.3(*a*).

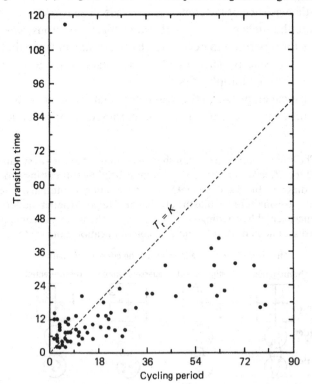

behaviour. For example, nets with $m = 0.1$ typically showed transients longer than 500 time units, while nets with $m = 0.3$ usually cycled trivially. Hence a suitable choice of m would be 0.15 to 0.2. Note that the typical maximum emphasis applied to local connectivity was 20, which is not extreme enough to bar many neurons from external connections. We define emphasis as the ratio m_{int}/m_{ext} of internal to external connection probabilities.

Transition times were *shorter* than cycling periods in 90% of runs on nets with local-emphasis netlet substructure. (See Fig. 22.3.) Cycles of period $K > 10$ were reached via transitions longer than K in only 2% of the cases. These relatively longer transitions all occurred in nets with parameters that would typically have produced much longer cycles.

Note that the couplings V_{ij} were restricted to -1, 0 and $+1$. The influence of architecture could be quite different if local emphasis were implemented by reducing the *magnitudes* of the strengths V_{ij} of internetlet connections, while not affecting the number of such connections.

22.4 Effect of the cutting prescription on transitions to cycling

As a counterpoint to the local-emphasis prescription for generating structured nets, we can, alternatively, study a given net all through a process of disassembly into many netlets, by severing small sets of links in succession. The kinds of structures created in the two cases are in fact quite different. In particular, cutting produces a black and white connection matrix, with no grey areas; hence certain neurons in each netlet are

Fig. 22.4. The relationship of transition time to period is shown, for individual nets reached during the cutting process. The maximum run time was 500 steps, and each dot represents one run. The line $K = T_t$ is a reminder that, in general, transitions are relatively short, but that some, usually within structured nets, are longer.

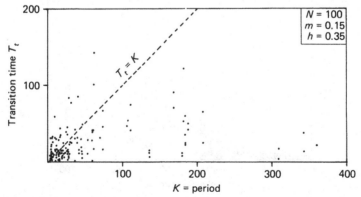

given the status of external communicators and all neurons are not equivalent. It should still be possible to draw close parallels as well as distinctions between the behaviours of the two types of structured nets. For example, Fig. 22.4, which gathers information on transition time versus cycling period for cut nets, is to be compared with Fig. 22.3.

In the cutting process, it was observed that even the smallest changes in the connections of the net, brought about by single 'cuts', generally resulted in very different cycles being accessible. This syndrome was most prominent in the middle stages of the process in some nets. When the netlets were already evident, but still very well connected to one another,

Fig. 22.5. (*a*) Cycling period versus eligibility, for nets of size $N = 100$. A neuron is considered to be eligible if it is neither always firing nor always silent, over the time interval of interest. Each square represents one or more occurrences of the same cycle. Varied combinations of net conditions (m, h, cuts) are included. Modes in which cycling was not evident over the maximum run time of 500 are plotted as close to the top of the graph as possible. In cases where cycling was overtly established during the run, eligibility refers to the cyclic phase; otherwise it refers to the full watching period including transient.

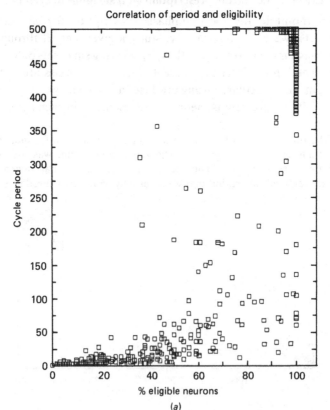

(*a*)

drastic changes in eligibility could be seen after cutting of certain (apparently vital) links.

The effect of cutting a net into netlets was to reduce the m-dependence of cyclic behaviour; for example, $N = 100$ nets were far more dependent on m in this respect than $N = 25$ nets. Thus, low-m nets (which often do not cycle during a reasonable watching period) and high-m nets (which often cycle trivially) could be made to converge to similar behaviour by the cutting procedure.

The lengths of cycles tended to fluctuate widely from one case to another and therefore proved to be an unsuitable gauge of complexity of behaviour. Instead, the degree of eligibility and the nature of the onset of cycling (or the rate of accumulation of cycling neurons) were found to be better indicators. An average of all runs showed maximum eligibility of 66% of the neurons after 15 out of 25 possible cuts have been made. The ratio of internal to external m-densities is then 6. This does not tell us anything about relative rates of transition to order. However, bringing a given net into a suitable eligibility range by cutting, typically reduced the number of trivial or virtually inaccessible cycles and correspondingly increased the number of disorder-to-order transitions warranting closer examination (cf. Fig. 22.5).

Fig. 22.5. (*b*) Magnified view of the lower-eligibility region of Fig. 22.5(*a*). Note that the long periods of cycles with participation less than 50% are a consequence of four independent netlets contributing to the common multiple of subperiods.

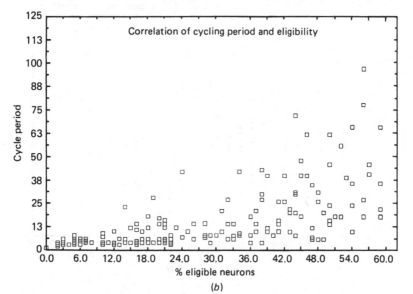

(*b*)

Subcycling was rarely found in nets that did not show cycling in 500 steps, in spite of the unusually long time available. This observation was unexpected in structured nets, but in homogeneous or mildly structured nets, distances are short enough (cf. Clark *et al.*, 1985) to make the possibility of independent subcycling remote.

For extremely lumpy architecture, the number of subcycles was limited because an uninterrupted subcycle would only be recorded once, and the transition loses its significance if each netlet has a different period. With minimal but vital communication channels open between netlets (a total of 3–7 for the 25 neurons of a netlet, after 18–22 cuts), repeated states in netlets persisted for longer and sometimes influenced other netlets, rendering slow transitions more likely. Fig. 22.6 presents information on the abundance of subcycling, while Fig. 22.7 gives an example of a net

Fig. 22.6. Repeated states. The various symbols indicate the numbers of repeated states found in netlets. Each column represents one net. All nets contain $N = 100$ neurons, but the netlet sizes are $N_s = 10, 25$ and 50 as shown. Netlet size is equal to the number of cuts necessary to completely sever the netlets. Large dots symbolise many repeated states (>50), and small dots about 15–50 repeated states. Crosses stand for independent uninterrupted repeated states in each netlet. Code numbers signify parameters m, h: (1–3): 0.075, 0.35; (4–6): 0.15, 0.35; (7–9): 0.2, 0.35; (10–11): 0.25, 0.35; (12–14): 0.3, 0.35; (15–17): 0.15, 0.35; (18–20): 0.3, 0.35; (21–29): 0.15, $h = 0.2$–0.3.

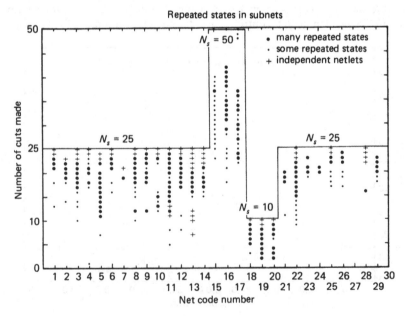

with some unusually long transitions in which the individual netlets acquire the cycle in succession.

22.5 Concluding remarks

It is all very well to divide a net into netlets and then to show that repetitions occur within the netlets, but how can one tell whether or not seemingly homogeneous nets have natural divisions into little groups of neurons in close communication? A series of earlier studies showed that frequently two or three neurons out of 60 would have the same period for a while during the transient, without 'precipitating' cycling. This find is not likely to be spurious and may relate to the many-to-one property that forces a rapid convergence toward stable, ordered modes. In the vast majority of cases, any inherent structure of sample nets, assembled

Fig. 22.7. Cooperation and competition in a particular net of size $N = 100$ at three different stages of cutting. The net is being divided, by cutting, into four netlets. The number of neurons participating non-trivially in the relevant cyclic mode is plotted against time to show the transition phase. A neuron is said to be *participating* (nontrivially) in a given cycle, incipient or established, if (a) it is neither steadily on nor steadily off and (b) its temporal pattern of firing is the same as it is in the fully established cycle. On the left the participation in *each netlet* is depicted on the same time scale, from 90 steps before cycling till the onset of cycling. The onset time indicated is actually the total transient time. *Total* participation in each cut net versus time (in units of the relevant cycle period) is sketched in the smaller graphs on the right, and the eligibility during cycling is indicated for the three cut nets on the vertical scale at the right edge of the figure.

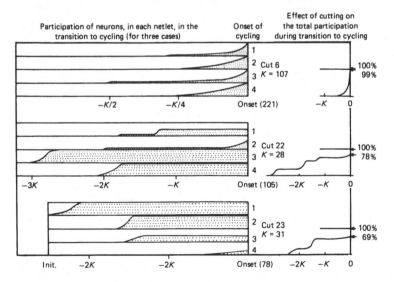

randomly according to a prescription involving uniform connection probability, was insufficient to produce relatively slow transition times for cycles of appreciable length. Such transitions only occurred with some frequency in the context of markedly structured nets operating with many eligible neurons.

Acknowledgements

Research support from the FRD and CSIR Bursary, RSA, and from the Condensed Matter Theory Programme of the Division of Materials Research of the U.S. National Science Foundation, under grant No. DMR-8519077, is greatly appreciated.

References

Clark, J. W., Rafelski, J. & Winston, J. V. (1985). 'Brain without mind: computer simulation of neural networks with modifiable neuronal interactions'. *Physics Reports*, **123**(4), 215–73.
Clark, J. W., Littlewort, G. C. & Rafelski, J. (1987). 'Topology, structure and distance in quasirandom neural networks'. These proceedings.
Littlewort, G. C. (1986). Phase Transitions in Neural Networks. M.Sc. Thesis, University of Cape Town.

23

Exemplification of chaotic activity in non-linear neural networks obeying a deterministic dynamics in continuous time

K. E. KÜRTEN and J. W. CLARK

23.1 Introduction

During the last decade, a conspicuous theme of experimental and theoretical efforts toward understanding the behavior of complex systems has been the identification and analysis of chaotic phenomena in a wide range of physical contexts where the underlying dynamical laws are considered to be deterministic (Schuster, 1984). Such chaotic activity has been examined in great detail in hydrodynamics, chemical reactions, Josephson junctions, semiconductors, and lasers, to mention just a few examples. Chaotic solutions of deterministic evolution equations are characterized by (i) irregular motion of the state variables, and (ii) extreme sensitivity to initial conditions. The latter feature implies that the future time development of the system is effectively unpredictable. An essential prerequisite for deterministic chaos is non-linear response; and although there are famous examples of chaos in relatively simple systems (e.g. Lorenz, 1963; Feigenbaum, 1978), we expect this kind of behavior to arise most naturally in systems of high complexity. Since biological nerve nets are notoriously non-linear and are perhaps the most complex of all known physical systems, it would be most surprising if the phenomena associated with deterministic chaos were irrelevant to neurobiology. Indeed, there has been a growing interest in the detection and verification of deterministic chaos in biological preparations consisting of few or many neurons. At one extreme we may point to the pioneering work of Guevara *et al.* (1981) on irregular dynamics observed in periodically stimulated cardiac cells; and, at the other, to the recent analysis by Babloyantz *et al.* (1985) of EEG data from the brains of human subjects during the sleep cycle, aimed at establishing the existence of chaotic attractors for sleep stages two and four. In such living nets there is the obvious problem of disentangling a deterministic component from ever-present background noise.

In this paper we turn instead to the search for chaotic solutions in non-linear mathematical models of neural networks. The model to be adopted, which is due to Stein *et al.* (1974*a,b*), has some claim to neurophysiological realism, at least within the confines of a nodal description in which structure and function are not probed below the whole-neuron level. To date, no instances of chaos have been uncovered in small systems of such model neurons, under conditions of constant external stimulus to a subset of cells. The examples to be presented here were discovered during computer explorations of the systematics of steady and periodic modes in moderately complex assemblies containing up to ~100 model neurons. In Section 23.2 the mathematical model is formulated and its roots in neuronal physiology are discussed. Section 23.3 is devoted to the demonstration and authentication of chaotic activity in sample networks from a class of model systems with randomly chosen synaptic interactions. These examples involve steady external input and hence do not rely on periodic forcing as a mechanism for chaos. We conclude, in Section 23.4, with a brief consideration of some of the neurobiological implications of deterministic chaos.

23.2 Nonlinear continuous-time network model

One of the challenges facing the brain theorist is the formulation of a model of single nerve cells which is simple enough to permit extensive analysis of the dynamical behavior of networks of model neurons, yet complicated enough to mimic the essential characteristics of real neurons. Thinking in this vein, Stein & coworkers (1974*a,b*) have developed a continuous-time model of single-neuron response and of neuronal networks which strikes a reasonable compromise between mathematical (or computational) tractability and physiological veracity. Their description is based on the assumption that the mean interval between action-potential pulses emitted by any neuron is short compared to the time scale for significant changes in the signal it is receiving. It then becomes meaningful to represent a pulse train by a continuous variable $x(t)$, the average firing rate of the neuron. The firing rates of the individual neurons provide the basic dynamical variables of the neural model of Stein *et al.* This model is in fact designed to embody a mean-rate code or *frequency coding* as the chief mechanism for transmission of information.

In many neurons (notably sensory neurons), a plot of firing rate x versus stimulus strength f shows a substantial range in which x increases linearly with f. Thus, although all action-potential pulses of a given neuron are essentially identical, a neuron is able to pass on the information that it is feeling a stronger stimulus by firing pulses at a greater rate (Stevens, 1966). As emphasized by Stevens, two prominent features of neuronal physiology may contribute to the observed increase of x with f. These are (i) the refractory properties of the axonal membrane, as reflected in the relaxation of the threshold from large values following an action potential, and (ii) the narrowing, with increasing stimulus strength, of the interval between the onset of superthreshold stimulus and the peak of the resulting action potential.

The response of a neuron has, of course, important non-linear aspects: for instance, there is often a significant mean firing rate even at zero input due to neuronal spontaneity, and the impulse frequency necessarily saturates at very high input due to the existence of an absolute refractory period.

In addition to the primary phenomena of frequency coding and of non-linear response at small and large stimuli, the model of Stein *et al.* is designed to incorporate a secondary characteristic of individual neuronal behavior which has important qualitative consequences in the functioning of neural networks. Suppose a neuron, initially undisturbed, is given a stimulus that turns on instantaneously at a superthreshold level which is maintained indefinitely. The output x of the neuron will rise rapidly (on a few-millisecond time scale) from zero to some peak value; thereafter the firing rate may stay at the peak value or it may *decline* (on a longer time scale) to a reduced constant level. This latter behavior, in which the neuron 'gets used to' an input signal, is called *accommodation* or *adaptation*; in effect, it is a kind of time-delayed self-inhibition.

A step-by-step heuristic construction of the equations of motion characterizing the model may be found in the papers of Stein *et al.* (1974*a,b*) and the thesis of Chen (1986). Here we merely write down the equations, define their ingredients, and motivate their structure *a posteriori*. The dynamical behavior of a system of N interconnected neurons is described in terms of the neuronal impulse frequencies x_i and adaptation variables y_i, $i = 1, \ldots, N$. The time development of these variables is governed by the set of equations

$$a_i^{-1} \frac{\mathrm{d}x_i}{\mathrm{d}t} = -x_i + r_i^{-1} S\left[f_i(t) - f_{0i} + \sum_{j=1}^{N} c_{ij}x_j + b_i y_i \right], \tag{1a}$$

$$\frac{\mathrm{d}y_i}{\mathrm{d}t} = x_i - p_i y_i, \tag{1b}$$

where a_i, r_i, f_{0i}, b_i, p_i and the c_{ij} are specified constants, The function $S(\zeta)$ is supposed to be of sigmoid shape, being monotonic over $-\infty < \zeta < \infty$, and approaching the limiting values 0 and 1, respectively, as the argument ζ goes to $-\infty$ and $+\infty$. To be definite, we take $S(\zeta) = [1 + \exp(-\zeta)]^{-1}$.

The quantities entering these equations may be interpreted as follows. The firing rate x_i serve as the principal variable and output of element i. The total input F_i to cell i is given by the sum of the first, third, and fourth terms in the argument of the S function. The first term, f_i, is the external stimulus or input; the third is the total synaptic input from all cells j of the net (including i); and the fourth (assuming $b_i < 0$) brings in an effective self-inhibition due to accommodation (or a self-excitation for $b_i > 0$). So far as single-neuron behavior is concerned, the proposed dynamical model may account for (a) the restricted range of firing rates due to an absolute refractory period (one parameter, r_i), (b) decreased sensitivity of neuronal response at large excitatory or inhibitory inputs (through the sigmoid shape of the function S which summarizes the accumulation and processing of stimuli), (c) spontaneous firing, i.e., firing in the absence of input (one parameter, f_{0i}), (d) response time for the increase of firing rate following a step increase of input (one parameter, a_i^{-1}, which lumps together synaptic delays, rise times of postsynaptic membrane potentials, time for passive spread of excitation to the point of initiation of action potentials, etc.) and (e) the phenomenon of accommodation of neuronal firing rate to maintained inputs (one variable y_i, one level parameter b_i and one rate constant p_i). Explicit reference to the refractory periods r_i may be eliminated by working with normalized, dimensionless impulse frequencies $\hat{x}_i \equiv r_i x_i$, lying between 0 and 1 and designated again simply as x_i. (Also, the spontaneity parameter f_{0i}, a threshold value of input at which the steady firing rate is $\frac{1}{2}$, may be absorbed into F_i in the interest of economy.) The topology of the neural network and the strengths of the interactions among the neurons are specified by the N^2 coupling coefficients c_{ij}. In particular, c_{ij} measures the effectiveness of the activity x_j of neuron j in producing input to neuron i, represented as $\Sigma_j c_{ij} x_j$. A positive (negative) coupling coefficient c_{ij} means that the postsynaptic effect on i, of active j, is excitatory (inhibitory), and of course $c_{ij} = 0$ if j has no synapses on i. In general, action and reaction are not equal and opposite in the nervous system: $c_{ij} \neq c_{ji}$.

This scheme may be readily generalized to include two or more adaptation processes, with specific level parameters and rate constants, as considered in Stein *et al.* (1974*a, b*) and Kürten & Clark (1986).

Mathematically, (1) presents us with a set of $2N$ coupled, first-order, ordinary, nonlinear differential equations. (Actually, only the first of the two equations for neuron i is nonlinear.) An obvious approach to any given system obeying the dynamical equations (1) is: *first*, enumeration of the steady-state solutions; *second*, linearization of the equations about these steady states and determination of their (local) stability or instability (by finding the eigenvalues of the linearized equations); *third*, direct numerical solution of the full equations for the time course of the firing rates, in interesting cases; and *fourth*, construction of input-output relations (where in the case of ordered behavior the output may be taken as the average of firing rate over time – generally over one period – and over all the neurons).

A preliminary intuitive understanding of this nodal description can be gained by first trimming it down, and then restoring various effects one at a time. Consider a single neuron (thus taking all the c couplings equal to zero), dispense with adaptation (thus setting the bs zero) and either assume immediate warm-up (a effectively infinite) or look for the steady state. Then the normalized firing rate is simply given by $x = S(f - f_0)$, dropping irrelevant indices. Three desirable features of this simplified model may be noted: (i) there is an appreciable intermediate range of input over which the response is approximately linear, (ii) as the input grows very large, the output saturates at the maximum possible firing rate of one pulse per refractory period r, and (iii) an average effect of spontaneous firing is simulated by a small positive value of x at zero input. Allowing a *finite* warm-up time, i.e., a^{-1} non-zero, the time development of the pulse frequency, following a step increase of input, will show first a linear rise from an initial value of zero and later an exponential approach to the steady rate $\frac{1}{2}$.

Reverting to the general formulation (1), focus next on the adaptation equation, the linear differential equation for y_i. We see that the adaptation variable is driven by the firing rate of neuron i; the larger x_i, the faster y_i grows. The larger y_i, the greater is the self-inhibition due to the corresponding $b_i < 0$ term in the input F_i. On the other hand, if neuron i is turned off, y_i just decays exponentially, with rate constant p_i. These are features we would expect from the proposed electrochemical mechanisms for accommodation (Stein *et al.*, 1974*b*).

Now return to the single-neuron case, and include accommodation. For $N = 1$ with b negative, it can easily be shown that for given steady input f there is a *unique* steady-state solution x^* for the firing rate, and moreover that this steady solution is *stable*. For arbitrary initial firing rate $x(0) = x_0$, the solution $x(t)$ will, after some transient period which depends on the initial conditions, eventually approach the steady value x^* exponentially.

With the accommodation mechanism in effect and $N = 2$ or more interacting neurons present, the system can in principle display a rich variety of behaviors. Asymptotically, it may approach an *ordered* condition, with each firing-rate variable in either a (locally) stable steady state or a (locally) stable condition of sustained periodic oscillation. We note that unstable steady states will ordinarily have short lifetimes in the presence of minimal noise. Generally, more than one ordered terminal mode may be reached in a given net, by changing the initial conditions. (A simple example of stable, periodic oscillations may be seen in the so-called *neural oscillator* (Stein *et al.*, 1974a; Chen, 1986) which consists of a pair of identical neurons acting on one another in a balanced, mutually inhibitory manner: $c_{12} = c_{21} > 0$.) In contrast to such ordered long-term behavior, the solution might instead correspond to *deterministic chaos* (Kürten & Clark, 1986; Choi & Hubermann, 1983); this possibility is opened by the non-linearity of the equations (1a). A chaotic solution of (1) will be characterized by aperiodic oscillatory motion and by sensitivity to the initial conditions which is so extreme that although the evolution is in principal deterministic, it is in practice unpredictable (Schuster, 1984).

The continuous-time neural-network model adopted here is complementary to the usual discrete-time nodal models, in the following sense. In the latter models (see e.g. Clark, Rafelski & Winston, 1985; Clark, Kürten & Rafelski, 1987) it is normally assumed that the decay time of postsynaptic potentials (PSPs) is *short* compared to the smallest possible interval between pulses (the spacing of the time grid or the absolute refractory period). In the continuous model of Stein *et al.*, it is in effect assumed that the time-integrated stimulus is sufficiently strong to produce firing within a time short compared to the PSP decay time, or, that the PSP decay time is *long* compared to the minimum interval between pulses. Thus, we expect that the common discrete models are more appropriate when the temporal distribution of pulses is sparse and, conversely, we expect the continuous model specified above to make better sense when the mean pulse rate is high.

Recently, the model of Stein *et al.* has been extended to achieve a description which is free from the assumption of long PSP decay times (Chen, 1986). In this scheme, the soma membrane potential u_i is intro-

duced as a *third* dynamical variable of neuron i, the time development of
this variable being governed by an *additional* differential equation which
is coupled to those for the firing rate x_i and the adaptation variable y_i. The
new dynamical equations read

$$a_{1i}^{-1} \frac{dx_i}{dt} = -x_i + r_i^{-1}S[u_i - u_{0i}], \tag{2a}$$

$$a_{2i}^{-1} \frac{du_i}{dt} = -(-u_i - u_{oi}) + f_i + \sum_{j=1}^{N} c_{ij}x_j + b_iy_i, \tag{2b}$$

$$\frac{dy_i}{dt} = x_i - p_iy_i. \tag{2c}$$

The membrane potential $u_i(t)$ is measured from the resting potential, and
the constant u_{oi} plays the role of threshold. The response times a_{1i}^{-1}
(analogous to a_i^{-1} of eqn (1a)) and a_{2i}^{-1} should be of the order of milliseconds to tens of milliseconds. We are now free to interpet a_{1i} as a
warm-up or response time at the output point (axon hillock) where the
firing decision is made and action potentials are generated, and a_{2i} as a
warm-up or response time on the input tree (associated with the time-
course of postsynaptic potentials as well as synaptic delay). Thus the
description becomes much clearer from the neurophysiological point of
view.

There are (at least) two limiting cases of interest:
(1) Let $a_{2i}^{-1} = 0$. This brings us back to eqns (1) and therefore to the
    formulation of Stein *et al.* with a single adaptation variable for each
    neuron. (Note that generalization to two or more adaptation vari-
    ables per neuron is straightforward.)
(2) Let $a_{1i}^{-1} = 0$. Set $b_i = 0$ and ignore the adaptation process. This
    gives us the continuous-time model of Hopfield (1984).

The behaviors attainable in the extended model (2) are presently being
explored in a number of contexts ranging from few-neuron networks to
cortical structures (Chen, 1986). However, the demonstrations recounted
in the next section are confined to the older model.

23.3 Complex behavior in randomly assembled model nets

The model of Stein *et al.*, as well as extensions of it to include explicit
synaptic time lags and to account for the finite decay time of postsynaptic
potentials, has been applied to biological nerve nets such as the retina
(Oğuztöreli, 1982) and the olfactory bulb (Chen, 1986). To date, no
definite evidence of chaotic activity has been found in these applications.
Here we shall concentrate on a rather more abstract problem which is of

considerable value in its own right within the general theoretical areas of neural networks and non-linear dynamics, namely, determination of the nature of solutions of the model equations for the case of *quasirandom* connectivity. The adjective 'quasirandom' signifies that although the connections are chosen randomly, they must be consistent with certain preordained gross network parameters, such as the number of neurons, the number of inputs per neuron, the number of inhibitory links, etc. Computer simulation is being used to map out the systematics of the locally stable and unstable steady-state solutions, as well as to explore the conditions for sustained, periodic oscillations, for systems of varying sizes and degrees of connectivity, with strength of the external input as the control parameter. In general, oscillatory modes are readily generated. In some cases a remarkable phenomenon has been observed (Kürten & Clark, 1986). Upon entering a certain range of input strength, the nature of the solution changes drastically; rather than achieving a locally stable steady state or a condition of sustained periodic oscillation, the motion assumes a chaotic appearance.

The class of randomly connected networks involved in these simulations has the following specifications.

(1) *Single-neuron properties*. All model neurons are taken to have the same intrinsic parameters: $f_{0i} = f_0 = 0, a_i = a = 100\,\mathrm{s}^{-1}, b_i = b = -200\,\mathrm{s}^{-1}$, $p_i = p = 10\,\mathrm{s}^{-1}$. These values produce a reasonable semblance of observed neuronal responses. In fact, they define a standard model (Stein *et al.*, 1974*a,b*) which has received extensive numerical documentation (see, e.g., Chen (1986)). The individual neuronal elements are inherently stable.

(2) *Network connectivity*. The pattern of synaptic connections, their signs, and their absolute strengths are decided with the aid of some random-number generators. (a) Each neuron i is assigned exactly M non-zero c_{ij}s, where $0 \le M \le N$, the distinct neurons j provided synaptic input to i being picked entirely at random and without bias from the N neurons of the pool. (b) A prescribed fraction h of the set of non-zero couplings c_{ij} is taken to be inhibitory, the choice of the NMh inhibitory links being likewise random and unbiased. (Note that any given neuron will not in general have Nh inhibitory inputs. Note further that the neurons are not divided into separate excitatory and inhibitory subsets.) (c) The magnitudes of the non-zero c_{ij}s are chosen by sampling a uniform distribution on the interval $(0, L]$. Typical values adopted for the gross network parameters (guided by studies of the basic circuit of the olfactory bulb and used in the cases cited below) are: $h = 0.5$ and $L = 90$. We have

considered N up to 80, and examples with M ranging from 1 (very sparsely connected) to N (fully connected net).

(3) *External input*. The network is stimulated by steady external inputs f_i to a randomly selected set of neurons i, N_s in number, with zero external input to the remainder. In the cases to be cited, $N_s/N = \frac{1}{2}$. We take all non-zero inputs to have the same value f and consider a wide range in this control parameter.

Within this class of quasirandom networks, we have been able to identify several specimens which show legitimate chaotic behavior. The example which has received the most attention has $N = 26$ neurons with $M = 7$ incoming connections per neuron. For this net, a thorough numerical search (using a damped Newton–Raphson method) revealed only one fixed point (steady state), which is unstable, while in some of the other sample networks as many as 30–40 fixed points may be found. Upon varying the external input f to the net in question, we observe instances of putatively chaotic output of a certain subset of 15 neurons when the driving force lies in the range $36 < f < 43$. (The limiting values stated are not meant to be precise.) These neurons, non-trivially active, are termed *eligible*; it is important to mention that they *do not* necessarily receive direct external input. Across the pertinent regime of the control parameter f, the other neurons of the system turn off asymptotically (impulse frequency drops to zero) or else lock into a condition of saturated activity (with firing rate unity). Increasing the stimulus f past the lower critical boundary, and examining long-term behavior, the eligible subset of neurons is seen to undergo a transition from simple periodic motion of the x_i, with two oscillations per period and a period of roughly 40 ms, to a condition resembling intermittency; increasing f through the upper boundary, there is a transition from apparent chaos to periodic motion. By $f = 42.8$ the solutions are already periodic, with exceptionally long transients in the existing runs. At $f = 42.8$, there are three oscillations per period; at $f = 44.8$, seven; and at $f = 46.8$, eleven (with a period of some 800 ms). By $f = 54.8$ we find once more a simple mode with two oscillations per period (and a period of about 40 ms). It seems that, depending on the initial conditions, different branches of a complex dynamical manifold can be reached, and different eligible neurons generally have time series of quite different structure. When periodic motion occurs, all neurons oscillate with the same frequency. Solutions for the individual-neuron firing rates have been computed as far out as 25 s. Fig. 23.1 displays a selection from such numerical solutions for a representative eligible neuron, in ranges of the control parameter corresponding to

K. E. Kürten & J. W. Clark

ordered, periodic behavior (plot (b)) and to apparent chaos (plots (a) and (c)).

We must interject here a reservation which is especially germane for systems of such high dimensionality (52 and 160, in the examples at hand). It may well happen that although the numerical solution of a dynamical problem looks chaotic, one is actually observing a very long transient, or a periodic motion of extremely long period, or multiperiodic motion on a torus. To eliminate these possibilities (or the chaotic alternative), one would like to have available the spectrum of Lyapunov exponents, which provides the most incisive dynamical diagnostic for chaotic systems. Lyapunov exponents are the average exponential rates of divergence or convergence of neighboring trajectories in phase space. Any motion having at least one positive Lyapunov exponent is by definition chaotic, and the magnitude of the positive exponent measures the time scale on which the evolution of the system ceases to be predictable. In practice, the

Fig. 23.1. Firing-rate time series for a representative eligible neuron at three values of the control parameter, viz. at external inputs (a) $f = 41.8$ (chaotic case), (b) $f = 46.8$ (periodic) and (c) $f = 36.3$ (chaotic).

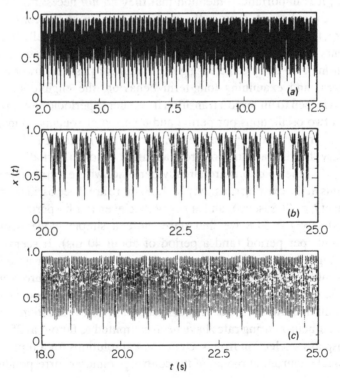

Lyapunov exponents may be directly determined by integration of the linearized equations of motion (Wolf *et al.*, 1985). Although quite demanding computationally, work in this direction is in progress. For the time being we must rely on more practicable diagnostics involving the examination of power spectra and the estimation of the fractal dimension of the attractor. While the Lyapunov spectrum is closely related to the fractal dimension of the associated strange attractor through the information dimension, calculation of the latter requires knowledge of all but the most negative Lyapunov exponents (Wolf *et al.*, 1985).

In authenticating a case of deterministic chaos it is also necessary to eliminate the possibility that one is merely seeing otherwise ordered behavior which is obscured by random noise. In the present context, the latter would have to be numerical or computational noise, since the basic equations have no stochastic ingredients. We can in fact rule out this possibility using the method developed by Grassberger & Procaccia (1983).

With these caveats in mind, let us resume consideration of the network example with $N = 26$ and $M = 7$. Two selected phase projections, in which the output of one eligible (neuron 1) is plotted against the simultaneous output of another eligible neuron (neuron 2), are shown in Fig. 23.2. Illustrative power spectra, based on 8000 data points, are compared in Fig. 23.3 (note the difference in vertical scales). The results in these diagrams are derived from the particular solutions sampled in Fig. 23.1(*a*) and Fig. 23.1(*b*). Looking again at Fig. 23.1, it appears that at $f = 36.3$ the system is operating just within the boundary of the chaotic regime, while the solution at $f = 46.9$ is definitely periodic. At $f = 41.8$ chaos

Fig. 23.2. Phase portraits at two values of the control parameter: (*a*) $f = 41.8$ (chaotic case) and (*b*) $f = 46.8$ (periodic). Impulse frequency $x_1(t)$ of eligible neuron 1 is plotted against impulse frequency $x_2(t)$ of eligible neuron 2. Transient not included in (*b*).

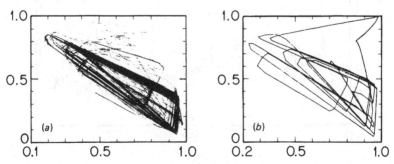

seems to be well developed. Indeed, for $f = 40.8$, in a run very similar to that of Fig. 23.1 at input 41.8, the existence of chaos has been verified rather convincingly by implementing the algorithm proposed by Grassberger & Procaccia (1983) for the characterization of an attractor using a single-variable time series. The correlation exponent ν (which is known to provide a generally tight lower bound on the fractal dimension D) is found to be 3.1, whereas the expected value of unity is obtained in the periodic case at $f = 46.8$. Further (though less compelling) evidence of the chaotic nature of these $f = 40.8$ and $f = 41.8$ solutions is furnished by the associated phase portraits and especially by the associated power spectra. Referring to Fig. 23.3(a), we see the characteristic broad continuum at low frequency. There is a clear contrast with the periodic example of Fig. 23.3(b), which is distinguished by the occurrence of sharp peaks. The power spectrum for the run at $f = 36.3$ – on the edge of the chaotic regime – has an intermediate appearance.

The high dimensionality of this example stands in the way of a deeper

Fig. 23.3. Power spectra at two values of the control parameter: (a) $f = 41.8$ (chaotic case) and (b) $f = 46.8$ (periodic). Here, $P(\omega) = \int_0^T \hat{x}(t) e^{i\omega t}\, dt$, where $\hat{x}(t) = x(t) - T^{-1} \int_0^T \hat{x}(u)\, du$ and T is the upper limit of the computed time series.

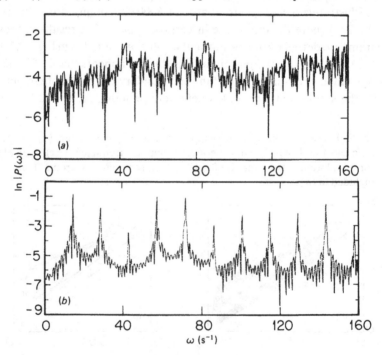

understanding of its mathematical nature, in terms of bifurcation routes to chaos. Nevertheless, it will be interesting to accumulate information – derived numerically or otherwise – on the fine structure of the chaotic domain and of the adjacent regions, on any windows of limit cycles which might be embedded in chaotic bands, on the occurrence of tangent bifurcation, on the number of changes of sign of Lyapunov characteristic exponents, etc.

At the same time it is important to discover other examples of quasi-random nets displaying chaotic behavior. In fact, numerous additional examples have been discovered in systems with 80 neurons and $M = 40$ incoming connections per neuron. Fig. 23.4 offers a sampling of solutions which rather obviously exhibit chaotic activity. However, in some cases the final certification has yet to be made on the basis of estimated fractal dimension (or, eventually, the Lyapunov spectrum).

23.4 Biological significance of chaotic dynamics

From our simulation experiments with randomly assembled model neural networks, described by a set of coupled non-linear differential equations implying deterministic evolution in continuous time, we expect that chaotic activity may not be uncommon in neural systems of sizeable dimension, although it may be difficult to authenticate.

There remains the important question of the biological implications of chaos in neural systems. In most situations, a tendency toward chaos would surely be harmful, an impediment to reliable response and to

Fig. 23.4. Selected chaotic firing-rate time series of eligible neurons in several quasirandom networks containing 80 neurons and 40 incoming connections per neuron.

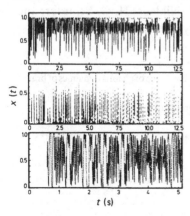
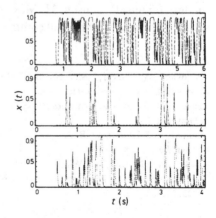

organized behavior conducive to survival. With regard to performance of the mature animal, there would accordingly be a need for some internal mechanism which suppresses chaotic behavior if the synaptic interactions (the c_{ij}) and other conditions of structure and stimulus permit it, by modifying the network parameters in some way. On the other hand, during development of the animal there would be a need for some mechanism for avoiding, insofar as is possible, the patterns of synaptic and neuroanatomical organization which are favorable to chaos. The latter end is presumably achieved, at least in part, by genetic programming.

While chaos would *usually* be harmful, we should not exclude the possibility that in some circumstances it could (in moderation!) be beneficial, especially in the context of higher mental processing where it is advantageous to be able to break out of rigid, stereotyped behavior. For extensive and perceptive commentary on the occurrence of chaos in neural systems and its role in neurobiology, the reader should consult Harth (1983) and Guevara *et al.* (1983).

In view of the intriguing implications for neural systems of the kind of unpredictability implied by deterministic chaos, it becomes of great interest to characterize the mathematical nature of the chaotic solutions of the neural-net equations, and in particular to reveal the bifurcation routes involved and to elucidate the conditions (on the connectivity, etc.) for the occurrence of such erratic modes of behavior.

Acknowledgments

This research was supported by the Condensed Matter Theory Program of the Division of Materials Research of the U.S. National Science Foundation, under Grant No. DMR-8519077. We thank J. W. Chen, U. an der Heiden, R. Jensen, H. Moraal, K. Niklaus, H. G. Schuster, and H. A. Wischmann for critical commentary and informative discussions.

References

Babloyantz, A., Salazar, J. M. & Nicolis, C. (1985). 'Evidence of chaotic dynamics of brain activity during the sleep cycle'. *Phys. Lett.*, **111A**, 152–6.

Chen, J. W. (1986). The Dynamics of Neural Systems. Ph.D. Thesis, Washington University.

Choi, M. Y. & Huberman, B. A. (1983). 'Dynamical behaviour of nonlinear networks'. *Phys. Rev. A*, **28**, 1204–6.

Clark, J. W., Rafelski, J. & Winston, J. V. (1985). 'Brain without mind: Computer simulation of neural networks with modifiable neuronal interactions'. *Physics Reports*, **123**, 215–73.

Clark, J. W., Kürten, K. E. & Rafelski, J. (1987). 'Access and stability of cyclic modes in quasirandom networks of threshold neurons obeying a deterministic synchronous dynamics'. These proceedings.

Feigenbaum, M. J. (1978). 'Quantitative universality for a class of non-linear transformations'. *J. Stat. Phys.*, **19**, 25–52.

Grassberger, P. & Procaccia, I. (1983). 'Measuring the strangeness of strange attractors'. *Physica*, **9D**, 189–208.

Guevara, M., Glass, L. & Shrier, A. (1981). 'Phase locking, period-doubling bifurcations, and irregular dynamics in periodically stimulated cardiac cells, *Science*, **214**, 1350–3.

Guevara, M. R., Glass, L., Mackey, M. C. & Shrier, A. (1983). 'Chaos in neurobiology'. *IEEE Trans. Syst. Man Cybern.*, *SMC-13*, **5**, 790–8.

Harth, E. (1983). 'Order and chaos in neural systems: an approach to the dynamics of higher brain functions'. *IEEE Trans. Syst. Man Cybern.*, *SMC-13*, **5**, 782–9.

Hopfield, J. J. (1984). 'Neurons with graded response have collective computational properties like those of two-state neurons'. *Proc. U.S. Nat. Acad. Sci.*, **81**, 3088–92.

Kürten, K. E. & Clark, J. W. (1986). 'Chaos in neural systems'. *Phys. Lett.*, **114A**, 413–18.

Lorentz, E. N. (1963). 'Deterministic nonperiodic flows'. *J. Atm. Sci.*, **20**, 130–41.

Oğuztöreli, M. N. (1982). 'Modelling and simulation of vertebrate primary visual system: basic network'. *IEEE Trans. Syst. Man Cybern.*, *SMC-13*, **5**, 765–81.

Schuster, H. G. (1984). *Deterministic Chaos: An Introduction*. Weilheim: Physik-Verlag.

Stein, R. B., Leung, K. V., Oğuztöreli, M. N. & Williams, D. W. (1974a). 'Properties of small neural networks'. *Kybernetik*, **14**, 223–30.

Stein, R. B., Leung, K. V., Mangeron, D. & Oğuztöreli, M. N. (1974b). 'Improved neuronal models for studying neural networks'. *Kybernetik*, **15**, 1–9 (1974).

Stevens, C. F. (1966). *Neurophysiology: A Primer*. New York: Academic Press.

Wolf, A., Swift, J. B., Swinney, H. L. & Vastano, J. A. (1985). 'Determining Lyapunov exponents from a time series'. *Physica*, **16D**, 285–317.

24

Computer simulation of the cerebellar cortex compartment with a special reference to the Purkinje cell dendrite structure

L. M. CHAJLAKHIAN, W. L. DUNIN-BARKOWSKI,
N. P. LARIONOVA and A. JU. VAVILINA

A huge amount of physiological research shows the importance of the role of the cerebellum in motor control (Ito, 1984; and many others). It is natural for physiologists to try to understand what the cerebellum function is and when and which corrections or other modifications of cerebral cortical motor programs are introduced by the cerebellum. It seems to us that in recent decades the most interesting hypotheses on cerebellar performance have been proposed by the late David Marr in 'A theory of cerebellar cortex' (Marr, 1969). According to Marr, the main operation of the cerebellar circuitry is the switching on of proper motor commands by the current sensory input and the automatic adaptive acquisition of such cerebellar network capability. The location of the cerebellum – in the crest of almost all the ascending and descending nervous tracts – is definitely strategic for such a function. The unique combination of tens of thousands of granular cells (GrCs) and one climbing fibre (CF) at one Purkinje cell seems to be crucial for it.

The kernel of Marr's theory is composed by the postulates of the GrC –PC synaptic modification due to simultaneous excitation of the climbing fibre (CF) and parallel fibres (PF). In other words, Marr supposed that the Purkinje cell memorizes the afferent conditions in which it ought to be active.

The main postulates of the theory were verified experimentally 18 years after its publication (review in Ito, 1984). In particular, the evidence of the PF–PC synaptic efficiency increased after the joint stimulation of CF and PFs in the frog cerebellum had been obtained (Chajlakhian *et al.*, 1980).

The experimental results of Chajlakhian *et al.* (1980) are presented in Table 24.1.

Table 24.1. *The results of electrophysiological investigations of the PC's plasticity in the frog cerebellum*

N/N n/n	Neuron type	Experiment duration (min)	Fin. ($\frac{1}{2}$) / Ini. ($\frac{1}{2}$)
1	+	140	0.76
2	+	200	0.51
3	+	150	0.68
4	+	305	0.38
5	+	155	1.00
6	+	200	0.76
7	+	165	0.61
8	+	125	0.93
Mean value			0.70
9	+/−	120	1.02
10	+/−	120	0.84
11	+/−	165	0.58
12	+/−	130	0.98
13	+/−	200	1.00
14	+/−	240	1.14
15	+/−	234	1.00
Mean value			0.94
16	−	140	0.97
17	−	160	0.96
18	−	140	1.04
Mean value			0.99

In Table 24.1 the ratio of a threshold current which elicited the monosynaptic PC response to the PF stimulation after the conditioning procedures and before them is presented. The guarantee of climbing fibre activation in conditioning procedures restricted to the '+' lines of the table; only in these lines can one see the PC monosynaptic response threshold decrease. These experiments now present the only evidence of the so-called 'positive' PC learning (an increase, but not decrease, of the PF–PC synaptic efficiency observed by Chajlakhian *et al.* (1980), in contrast to (Ito, 1984)). There are no other positive data on the possibility of the cerebellar learning *in vitro*.

So the main operational principle of the cerebellum as a device for a movement correction is the PC ability to make clear distinction between the learned and unlearned pools of excited granule cells. It is obvious that there is some optimal number of the learned GrC pools. When this number, n, is small, the functional potential of a single PC is highly restricted. The ability of PC to discriminate learned and unlearned pools becomes less with the increase of n. These are the objectives for a quantitative analysis of the situation. In addition, it is interesting to note the dependence of the 'optimal' value of n on the 'global' structural properties of the MF–GrC afferent input to PC, as well as PC excitation dependence on its synaptic inputs. To answer these questions a computer simulation of a cerebellar cortex compartment was undertaken.

The cerebellar cortex compartment model consisted of (i) one PC, (ii) 20 000 granule cells, and (iii) 700 mossy fibres (MF). These data approximately correspond to the rat cerebellum. A mean number 5, of MFs converging to a single GrC was chosen. This meant that the mean number of GrCs per 1 MF was approximately 143. There is freedom in the choice of non-local geometry of MF–GrC connections under the local numerical limitation described above. We considered only the four basic variants of these connections (Fig. 24.1):

(1) The P-scheme. The connections between any MFs and GrCs are random (the decision to have a given connection or not to have is determined by the random number generator) with the only limitation of mean numbers of GrC and MF connections.
(2) The B-scheme. The same as the P-scheme but every GrC has exactly five connections with different MFs.
(3) The D-scheme. This is the deteriorated deterministic scheme. It is formed by the partition of the mossy fibres into 140 sets, each of five MFs; 143 identical granule cells are ascribed to each MF set.
(4) The DR-scheme. The difference here from the D-scheme is that one of the five connections of each of 143 GrCs of a given MF set is connected with another MF set.

The difference between the schemes is evident if one looks at the probability distribution functions of excited GrCs when different randomly chosen sets of mossy fibres are excited. In Fig. 24.2 one can see these probability distribution functions which were obtained in different scheme types when random sets of equal numbers (357) of mossy fibres were excited for each random sampling with threshold value equal to five for all the GrCs.

One should note that the distribution is lattice-like for a deterministic

D-scheme because of the fact that the number of active granule cells in this case is equal to 143, multiplied by a small integer; the DR obeys a 'continuous' (non-lattice-like) law of an active-cell distribution. However, the distribution dispersions for D- and DR-schemes are almost equal. In contrast, the B-scheme distribution dispersion is significantly less, despite the fact that the mean number of excited GrCs for this scheme is in fact the same as for the D- and DR-schemes. The mean

Fig. 24.1. The connection graphs of the undeterministic schemes P, B, the deteriorated deterministic schemes D and improved deteriorated scheme DR. MF – mossy fibres, GrC – granular cell, PC – Purkinje cell.

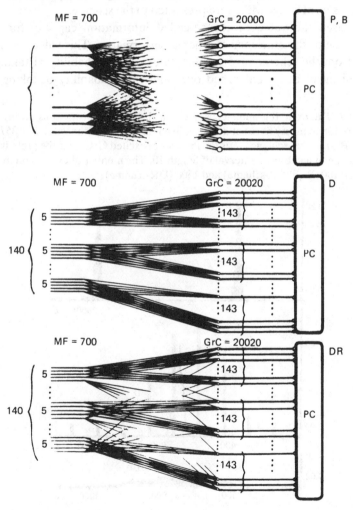

number of excited GrCs for the P-scheme is three times that of the B-scheme. This results from the fact that the local parameters of this scheme differ from the local parameters of the other schemes.

There were two distinct procedures used in the simulation: (1) the recording of excited MF sets, and (2) the recall of recorded information. During the RECORD procedure the synapses of those granule cells which were excited by each recorded set of active mossy fibres were modified, i.e., they became 'learned' synapses. It was consequently supposed that the climbing fibre was excited during the recorded MF set's action on the PC.

During the RECALL procedure either the previously recorded or random sets of active MFs were presented to the scheme.

We used the value of the so-called information capacity for the evaluation of the efficiency of scheme performance. This value is calculated from the scheme error probabilities – the probability of taking a learned event as an unlearned one, and the probability of taking an

Fig. 24.2. The excited granule cells' number distribution histograms during the prescutation to mossy fibres of different fixed size events of the value $L = 357$ for the P-, B-, D-, DR-schemes. L is the number of excited GrCs, p is the probability of L falling in an abscissa interval of length 10. The number of events counted is between 100 (B-, P-, D-scheme) and 1500 (DR-scheme).

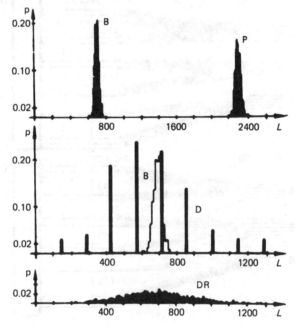

unlearned event as a learned one (Dunin-Barkowski & Larionova, 1985). The information capacity is indeed useful due to the fact that it gives us absolute information on the efficiency of the scheme in terms of the number of bits stored per number of bits which could be stored, should the scheme be absolutely effective:

$$E = I/N \times \log_2 q,$$

where I is information capacity, N is the number of modifiable synapses, and q is the number of synaptic efficiency states (in our model $q = 2$ – each PF–PC synapse is either 'learned' or 'unlearned'). It is obvious that, in any case, $E < 1$ (Dunin-Barkowski, 1978).

Fig. 24.3 presents the results of an information content evaluation for different schemes and different PC excitation rules. The information content is given as a function of the MF learned sets, n. The data, denoted by numerals 1, 2, 3, are for the B-schemes; 1 – for the case when the learned synapse excites the PC and the unlearned has no action on it; 2 – the learned synapse excites the PC and the unlearned one inhibits it; 3 – the same as 2, but the PC threshold is tuned to optimal value. The uppermost smooth curve is the limit of the so-called simple theory of cerebellar compartment (Dunin-Barkowski, 1978).

Fig. 24.3. The PC efficiency (in bits per one binary PF–PC synapse) vs. the learned event number for different connection types between MFs and GrCs and some PC excitation laws. A, the B-scheme: (1) $I = 0$, optimal h; (2) $I = -N$, $h = 0$; (3) same as in 2 but at optimal h. B (in the dashed circle): $I = 0$; (4) the D-scheme; (5) the DR-scheme. T is the theoretical curve (A) (Dunin-Barkowski & Larionova, 1985).

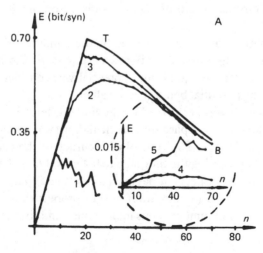

The data for information capacity of the D- and DR-schemes are small compared with the data obtained for the B-scheme; they are presented in Fig. 24.3 on a magnified scale.

The following properties of the data obtained in computer simulation are felt to be substantial for further research:

(1) The maximum efficiency of the memorizing scheme is 0.6 bit per binary synapse, which is only slightly less than the theoretical limit: ln 2 = 0.693 bit/synapse (analytic results of Longuet-Higgins, Willshaw & Buneman, 1970; Dunin-Barkowski, 1978; and others).

(2) This upper limit of the information efficiency is attained when the unlearned synapse weight is opposite in sign and many times greater than the learned synapse weight.

(3) The 'good' performance characteristics are demonstrated by schemes with random connections between MFs and GrCs. The schemes with a high correlation of different GrC excitation are highly ineffective.

Our simulation made use of a standard McCulloch–Pitts model neuron. In this model the individual synapses have no other effective parameters than their synaptic weight. It is well-known, however, that the synapses at the real neuron are in fact linked together by their neighbourhoodness in the cell dendrite. So the result of the synaptic action on the postsynaptic neuron may depend on the active synaptic configuration at a given moment (Arshavsky *et al.*, 1971; Rall & Segev, 1986). For the evaluation of membrane inhomogeneity and the dependence of neuron reaction upon the relative position of the activated synapses, we studied the PC integration properties discounting its real dendritic structure.

The geometric structure of a model was based on the rat PC data (Shelton, 1985).

The cell performance was modelled by the numerical decision of the cable equation. The synaptic activities were modelled as ionic conductance changes. An ion equilibrium potential was considered to be +80 mV, the resting potential being at zero value.

The calculation was performed by the finite differences method. The minimal cable piece (the space step in calculation) was equal to 3 mks, the time step being 1 mks. The control of accuracy of the calculation was performed by decreasing the time step to 0.4 mks. Our calculations were associated with two aspects of passive (electrotonic) potential propagation. We investigated (a) the difference in properties of neurons with homogeneous and inhomogeneous membranes, and (b) the difference in the non-linearity of summation influences at the site of the synapse location and in the soma region.

Fig. 24.4 presents the response in the dendrite in the soma region to the activation of one synapse at a thin distal dendritic branch, for homogeneous and inhomogeneous neuron membranes. It is evident that the cell with a homogeneous membrane 7–9 ms after the beginning of synaptic action becomes isopotential and the potential reduction everywhere in the cell is exponential (with the time constant $R_m \times C_m$). For the cell with an inhomogeneous membrane the EPSP decrease also becomes exponential 9–10 ms after the beginning of synaptic activation, but the ratio of potential values between the site of synapse action and soma remains constant. This result permits the proposal of a simple experiment for the evaluation of the neuron membrane inhomogeneity. The electro-excitability of a neuron in the experiment must be inactivated. The response of a neuron to a short impulse of PF activation must be recorded by three microelectrodes: one intracellular electrode (in the soma region) and two extracellular ones, one near the soma and the other near the dendrites. In the case of homogeneous neuron membrane the potential difference between extracellular electrodes will show a much more prompt potential reduction than the potential of the intracellular electrode. In the case of the inhomogeneous membrane the time course of intracellular potential and the potential difference between extracellular electrodes would be similar.

Fig. 24.5 presents the calculated values of potentials in the soma and in the dendrites when three different synapses were simultaneously activated at one thin dendrite branch. It is evident that the increase in the maximal conductance of synapses (three times) causes an increase in maximum of potential both in dendrites (Fig. 24.5(*a*)) and in the soma (Fig. 24.5(*b*)). The absolute value of this increase in the dendrites is more than that in the soma. Nevertheless, the relative changes of synaptic potentials are more pronounced in the soma.

These results can explain the facts, obtained in Ito's laboratory (Ekerot, Ito & Kano, 1983) which were observed in PC synaptic plasticity experiments. In these experiments there were only small changes of the PC extracellular postsynaptic potentials after climbing fibre 'learning' procedure, but changes in PC impulse response in similar conditions were more prominent. That is, the discrepancy – the presence of change at the PC soma level and its near absence in PC dendrites – which has been noted by Ekerot *et al.*, 1983 may not be a discrepancy at all. Our data show that

Fig. 24.4. The potential changing after a single synaptic activation. Upper curve – potential at the locus of activation. Bottom curve – the potential at soma. (*a*) Homoheneous neuron membrane. (*b*) Inhomogeneous neuron membrane. Abscissa – time. Ordinate – logarithm of potential.

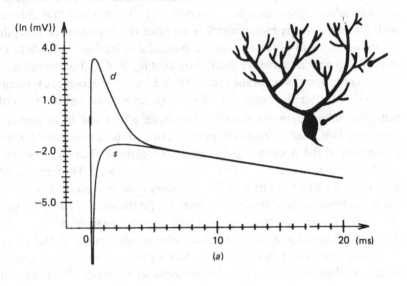

(*a*)

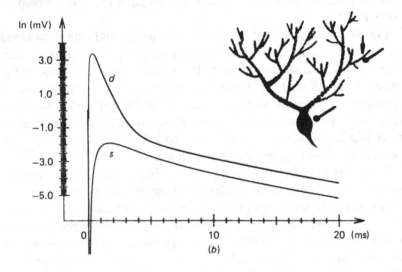

(*b*)

Fig. 24.5. The potential changing after single activation of three synapses. Upper curve – $g = 0.3$ Sm. Bottom curve – $g = 0.1$ Sm. (*a*) Potential at locus of activated synapses. (*b*) Potential at soma. Abscissa – time. Ordinate – potential.

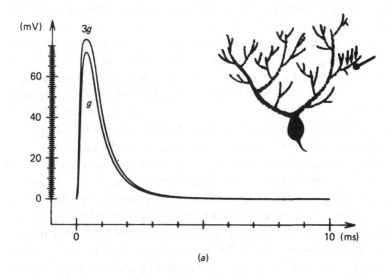

(*a*)

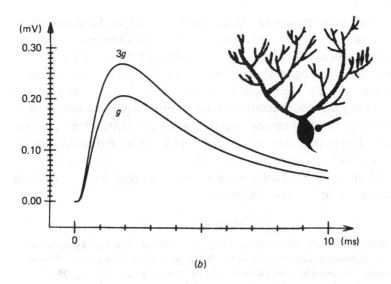

(*b*)

the difference between dendrite and soma potentials may be due to the fact that synaptic action at dendrites is due primarily to the increase of membrane conductance.

In conclusion we would like to elucidate one rather general aspect of the synaptic action on the neuron.

First of all, let us define the synaptic cooperativity function as a function of the difference between the sum of the effects of single activated synapses and the effect of jointly activated synapses versus the distance between the synapses. The following seems to be of certain importance: (1) if the whole dendrite membrane is passive the cooperativity of adjacent synapses is negative (our data, Fig. 24.5, and many others); (2) if the dendrite membrane has the same properties as the axon membrane, the cooperativity of adjacent synapses is highly positive (Arshawsky *et al.*, 1971). It follows that 'intermediate' dendrite membrane properties can exist in reality, which provides zero cooperativity. It ought to be noted that there are indeed data on the PC dendrite membrane inter-mediate properties, i.e., not pure not passive and not fully active proper-ties (Llinas, Sugimory, 1980). Then, logically, it could be asked if there are any data on preferably cooperative synaptic action at the PC input? The answer is negative because the synapses of the same function inputs to the cerebellar cortex may be located in any part of the PC dendrites (Ito, 1984).

In conclusion, we would like to point out that we have reasons to suggest that the PC dendritic membrane peculiarities and a concrete organization of the afferents to the cerebellar cortex are arranged so as to provide 'zero topological cooperativity' of the PC synapses. According to this view, the PC information characteristic analysis based on the McCulloch–Pitts model neuron is indeed correct. Also, it is easy to show that any sign of PC synapses' 'topological cooperativity' (both negative and positive) in the frames of our model of PC memorizing information properties will act as a 'noise', reducing the information capacity of the memorizing structure. That is, the absence of PC synaptic cooperativity is a beneficial factor of natural selection.

References

Arshawsky, Yu. J. *et al.* (1971). 'An analysis of the functional properties of dendrites in relation to their structure'. In *Models of the Structural–functional Organisation of Several Biological Systems*, eds. J. M. Gelfand, S. V. Phomin and M. L. Cetlin, pp. 25–77. Cambridge: M.I.T. Press.
Chajlakhian, L. M. *et al.* (1980). 'An analysis of the synaptic plasticity in the frog cerebellum

in vitro'. In *Synaptic Constituents in Health and Disease*, ed. M. Brzin *et al.*, p. 423. Ljubliana: Mladinska Khiga.

Dunin-Barkowski, W. L. (1978). *Information Processes in Neural Structures*, ed. L. M. Chailakhian. Moscow: Nauka (in Russian).

Dunin-Barkowski, W. L. & Larionova, N. P. (1985). 'Computer simulation of a cerebellar cortex compartment I, II'. *Biological Cybernetics*, **51**, 399–415.

Ekerot, C.-F., Ito, M. & Kano, M. (1983). 'Long-lasting depression of PF–P-cell transmission caused by conjunctive stimulation of PF and CF'. *Neuroscience Letters. Supplement*, **13**, 25.

Ito, M. (1984). *The Cerebellum and Neural Control*, 580 p. New York: Raven Press.

Llinas, M. & Sugimory, M. (1980). 'Electrophysiological properties of in vitro Purkinje cell dendrites mammalian cerebellum slices'. *Journal of Physiology*, **305**, 197–214.

Longuet-Higgins, H. C., Willshaw, D. J. & Buneman, O. P. (1970). 'Theories of associative recall'. *Quarterly Reviews of Biophysics*, **3**, 223–44.

Marr, D. (1969). 'A theory of cerebellar cortex'. *Journal of Physiology*, **202**, 437–70.

Rall, W. & Segev, I. (1986). 'Excitable dendritic spine clusters: non-linear synaptic processing' (this volume).

Shelton, D. P. (1985). 'Membrane resistivity estimated for the Purkinje neuron by means of a passive computer model'. *Journal of Neuroscience*, **14**, 111–31.

25

Modeling the electrical behavior of cortical neurons – simulation of hippocampal pyramidal cells

LYLE J. BORG-GRAHAM

25.1 Introduction

Modeling the brain requires some *a priori* description of its functional computing elements. The sophistication of this description depends on the goal of the model, but it is clear that describing single neurons as simple 'leaky-integrators' with a non-linear threshold has limited utility in exploring the capability of the neural net for processing information. In fact, cortical pyramidal neurons are functionally quite complicated, both in terms of how their complex geometry determines their electrotonic structure, and in terms of the active currents that modulate the linear response of these cells.

Over the past several years investigators have uncovered a plethora of currents in one type of cortical pyramidal neuron, the hippocampal pyramidal cell. The currents, which presumably are mediated by distinct ion channels, include the classical fast sodium current (I_{Na}), a persistent sodium current (I_{NaP}) (French & Gage, 1985), a delayed-rectifier potassium current (I_{DR}) (Segal & Barker, 1984), a calcium current (I_{Ca}) (Halliwell, 1983), a slow calcium current (I_{CaS}) (Johnston *et al.*, 1980), a fast transient calcium-mediated potassium current (I_C) (Brown & Griffith, 1983), an after-hyperpolarization calcium-mediated potassium current (I_{AHP}) (Lancaster & Adams, 1986), a muscarine-inhibited potassium current (I_M) (Halliwell & Adams, 1982), a transient potassium current (I_A) (Gustafsson *et al.*, 1982), a chloride current ($I_{Cl(v)}$) (Madison *et al.*, 1986), and a possibly mixed carrier anomalous rectifier current (I_Q) (Halliwell & Adams, 1982). Each current has a unique time- and voltage-dependence, and some currents are sensitive to constituents in the extra- or intra-cellular environment, for example free Ca^{++} or muscarinic agonists.

Given that regenerative transmission of electrical signals in the nervous system can be accomplished with only a single active conductance, the question arises as to why certain cells have such large families of active currents, interwoven as they are in a complex that reflects an assortment of temporal, chemical, and voltage-dependencies. Accurate modeling of the interaction between the currents and the morphology of hippocampal pyramidal cells is a step towards answering this question.

The development of the model described here includes determination of the electronic structure of hippocampal pyramidal cells and the cataloging and integration of electrophysiological data on the conductances found in these cells (Borg-Graham, 1987).

A substantial amount of effort was invested in the user interface of the model, which was implemented on a Symbolics 3600 LISP machine. Input to the program is with a menu system that allows efficient manipulation of the relevant parameters and a subsequently rapid set-up for a given simulation. Output of the model is both graphical and numerical. Manipulation of simulation results is straightforward and non-displayed parameters are easily accessible. This user interface allows the model to be used in an interactive, self-documenting fashion.

25.2 Simulation of hippocampal neurons based on intracellular data

Quantitative data on the kinetics of active membrane currents is often not complete because the small size and complex electrotonic structure of the cells make intracellular measurements of them difficult. In particular, some currents are either too fast or too large for resolution with present microelectrode voltage clamp techniques. In the literature the kinetics of some currents have been partially fitted to those described by the Hodgkin & Huxley (HH) model (Hodgkin & Huxley, 1952), while for others only the general behavior under various stimuli (typically current clamp) and different pharmacological and chemical conditions has been documented. In order to understand these currents and their possible functions better, simulations are used in an iterative fashion to augment the sparse data.

An extension of the HH model for the voltage- and time-dependence of active currents in squid axon is the basis for the current kinetics used in the model. In summary, this description assumes that the conductance of the channel protein responsible for a given current is governed by one or more types of 'gating particles'. These particles can be thought of as distinct regions of the channel protein, each of which can be in one of two stable conformations or states, conducting (open) or non-conducting (closed). For a given channel to conduct, all of its gating particles must be in the open state. The transitions of the particles between states are governed by first-order kinetics. Each state or conformation corresponds to a free-energy well, with a single high-energy rate-determining barrier between the two states. Movement of the grating particles between states is assumed to be accompanied by a movement of charge, thus causing the state-transition kinetics to be dependent on the membrane voltage. The magnitude of the voltage-dependence is derived from the Boltzmann equation which specifies the probabilities of state occupancies according to the free energies of the states. It proved useful to incorporate in our model an additional assumption of a voltage-independent, rate-limiting mechanism, e.g., drag on the gating portion of the protein as it changes conformation, which places an upper limit on the rate constants of the gating transitions.

In practice, voltage clamp protocols, in which the membrane relaxation currents are measured as the cell membrane is 'clamped' at different potentials with a microelectrode, are used to measure the kinetics of the various currents. This technique assumes that the kinetics of different currents can be measured independently, either because different currents are activated over non-overlapping membrane voltages, the time courses are distinct, or because the currents have distinct pharmacological sensitivities. Implicit in this approach is the assumption that different currents interact only through the membrane voltage. The exception being those currents which are dependent on the movement of Ca^{++} into the cell. The independence of the currents is exploited by the electrophysiologist as he devises protocols for intracellular measurements.

A typical strategy for our simulations is to evaluate as many parameters as possible under orthogonal or nearly orthogonal protocols, thereby mimicking the electrophysiologist's approach. Careful attention is made when protocols initiate events with overlapping kinetics, particularly when superposition does not hold (when superposition does hold, it then may be exploited to extract relevant parameters from the total response). It is in these gray areas where the model is later used to try out speculations regarding the underlying mechanisms.

25.3 Data base of the model

25.3.1 Voltage clamp and current clamp data

Model data includes voltage clamp and current clamp data from hippocampal CA1 and CA3 pyramidal cells, from both slice and culture preparations. In some cases, voltage clamp data from pyramidal cells from other cortical regions or from other mammalian neurons were consulted when the corresponding data from hippocampal preparations was not available. For the hippocampal data, I currently do not distinguish between cells from slice or culture preparations, or from CA1 or CA3 pyramidal cells, although it is possible that cells from these different sources differ non-trivially in the distribution, kinetics, or presence of some currents. For example, the muscarinic potassium current has yet to be conclusively demonstrated in cultured cells (Segal, personal communication). As more electrophysiological data from the hippocampus becomes available, different versions of the model will be developed, each being specific as to the hippocampal subfield from which the target cells originate and to the preparation technique.

Voltage clamp data were used whenever possible since this protocol measures the HH model parameters directly. If such data were not available current clamp data were used to converge on a kinetic description. This approach is a qualitative one since it is not possible to verify that a solution obtained in this way is the correct one. However, one of the main strengths of the computer model technique is that the limited voltage clamp data can be incorporated in an iterative fashion with current clamp data, yielding either the best estimate possible or, in some cases, an indication that a valid estimate cannot be made (e.g., certain characteristics of firing not simulated accurately). In the latter case, this caused us to re-examine the original data and the assumptions and conditions under which they were taken.

25.3.2 Approximation of the pyramidal cell

Our model is mainly intended to examine the several soma currents that have been reported and the contribution of the dendritic tree to somatic electrical behavior. The model is based on a compartmental approximation of the pyramidal cell that is similar to that used in other studies (Traub & Llinas, 1979). A spherical isopotential soma is attached to one or more cables, each of which may represent either part of the dendritic tree or the proximal part of the axon. The cable approximation of the dendritic tree structure is based on the equivalent cylinder approximation developed by Rall (Jack, Noble & Tsien, 1977). The cables, in turn, are approximated by a series of isopotential compartments. Typically, our simulations were run using the simple geometry of a single dendritic cable and soma with no axon, as illustrated in Fig. 25.1. This configuration gave a reasonable tradeoff between the accuracy of a simplified electronic structure and the associated reduction in the execution time.

25.4 Modeling strategy

25.4.1 Estimation of passive properties and factors governing the resting potential

We began constructing the model by considering the linear characteristics of the cells. The data used for the model included measurements of hippocampal pyramidal cell geometry using histological techniques, the linear electrical response of hippocampal pyramidal cells taken from intracellular measurements, and known or estimated passive characteristics of biological membranes in general.

It was very important to begin constructing the model with a good estimate of the cells' linear properties, since the linear structure provides a base from which to develop estimates of the subtle, non-linear characteristics of the cells. In fact, without a valid linear description, there is little hope of deriving estimates of the non-linear properties with the model. The simulations demonstrated that small changes in linear properties can have large effects on the behavior of the non-linear conductances of the cell.

For example, in our analysis of the Na^+ current kinetics, the magnitude and reversal potential of the leak conductance had a strong effect on the Na^+-only spike simulations, because in this case repolarization of a spike is completely due to Na^+ current inactivation and leak current.

The linear cell properties are an important factor in maintaining the resting potential, and thus determining the stability of the cell in the presence of active conductances. The distribution of the leak conductance (membrane resistivity) is also important in setting the electrotonic dimensions of the dendritic tree which, in turn, determines the relationship

Fig. 25.1. Typical geometry of simulation, including soma sphere and dendritic compartments and current injection into the soma. The extracellular medium and each compartment are isopotential.

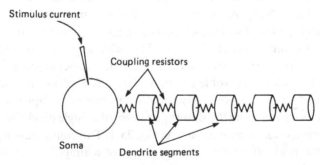

between the location of dendritic input and the effectiveness of that input in triggering action potentials.

The model allowed us to adjust somatic membrane resistivity (somatic leak conductance), dendritic membrane resistivity (dendritic leak conductance), cytoplasmic resistivity, and the reversal potential for the leak conductances in order to match the observed linear response of the cell, including the somatic input resistance, while maintaining the dimensions of cell (soma diameter, diameter and length of equivalent dendritic cable) that were estimated from histological data. In addition, the contribution of the non-specific leak introduced by the recording electrode was modeled.

25.4.2 *Simulation of voltage clamp data*

Once the linear parameters had been estimated, fitting parameters of active conductances into the model began with the simulation of voltage clamp data. This step allowed us to investigate the effect of non-perfect voltage clamp (i.e., non-ideal space clamp) on the voltage-clamp data reported in the literature. It is important to know how the extensive electrotonic structure of the pyramidal neurons contributes to error in kinetics and conductances derived from voltage-clamp data.

25.4.3 *Simulation of current clamp data*

Once all the available voltage clamp data had been incorporated, the next step was the simulation of current clamp data and concurrent adjustment of the relevant parameters to better match the data. This stage was the most difficult, since it was not always obvious how the parameters should be adjusted from run to run. Often it was necessary to return to the original voltage clamp data when a solution proves intractable, so that any inconsistencies could be estimated and resolved.

25.5 Estimating fast Na$^+$ parameters

One of the first applications of the model has been the estimation of the Na$^+$ currents in hippocampal pyramidal cells, including those which underlie the depolarizing phase of the action potential. A quantitative description of the Na$^+$ currents is vital because these currents, as one of the basic determinants of neuronal function, are the progenitors of the action potential. Also the activation/inactivation properties of the Na$^+$ currents set the stage for the entrance of the numerous outward currents.

Specifically, I have attempted to derive channel kinetics that are consistent with current clamp records of Na$^+$-only spikes (Storm, personal communication), the steady-state Na^+ dependent current–voltage characteristic (French & Gage, *ibid*; Storm, *ibid*), and current clamp records of normal action potentials obtained under various conditions.

There is little voltage clamp data for Na^+ currents since these currents are typically large and fast, exceeding the current sourcing ability and the temporal response of the single-electrode clamp circuit used to make the measurements. Since the data are not complete, it was necessary to look to sources of data other than those from hippocampal preparations. These included estimations of the kinetics of a fast Na^+ current in the rabbit node of Ranvier (Chiu *et al.*, 1979) and in the bullfrog (Koch & Adams (bullfrog sympathetic ganglion simulations) personal communication). In addition parameters used in other neuron simulations were consulted (Traub & Llinas, *ibid* (hippocampal simulations)).

Again, I have assumed that any channels that conduct Na^+ may be described by the HH-like kinetics described earlier and, further, that each channel may have one or two types of gating particles. Thus our task was to try to fit the behavior of this class of voltage-dependent channels to the data. I began by considering the Na^+-only spike.

25.5.1 Implications of Na^+-only spike

Current clamp records taken using hippocampal slices which had been treated with agents that blocked all potassium and calcium currents enables one to look at the behavior of the Na^+ currents and, presumably, the leak conductance in isolation. Such protocols assume that (1) all active currents other than Na^+ currents may be blocked, and (2) such treatment leaves the leak conductance unscathed. Fig. 25.2 shows a record of a Na^+-only spike under such conditions.

Several features of this spike yield clues as to the nature of possible Na^+ currents. The first feature of note is that the spike threshold is quite sharp. Note also that the subthreshold response seems to show very little activation of inward current. This implies that the activation curve for the fast Na^+ current is steep, and that its foot is at about -55 mV.

The second feature is the biphasic repolarization of the spike. The trajectory of the spike repolarization under these conditions is due to the inactivation of the Na^+ current(s) and the linear leak of the membrane. Initially, the spike repolarizes rapidly. Assuming that the major portion of the spike is due to a Na^+ current similar to the classical fast Na^+ current described in squid axon, this initial repolarization is consistent with the rapid inactivation of the channel with depolarization. Thus at depolarized membrane potentials, the time constant for inactivation is on the order of a few milliseconds. However, approximately 7 ms after the spike peak the repolarization slows drastically. This slow phase of the repolarization, which commences when the membrane voltage is about -20 mV, lasts approximately 60 ms. Since this decay is too slow to be accounted for by the time constant of the cell, we propose that the long tail is due to an active (Na^+) inward current.

Considering regular action potentials, we can determine whether it is likely that a Na^+ tail current is present during the actively repolarized spike. The action potential is repolarized by K^+ currents, in addition to the leak conductance and the inactivation of the Na^+ currents. If any Na^+ tail current has been activated during the fast spike, then it must be cancelled by a slow residual component of the outward currents, since no long-lasting depolarized tail is observed. Thus during a normal action potential there is either a completely activated slow component of the fast Na^+ current that is cancelled by a slow K^+ current(s), or there is a separate slow Na^+ current that has not had a chance to be activated during the short spike, or there is some middle ground where an incompletely activated inward current is cancelled by a residual outward current.

In order to estimate the current during a Na^+-only spike, the time course of the actual spike was used as the clamp voltage in a voltage clamp simulation using the passive cell. The resulting simulated clamp current revealed the total current that must be supplied by active conductances during the spike. The time course of this current implied that the active

Fig. 25.2. Na^+-only spike–current clamp protocol with cesium chloride electrode, TEA, 4AP, and Mn^{++} added to block the calcium and potassium currents. Stimulus current is top trace. From Storm, unpublished data.

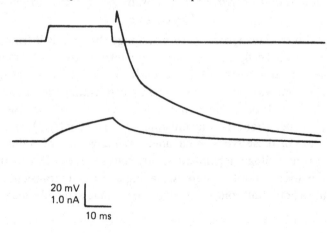

20 mV
1.0 nA
10 ms

mechanisms underlying the spike had at least two distinct components. Incidentally, this protocol was an example of the power of the simulation technique, since it is often not possible to control an actual microelectrode voltage clamp with such a fast time-varying signal.

The two possible mechanisms that I therefore considered for the repolarizing tail were an abrupt slowing of inactivation of the fast Na^+ current underlying the spike, or the presence of another kind of Na^+ channel. The first possibility was discounted when I could not derive a function for the voltage-dependent time-constant for inactivation for the fast Na^+ that was consistent with the single-barrier gating assumptions and that had the necessary sharp increase at the appropriate voltage. In considering the possibility of a distinct tail current, the important characteristics of this current was that it had to have a high threshold and a slow onset, consistent with the lack of a long after-depolarization in normal spikes. For example, if this current had a threshold of approximately -10 mV with a slow activation time-constant, i.e. 4 ms, then during a normal spike this current will not have time to activate fully. On the other hand, during the slower repolarization that occurs without active outward currents, this tail current will have time during the peak of the spike to activate more, and thereby contribute to a long repolarization. I called this current $I_{Na\text{-}tail}$. I attempted to adapt the activation data for I_{NaP} (discussed next) to account for the action of the so-called $I_{Na\text{-}tail}$, but this has been unsuccessful to date. This is primarily because the low threshold of the activation curve for I_{NaP} has thwarted attempts at deriving a function for the time-constant of activation that is consistent with the single-barrier model and which in turn reproduces the Na^+-only spike.

25.5.2 *Implications of tetrodotoxin sensitive steady state current-voltage characteristic*

Fig. 25.3 shows a steady-state current–voltage characteristic from hippocampal pyramidal cells that demonstrates a tetrodotoxin (TTX) sensitive inward-rectification (French & Gage, *ibid*). Assuming that a sensitivity to TTX means that Na^+ currents underlie this rectification, the characteristic can be accounted for by either the 'window current' of a transient Na^+ current, by a persistent (non-inactivating) Na^+ current (I_{NaP}), or by some combination of these types of channels. Window current is due to any overlap in the voltage-dependent steady-states curves of the activation and inactivation variables, thereby making a normally transient current contribute a persistent component over some range of membrane voltage.

Since any overlap in the activation and inactivation curves will be limited, rectification due to a window current alone would disappear at depolarized membrane voltages. The steady-state current voltage characteristic would then continue the linear characteristic established prior to the onset of rectification. The data for this cell, however, would not necessarily demonstrate a depolarized removal of rectification since the steady-state current–voltage curve was only measured to -35 mV.

25.5.3 Implications of Na$^+$-only repetitive firing

Repetitive firing elicited in cells in which all currents except Na$^+$ have been blocked offers additional clues as to the nature of the Na$^+$ currents in hippocampal pyramidal cells. Fig. 25.4 illustrates such a record. The key features of these voltage traces are (1) higher threshold of spikes following initial spike, (2) reduced amplitude of repetitive spikes, (3) reduction of spike amplitude with increasing stimulus, and (4) repetitive firing elicited only in a narrow range of membrane voltages.

Na$^+$ mediated repetitive firing in cells depolarized from the resting potential implies that the inactivation curve for the current underlying the higher threshold spikes is non-zero at the depolarized level. However, since there is no inward-rectification at the lower threshold, this contradicts the earlier conclusion that the activation curve for the fast Na$^+$

Fig. 25.3. Inward Rectification by Na$^+$. Curve derived from steady-state activation of a persistent Na$^+$ current, I_{NaP} (derived from French & Gage, *ibid*).

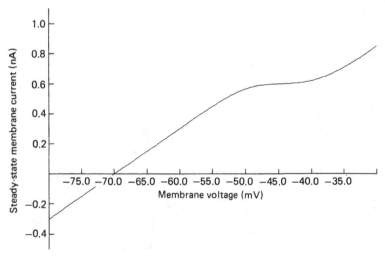

current is steep at the lower threshold. A steep activation curve at the lower threshold taken with the non-zero inactivation at depolarized membrane potentials would result in an appreciable window current. This window current in turn would contribute to inward rectification starting at the lower spike threshold of 55 mV.

To explain these phenomena, I suggest that there is an additional fast Na^+ channel whose threshold for firing is depolarized from that of the original fast Na^+ channel, and whose activation and inactivation kinetics are such that it might mediate Na^+-only repetitive firing. In the absence of active repolarization from any outward currents, our simulations indicated that there must be a finite overlap of the activation and inactivation curves of any HH-like Na^+ channel that can mediate repetitive firing. This overlap will result in a finite window current, and thus steady-state inward rectification and I was able to adjust this rectification to qualitatively reproduce the onset of the observed rectification discussed earlier. Because it mediates repetitive Na^+-only spikes, I named the high threshold current I_{Na-rep}. Since I deduced that the original fast Na^+ current had a sensitive, low threshold for initiating the action potential, I called this current $I_{Na-trig}$.

Fig. 25.4. Na^+-only repetitive spiking–current clamp protocol under same conditions as Fig. 25.2. Current stimuli is bottom trace (from Storm, unpublished data).

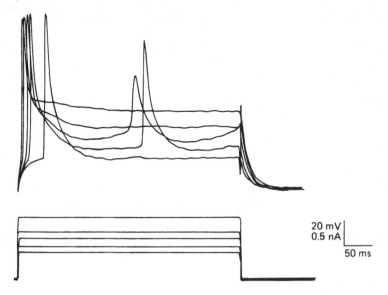

20 mV
0.5 nA

50 ms

25.5.4 Strategy for determining Na^+ current kinetics

Once it was determined that three Na^+ currents might model the observed behavior, the strategy used to derive their kinetics was as follows:

(1) Estimate the absolute Na^+ conductance for the fast Na^+ currents ($I_{Na\text{-trig}}$ and $I_{Na\text{-rep}}$) by calculating the current necessary to generate the rising phase of the Na^+-only spike. This current in turn depended on the electrotonic structure and estimates were verified with current clamp simulations of the response of the passive cell to current pulses.

(2) A reasonable set of equations governing the kinetics (backward and forward rate constants for the activation gating particle m and inactivation gating particle h) for the three putative Na^+ currents was determined. The free parameters for each function include the free energy changes between the stable states and the transition state, the location of the transition state within the membrane, and the effective valence of the gating particle. Voltage-dependent functions of the time-constants and steady-state values of the gating particles are then derived from the appropriate rate functions.

(3) Run (current clamp) simulations of the Na^+-only single and repetitive spike protocols.

(4) Compare the simulations with the data.

(5) Adjust the appropriate rate-constant functions and repeat the simulations.

(6) Once a good match between the current clamp simulations and the data was reached, the steady-state current–voltage characteristic of the cell with all three Na^+ currents activated was derived to measure the inward-rectification generated by the estimated currents.

(7) This characteristic was compared with that of one from the model with the derived Na^+ current replaced by the reported persistent Na^+ current.

(8) If needed, return to step 5 in order to obtain a good fit to all the available data.

This process eventually converged to yield a model description that was in good qualitative agreement with the data pertaining to Na^+ behavior. The derived Na^+ currents were then tested by running simulations in which various K^+ currents were added. This would often cause us to modify some of the parameters of the Na^+ currents while preserving the Na^+-only behavior. The entire process is one of adding one piece of information at a time to the model, and then running simulations to find out how the new data affect the model's behavior. The model is thus continually evolving as more data become available for these cells.

25.6 Results

25.6.1 Estimation of soma and dendritic membrane resistivity

One result of the simulations was that a low soma membrane resistivity was required in order for Na^+-only spikes to repolarize as quickly as they did without the help of active outward currents. The soma membrane resistivity in the model was of the order of 1000 Ωcm^2, assuming a parallel 100 $M\Omega$ electrode shunt resistance in the soma. This value meant that the dendritic membrane resistivity had to be significantly higher (typically 20–40 $k\Omega cm^2$, assuming a cytoplasmic resistivity of 100 Ωcm), in order to give the observed soma input resistance (typically 30–60 $M\Omega$). A similar distribution of membrane resistivity has been suggested in modeling studies of the Purkinje neuron (Shelton, 1985). The possibility of a non-homogeneous membrane time constant caused us to re-examine published data on the passive characteristics of hippocampal cells (e.g. Brown *et al.*, 1981). Typically in these studies, the (assumed) linear response to a hyperpolarizing current step is examined in order to derive the cell's passive parameters. These derivatives are often based on the calculated response of a soma-cable approximation of the cell, with the assumption of a homogeneous membrane time-constant (e.g., homogeneous specific membrane resistivity and capacitance). However, it can be shown that the introduction of distance soma and dendritic membrane time-constants via distinct membrane resistivities, as our simulations suggest, changes the soma step response so as to alter derivations of parameters such as dendritic–somatic conductance ratio (ϱ), and the electrotonic length of the dendritic cable (L). One implication of these findings is that the dendritic tree of hippocampal pyramidal cells may be more electrically compact than previously thought.

25.6.2 Simulation of Na^+-mediated inward-rectification and spikes

Fig. 25.5 compares the steady-state current–voltage characteristic of the model with (1) the reported I_{NaP}, and (2) the $I_{Na\text{-}trig}$, $I_{Na\text{-}tail}$, $I_{Na\text{-}rep}$ currents. The model currents cause an onset of inward rectification that is in qualitative agreement with the published data. However, since this steady-state inward current is mainly due to the transient $I_{Na\text{-}rep}$ window current, the rectification only occurs over a limited range of membrane voltages. This is not necessarily inconsistent with the characteristic of I_{NaP} because of the limited range over which this current was measured, as explained earlier. It is possible that the so-called persistent Na^+ current is actually a transient current which would demonstrate removal of inward-rectification at more depolarized membrane potentials. Given more data, it is also possible that the derived characteristics of the so-called $I_{Na\text{-rep}}$ might be adjusted to better match the steady-state current–voltage relationship of the model.

Fig. 25.6 illustrates a simulation of the Na^+-only single spike. The model's behavior is in good agreement with the data, in particular in regards to the sharp threshold of the spike, the time course of the depolarizing phase, the initial fast repolarization, and the slower late repolarization. Also in the diagram are the three model Na^+ currents that underline the Na^+-only spike. Note the initial activation of $I_{Na\text{-trig}}$, the subsequent recruitment of the higher threshold $I_{Na\text{-rep}}$, and the slow time course of $I_{Na\text{-tail}}$ after the first two currents have inactivated.

Fig. 25.7 illustrates a simulation of Na^+-only repetitive firing under different constant current inputs. At the bottom of the diagram are the Na^+ currents underlying the marked spike train. Note that after the first spike, the initiation of later spikes is mediated completely by $I_{Na\text{-rep}}$.

Fig. 25.5. Current–voltage characteristics of model showing inward-rectification mediated by I_{NaP} and by $I_{Na\text{-trig}}$, $I_{Na\text{-tail}}$, and $I_{Na\text{-rep}}$ currents.

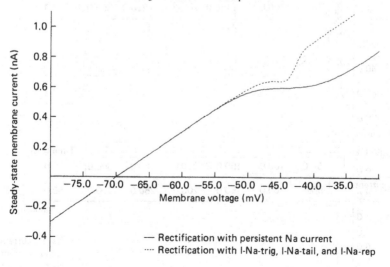

Fig. 25.6. Current clamp simulation of Na$^+$-only single spike and sub-threshold protocol. Spike stimulus − 0.39 nA. Subthreshold stimulus − 0.38 nA. $I_{Na\text{-}trig}$, $I_{Na\text{-}tail}$, $I_{Na\text{-}rep}$ currents during spike.

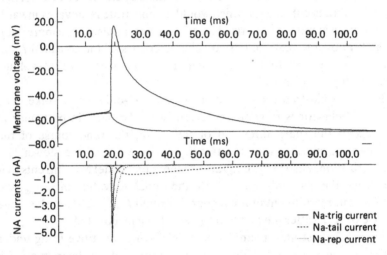

Fig. 25.7. Current clamp simulation of Na$^+$-only repetitive spike protocol. Tonic stimulus − 0.5 nA. $I_{Na\text{-}trig}$, $I_{Na\text{-}tail}$, $I_{Na\text{-}rep}$ currents during trace marked with the arrow.

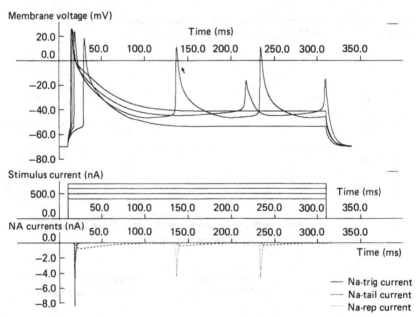

25.6.3 Simulation of single action potential

With the derived Na$^+$ currents in place, the model is then tested with the addition of preliminary descriptions of the various K$^+$ currents and Ca^{++} currents that have been described for this class of cell. Fig. 25.8 illustrates the simulation of a single action potential. Note in particular the more rapid time course of this spike as compared to the Na$^+$-only spike, due to the active repolarization of the two K$^+$ currents.

25.6.4 Discussion of functional role of the proposed Na$^+$ currents

Once we have constructed the three model currents that successfully reproduce the data, it is important to ask what roles these currents might play in the pyramidal cell. Consider $I_{\text{Na-trig}}$. The characteristics of this current allow for a sharp firing threshold from resting potential. The advantage of this is that the neuron is more tuned to a specific input firing level; there is a higher noise margin with regard to the firing efficacy of a given pattern of synaptic input. In addition, the lack of a window current for $I_{\text{Na-trig}}$ means that at rest or at subthreshold membrane potentials there will be little 'wasted' Na$^+$ current. This is metabolically favorable as the

Fig. 25.8. Current clamp simulation of single action potential. Some of the major currents during the single spike are on the left, including $I_{\text{Na-trig}}$, $I_{\text{Na-tail}}$, $I_{\text{Na-rep}}$, I_{DR}, I_{C}, and the soma–dendrite current. Note the fast after-hyperpolarization (fAHP) (arrow) caused by the activation of I_{C} (Storm, 1986). In this simulation the after-depolarization (ADP) immediately following the fAHP is due to both residual $I_{\text{Na-tail}}$, and passive charge redistribution from the dendrite (soma–dendrite current). Stimulus is 1.0 nA pulse for 2 ms.

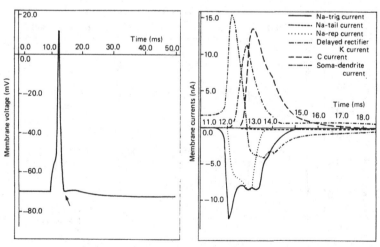

cell does not have to remove the buildup of Na$^+$ resulting from such a background current. Likewise, any constant inward current at rest would have to be balanced by an outward (presumably K$^+$) current in order to maintain the resting potential. Again, this loss adds to the energy requirements of the cell at 'rest'.

What could be the advantage of a second, higher threshold Na$^+$ current that is capable of Na$^+$-only repetitive firing? Such a higher threshold Na$^+$ current on top of a sharp, lower threshold Na$^+$ current could relax the requirements of the repolarization mechanism during a train of spikes in response to some tonic depolarization. An $I_{\text{Na-rep}}$-type current could mediate later action potentials without the requirement that the cell repolarize to below the threshold of an $I_{\text{Na-trig}}$-type current – all that is needed is that the cell repolarize to somewhere below the threshold of $I_{\text{Na-rep}}$. Simulation of repetitive firing (Fig. 25.9) shows how $I_{\text{Na-rep}}$ could furnish the major portion of depolarizing current for spikes after the first spike of a train.

Allowing the cell to fire again from a higher threshold reduces the amount of outward current needed to sustain multiple spikes, which in turn impose less of a burden on the cell's machinery for maintaining the K$^+$ concentration gradient. In addition, the overlap of the activation and

Fig. 25.9. Current clamp simulation of normal repetitive firing in response to 0.5 nA 300-ms pulse. Note fast after-hyperpolarization (fAHP) after first spike, mediated by I_C (Storm, *ibid*). In lower part of figure are the $I_{\text{Na-trig}}$, $I_{\text{Na-tail}}$, $I_{\text{Na-rep}}$ currents during the train.

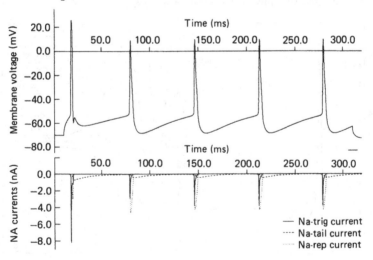

inactivation curves of I_{Na-rep} results in an ill-defined threshold for repetitive firing, allowing for a greater flexibility in modulating the frequency of firing by other mechanisms, e.g. distinct actions of the various K^+ currents.

What about the proposed $I_{Na-tail}$? As constructed, this current contributes to a small after-depolarization during a normal spike that must be countered by an outward current. In our simulations, this is accomplished by I_{DR}. For now it is not clear what function this slowly inactivating Na^+ current would have. Perhaps this current may be inhibited in certain circumstances, thus allowing it to play a role in mediating repetitive firing. Such speculation awaits further evidence of such a $I_{Na-tail}$ in actual cells.

25.6.5 Interpreting the model's behavior

A key consideration in our work is that of evaluating the validity of the simulations since there will not be a unique solution for many of the simulated protocols. The complex non-linearity of the problem means that non-physiological descriptions of the kinetics may enable the model to still behave 'reasonably'. Also, the HH description of ion channel kinetics is primarily an empirical description of the mechanisms underlying macroscopic currents. However, the simulation test-bed allows the exercising of a given solution with a range of different parameters in order to evaluate the confidence of that solution.

Clearly, modeling of the brain at a higher level can be accomplished without a detailed description of the individual computing elements, but it is imperative that any description of those elements be made without unwarranted simplification. Subtleties in the transfer function of single neurons can have profound implications in the information processing function of the neuronal ensemble. Since intracellular measurements of cortical neurons are difficult, computer simulations can be used in conjunction with the available data to build a description of the biophysical mechanisms mediating the electrical activity of the single cell.

Acknowledgments

The parameters for the model, including the kinetics of the active currents and the passive characteristics of hippocampal pyramidal cells, were derived either from the literature or from consultation with Prof. Paul Adams and Dr Johan Storm, both of the Department of Neurobiology and Behavior, State University of New York at Stony Brook, and Prof. Christof Koch, of the Division of Biology, California Institute of Technology. The neural modeling work of Profs. Koch and Adams provided the impetus for the model described here, and in the case of Prof. Adams and Dr Storm, their input as experimentalists was invaluable in the development of the model and in the interpretation of measurements of hippocampal pyramidal neurons. I would also like to thank Prof. Tomaso Poggio, Dr Storm and John Sliney for their review of this paper, Dr Storm for providing the data of Na^+-only behavior, and Prof. Poggio for the support of this research.

Appendix: model algorithm

In our model a spherical-soma/dendritic-cable approximation of the pyramidal cell is reduced to an electrical network. The program calculates the time response of the network using a predictor-corrector scheme similar to that used by previous investigators (Cooley & Dodge, 1966). The components of the network include:

   active conductances in series with voltage sources representing the appropriate reversal potentials;

   membrane capacitance;

   current injected into the compartments, modeling that injected via microelectrodes;

   controlled voltage source across the soma membrane for voltage clamp simulations.

The outputs of the network include:

   voltage and the derivative of the voltage for each compartment;

   state variable values and their derivatives for all the active conductances;

   currents through all the network elements.

The program first calculates the steady state of the network if it exists for the current set of simulation conditions. If a steady state does not exist (e.g., the cell fires spontaneously) a quasi-steady-state solution is used as the initial values for the simulation. The algorithm then proceeds as follows for each time increment.

(1) Estimate the voltage of each compartment by an open integration formula, based on the voltage at the last time step, the derivative of the voltage at the last time step, and the length of the time step.

(2) Estimate the steady state values of the state variables and their time constants as a function of the estimated voltage at the current time.

(3) Estimate the present value for the state variables by trapezoidal approximation, using the old values for the state variables and their derivatives, the estimates for their current steady state value, and the estimates for their time constants.

(4) The conductances are estimated from the appropriate state variable estimates.

(5) Conservation of current (KCL) and the current–voltage branch equations are used to estimate the capacitive current for each compartment. From this the derivative of the compartment voltages are derived. Thus the derivative of the compartment voltages are a function of the estimated conductances, the estimates for the voltages in adjacent compartments, and the injected current (if any) into the compartments.

(6) A second estimate of the compartment voltages is made with a trapezoidal approximation, based on the previous values of the compartment voltages and their derivatives, and the estimate for the present derivative of the compartment voltages.

(7) The new voltage estimates are compared with the previous voltage estimates for all the compartments. If any of these estimates is not within some convergence criterion ε, then return to step 2 using the mean of the previous and present voltage estimates.

(8) If all the voltage estimates are within the convergence criteria then these estimates are stored as the present values for the compartment voltages. A final estimate of the state variables and the derivatives of the voltages are then calculated, once again using steps 2 through 6. The derivatives of the state variables are also calculated using the appropriate differential equations. These values are also stored as part of present state of the network.

(9) Increment the time and continue simulation.

The stability of the algorithm was primarily a function of the time-step and the state variable with the fastest kinetics. Runs or a given simulation were done with the largest time-step that resulted in a convergent solution. Typically simulations were run with a time-step of 0.05 ms, and an ε of 0.1 mV. The accuracy of key simulations was checked by rerunning the simulation with a small time-step and a small epsilon (typically 0.01 ms and 0.01 mV respectively). Running time for simulations with a 0.05-ms time-step and an ε of 0.1 mV was approximately 0.5 s per ms of simulation.

References

Borg-Graham, L. (1987). Modelling of the somatic electrical response of hippocampal pyramidal neurons. S.M. thesis, Massachusetts Institute of Technology, Dept of Electrical Engineering and Computer Science.

Brown, D. & Griffith, W. (1983). 'Calcium activated outward current in voltage clamped hippocampal neurons of the guinea pig'. *J. of Physiol.*, **337**, 287–301.

Brown, T., Fricke, R. & Perkel, D. (1981). 'Passive electrical constants in three classes of hippocampal neurones (CA1, CA3 and granular cells)'. *J. of Neurophysiol.*, **46**(4), 812–27.

Chiu, S. Y., Ritchie, J. M., Rogart, R. B. & Stagg, D. (1979). 'A quantitative description of membrane currents in rabbit myelinated nerve'. *J. Physiol. (London)*, **309**, 499–519.

Cooley, J. & Dodge, F. (1966). 'Digital computer solutions for excitation and propagation of the nerve impulse'. *Biophys. J.*, **6**, 583–99.

French, C. & Gage, P. (1985). 'A threshold sodium current in pyramidal cells in rat hippocampus', *Neurosci. Lett.*, **56**, 289–93.

Gustafsson, B., Galvan, M. & Grafe, P. (1982). 'A transient outward current in a mammalian central neurone blocked by 4-aminopyridine'. *Nature*, **299**, 252–54.

Halliwell, J. & Adams, P. (1982). Voltage clamp analysis of muscarinic excitation in hippocampal neurons'. *Brain Res.*, **250**, 71–92.

Halliwell, J. (1983). 'Caesium loading reveals two distinct Ca-currents in voltage clamped guinea pig hippocampal neurones in vitro'. *J. Physiol. (Proc. of the Physiol. Soc.)*, pp. 10P–11P.

Hodgkin, A. L. & Huxley, A. F. (1952). 'A quantitative description of membrane current and its application to conduction and excitation in nerve. *J. Physiol. (Lond.)*, **116**, 500–44.

Jack, J. J. B., Noble, D. & Tsien, R. W. (1977). *Electric Current Flow in Excitable Cells*. Oxford University Press, London, 518 pp.

Johnston, D., Hablitz, J. & Wilson, W. (1980). 'Voltage clamp discloses slow inward current in hippocampal burst-firing neurones'. *Nature*, 286.

Lancaster, B. & Adams, P. (1986). 'Calcium dependent current generating the afterhyperpolarisation of hippocampal neurons'. *J. of Neurophys.*, **55**, 1268–82.

Madison, D., Malenka, R & Nicoll, R. (1986). 'Phorbol esters block a voltage-sensitive chloride current in hippocampal pyramidal cells'. *Nature*, **321**, 695–7.

Segal, M. & Baker, J. (1984). 'Rat hippocampal neurons in culture: potassium conductances'. *J. of Neurophys.*, **51**(6), 1409–33.

Shelton, D. P. (1985). 'Membrane resistivity estimated for the Purkinje neuron by means of a passive computer model'. *Neurosci.*, **14**(1), 111–31.

Storm, J. (1986). 'A-current and Ca-dependent transient outward current control the initial repetitive firing in hippocampal neurons'. *Biophysical J.*, **49**, 369a.

Traub, R. & Llinas, R. (1979). 'Hippocampal pyramidal cells: significance of dendritic ionic conductances for neuronal function and epileptogenesis'. *J. of Neurophysiol.*, **42**(2), 476–96.

26

Neural computations and neural systems

J. J. HOPFIELD

In deciding on a chapter for this book I had to choose between my interests in bringing ideas from biology to computational hardware, and in trying to bring computational ideas towards the biological wetware. I chose the direction of biological wetware, but it is instructive to begin with a few words about VLSI 'neural' networks.

There have been sizeable associative memories built out of the VLSI kinds of hardware. A first effort succeeded in building a 22 neuron circuit (1). A 54-neuron circuit with its 3000 connections has been made at Bell Laboratories (2) and a 512-neuron circuit with its 256 000 intersections has been fabricated, but not yet made to work (3). An interesting and significant feature which emerges from looking at these chips is the degree to which, although the idea of an associative memory is very simple, a large fraction of the devices and area on the chip are doing things which are essential to the overall function of the chip, but which seem peripheral to the *idea* of associative memory. I will describe a similar facet in the biological case, in going from the abstract idea of an associative task toward a complete neural system. Much paraphernalia must be added and many changes made in order that an elementary associative memory can perform a biological task.

I will use the example of olfaction. You might well ask why choose the sense of smell – isn't it a rather difficult sense to work with? But consider the biological problem. The purpose of most sensory systems is to learn about and to identify what might be called external objects. Vision (which many would view as the most highly understood sensory system) and smell are very different in important regards with respect to this biological function. When you look at a particular person there will be 50 cells in the retina which are much more active than any of the other retinal cells.

When you smell a particular odour there will be 50 cells in the sensory epithelium of the nose which are more active than any other such cells. In the case of vision, if the lighting is changed a little, or if a highlight moves somewhere else in the scene, or if the person moves, the retinal cells which are most strongly driven completely change. In the case of vision, the 50 most intensely driven cells actually say nothing very useful about the nature of objects 'out there'. On the other hand, in olfaction, the sensory cells are somewhat chemically selective. As a result, the 50 most intensely excited cells are describing something very explicit about the world 'out there'. There are molecules which have come from 'there' to the sensory epithelium, and which are now bound by chemoreceptors. The structure of the molecules of the distal sensory object itself is being measured by the chemical binding and 'fit' to the site. Thus, already in the earliest stage of olfactory processing, the nervous system acquires details of particular objects. The visual nervous system is dominated by proprocessing designed to generate equally meaningful details about visual objects from the original sensory input. One loses track of what is going on in the visual system long before arriving at an ability to understand computationally how objects are perceived. So olfaction is really a simpler system than vision, and fortunately is being increasingly studied.

We will chiefly consider a 'sample' system, the garden slug, *Limax maximus*, which has been extensively studied by Gelperin (4), Sahley (5), and their students. The simplest learning paradigm (6) which olfactory systems show is first-order conditioning. In this paradigm an odour *A* which is initially attractive to the animal is followed in time by a noxious stimulus. *Limax* learns, and after that paired exposure *Limax* no longer finds *A* attractive. Instead it finds *A* repellent (exhibits aversive behaviour), whereas some other initially attractive stimulus odour, *B*, which was not paired with the noxious stimulus, is still found to be attractive. Apetitive conditioning, in which the attraction to an odour is positively reinforced by reward, can also take place. *Limax* also displays second-order conditioning, in which having learned (by such a paired aversive training) not to like *A*, a *Limax* can now use its dislike of *A* (which is intrinsically a harmless substance) to do further learning. A presentation of *B*, a stimulus which is weakly attractive, followed by *A* (which it has previously learned to dislike) results in an aversive behaviour for both *A* and *B*. Additional important learning paradigms displayed by *Limax* include extinction and blocking. These are the typical learning paradigms of Pavlovian conditioning. Dogs and humans both display these learning behaviours, and the same learning paradigms apparently go on even at very low levels in the animal kingdom.

The simplest concept of a network which can perform this sort of processing is shown below (6). First, there are receptive cells labelled T which in turn drive some categoriser and memory neurons S. All the tasks of Pavlovian conditioning described above are really tasks of association, so this categoriser/memory should be a form of associative memory. Next, to make a complete system which can be functionally examined, one must connect the categoriser/memory to an additional system which generates behavioural outputs. In the simplest experiment protocol, the subject is forced to make a binary choice. For typical *Limax* experiments, the choice is one of eating (or choosing to go toward a substance), or not eating (choosing to move away from it). These will be labelled 'eat' and 'flee'. If there are only two possible motor behaviours, the possibility of those two behaviours can be modelled by two different cells which are mutually cross-inhibited so that, at any time, at most one of these can be active. The outputs of these two cells drive the two motor behaviours. The existence of such cells driving the jaw muscles in *Limax* is well known, and an electrical signal 'eat' (feeding motor program) can be identified in a nerve even in a dissected preparation which has removed the jaw, muscles, and virtually all of the rest of the animal (7).

There is direct sensory input to the sensory memory in Fig. 26.1. The

Fig. 26.1.

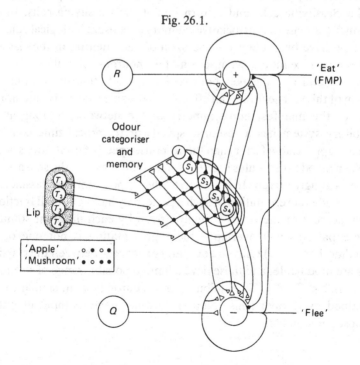

memory also serves as a classifier in this neural circuit. (Some kind of preprocessor between sensory cells and the memory system may be necessary – see below.) The last feature needed to complete the system are the two additional *labelled* inputs. R (reward) is an input from a stimulus which is intrinsically attractive and non-modifiable, and always results in the behaviour 'eat'. The second special input labelled Q (quinine) represents input from a receptor driven by an intrinsically noxious stimulus. (*Limax* cannot be trained to like quinine.) This kind of built-in unmodifiable connection to special genetically determined chemoreceptors is necessary because a learning system must have a fundamental reference. There is no way of *learning* which category is which from neural electrical signals alone, since good and bad are merely two different electrical signals. This fundamental reference for what is good and what is evil, as it were, can come only from inheritance and genetics, by linking a particular sensory stimulus with some determined neurons or behaviours.

Several more things must be added to make this system actually function. First, inhibition is needed in the classifier. The classifying cells receive excitatory inputs from the sensory system, and in addition have mutual excitatory connections between themselves. Inhibition comes from inhibitory interneurons *I* which receive excitatory inputs from each of the classifying cells and in turn inhibit the classifying cells. In this classifier (in reality an associative memory) the usual biological rules for cell type have been obeyed – the axon of each neuron in the classifier makes either excitatory synapses on other neurons, or makes inhibitory synapses, and never makes both types. The addition of an inhibitory system of this sort generates an effective and stable associative memory in spite of the manifest non-symmetry of the network, as long as the inhibitory system has a response speed (or reciprocal time constant) which is appreciably faster than the response speed of excitatory system.

When an odour stimulus is given, some small subset of the sensory cells will be strongly driven. In considering the response of the classifier, we used a crude representation of such a pattern by having a small fraction f, a few percent of the total, strongly driven by each different stimulus. (These patterns will overlap – the representation is not one of the 'grandmother cells'.) Only the excitatory synapses between the classifier cells are modifiable, and these have a limited possible range of strengths, taken as $0 < T_{ij} < 1$. The inhibitory interneuron system, similar to that described by Cooper (this volume) does not have its input or output synapses modifiable.

The classifier/memory neurons S also drive the neurons + and − which drive the two motor behaviours. The set of synapses connecting these cells are also modifiable, with the same rules as for the excitatory connections between neurons S.

This network is capable of performing associative memory tasks. Interestingly, by moving toward biology (0-1 neurons, separate excitatory and inhibitory neurons, limited range synapses, low mean activity level) and away from the mathematically simpler network which Peretto was using (this volume), one avoids some of the difficulties for which Peretto found additional hardware was needed. For example, because excitation and inhibition play quite different roles in our system, it is capable of learning a new memory and having that new exposure continue for a very long period of time without having all its previous memories made inaccessible because of that unbalanced experience. (The control of learning is a major problem for any system which learns while it functions. Many computer learning systems require an external control network to avoid over-learning, or to provide instruction about the 'objects' of the world.)

The learning algorithm which is needed can symbolically be written as

$$\frac{\Delta T_{ij}}{\Delta t} = \propto V_i V_j - forgetting,$$

$$\sum_j T_{ij} = constant,$$

and combines a Hebbian term increasing excitatory connections with a forgetting term which keeps the total synaptic strength of a cell approximately constant by weakening somewhat other synapses when specific synapses are being strengthened.

One of the new findings from comparing the capabilities of this model network with the behaviours of the real animal, is that this synapse modification rule is not adequate. It fails to be appropriate in a way which is very different from the failures which were discussed by Cooper and by Peretto. In the laboratory, two different first-order conditioning experiments can be done. In forward conditioning the odour is given first, and then the aversive stimulus (quinine). A slug − or a dog, or a human − learns well not to eat this food a second time. In backward conditioning the noxious stimulus begins before the food odour. In this case there is very little learning.

In the synaptic change algorithm described above, the duration of the time of overlap between the odour and the aversive stimulus is the quantity of importance. The question of which one began first does not enter. By contrast, in biology there is a strong sense of time order, and all biological systems show a very strong difference in learning between forward and backward conditioning. In some sense biology believes *post hoc ergo propter hoc*, or perhaps *ante hoc ergo non propter hoc*. You have an extreme sense of time yourself. What is the significance of the number 95 141.3? Do you recognise it as π? Because of the direction in which you read English, you see this stimulus in a particular time order, the reverse of the one which would readily identify it. A change in the synaptic modification rule is needed in order to obtain the appropriate effect of time order in the system. The required minor alteration removes the symmetry between the pre- and post-synaptic cell potentials in the synapse change algorithm, by introducing a time lag between the two sides. Such a modification could be readily generated by biochemical dynamics, and preserves the locality of the Hebbian modification algorithm. An appropriate change is described in detail in Gelperin *et al.* (6). In general, such new ideas and constructs always turn out to be necessary whenever one tries to make a model system *really* process information and not merely *appear* to be adequate to do so. The new modification rule would also generate exactly the kind of connections necessary to learn *sequences* in associative memories (8).

The next task to be considered is that of trying to recognise a weak signal. One of the intrinsic problems an organism has in nature is that if there is food a long distance away, only a weak scent of it is available. The first thing the organism should compute is: 'What food is it that I am smelling?' in order to make a further computation and the appropriate behavioural choice of the direction of locomotion. A biological system needs to be able to recognise weak signals.

The generic way to recognise weak signals might be described as follows. Set up a dynamic computational neural circuit with multiple stable states representing different known odours. Start this system at an unstable dynamical point (saddle point or maximum). The weak input being received is an effective force on the dynamic system. The state of the neural system will then move from the unstable point to that stable point which is most nearly in the direction of the effective force vector from the input. This kind of procedure is necessary in order to have both high sensitivity and the ability to make a *decision* about a weak stimulus. The situation must be set up by an appropriate manipulation in time during the decision process – the system must go from an unstable to a stable condition while being exposed to the effective force due to the stimulus input. The easiest way to accomplish this is to change the overall gain or threshold of the system as a function of time. The dynamical system will then evolve from a condition of having only one stable point, through a critical domain, to a condition of having unstable points and multiple stable points. If a weak input is present at the critical time, a decision is made as to which minimum to go to on the basis of the weak force on the system when the local potential surface goes flat at the critical time. If the decision is made somewhat sequentially, there may be several serial critical times and configuration regions. The basic idea concerns evolving the dynamical system from a single stable point to multiple stable points by changing the parameters of the dynamical system with time.

A simple and biologically plausible way of doing this it to let the inhibitory network of cells I have a cyclic activity. Alternatively, the input–output relation of the processing neurons could be cyclically altered by a *modulatory* system which changes the excitability of cells on the efficacy of synapses. In either case, one of the expected aspects of a sensitive classifier is that it will be an oscillatory system. Unfortunately, there are so many oscillators and rhythms in most neural systems that the prediction that a particular set of cells should be oscillatory is almost not a prediction (9, 10). Often, as in these cases, one does not understand the *function* of the oscillation – what is the oscillation accomplishing that could not as well or more easily be done without oscillation. Here we see one particular information processing role to such oscillations, namely helping to make firm decisions on the basis of weak inputs. The modulation produces a shift from a situation where the neurons are input-dominated to a situation where the input is no longer relevant (network is then internally dominated) but when the *state* of the system now depends upon the input during the transit of the transition region.

A second problem – and one which again involves more hardware – has to do with the question of making appropriate categories of foods. In the modelling described earlier, each food simply drove a collection of sensory cells with different strengths, and the input pattern had some small fraction of these cells strongly driven while others were weakly driven. A pattern which had a few cells active and most cell inactive was abstracted, and that information was sent on directly to the memory network. This is one of many possible forms of input to a processing system.

There are two contending attitudes towards olfaction and other complex sensory modalities, sometimes referred to as the analytic and synthetic viewpoints (11). In the analytic view of olfaction (or another sense, *mutatis mutandis*) information about sub-components of the odour tends to be retained. If sensory cells are directly coupled in an elementary way to the memory cells, the chemical information present at the sensory cell level is to some extent available later in the network. This leads to the possibility of resolving the components of an odour in the same sense that the individual notes of a two-note chord (played simultaneously on a piano) can be resolved and both frequencies identified. The chord does not sound like 'one thing', two separate frequencies can be identified. We have an analytic ability in this perception of two tones. Similarly, the olfaction system described up to now in this paper is highly analytic in that the neurons of the categoriser/memory can be given chemical meaning.

The odour system with no preprocessing before the memory generalises very well. Stimuli which are similar chemically will produce very similar patterns of input excitation to the memory/categoriser, and thus tend to produce the same behaviours. This system over-generalises, tends to put too many things in one category, and fails to be able to make behavioural discriminations between chemically similar odours.

The network shown in Fig. 26.2 is a categoriser which can be inserted between the sensory cells and the memory network. It has an array of processing neurons, C, and all neurons in a row of the array are equally excited by a single sensory cell. Inhibitory interneurons are also present. Interneurons i provide a mutual inhibition path for neurons within a single row of the network. Inhibitory interneurons I provide inhibitory

Fig. 26.2.

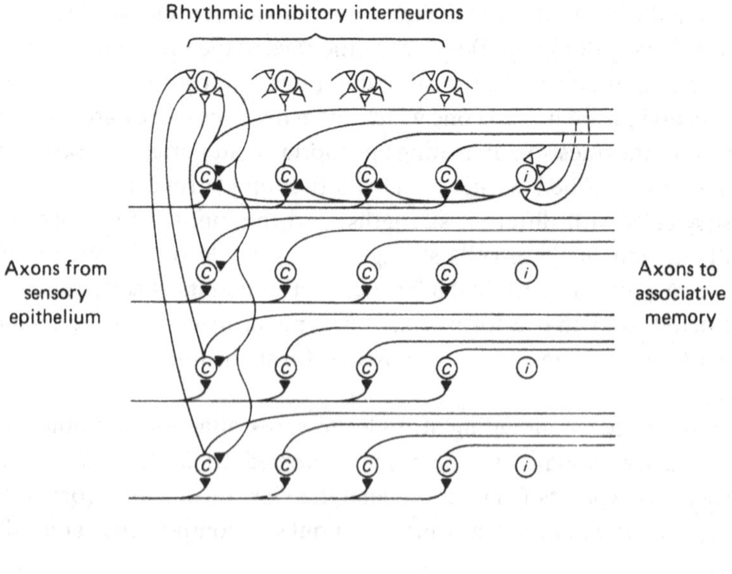

interactions within a single column of categoriser neurons, C. This network is unlike the memory/categoriser network of Fig. 26.1 in that it has no internal excitatory connections. Excitation is proved by the sensory cells. The output of this processor is then sent on to the previous memory/categoriser network.

The thresholds (or inhibition) in the interneurons I of this processing network are also periodic in time with different columns of the processing array in different temporal phases. The ability of neurons to be active is turned on sequentially, so that first one, then the second, etc., columns become able to be activated by the input. If the inhibition is appropriately chosen so that only one of a set of the mutually inhibiting (*via* the interneurons) neurons C can be strongly active at once, this network will settle into a pattern of excitation which *reflects the relative strengths of excitation of the sensory cells*. It 'makes a computation' and generates an output pattern on the basis of these relative strengths. The pattern of excitation which results is *completely* changed if the input from the strongest-driven sensory neuron is eliminated. This kind of response might be associated with a 'synthetic' system because total changes in pattern can sometimes result from a small change in the stimulus pattern. By contrast, the pattern of excitation in the earlier 'analytic' system was very little changed (changed in only one neuron) if the input from the strongest-driven sensory neuron was eliminated. This new processor reflects relative analogue strengths in a biologically relevant way, in that it can separate the categories of odours which are different in relative analogue strengths of their strongest component parts. This network has a weaker capacity for generalisation than the original system, but is good for doing specific recognitions. An effective olfactory system might well have elements of each of these systems. It is important to realise that the major difference between an analytic and a synthetic sense cannot necessarily be seen in the neuroanatomy. This difference between analytic and synthetic in our model circuit has a great deal to do with the oscillation cycle which takes place in the set of inhibitory interneurons. (The particular classifier network described is illustrative only, and there is no present knowledge of how a classifier in *Limax* might be constructed.)

Recent experiments have shown that *Limax* can distinguish between partially and completely mixed odours (12). Two 'mixture' experiments have been performed when *Limax* is foraging on a screen about 5 mm above the bottom of a Petri dish. In one, a physical mixture of odourants

A and *B* is placed on the bottom of the dish. In the other, alternate stripes 2 mm wide of *A* and *B* are painted on the bottom of the dish. There is little control of air flow – 'still room air' – with normal convective currents is present. Nonetheless, in the former case, *Limax* learns to avoid (with an appropriate conditioning) the physical mixtures (*AB*), while it still is attracted to the individual components *A* and *B*. In the latter case, it learns to avoid *A*, *B*, and the physical mixture, *AB*.

The second of these experiments reflects a problem present in the natural environment. Convectively moving air is not well mixed, and individual 'packets' of air moving sequentially by the antennae of *Limax* convey a much more detailed picture of the objects of the odour world than would completely mixed air. *Limax* should be chiefly concerned with trying to reconstruct the nature of the distal odour objects, and for this the analysis of the time fluctuations due to the only partially mixed air is an invaluable information source. In this context, the learning and discrimination exhibited in the stripe experiment exemplify an important aspect of *Limax* perception. *Limax* must be able to process and compare odourant fluctuations which occur on the time scale of one second or so in order to make the observed discriminations. An ability to use the fluctuations in time of the odour on a similar time scale is also essential to determining the direction of an odour source by a headwaving behaviour. The temporal nature of this directional olfaction problem must require an appropriate temporal character to the *Limax* nervous system processing in order that appropriate abstractions are made from time-dependent signals.

Thus in going from an idea of association to a real system, even in a simple problem like olfaction, many new issues arise, whose analysis requires additional details and wetware. There seems to be great importance to time dependences, oscillation, and the ability to process signals in time. I was originally mystified by the work of Walter Freeman, which emphasised the oscillatory character of the olfactory bulb of mammals. But the use of time appears a natural and simple way to deal with some of the real computational and hardware problems which characterise an olfactory environment.

Note added in proof

For reviews of this style of modeling and computation, see Hopfield, J. J. & Tank, D. W., *Science*, **233**, 625 (1986); and D. W. Tank & J. J. Hopfield, *Scientific Am.*, **257**, 104 (1987).

Acknowledgement

The author thanks Alan Gelperin and Jessica Hopfield for conversations on this problem. The manuscript was prepared while the author was visiting the Institute for Theoretical Physics (UCSB). The research was supported in part by NSF #PCM8406049.

References

(1) Sivilotti, M., Emmerling, M. & Mead, C. A., *1985 Conference on Very Large Scale Integration*, H. Fuchs, ed., Computer Science Press, Rockville, Maryland, p. 329 (1985).

(2) Graf, H. P. & DeVegvar, P., *Proceedings of the ISSCC*, New York, February (1987).

(3) Graf, H. P., Jackel, L., Howard, R., Staughn, B., Denker, J., Hubbard, W., Tennant, D. & Schwartz, D., *Proceedings of the Snowbird Conference*, 'Neural networks for computing,' J. Denker, ed., American Institute of Physics (1986).

(4) Gelperin, A., *Science*, **189**, 567 (1975), in *Neuroethology and Behavioral Physiology*, F. Huber & M. Markl, eds., Springer-Verlag, p. 189 (1983). Culligan, N. & Gelperin, A., *Brain Research*, **304**, 207 (1984).

(5) Sahley, C. L., Gelperin, A. & Rudy, J. W., *Proc. Natl. Acad. Sci. USA*, **78**, 640 (1981). Sahley, C. L., Rudy, J. W. & Gelperin, A., *J. Comp. Physiol.*, **144**, 1 (1981).

(6) This work is reviewed in Gelperin, A., Hopfield, J. J. & Tank, D. W., in *Model Neural Networks and Behavior*, A. I. Selverston, ed. Plenum Press, New York (1985).

(7) A much more detailed understanding of the neuroanatomical basis for behavioural choices is available in the simpler *mollusc Pleurobranchaea californica*. See London, J. A. & Gillette, R., *Proc. Natl. Acad. Sci., USA*, **83**, 4058 (1986); also Mpitsos, G. J. & Cohan, C. S., *J. Neurobiol.* (in press).

(8) Hopfield, J. J., *Proc. Natl. Acad. Sci. USA*, **79**, 2554 (1982); Sompolinsky, H. & Kanter, I., *Phys. Rev. Lett.*, **57**, 2861 (1986); Kleinfeld, D., *Proc. Natl. Acad. Sci., USA*, **83**, 9469 (1986).

(9) There are extensive rhythms in mammalian olfactory processing systems, both in the olfactory bulb (see, for example, reviews by Freeman of his own and others' research in *Perspectives in Biology and Medicine*, **24**, 561 (1981), and in *Brain Theory*, Palm, J. G. & Actsen, A., eds. (1986)), and in olfactory prepiriform cortex (see, for example, Haberley, L. B. and Shepherd, G. M., *Neurophysiology*, **36**, 789 (1973); Haberley, L. B. and Bower, J. M., *J. Neurophysiol.*, **51**, 90 (1984)).

(10) Recent modelling work (Shaw, G. L., Silverman, D. J. & Pearson, J. C., *Proc. Natl. Acad. Sci., USA*, **82**, 2364 (1985), based on cortical electrophysiology, has emphasised the properties of cyclic patterns for memory and recall but has not yet coupled these patterns to a particular biological computational system.

(11) A discussion of the analytical abilities of human olfaction may be found in Beets, M. G. J., *Structure-Activity Relationships in Human Chemoreception*, Applied Science Publishers, London (1978); Some discussions of specificity (analytic) versus patterning (synthetic) views can be found by Doving, K. B., in *Taste and Smell in Vertebrates*, G. E. W. Wolfstenholm & J. Knight, eds. J. A. Churchill, Pub., London (1970), 197 ff; pp. 221–2; Dzendolet, E., in *Olfaction and Taste* III, C. Pfefferman, ed., Rockefeller Univ. Press, New York (1969), 420 ff.

(12) Gelperin, A. & Hopfield, J. F. (private communication).

27

Development of feature-analyzing cells and their columnar organization in a layered self-adaptive network

RALPH LINSKER

27.1 Introduction

Many features of the functional architecture of the mammalian visual system have been experimentally identified during the past 25 years. Among the most striking of these features is the presence of layers of orientation-selective cells – cells whose response to an edge or bar in the appropriate portion of visual field is sensitive to the local orientation of the input. These cells are organized in bands or 'columns' of cells of the same or similar orientation preference. The preferred orientation varies roughly monotonically, but with frequent breaks and reversals, as one traverses the cell layer. Orientation-selective cells, organized in this fashion, are found in cat, monkey, and other mammalian systems. In macaque monkey, they are present at birth.

I have found that several salient features of mammalian visual system architecture – including orientation-selective cells and columns – emerge in a multilayered network of cells whose connections develop, one layer at a time, according to a synaptic modification rule of Hebb type. The theoretical base is biologically plausible, none of the assumptions is specific to visual processing, no orientation preferences are specified to the system at any stage, and the features emerge even in the absence of environmental input.

The development of this system is discussed in detail, and references to experimental work are provided, in a series of three papers (Linsker, 1986*a*,*b*,*c*). Here, I shall briefly review the network description and results, and shall illustrate and discuss a few of the features in more detail than has previously appeared. Very little mathematics is required to follow the discussion; the exception is the section, 'Connection with physical systems,' which is largely self-contained.

27.2 A modular (layered) self-adaptive network

The network consists of several layers $(A, B, \ldots)$ of cells. Each cell of layer M $(M = B, C, \ldots)$ receives synaptic inputs from an overlying neighborhood of cells of the previous layer L. The positions (in layer L) of the N_M synaptic inputs to each M-cell are randomly chosen from a distribution whose synaptic density decreases monotonically with distance r from the point overlying the cell's location. A Gaussian synaptic density, exp $(-r^2/r_M^2)$, is used for calculations. Each cell has a linear-summation response function. That is, the output activity $F_n^{M\pi}$ of an M-cell (the cell is indexed by n) is a linear function of its input activities, with the input activity $F_{\text{pre}(ni)}^{L\pi}$ at the ith synapse of cell n being weighted by a connection strength c_{ni};

$$F_n^{M\pi} = R_a + R_b \sum_i c_{ni} F_{\text{pre}(ni)}^{L\pi}. \tag{1}$$

Here $R_{a,b}$ are constants $(R_b > 0)$, and π (for 'presentation') labels the particular set of input activities at a given time, and the resulting response.

The c-values change with time according to a Hebb-type rule that 'rewards' correlations between pre- and postsynaptic activity:

$$(\Delta c_{ni})^\pi = k_a + k_b \times (F_n^{M\pi} - F_0^M) \times (F_{\text{pre}(ni)}^{L\pi} - F_0^L), \tag{2}$$

where $k_{a,b}$, F_0^M, and F_0^L are constants $(k_b > 0)$. We assume that the connection strength changes very little with each presentation.

Each c-value is, in addition, constrained to lie within an allowed range, and saturates at its extreme value if the modification rule (eqn (3)) would otherwise drive it beyond this value (at a given time step). The allowed range is either taken to be (i) $(0, 1)$ for the fraction n_{EM} of synapses that are excitatory and $(-1, 0)$ for the remaining, inhibitory, synapses; or (ii) $(n_{EM} - 1, n_{EM})$ for all synapses. Both cases lead to development of the same cell types and organization; the first is more biologically realistic.

From this base we have derived (Linsker, 1986a) a differential equation for the development of the c-values. Each M-cell (indexed by n) develops independently of the others, since at this stage there is no lateral coupling between M-cells. We have:

$$\dot{c}_{ni} = k_1 + (1/N_M) \sum_j (Q_{\text{pre}(ni),\text{pre}(nj)}^L + k_2) c_{nj}, \tag{3}$$

where 'pre(ni)' denotes the L-cell that is presynaptic to the ith synapse of postsynaptic M-cell n, and Q_{ab}^L is proportional to the two-point autocorrelation function of layer-L activity at the L-cells a and b. We have shown (Linsker, 1986b) that

$$Q_{nm}^M \propto \sum_i \sum_j Q_{\text{pre}(ni),\text{pre}(mj)}^L c_{ni} c_{mj}; \tag{4}$$

this allows us to compute Q^M once we know Q^L and the transfer function (given by the $\{c_{ni}\}$) from layer L to M.

We start with layer-A activity that is random, spontaneous, and spatially uncorrelated (from cell to cell). The Q_{ab}^A function for such an activity ensemble is 1 if a and b are the same cell, and 0 otherwise. This is an appropriate starting point in the absence of visual input to the system. We consider this case in order to understand a possible basis for the prenatal emergence of orientation-selective cells in certain primates. (See Linsker (1986a) for details.) If environmental input is present during maturation, the ensemble of such inputs is used to compute the appropriate Q^A function.

Our procedure for calculating the mature c-values for a set (layer) of M-cells, given the Q^L function, is as follows: (1) Choose parameter values k_1, k_2, n_{EM}, and r_M for the layer. (2) For each cell, randomly choose synaptic positions according to the Gaussian density distribution $\exp(-r^2/r_M^2)$. (If we take a fraction of the synapses to be excitatory, and the rest inhibitory, we assume the same arborization radius r_M applies to both. This is to avoid introducing more parameter dependencies than necessary at this stage of the analysis.) (3) For each cell, randomly choose an initial c-value for each synapse. (4) Solve eqn (3) (subject to the saturation limits on the c-values) for the time development of the cs, until all cs have reached their final values; these values define the 'mature morphology' of the cells. (5) Study the random cell-to-cell variations in mature morphology. If the morphology is robust against the random choices of synaptic position and c-value – that is, if the M-layer is of substantially uniform morphology – then we proceed to calculate Q^M and to repeat the procedure for the next layer. Computations are greatly simplified, and theoretical understanding enhanced, when it is possible to use the idealization – for calculating Q^M – that all M-cells are of identical, rather than merely similar, morphology. We find that the possible mature morphologies, for each layer as it matures in turn, are quite limited, and that there are parameter regimes within which the mature morphology is substantially determined by the set of four parameter values (i.e., is uniform for the cells of a layer, when the parameter values are substantially the same for all cells of the layer).

27.3 Emergence of spatial-opponent cells

For the A-to-B connections, the morphologic options are: (1) All cs reach their excitatory limit (all B-cells are 'all-excitatory'). (2) All B-cells become 'all-inhibitory'. (3) For each B-cell, some cs reach their excitatory limit, and the others reach their inhibitory limit ('mixed' case), with no segregation of the arborization into excitatory and inhibitory spatial regions. (A fourth case, leading to a nonuniform B-layer, is discussed in Linsker 1986a.)

Suppose we choose the parameter regime corresponding to the first ('all-excitatory') choice. (The argument is identical for the 'all-inhibitory' case. If the 'mixed' case is chosen, layer-B activity will be random and uncorrelated from cell to cell, like that of layer A, and the above analysis will substantially repeat itself when we pass to layer C.) Then, apart from random fluctuations discussed in Linsker, 1986a, Q_{nm}^B is a Gaussian function $Q^B(s) = \exp(-s^2/2r_B^2)$ of the separation s between cells n and m.

We now solve for the development of the B-to-C connections (i.e., $L = B, M = C$) by the same procedure. The possible morphologic options for the cells of layer C are: (1) All-excitatory or all-inhibitory, as in layer B. (2) Circularly-symmetric cells with excitatory core and inhibitory surround (the 'ON-center' spatial-opponent cell), or with inhibitory core and excitatory surround ('OFF-center' cell). (3) An eccentric excitatory core with inhibitory surround (or the reverse). (4) An extreme form of case 3 in which the boundary between the two regions is an arc, or a straight line, passing near or through the cell's center.

Cells whose receptive field is of spatial-opponent type are well-known experimentally, and are found first in the bipolar-cell layer of retina. Our purpose here is not to provide a detailed model of retinal development; for example, the retinal gross architecture is more complicated than the A-to-B-to-C connectivity of our network. Our goal is rather to explore how feature-analyzing cells that are observed biologically, and have functional significance, can emerge even in a simple network of the class we call 'modular (layered) self-adaptive networks' (Linsker, 1986a). The feature-analyzing property in the case of spatial-opponent cells is spot contrast: an 'ON-center' cell responds maximally to a centered spot of illumination against a dark background.

Fig. 27.1 shows a time sequence of 'snapshots' of an 'ON-center' cell at different stages in its development, starting with random c-values, then showing the emergence of an enlarging excitatory core, and finally the mature excitatory core and inhibitory surround. The reason why this segregation of regions occurs, is discussed in Linsker, 1986a. Also, note that all c-values (or – a technical point that is unimportant here – all but one c-value per cell) mature to reach an extreme value – either the

excitatory or inhibitory limit for each synapse – rather than an intermediate value. This is a general feature of the development eqn (3), and
is proved in Linsker, 1986a.

There is a parameter regime for 'ON-center' cell formation, such that
essentially all C-cells sharing the same parameter values will become
'ON-center' cells, provided there are at least several hundred synaptic

Fig. 27.1. Development of an 'ON-center' layer-C cell. Parameters are $n_{EC} = 0.5$,
$r_C/r_B = \sqrt{5}$, $k_1 = 0.35$, $k_2 = -3$. $N_C = 800$ synapses (400 each excitatory and
inhibitory) are randomly placed according to a Gaussian distribution, and symbols
indicate their c-values: $-1 < c < -0.9$ ('O'); $-0.9 < c < -0.5$ (midsized circle);
$-0.5 < c < -0.05$ (small circle); $0.05 < c < 0.5$ ('+'); $0.5 < c < 0.9$ ('x');
$0.9 < c < 1$ (dot). Synapses with small $|c|$ (less than 0.05) are not plotted.
(a) Initial connection strengths (random, from normal distribution with mean =
0.5 for excitatory synapses and -0.5 for inhibitory synapses; s.d. = 0.2).
(b, c) Intermediate stages of development. Central synapses reach excitatory
limit, and this 'core' region expands. (d) Mature state.

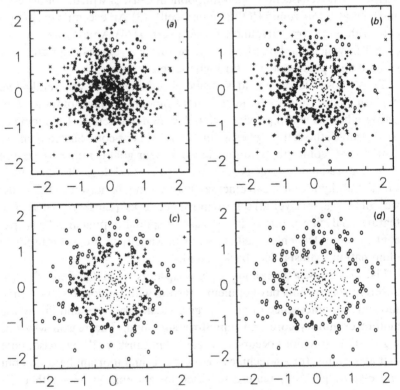

inputs per cell. That is, the mature morphology is uniform across the layer, despite cell-to-cell random variations in initial conditions. Cases in which different subsets of cells within the same layer have different sets of parameter values can be treated within our framework, but are not considered here.

27.4 Emergence of orientation-selective cells

Let us choose layer C to consist of 'ON-center' cells. Then we find that the Q^C function is of 'Mexican-hat' form (Fig. 27.2). The morphologic options for postsynaptic cell development under the influence of a 'Mexican-hat' Q-function include: (1) cells having alternating striped excitatory and inhibitory regions (running across the input arborization of the postsynaptic cell) with the stripes running in a direction that is arbitrary for each postsynaptic cell, and with a stripe boundary passing near or through the cell's center (Fig. 1 of Linsker, 1986b); (2) cells having a central excitatory band flanked by two inhibitory lobes (or the reverse)

Fig. 27.2. Activity autocorrelation functions $Q^{C,D,E,F}$ (s) (shallow solid curve, dotted curve, light dashed curve, and bold dot-dashed curve, respectively), and the Bessel function J_0 $(1.92s)$ (solid curve with deep minimum), versus the distance s between the two cells. Note progressive deepening of Mexican-hat minimum from Q^C to Q^F. The Bessel function would be the activity autocorrelation function for an ensemble of patterns each of which is a regular sinusoidal grating of arbitrary orientation and phase. See Linsker, 1986b for significance of the Bessel function, and for parameter values used to derive $Q^{C,D,E,F}$.

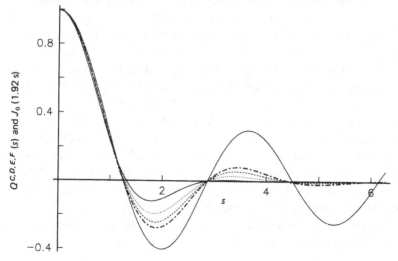

– we call these 'bilobed' cells (Fig. 27.3(*c*)); (3) 'ON-' and 'OFF-center' cells as in layer C; (4) cells with excitatory and inhibitory regions with a boundary passing through or near the cell's center, as in layer C; (5) circularly symmetric cells with excitatory core, inhibitory surrounding annulus, and excitatory outer region, or the reverse; (6) morphologies having an intermediate degree of striped (or banded) vs. circularly-symmetric character; e.g., cells of type 5 that have an ovoid core, or a core that 'breaks through' to the outer region, resulting in a 'C'-shaped inhibitory ring against an excitatory background; (7) cells with more than two inhibitory 'islands' (often three, hence 'trilobed' cells) in an excitatory 'sea', or the reverse.

The 'bilobed' cell type, and the type having excitatory and inhibitory regions separated by a straight boundary through the cell's center, give receptive fields (patterns of response to point illumination in layer A) similar to those described by Hubel & Wiesel (1962) for 'simple cells' in the cat.

Suppose the 'Mexican hat' Q-function has a shallow minimum – as in the case of Q^C in Fig. 27.2. Then only some of the morphologic options listed above may be available, and others may not be robust against random cell-to-cell variations (e.g., one can see an admixture of 'bilobed' and 'trilobed' cells, or of 'bilobed' and 'type 5' cells, in the mature layer). However, the 'ON-' and 'OFF-center' regimes are robust and lead to a layer of uniform morphology, even for the relatively shallow Q^C-function.

There is a way that our system can develop a uniform layer of 'bilobed' cells, robust against random variations. Choose parameter values for layer D to lie in the regime that produces 'ON-center' opponent D-cells. Then the Q^D function is again of 'Mexican-hat' form, but has a deeper minimum (relative to its peak) than does Q^C. This process can be repeated (Fig. 27.2). The Q^F function (resulting from a series of four 'ON-center' layers) is of sufficiently pronounced 'Mexican-hat' character that we obtain – in layer G – 'bilobed' and other cell types whose morphology is robust against random cell-to-cell variations. Figs. 27.3–27.5 (to be discussed) are based on calculations using this Q^F function. Fig. 27.3 shows a time sequence of developmental 'snapshots' for a cell in the bilobed regime. This sequence is analogous to that of Fig. 27.1 for an 'ON-center' cell in the earlier layer C, but we have omitted the initial (random-*c*-value) figure of the series.

It is interesting to note that some of the intermediate configurations (Figs. 27.3(*a,b*)) en route to the mature 'bilobed' cell themselves resemble other allowed mature cell types for this layer (in different parameter regimes). Fig. 27.3(a) is of 'type 5' (above), and Fig. 27.3(b) is of 'type 6'. In this case, at least, ontogeny recapitulates the sequence of mature states that would arise if we increased one of the parameters (k_1), holding the other parameters fixed.

Fig. 27.3. Development of a 'bilobed' orientation-selective layer-G cell. Parameters are $n_{EG} = 0.5$, $r_G/r_F = 1.8$, $k_1 = 0.6$, $k_2 = -3$. Here c-value limits are $(-0.5, +0.5)$ for all 800 synapses (same 'bilobed' arrangement also emerges if there are 400 synapses each of excitatory and of inhibitory type, as in Fig. 27.1). Symbols are as in Fig. 27.1, except that values of $2c$ rather than c are plotted (note $2c$ ranges from -1 to $+1$). Synaptic positions same as in Fig. 27.1. Initial c-values (not shown) are random normal values with mean = 0, s.d. = 0.2. (a) Early stage of development; excitatory central region, inhibitory ring, excitatory outer region. (b) Intermediate stage; central and outermost regions join to form 'C'-shaped excitatory region. (c) Mature state.

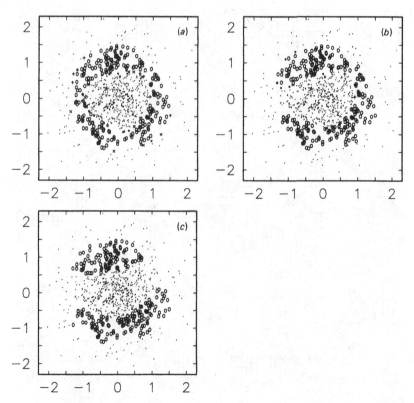

424 *Ralph Linsker*

27.5 Emergence of orientation columns

Let us now repeat the development of layer G, but with lateral G-to-G connections as well as feedforward F-to-G connections. We have found that if the lateral connections are excitatory and form prior to the feedforward connections, then (under certain conditions discussed in Linsker, 1986c) the resulting G-layer consists of 'bilobed' orientation-selective cells organized into regions of similar orientation preference.

Fig. 27.4. Orientation columns obtained by near-minimizing eqn (9) on an 80 × 80 square array with periodic boundary conditions. Each site of the array is 'stained' as follows, according to the orientation preference θ (measured counterclockwise from the vertical) of the cells at that site: θ between 9–45° (dot); 45–81° (circle); 81–117° (+); 117–153° (X); 153–189° (blank). The Q^G and $\varrho(d)$ functions used, and the distance (relative to r_G) between adjacent grid positions, are the same as for Fig. 2 of Linsker, 1986c. The random starting conditions (as well as the array size) are different, so we obtain a different, but qualitatively similar and also globally near-optimal, pattern here.

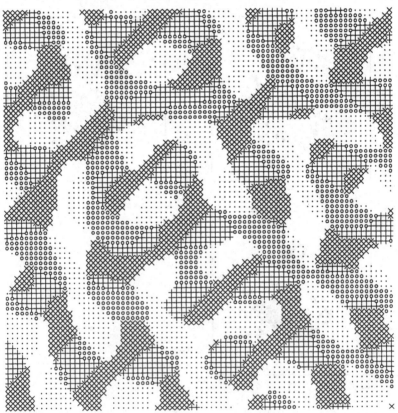

An example of this computed columnar organization is shown in Figs. 27.4 and Fig. 27.5, and agrees qualitatively with experimental findings in macaque monkey.

The method by which Figs. 27.4 and 27.5 are computed is described in detail in Linsker, 1986c, and the parameter values used here are the same as in that reference. The random initial conditions are different, leading to a pattern of orientation columns that differs in detail from the pattern shown in Linsker, 1986c, but has the same qualitative features.

Fig. 27.5. 'Needle' plot of orientations for the same pattern as Fig. 27.4. Any of ten θ values (spaced by 18°) are allowed at each site. In addition to the orientation 'needle' at each site, a line segment is interposed as a marker wherever two adjacent sites (one on either side of the marker segment) have orientations differing by at least 54°. Most of the short markers (those that traverse one to a few sites) indicate the positions of vortices (see text). The longer markers indicate linear 'fractures' across which the orientation changes discontinuously.

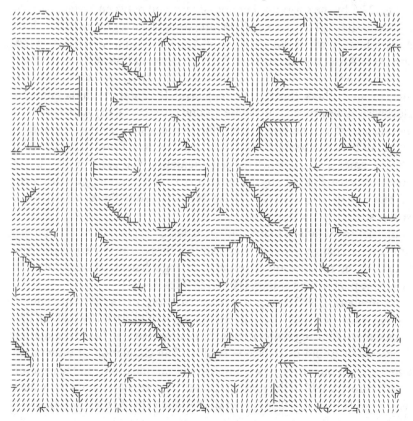

Fig. 27.4 shows an assembly of mature *G*-cells that have been 'stained' to indicate the orientation of the 'bilobed' cell axis for each *G*-cell. This axis orientation is the same as the local orientation of a bar or edge test stimulus that would evoke the maximum response from the given cell (Linsker, 1986*b,c*).

Fig. 27.5 shows explicitly (as an array of oriented 'needles') the cell orientations at each site in the same assembly of mature G-cells whose 'staining' pattern was indicated in Fig. 27.4. Using these two forms of presentation (the 'stain' and 'needle' maps) we can see that : (1) There are iso-orientation regions. Some of these regions are elongated along the direction of their preferred cell orientation (Linsker, 1986*c*); some are more blob-like in shape. (2) Adjacent regions are generally of similar cell orientation. (3) There are points (or small regions comprising a few adjacent sites) about which the orientation varies rapidly – through 180° as we trace a circle of 360° around the point. We call these points 'vortices' to indicate the form of this 'flow'. The locations of vortices are identified in Fig. 27.5 by the short marker lines interposed between certain pairs of adjacent sites. (The marker lines are straight or zigzagged; the short marker lines to which we are referring run for a distance of one to a few sites.) (4) Around some vortices the flow of orientation angle is 'positive' (orientation shifts clockwise as we proceed clockwise around the vortex), and around others the flow is 'negative' (orientation shifts counter-clockwise as we proceed clockwise around the vortex). (5) As we proceed around an iso-orientation region, the vortices we encounter generally alternate between being positive and negative. (6) There are occasional linear segments across which the cell orientation changes abruptly. These are identified in Fig. 27.5 by the longer marker lines (running for distances of more than a few sites). These segments sometimes connect two vortices.

Blasdel & Salama (1986) find such linear segments of abrupt cell orientation change – which they call 'fractures' – in their images, and breaks in the progression of orientation angle have long been found in electrode penetration studies (Hubel & Wiesel, 1977).

Braitenberg (1985) proposed that an array of organizing centers, around each of which the cell orientation would vary (by 360° as one circled the organizing center), could be arranged so as to fit the orientation progressions found in electrode studies. The circulation of orientation about each of our vortices is reminiscent of this idea, though the rotation is only through 180° in the present case. (The particular parameter values used here (Linsker, 1986*c*) generate bilobed cells that are substantially bilaterally symmetric, so that rotation of the cell axis through 180° maps a cell onto itself.) The more important distinction between our results and Braitenberg's proposal is that we have introduced no 'organizing centers' into the layer – *all* of the structure has emerged, in an initially featureless isotropic and homogeneous layer, by a symmetry-breaking mechanism.

27.6 Connection with physical systems – an energy formulation, globally near-optimal states, and spin lattices

Starting with the development eqn (3), let us define an 'energy' or 'objective function' for the connections to a single postsynaptic M-cell indexed by n:

$$E_n = E_n^k + E_n^Q, \tag{5}$$

where

$$E_n^k \equiv -k_1 g_n - (k_2/2) g_n^2, \tag{6}$$

$$E_n^Q \equiv -(1/2N_M^2) \sum_i \sum_j Q_{\mathrm{pre}(ni),\mathrm{pre}(nj)}^L \, c_{ni} \, c_{nj}, \tag{7}$$

and

$$g_n \equiv \left(\sum_j c_{nj} \right) / N_M .$$

Then E_n is a function of $\{c_{n1}, c_{n2}, \ldots\}$ such that

$$\dot{c}_{ni} = -N_M \, \partial E_n / \partial c_{ni} \tag{8}$$

for all i.

The 'configuration space' for a single M-cell is, by definition, the abstract space having N_M dimensions, one for each synaptic input. Any set of values $\{c_{n1}, c_{n2}, \ldots\}$ is represented by a point in this space whose ith coordinate has value c_{ni}. During development, the M-cell thus traces a path in the configuration space. The significance of eqn (8) is that it shows that this path is the path of locally steepest descent – i.e., of gradient descent – of the E_n function, at all times. This ensures that the final state of the system is a local minimum of the E_n function.

As we noted above, all (or all but one) mature c-values for each cell are extremal; that is, lie at their excitatory or inhibitory limit. Thus the mature state of the M-cell is guaranteed to lie essentially at a vertex of the configuration space, and at a local minimum of E_n.

We have further found empirically (with an exception when $k_2 > 0$ (Linsker, 1986b)) that the mature states calculated using eqn (3) are not only local minima of E_n, but are *globally* near-minimal as well. This means that the same mature morphology is obtained whether we solve

eqn (3) for the explicit development (starting with various random
c-values) or instead compute the global near-minima of E_n over all
configurations whose c-values are extremal. Near the boundary between
two morphologic regimes (in parameter space), both morphologies are
found to have similar, and near-minimal, energy.

Thus there is a detailed correspondence between the computation of
mature cell morphology and the computation of the ground states of a
spin lattice whose allowed spins have values $n_{EM} - 1$ and n_{EM}, and whose
sites (corresponding to synaptic positions for a single postsynaptic cell)
are placed according to a Gaussian density distribution. The E_n^k term
depends upon the spin configuration (the choice of cs) only through the
average value g_n of the cs; hence it plays a role similar to an external
magnetic field interaction energy (although E_n^k contains terms quadratic,
as well as linear, in g_n). When $k_{1,2}$ are such that E_n^k dominates the total
energy E_n, then E_n^k-minimization essentially sets the mature value of g_n,
and the mature morphology is that arrangement of c-values that
minimizes E_n^0 subject to this constraint on g_n.

Some features of the mature morphologies we have found can be
readily understood in terms of global energy minimization. In layer C
(formation of 'ON-center' opponent cells), the E_n^Q term acts like a surface
tension term, at least when r_C/r_B is large, so that the spatial scale
(proportional to r_B) of the Gaussian $Q^B(s)$ is small compared with the
arborization radius r_C. That is, E_n^Q is minimized by decreasing the number
of pairs of nearby unlike spins (for the case $n_{EC} = 0.5$). This is an
isoperimetric problem, similar to minimizing the boundary of a soap
bubble (in two dimensions) of a given area – except complicated by the
fact that the area contributions are weighted by the synaptic density
$\exp(-r^2/r_c^2)$, and the boundary term is weighted by the square of the
synaptic density (E_n^Q is quadratic in the cs). The 'bubble' in the case of an
'ON-center' cell is the excitatory core.

In the case of orientation-selective cells, the mature state has various
degrees of circularly-symmetric and striped (or banded) character,
depending upon the parameter regime. This is explained in terms of
energy minimization in Linsker, 1986b.

Finally, the pattern of orientation columns results from the global
near-minimization of a function that has the form

$$E = -\sum_{\mathbf{x}} \sum_{\mathbf{y}} \varrho(|\mathbf{x} - \mathbf{y}|)Q^G(\theta_{\mathbf{x}}, \theta_{\mathbf{y}}, \mathbf{y} - \mathbf{x}). \qquad (9)$$

(See Linsker, 1986c for derivation and details.) Here the configuration is
characterized by the values of orientation angle $\theta_{\mathbf{x}}$ at each site $\mathbf{x}$ on a

square lattice, and $\varrho(d)$ is the density of lateral connections of length d. The function $Q^G(\theta, \theta', \mathbf{d})$ is a complicated function, derived explicitly from our network development rules (Linsker, 1986c), that (given θ) favors θ' to be: similar to θ when $\mathbf{d}$ is parallel to the orientation θ; similar to θ when $\mathbf{d}$ is orthogonal to θ but small in magnitude (i.e., near-neighbor case); and orthogonal to θ when $\mathbf{d}$ is orthogonal to θ and of intermediate magnitude (i.e., midrange-neighbor case). This Q^G behavior (as a function of θ' and $\mathbf{d}$ for fixed θ) can be loosely described as 'Mexican-hat'-like in the direction orthogonal to θ, and Gaussian in the direction parallel to θ (Linsker, 1986c). The physical analogue of this network development problem is thus the problem of computing ground states in a spin lattice with a particular type of orientation-dependent interaction Hamiltonian (energy function). The interaction energy between two sites (at given $\mathbf{d}$) is qualitatively similar to a $\cos^2(\theta - \theta')$ coupling, but depends upon the angles between the displacement $\mathbf{d}$ and the orientations θ and θ' as well.

27.7 Why the Hebb rule induces formation of feature-analyzing cells: A principle of constrained optimal inference

The Hebb-type rule causes the c-values to develop so as to minimize E_n^Q for given g_n (eqns (5–7)). What does this mean from an information processing standpoint? The statistical variance of the postsynaptic activity $F_n^{M\pi}$ is $\langle (F_n^{M\pi} - \bar{F}_n^M)^2 \rangle_\pi \propto Q_{nn}^M \propto -E_n^Q$, where we use eqns (4) and (7) and where the overbar and $\langle \ldots \rangle_\pi$ both denote the average over an ensemble of presentations. Therefore, minimizing E_n^Q means maximizing the output activity variance for given g_n, subject to the c-value limits.

In statistics, the method of principal component analysis consists of choosing values c_i (subject to $\Sigma c_i^2 = 1$) such that, for a given ensemble of input vectors $\{\mathbf{F}^{L\pi}\}$ (where each $\mathbf{F}^{L\pi}$ stands for the vector $(F_1^{L\pi}, F_2^{L\pi}, \ldots)$), the variance of the projected value $F^{M\pi} = \Sigma F_i^{L\pi} c_i$ is maximized. For data exhibiting structure (e.g., clustering), this choice of projection can tend to highlight 'interesting' features of the data. Our Hebb-type rule is performing a very similar role – the only difference is in the constraint subject to which the output activity variance is being maximized. (Oja (1982) has described a neural model that is explicitly designed to perform principal component analysis.)

Furthermore, suppose we make an estimate of the values of the inputs $\{F_i^{L\pi}\}$ (for each π), given the output $F^{M\pi}$ and otherwise knowing only the ensemble-averaged values $\bar{F}_i^L$. (For notational ease, we have dropped the M-cell index n here, and refer to $F_{\text{pre}(ni)}^{L\pi}$ simply as $F_i^{L\pi}$.) We know the value of the projection of the $\mathbf{F}^{L\pi}$ vector in the direction of the $\mathbf{c}$

vector; it is a linear function of $F^{M\pi}$ (eqn (1)). Let us estimate the projection of the $\mathbf{F}^{L\pi}$ vector onto the plane normal to the $\mathbf{c}$ vector, to be just the projection of the mean vector $\overline{\mathbf{F}}^L$ onto the same plane (this treatment is oversimplified). What is the mean-squared error incurred by this method of estimation? It is just the variance of the projection of the $\mathbf{F}^{L\pi}$ vector onto this plane. That quantity equals $\langle|(\mathbf{F}^{L\pi} - \overline{\mathbf{F}}^L)|^2\rangle$ (which is independent of the choice of $\mathbf{c}$ vector) minus a quantity proportional (for the cases discussed in this paper) to the variance of $F^{M\pi}$ (eqn (1)). We conclude that because the Hebb-type rule generates a cell whose c-values *maximize* the variance of $F^{M\pi}$ (subject to the stated constraint), the mature c-values also *minimize* the mean-squared error resulting from estimating the vector of input activities from the output activity in this way.

A more detailed analysis using optimal estimation theory shows that the minimum possible mean-squared inference error is achieved when the cell's output activity variance is maximized subject to $\Sigma\,c_i^2 = 1$. A suitable Hebb rule thus generates a cell whose output allows one to optimally infer its input activity values. This result may provide insight into the role the Hebb rule play with respect to information processing in networks.

27.8 Concluding remarks

The excitement of the present enterprise arises not only from its success in generating some of the key features of the observed functional architecture of the mammalian visual system, but also from the possibility that we may be far from exhausting the capacity of a simple, and biologically plausible, developmental program to generate architectural structures that have useful information-processing function and that match biological observations.

It is certain that some of the simplifying features of the network analyzed here will have to be modified. Non-linear cell response is known to be biologically significant, and the functioning of certain cell types (e.g., Hubel–Wiesel 'complex' cells) may demand this property. Gross architectures more complicated than our simple 'A-to-B-to-C . . .' form will need to be analyzed. Whatever rules are found to govern synaptic modification in biological systems will undoubtedly be more complicated than the one we have considered here, although the key feature of modifying connection strengths in relation to correlations between signaling activities may well survive. All of these types of complications can be incorporated within our modular self-adaptive network approach.

Also, it is possible that some features whose activity-dependent emergence we have demonstrated in our system, may have more of a 'hard-wired' (prespecified) character in certain biological systems. For example, one could obtain 'ON-center' cells by prespecifying the arborization to be broader for inhibitory than for excitatory synaptic inputs. An attractive feature of our approach (for substantially feedforward gross architectures) is that the development of a later layer depends only upon the ensemble statistical properties of activity in the preceding layer – and not upon the means by which these properties arise. Thus the emergence of orientation-selective cells and columns can occur as described here, regardless of how the Mexican-hat Q-function is produced within the previous layer.

What is striking is the power of this approach to generate many of the observed salient features of visual system architecture – in even the simplest incarnation of a modular self-adaptive network. Furthermore, since none of our assumptions is specific to visual processing, we may expect the same sets of morphologic options to apply to at least the early stages of perceptual systems other than the visual. How far the ideas developed here can take us toward understanding the development and mature state of neural networks within and beyond the first several stages of a perceptual system is an exciting question for future work.

References

Blasdel, G. G. & Salama, G. (1986). 'Voltage-sensitive dyes reveal a modular organization in monkey striate cortex.' *Nature*, **321**, 579–85.

Braitenberg, V. (1985). 'Charting the visual cortex.' In *Cerebral Cortex*, vol. 3, eds. E. G. Jones & A. Peters, pp. 379–414. New York: Plenum Press.

Hubel, D. H. & Wiesel, T. N. (1962). 'Receptive fields, binocular interaction and functional architecture in the cat's visual cortex.' *Journal of Physiology*, **160**, 106–54.

Hubel, D. H. & Wiesel, T. N. (1977). 'Functional architecture of macaque monkey visual cortex (Ferrier lecture).' *Proceedings of the Royal Society (London)*, **B 198**, 1–59.

Linsker, R. (1986a). 'From basic network principles to neural architecture: emergence of spatial-opponent cells.' *Proceedings of the National Academy of Sciences (USA)*, **83**, 7508–12.

Linsker, R. (1986b). 'From basic network principles to neural architecture: emergence of orientation-selective cells.' *Proceedings of the National Academy of Sciences (USA)*, **83**, 8390–94.

Linsker, R. (1986c). 'From basic network principles to neural architecture: emergence of orientation columns.' *Proceedings of the National Academy of Sciences (USA)*, **83**, 8779–83 .

Oja, E. (1982). 'A simplified neuron model as a principal component analyzer.' *Journal of Mathematical Biology*, **15**, 267–73.

28

Reafferent stimulation: a mechanism for late vision and cognitive processes

E. HARTH, K. P. UNNIKRISHNAN, and A. S. PANDYA

28.1 Introduction

Cognition, according to Ulric Neisser, 'refers to all processes by which the sensory input is transformed, reduced, elaborated, stored, recovered, and used. It is concerned with these processes even when they operate in the absence of relevent stimulation, as in images and hallucinations' (Neisser, 1966). To discover some of the neural mechanisms operating in these processes remains one of the great challenges of neuroscience.

Significant progress has been made in analyzing the mapping and coding processes that occur in the first few stages of mammalian vision. These processes of so-called *early vision* involve neural mechanisms that sort out geometrical features, heighten contrast, emphasize contours, and help determine shape and motion of objects (Marr & Poggio, 1979; Marr & Hildreth, 1980; Marr, 1982).

Cognition, as Neisser defines it, must go beyond these early processes, utilizing not only innate circuitry, but bringing the full richness of stored experience to bear on the new sensory information. The time scale of such processes must extend from the order of a hundred milliseconds to seconds and beyond.

28.1.1 Cognition and reafference

These *higher* and later cognitive processes are usually relegated to cortical association areas. In the present model, however, we assume that significant changes in the afferent sensory information are brought about at relatively peripheral sensory levels – the lateral geniculate nucleus in the case of vision – and that these changes play an important role in the *transformation*, *reduction*, and *elaboration* of the sensory input.

This model is in part suggested by the extensive feedback pathways, known since the days of Ramon y Cajal, and by the ascending pathways that lead from the brainstem reticular formation to areas in the cortex and neurons in the geniculate and perigeniculate areas. It is difficult to avoid the conclusion that cortical and brainstem information, thus carried to a sensory relay, must in some way *transform* the afferent sensory information. The question is only, how *specific* these transformations are, and whether they go beyond a simple raising and lowering of the general level of transmission between retina and the visual cortex.

Modification of sensory input by higher neuronal centers was first described by v. Holst & Mittelstaedt (1950) who spoke of a *principle of re-afference*. The anatomical requisites for such processes have been amply demonstrated in the corticofugal fibers connecting striate cortex to neurons in the dorsal lateral geniculate nucleus (dLGN) (Lund *et al.*, 1975; Singer, 1977; Morocco, McClurkin & Young, 1982). Other *reafferent* connections lead from perigeniculate neurons to dLGN (Ahlsén, Lindstrom & Lo, 1984; Montero & Singer, 1985) and from brainstem reticular formation back to thalamic centers (Singer, 1977; Steriade *et al.*, 1980; Ahlsén & Lo, 1982; Hughes & Mulliken, 1984). The mesencephalic reticular core also excerts strong influence on the cortex (Singer, Tretter & Cynader, 1976). Gibbs, Cohen & Broyles (1986) report direct observations of changes in the activities of retinoreceptive cells in the avian homolog of the dLGN following visual learning. Steriade, Domich & Oakson (1986) described activity changes in neurons of the nucleus reticularis thalami as well as thalamo-cortical neurons depending on the state of alertness.

These findings demonstrate that the thalamic sensory nuclei, specifically the dLGN, are more than passive relays between peripheral sensors and cortical projection areas.

28.1.2 Imagery vs abstraction

Since receptive fields of dLGN neurons are known to form a retinotopic mosaic, dLGN activity closely matches retinal images. The representation at that level may be termed *imagistic*. This is true to a lesser extent at cortical visual areas where feature analyzing systems extract various types of specific information. The representation is thus shifted from a purely *imagistic* to a more or less *propositional* character.

Cognitive psychologists are in disagreement over the degree to which imagistic or propositional codes are involved in mental activities involving recall and manipulation of remembered events. In his *six-code theory*, Owen Flanagan proposes that mental activity uses neural representations that are, to varying degrees, imagistic (using any one of the five exterosensory modalities) and sometimes purely 'abstract, propositional and quasi-linguistic' (Flanagan, 1984). This is contrasted by the *unified-code* model according to which mental representations occur solely in the abstract mode, and any subjective sensations of mentally manipulating images are the result of an *introspective trap*. Discussions of this controversy are found in Neisser (1976), Kosslyn (1980), Block (1981) and Flanagan (1984). Flanagan cites the experiments of Shepard & Metzler (1971) in support of a theory in which at least some mental activities are imagistic.

28.1.3 Assumptions of the model

We present below a model of late vision and visual imagery which is an extension of previous work (Harth, 1976; Harth & Unnikrishnan, 1985; Harth, Pandya & Unnikrishnan, 1986), together with results of computer simulations. The model is based on the following set of assumptions:

(1) Imagery and propositional representations are used to varying degrees depending on the character of the mental task; this is analogous to Flanagan's six-code theory.

(2) The neural centers involved in a mental task are principally those in which information is encoded in the appropriate representation (i.e., peripheral sensory areas in the manipulation of images such as the task reported by Shepard & Metzler (1971), speech centers in purely linguistic tasks).

(3) Activity at a given neural level is generated either by sensory inputs or by reafferent stimulation from higher cognitive centers. In general it will be a superposition of both.

(4) Neural representations elicited at a given level by *reafferent stimulation* resemble those caused by sensory input. Thus the recall of a visual stimulus will reproduce quasi-sensory activity at a neural level selected according to the degree of realism or abstractness of such recall.

(5) Some of the feedback pathways are involved in a process we have termed *Alopex* † (Harth & Tzanakou, 1974; Tzanakou, Michalak & Harth, 1979) which has the novel character that a *global scalar feedback* is able to simulate specific input patterns or modify inputs in feature-specific ways.

† Acronym for *Al*gorithm *of* *P*attern *Ex*traction.

Assumption (5) provides the actual mechanism that implements the other assumptions in the model. We will show that it provides the system with the ability to shift attention to specific features of sensory input, to enhance and suppress features, and to generate images at various levels of abstraction even 'in the absence of relevant stimulation'.

28.2 The *Alopex* algorithms in optimization problems

28.2.1 Studies of visual receptive fields

This method was originally devised (Harth & Tzanakou, 1974; Tzanakou *et al.*, 1979) for the purpose of experimentally determining receptive fields of individual neurons in the visual pathway. The problem there was to find the visual pattern (an array of light intensities) for which the recorded neural response is a maximum. Thus if the visual field is a matrix of $N \times N$ elements, any stimulus pattern is expressible as a vector $\mathbf{y} = (y_1, \ldots, y_{N^2})$. The neural *response* R was taken to be the number of spikes recorded over a given interval of time following presentation of the stimulus. Since R is determined by the stimulus pattern, the problem of finding the receptive field of the cell becomes one of maximizing

$$R = R(y_1, \ldots, y_{N^2}). \tag{1}$$

The form of this function is generally unknown, but values of R are determined experimentally by presenting different stimuli to an animal while recording R. In the past the experimental procedure has been to assume R to peak for some simple geometrical shapes, and then to locate the extremal values by varying a small number of parameters.

In the *Alopex* method patterns $\mathbf{y}$ were chosen iteratively according to an algorithm in which *each* element y_i is changed by an amount that depended on previous changes as well as on the corresponding changes of the *global* response R, according to

$$y_i(n) = y_i(n - 1) + \Delta y_i(n), \tag{2a}$$

where

$$\Delta y_i(n) = \gamma[y_i(n - 1) - y_i(n - 2)][R(n - 1) - R(n - 2)] + g_i(n) \tag{2b}$$

Here $y_i(n)$, $R(n)$ are the values of intensities and response in the nth iteration; $g(n)$ is a gaussian distributed random variable with a mean of zero and standard deviation σ. Unlimited growth of the intensities $y_i(n)$ is prevented by *normalizing* the total intensity $Y = \Sigma_i y_i$ to some fixed value.

The block diagram Fig. 28.1 depicts the flow of information in this process. Here the unit A generates a pattern $\mathbf{y}$ in accordance with the

Alopex algorithm and using the scalar feedback R. The unit B is a *pattern analyzer* that responds with R according to the resemblance of **y** to the *trigger feature* of B.

The algorithm defined by eqns (2) differs from the other currently used optimization procedures (Kirkpatrick, Gelatt & Vecchi, 1983; Hinton & Sejnowski, 1983; Kirkpatrick, 1984), which are based on a method suggested by Metropolis *et al.* (1953). In all these procedures, parameters are changed *one at a time* in a random fashion, and the change is accepted or rejected in accordance with the observed changes in the *cost* function. By contrast, *all* parameters are changed simultaneously in our algorithm, and all changes are accepted, i.e., they become the starting point for the next iteration. The changes depend on the correlation between previous changes, changes in the cost function, and on the *noise* term $g_i(n)$ (see eqn (2b)).

In the formulation (eqn (2)) of our algorithm, each parameter y_i is subject to two competing processes: a *diffusion* away from its starting value and a process that tend to drive y_i in the direction of increasing R. Good convergence of the pattern has been obtained in receptive field studies (Tzanakou *et al.*, 1979) and models of visual perception (Harth & Unnikrishnan, 1985) by choosing values for σ and γ which make the RMS value of the *feedback* term in eqn (2b) about equal to σ. The noise term $g_i(n)$ is analogous to a thermal agitation of the system and is necessary to prevent trapping in local extrema. Tzanakou *et al.* (1979) found that a lowering of σ as the run progresses generally improves convergence. This effect is related to what Kirkpatrick *et al.* (1983) have called *simulated annealing*.

In an alternate formulation of our algorithm we have chosen the changes $\Delta y_i(n)$ to be given by

$$\Delta y_i(n) = \begin{cases} +\delta(n) \text{ with a probability } p_i^+(n), \\ -\delta(n) \text{ with a probability } (1 - p_i^+(n)), \end{cases} \quad (3a)$$

Fig. 28.1. Schematic of information flow in receptive field study. Unit A generates a pattern **y** (broad arrow) which is *analyzed* in B causing a scalar (simple arrow) response R.

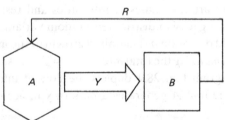

where

$$p_i^+(n) = 1/\{1 + \exp[-\Delta_i(n)/T(n)]\} \tag{3b}$$

and

$$\Delta_i(n) = [y_i(n-1) - y_i(n-2)][R(n-1) - R(n-2)]. \tag{3c}$$

The formulation expressed by eqns (2a) and (3) uses an algorithm described by Hinton & Sejnowski (1983) in which a probability is computed using the eqn (3b) involving a *temperature*. Expressions (3) turn out to be computationally simpler than the original formulation (eqn (2b)), but otherwise lead to very similar results. There are again two parameters to be chosen; the temperature T and the *step size* δ. Allowance is made for reducing both temperature and step size during a run.

28.2.2 *Other optimization problems*

We have used algorithms described in eqns (2) and (3) successfully in a variety of optimization problems (Harth *et al.*, 1986). In general, a *cost function* depends on a number of parameters; the dependence is often non-linear, and the number of parameters may be large. The problem consists of finding the parameter set that minimizes (or maximizes) the cost function. Steepest descent methods generally will not find the global extremum of the cost function when multiple extremals exist.

The *Alopex* algorithm applied to the parameter set usually leads to good convergence of the cost function to its global extremum. In Fig. 28.2 we show the dependence of the value of chi-square as a function of two out of four parameters that determine a damped sine wave; these are amplitude, logarithmic decrement, frequency, and phase. Multiple minima are clearly evident in the figure. A set of data points known to be normally distributed about a damped sine wave was used to determine the chi-square fit for an arbitrary initial set of four parameters. Fig. 28.3 shows the *optimization* of chi-square achieved by varying the four parameters according to the *Alopex* algorithm. The best set of parameters was reached in little over a 100 iterations and was in excellent agreement with the known parameters (Harth *et al.*, 1986).

28.3 Visual perception as an optimization process

We propose as a paradigm of perception a process in which the representation of sensory events at a particular neural level is modified in ways that tend to maximize some global response determined from higher neural levels.

In the original formulation of this idea (Harth, 1976), the dLGN was taken to be the level at which this modification took place, and a single response, derived from the combination of sets of responses of (cortical) feature analyzers, was the *cost function* to be maximized. This idea was further developed (Harth & Unnikrishnan, 1985) by considering cortical and brainstem feedback to the dLGN. Although dLGN was singled out in these papers as the locus of the process, it should be emphasized that such modification may take place at various levels of visual information processing, hence at various stages of neural coding.

The block diagram in Fig. 28.4 shows schematically the proposed functioning of the system. Here A is a sensory *relay* which modifies an incoming pattern **x** to **y**. The modification is carried out with an *Alopex* algorithm using the feedback R which is treated as the cost function. The modified pattern **y** is received simultaneously by a number of analyzers $B_1, B_2, \ldots$, whose responses $r_1, r_2, \ldots$ reflect the degree of presence of particular features in the input **y**.

Fig. 28.2. x^2 surface as function of frequency and phase for problem in which the four parameters of a damped sine wave are to be fitted to a set of data points.

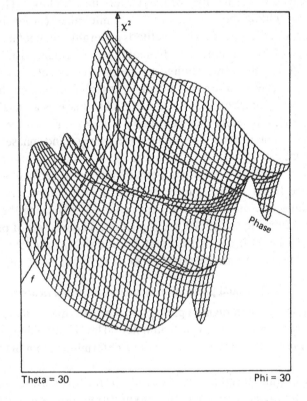

Theta = 30   Phi = 30

Fig. 28.3. Convergence of x^2 fit of parameter set for damped sine wave using *Alopex* optimization. (From Harth *et al.*, 1986.)

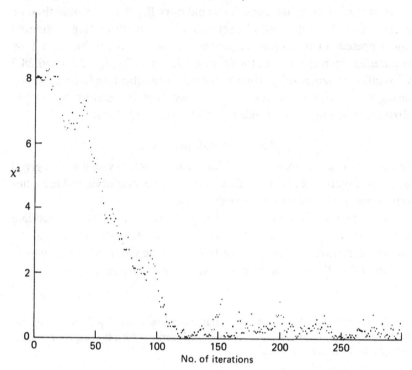

Fig. 28.4. Schematic of single stage model of perception. Sensory input **x** is received by A and a modified pattern **y** is transmitted to a bank of feature analyzers $B_1, B_2, \ldots, B_k$. The responses $r_1, r_2, \ldots, r_k$ are combined in S to produce the global feedback R.

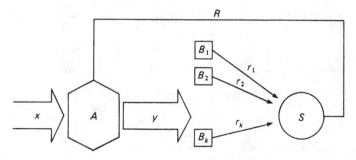

As an example, if we consider A to be the dLGN, x would represent the *raw* visual input as received from the retina and y the output of the thalamocortical relay neurons. The analyzers $B_1, B_2, \ldots$ would then be cortical circuits that respond preferentially to features (e.g., oriented lines) present in the input. A *global* response R is produced in S by combining the responses of the feature analyzers. In Figs. 28.4 and 28.7 we symbolize *neural relays* (in which pattern modification takes place) by hexagons, *analyzers* by squares, and response integrators by circles. Broad arrows are arrays, single arrows (scalar) responses.

28.3.1 A simple prototype

In one set of simulations we consider a small patch of visual space, given by a 4×4 matrix, x and y are then 16-element arrays of neural activities retinotopically representing the visual space.

Fig. 28.5 shows the *templates*, or trigger features, T_1–T_{16} corresponding to the cortical analyzers B_1–B_{16} which we have chosen in analogy to the analyzers of oriented lines known to exist in the visual cortex. *Complex features* (T_{17}–T_{20}) may be constructed by combining the responses of the

Fig. 28.5. Feature analyzers for a 4×4 patch of visual space. T_1–T_{16} are templates for *simple* analyzers. B_{17}–B_{20} are *complex* analyzers in which the responses of four simple analyzers are combined.

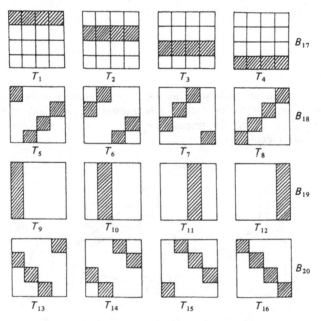

simple analyzers. Thus B_{17} combines the responses r_1–r_4 of the *horizontal* analyzers and will give a strong response r_{17} to *any* horizontal line in the patch.

28.3.2 Generation of responses

Simple responses. The simple responses r_1–r_{16} are obtained by combining the modified input **y** with the appropriate templates T_1–T_{16}. The latter are taken as 16-element arrays in which the dark squares (Fig. 28.5) are given values of 1, the blank squares are zeroes.

We define the *simple* response r_i, $(1 \leq i \leq 16)$ as

$$r_i = s_i \left[\sum_{j=1}^{16} (T_{ij} y_j)^a \right]^{1/a}, \tag{4}$$

where T_{ij} is the jth component of the ith template and s_i is the *sensitivity* of the ith template.

With the parameter a in eqn (4) chosen to be less than 1.0, the analyzer is designed to favor an even distribution of activity across the non-zero portions of the template. Thus,

$$a = 0.5 \quad \text{and} \quad \mathbf{y} = \begin{Bmatrix} 1 & 1 & 1 & 1 \\ 0 & 0 & 0 & 0 \\ 0 & 0 & 0 & 0 \\ 0 & 0 & 0 & 0 \end{Bmatrix} \quad \text{gives } r_1 = 16,$$

$$\text{while } a = 0.5 \quad \text{and} \quad \mathbf{y} = \begin{Bmatrix} 4 & 0 & 0 & 0 \\ 0 & 0 & 0 & 0 \\ 0 & 0 & 0 & 0 \\ 0 & 0 & 0 & 0 \end{Bmatrix} \quad \text{gives } r_1 = 4.$$

Complex responses. The complex responses r_k, $(17 \leq k \leq 20)$ are generated as follows:

$$r_k = \left(\sum_c r_i^b \right)^{1/b} \quad (17 \leq k \leq 20; \quad 1 \leq i \leq 16), \tag{5}$$

where Σ_c denotes summation over the four simple responses that define a complex response. It is seen that eqn (5) defines the complex analyzer in such a way that for $b > 1.0$, r_k will be largest if the input **y** favors just one of the four simple features.

Global response. The 20 responses r_i are combined in S (Fig. 28.4) in such a way that R is largest when any simple feature appears in **y**. This is achieved by defining R as

$$R = \left(\sum_{i=1}^{20} r_i^c \right)^{1/c}, \tag{6}$$

with $c > 1.0$. We have generally chosen $a = 0.5$, $b = c = 2.0$ in most of our simulations.

28.3.3 Application of Alopex algorithm

With the above choice of analyzer responses, and using R in an *Alopex* algorithm in A (Fig. 28.4) the system will tend to modify the relayed sensory input y so as to enhance simple features that may be suggested in x.

To take into account the visual input x, eqn (2a) must be modified to read

$$y_i(n) = \alpha x_i(n) + \beta y_i(n - 1) + \Delta y_i(n). \tag{7}$$

Here the coefficients α and β denote stimulus strength and reverberation strength, i.e., they determine to what extent the relayed pattern y is influenced by the raw stimulus x and the preceding pattern. The last term in eqn (7) is again given either by eqn (2b) or eqns (3).

In a series of simulations, Harth & Unnikrishnan (1985) obtained good convergence on simple features of the type shown in Fig. 28.5 and on patterns combining pairs of such features. In these runs the inputs x in eqn (7) were either zero, or consisted of brief stimuli, lasting for a few iterations. The algorithms were less effective in modifying a *sustained* input x, unless the stimulus strength α was made very small. We take this as analogous to the low probability of hallucinatory events in the normal brain under conditions of sensory input.

Under certain conditions, however, such as the hierarchical system of sensory perception discussed below, it may be desirable to bring about substantial changes in a sustained input pattern. This may be achieved by replacing the *additive* pattern modification exemplified in eqn (7) by a multiplicative correction of the type

$$y_i(n) = k_i(n)x_i(n), \tag{8}$$

and, using an optimizing algorithm,

$$k_i(n) = k_i(n - 1) + \Delta k_i(n) \tag{9a}$$

$$\Delta k_i = \begin{cases} +\delta \text{ with probability } \varrho_i^+(n) \\ -\delta \text{ with probability } [1 - \varrho_i^+(n)], \end{cases} \tag{9b}$$

$$\varrho_i^+(n) = 1/[1 + \exp(-\Delta_i(n)/T)], \tag{9c}$$

with $\Delta_i(n)$ given again by eqn (3c).

Eqn (8) is interpreted as describing a *filter* on the input x which at the ith location has a *transmissivity* k_i. This transmissivity is changed in a cumulative fashion, using eqn (9), with increments chosen according to an *Alopex* algorithm.

28.3.4 Neural circuitry

If feature-specific input modifications occur at the level of the dLGN, they must be explainable in terms of reafferent pathways that are diffuse and stereotypic. Crick (1984) proposed a mechanism in which the so-called reticular complex, which receives collateral input from both ascending and descending thalamocortical fibers, is able to cause brief enhancement of activity in the sensory relay neurons, followed by extended inhibition. The result is an internal attentional *searchlight* whose trajectory is guided by 'vertical' transient cell assemblies.

The processes we envision here are considerably slower, cumulative and capable of supplying considerable pictorial detail.

The neuronal requirements for carrying out the appropriate algorithms turn out to be minimal. A number of circuits can easily be devised which implement the *Alopex* process. Since the algorithms are guided by *changes* in activity levels at inputs and responses (eqn (3c)), the neural system (which is particularly sensitive to changes) is well suited for the task.

A simple circuit (Fig. 28.6) is shown here only for the purpose of illustrating how such processes can arise in a very natural way. The diagram represents a single picture element in the thalamic representation

Fig. 28.6. Schematic of a simple neural circuit representing a single element in a relay that executes an optimization algorithm. Retinal input x_i and thalamocortical signal y_i are shown by dotted arrows. T^+, T^- and S are transient ON, transient OFF and sustained relay neurons. Interneurons 1 and 2 are inhibited by reafferent fibers signalling increase (R^+) and decrease (R^-) in global response R (arrows are excitatory and dots are inhibitory synapses).

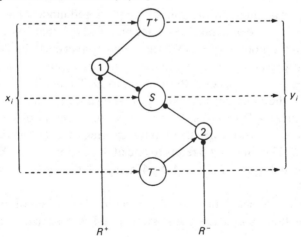

of visual input. It consists of three relay cells: transient ON (T^+), transient OFF (T^-) and sustained (S). They receive excitatory retinal input x_i (dotted lines from left) and relay similar excitatory activity y_i to the visual cortex (dotted arrows to right). Two interneurons receive excitatory inputs from within the local net as shown, and inhibitory inputs R^+ and R^-. These two reafferent stimulations signal increases and decreases in a global response, respectively and are diffusely distributed over all picture elements.

Analysis of the circuit in Fig. 28.6 shows that an increase in x_i (heightened activity in S, transient activity in T^+) will be sustained in y_i provided it is accompanied by activity in R^+, otherwise it will be inhibited. On the other hand a decrease in activity in S will be enhanced if accompanied by activity on R^-.

28.4 Hierarchic model of visual processing

28.4.1 Structure of the system

The prototype shown in Fig. 28.4 and its receptive fields (Fig. 28.5) are used as building blocks (pixels) to make up a visual field composed of 25 identical pixels, each receiving individual feedbacks that tend to enhance one of its trigger features. In a second stage the 500 responses of all feature analyzers (20 per pixel) are relayed to a set of analyzers designed to select patterns in the 25 pixel field. The responses of these pattern analyzers are finally combined to generate a single global response. *Alopex* algorithms are employed at the first level using the individual combined pixel responses as well as the global response; at relays of the second level the responses of the feature analyzers are modified by the global R.

Fig. 28.7 is a schematic diagram of the proposed model. The 'retinal' input $\mathbf{X}$ is composed of 25 pixels $\mathbf{X}_p$, each modified by a thalamic relay unit A_p. Each of the modified pixels $\mathbf{Y}_p$ is analyzed by a set of 20 simple feature analyzers represented by B_p whose 20 responses $\mathbf{Z}_p$ are again modified and relayed (W_p) to a set of pattern analyzers D. To simplify the diagram only one of the pixel units A_p, B_p, C_p is shown here. The single set of pattern analyzers D receives the 500 responses from all pixels. Superposition of responses is carried out in the 25 integrators S_p and the global integrator S. The subscript p refers to one of the 25 pixels, each $\mathbf{X}_p$ and its modified counterpart $\mathbf{Y}_p$ is a 4×4 array of the type described in Section 28.3.

The model depicted in Fig. 28.7 contains a number of structural features of the mammalian visual system and is designed to simulate feature and pattern modifications presumed to occur in cognitive processes. Here the relay units A_p are analogous to a mosaic of thalamocortical relays in the dLGN. Excitatory retinotopic feedback pathways R_p originate in the visual cortex. These terminate either on geniculate interneurons or on perigeniculate neurons which in turn are inhibitory on relay neurons. The global feedback R, which is diffusely distributed to all pixels in dLGN and visual cortex, is analogous to ascending fibers from areas in brainstem reticular formation.

28.4.2 Function

Functioning of the system is envisioned as follows: the *Alopex* relays A_p will tend to modify their individual inputs to enhance particular (linear) features of the type shown in Fig. 28.5. If the input X_p already *suggests* a particular line element, the process will cause strengthening of this feature. On the other hand, since the feedback R_p is influenced by the higher order *Alopex* process in C_p (which is guided by patterns analyzed in D), we may expect enhancement of those linear features in A_p which contribute to the appropriate pattern. This effect is further strengthened by the global feedback R on A_p.

The modified feature responses from all pixels are received in D by a number of pattern analyzers, which have again *templates*, but in a space

Fig. 28.7. Hierarchic model of visual processing. Retinal input X consists of 25 pixels with 16 elements each. A_p are thalamic relays; B_p cortical analyzers; C_p relays of cortical responses; D higher level pattern analyzers receiving feature responses W and generating pattern responses U, S_p and S are response integrators producing the *scalar* quantities R_p and R respectively.

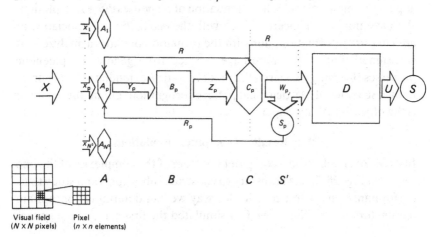

which is no longer simply retinotopic. The box D may also contain *association matrices*, linking patterns into more complex patterns or *scenes*, by mutual strengthening of their responses. Negative matrix elements can be used to provide mutual suppression between patterns.

28.4.3 Sequencing of patterns

Another feature that can easily be built into the unit D is a temporal association, or an *anticipation matrix*, which provides for lowering or raising of the sensitivities of pattern analyzers depending on preceding pattern responses. Thus if a pattern W' is *expected* to follow W, this fact would be encoded in D as the signal to raise the sensitivity of the analyzer for W' whenever the W analyzer registers a high response. The increase in global response resulting from the appearance of W' is now strongly correlated with the changes in W, hence the *Alopex* process in C is expected to cause an *immediate* further enhancement of the pattern. Unlike the quasi-static processes described before, in which changes in individual elements of the pattern are stochastic and weakly correlated with response changes, the dynamic changes brought about by temporal associations are fast and can be made quite strong. We should point out that it is also possible to *reduce* the sensitivity for the *expected* pattern. An expected sequence of input states would then elicit rather weak global responses, while an unexpected event would produce a strong 'startle' response and consequent enhancement of that state.

We like to emphasize, finally, that, while we are principally concerned here with the dynamic aspects brought about by the application of *Alopex* processes at the relays A_p and C_p, considerable richness can be built into the system by defining association and anticipation matrices in D as well as prescribing simple rules for attenuation of responses due to adaptation. We have not been concerned here with the *acquisition* of associative or anticipatory information, nor with the formation of pattern analyzers. It is assumed simply that these have resulted from genetic or epigenetic processes (learning). Clearly, the model could be extended to incorporate known schemes of plasticity and pattern recognition, but neither of these is the objective of this paper.

28.5 Results of computer simulations

In order to simulate on a computer a system of the complexity of the one shown in Fig. 28.7, it is necessary to construct subsystems and study their performance characteristics. In this way we can determine appropriate parameters. Accordingly, we first simulated the first stage of the system consisting of one unit A_p and its set of feature analyzers. Only 16 analyzers were used here; the four complex analyzers were discarded. The inputs X_p were either brief stimuli, *suggesting* one of the linear features, or random patterns, or blank fields. In the last case, the outcome is generally unpredictable, the convergence of Y_p onto one of the 16 features begins after a few tens of iterations. When the initial stimulus X_p has a *resemblance* to one of the features, i.e., when one of the feature responses is initially higher, convergence continues to improve that feature. Also, a particular feature can be elicited by increasing the sensitivity (see eqn (4)) of the corresponding analyzer.

Fig. 28.8 shows the results of a typical simulation experiment using eqns (2a) and (3). The sum of the 16 components of Y_p were *normalized* after each iteration to a value 4.0. Other parameters were $\delta(1) = 0.008$, $T(1) = 0.004$. In Fig. 28.8(a) step size and temperature T were held constant throughout the run. The uppermost curve in the diagram is the total feedback response obtained by combining the 16 feature responses using eqn (6), with $c = 5$. The 16 lower traces are the feature responses as a function of the iteration number. Since a blank initial input was used, all feature responses start at the same value. After a few tens of iterations, one of the feature analyzers gains control of the process; its response rises rapidly, and by the 100th iteration virtually all of the global response is due to that feature. Normalization causes all other features to be reduced.

Fig. 28.8. Simulation of feature generation by reafferent stimulation in a 4 × 4 visual *relay*. Upper trace: global response R; lower traces: 16 feature responses. The initial state is a blank field. (*a*) Constant temperature and step size. (*b*) Temperature and step size reduced by 0.998 in each iteration.

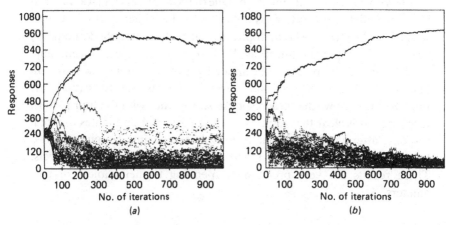

A steady state is achieved after about 400 iterations with no further improvement in the selected feature.

In Fig. 28.8(*b*) we show the results of a run started under similar conditions ($\delta(1)$ = 0.016, $T(1)$ = 0.004). However, in this experiment both step size and temperature T are gradually lowered by reducing them by a factor of 0.998 in every iteration. This process is similar to what Kirkpatrick *et al.* (1983) called *simulated annealing*, i.e., the progressive lowering of T and improved convergence. We note that the temperature reached in the 200th iteration (0.67 of the starting value) would *not* have made a good starting value.

Fig. 28.9 shows the results of simulating the simultaneous convergence of Y_p in the 25 relays A_p under the influence of their own feedbacks R_p (Fig. 28.7) without control from a higher level. As expected, each pixel Y_p converges on one of the linear features defined in Fig. 28.5. The convergence after 300 iterations is shown here in two representations. Fig. 28.9(*c*) shows the retinotopic representation in the 20 × 20 visual space. Fig. 28.9(*d*) shows the same result in the *abstract* space of feature responses. Here each of the 25 rows of boxes represents the 16 feature responses of one of the 25 pixels. Thus the black box in the 14th location of the 2nd row in Fig. 28.9(*d*) denotes the strong resemblance of Y_2 to the template T_{14} in Fig. 28.5.

Fig. 28.10 shows some typical *patterns* (and their representations in response space) for which we have designed analyzers in the second level of our system. As in the case of the first level, we have carried out computer simulations of this part in isolation.

Fig. 28.11 shows the result of a set of simulations involving the second level alone. Pattern analyzers with templates A, B, F and G were used in unit D with weak mutual inhibition. One of the analyzers (A) was favored by slightly higher sensitivity (as indicated by the higher starting value of R_A in Fig. 28.11(*b*)). The multiplicative algorithm described in eqn (9) was used for input modification. With featureless input, considerable modification takes place to the input by 1000 iterations, as shown in Fig. 28.11(*a*). Arrows indicate boxes corresponding to pattern A. Fig. 28.11(*b*) shows the total response R, together with the four pattern responses. It is clear that response for the pattern A dominates the total response after a few hundred iterations. In recent runs, coupling the two levels together, we have observed some convergence at both levels. These results are very preliminary, pending further choices of parameters.

Fig. 28.9. Test of the lower stage of hierarchic model shown in Fig. 28.7. (*a*) Initial blank pattern **Y**(1). (*b*) Its representation in the response space. (*c*) Final pattern **Y**(300) showing random convergence of features defined in Fig. 28.5. (*d*) Its representation in response space. In the response space each row of boxes represents the 16 simple feature responses for one of the 25 pixels.

Iteration no: 1

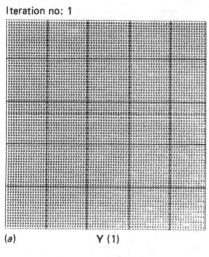

(*a*) Y (1)

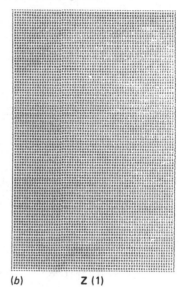

(*b*) Z (1)

Iteration no: 300

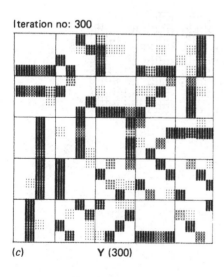

(*c*) Y (300)

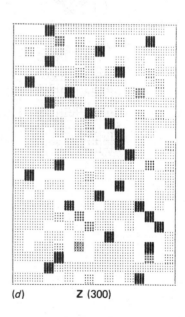

(*d*) Z (300)

Fig. 28.10. Seven different pattern analyzers used at the second level. The top row shows the patterns at the input level. The bottom row shows their corresponding representations in response space. The twenty columns used here represent 16 simple and 4 complex analyzers for each of the 25 pixels (rows).

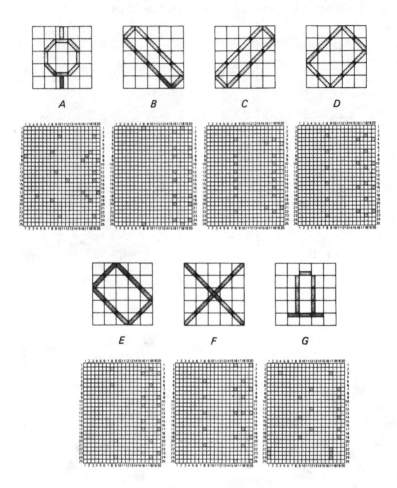

Fig. 28.11. Test of the upper stage of the model shown in Fig. 28.7. (*a*) Final pattern *W* in response space showing only the 16 *simple* analyzer responses. Arrows point to strong responses in common with pattern *A* in Fig. 28.10. (*b*) Four pattern responses U_A, U_B, U_F, U_G, together with *global* response *R*.

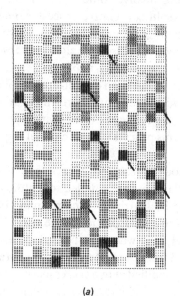

(*a*)

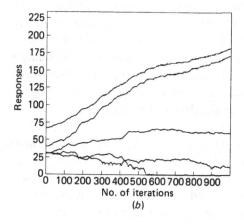

(*b*)

452   *E. Harth, K. P. Unnikrishnan & A. S. Pandya*

28.6 Summary and discussion

We have proposed a hierarchic model of visual information processing
that goes beyond the mapping processes in so called 'early vision', and
considers perception to involve some of the richness of stored sensory
information. In the resulting cognitive processes, neural representations
of sensory events appear at different levels of abstraction. It is assumed
that *reafferent* pathways which are ubiquitous in sensory systems, modify
these representations in ways which maximize responses at higher levels.
The process is thus reducible to an optimization problem.

In the model, modifications are performed at sensory relays; the
process is envisioned as a stochastic optimization process, called *Alopex*.
We have shown that this process places minimal requirements on details
of neural circuitry.

The hierarchic model presented here is composed of a mosaic of
prototype sensory relays that are coupled to feature analyzers, similar to
the system described by Harth & Unnikrishnan (1985). Each of these
modules corresponds to a small portion of the visual field. This is followed
by higher level analyzers whose responses depend on the array of
responses transmitted from the first stage. The neural representations of
the sensory input are modified at two successive *relays* by scalar feedbacks
derived from a superposition of responses at higher levels of processing.

Computer simulations show that at both relays, in the absence of
patterned input, the feedback will cause the modified patterns to converge
in a matter of a few hundred iterations on one of the features, or patterns,
that causes maximal response. Final patterns may thus be selected by
biasing, or increasing the sensitivity of the corresponding analyzer. If the
input bears a resemblance to one of the *trigger features*, the system will
enhance that feature, or – in the case of the second stage – that *pattern* of
features. Computer simulations involving the entire system are now in
progress.

The system shown in Fig. 28.7 is designed to bear an analogy to parts of
the mammalian visual system. Thus the *relays* A_p represent regions in the
dLGN receiving retinal inputs X_p and cortico-thalamic reafferents R_p
derived from simple and complex feature analyzers B_p in the visual
cortex. Other relays modify the responses of these feature analyzers
under control of a *global* response derived from higher level *pattern*
analyzers.

Considerable amount of flexibility may be built into the unit labeled D
in Fig. 28.7. Sensitivities of pattern analyzers may be biased or linked
together by association matrices. In this way the system can be made to be

sensitive to combinations of patterns. Negative matrix elements can be used to simulate mutual avoidance of patterns, and delayed associations can be made to produce fast enhancements and thus guide the flow of sensory information in a variety of cognitive tasks.

Acknowledgements

This research was supported by research contract No. DAAG 29-83-K-0167 of the Army Research Office and BRSG grant S07 RR077068-21 of the Biomedical Research Support Grant Program, NIH. One of the authors (E.H.) wishes to thank the Aspen Center for Physics for its hospitality during the preparation of the manuscript.

References

Ahlsén, G. & Lo, F. S. (1982). 'Projection of brainstem neurones to the perigeniculatenucleus and the lateral geniculate nucleus in the cat.' *Brain Research*, **238**, 433–8.

Ahlsén, G., Lindstrom, S. & Lo, F. S. (1984). 'Inhibition from the brainstem of inhibitory interneurones of the cat's dorsal lateral geniculate nucleus.' *Journal of Physiology* (*London*), **347**, 593–609.

Block, N. (1981). *Imagery*. Cambridge: MIT/Bradford Books.

Crick, F. H. C. (1984). 'Function of the thalamic reticular complex: the searchlight hypothesis.' *Proceedings National Academy of Science, USA*, **81**, 4586–90.

Flanagan, O. J. Jr. (1984). *The Science of the Mind*, p. 188. Cambridge: MIT/Bradford Books.

Gibbs, C. M., Cohen, D. H. & Broyles, J. L. (1986). 'Modification of the discharge of lateral geniculate neurons during visual learning.' *Journal of Neuroscience*, **6**, 627–36.

Harth, E. (1976). 'Visual perception: a dynamic theory.' *Biological Cybernetics*, **22**, 169–80.

Harth, E., Pandya, A. S. & Unnikrishnan, K. P. (1986). 'Perception as an optimization process.' In *Proceedings of IEEE Computer Society Conference on Computer Vision and Pattern Recognition*, pp. 662–5. Washington D.C.: IEEE Computer Society Press.

Harth, E. & Tzanakou, E. (1974). 'Alopex: a stochastic method for determining visual receptive fields.' *Vision Research*, **14**, 1475–82.

Harth, E. & Unnikrishnan, K. P. (1985). 'Brainstem control of sensory information: a mechanism for perception.' *International Journal of Psychophysiology*, **3**, 101–19.

Hinton, G. E. & Sejnowski, T. J. (1983). 'Optimal perceptual inference.' In *Proceedings of IEEE Computer Society Conference on Computer Vision and Pattern Recognition*, pp. 448–53. Washington D.C.: IEEE Computer Society Press.

Holst, E. V. & Mittelstaedt, H. (1950). 'Das Reafferenzprinzip.' *Naturwissenschaften*, **37**, 464–76.

Hughes, H. C. & Mullikin, W. H. (1984). 'Brainstem afferents to the lateral geniculate nucleus in the cat.' *Experimental Brain Research*, **54**, 253–8.

Kirkpatrick, S. (1984). 'Optimization by simulated annealing: quantitative studies.' *Journal of Statistical Physics*, **34**, 975–86.

Kirkpatrick, S., Gelatt, C. D. & Vecchi, M. P. (1983). 'Optimization by simulated annealing.' *Science*, **220**, 671–80.

Kosslyn, S. M. (1980). *Image and mind*. Cambridge: Harvard.

Lund, J. S., Lund, R. D., Hendrickson, A. E., Hunt, A. H. & Fuchs, A. F. (1975). 'The origin of efferent pathways from the primary visual cortex, area 17, of the macaque monkey as shown by horseradish peroxidase.' *Journal of Comparative Neurology*, **164**, 287–304.

Marr, D. (1982). *Vision*. San Francisco: Freeman.

Marr, D. & Hildreth, E. C. (1980). 'Theory of edge detection.' *Proceedings of Royal Society (London)*, **B207**, 187–217.

Marr, D. & Poggio, T. (1979). 'A computational theory of human stereo vision'. *Proceedings of Royal Society (London)*, **B204**, 301–28.

Metropolis, N., Rosenbluth, A. W., Rosenbluth, M. N., Teller, A. H. & Teller, E. (1953). 'Equation of state calculations by fast computing machines.' *Journal of Chemical Physics*, **21**, 1087–92.

Montero, V. M. & Singer, W. (1985). 'Ultrastructural identification of somata and neural processes immunoreactive to antibodies against glutamic acid decarboxylase (GAD) in the dorsal lateral geniculate nucleus of the cat.' *Experimental Brain Research*, **59**, 151–65.

Morocco, R. T., McClurkin, J. W. & Young, R. A. (1982). 'Modulation of lateral geniculate nucleus cell responsiveness by visual activation of the croticogeniculate pathway.' *Journal of Neuroscience*, **2**, 256–63.

Neisser, U. (1966). *Cognitive Psychology*, p. 4. New York: Appleton-Century-Crofts.

Neisser, U. (1976). *Cognition and reality*. San Francisco: Freeman.

Shepard, R. N. & Metzler, J. (1971). 'Mental rotation of three-dimensional objects.' *Science*, **171**, 701–3.

Singer, W. (1977). 'Control of thalamic transmission by corticofugal and ascending reticular pathways in the visual system.' *Physiological Reviews*, **57**, 386–420.

Singer, W., Tretter, F. & Cynader, M. (1976). 'The effect of reticular stimulation on spontaneous and evoked activity in the cat visual cortex.' *Brain Research*, **102**, 71–90.

Steriade, M., Domich, L. & Oakson, G. (1986). 'Reticularis thalami neurons revisited: activity changes during shifts in states of vigilance.' *Journal of Neuroscience*, **6**, 68–81.

Steriade, M., Ropert, N., Kitsikis, A. & Oakson, G. (1980). 'Ascending activating neuronal networks in midbrain reticular core and related rostral systems.' In *The reticular formation revisited*, eds. J. A. Hobson & M. A. B. Brazier, pp. 125–67, New York: Raven Press.

Tzanakou, E., Michalak, R. & Harth, E. (1979). 'The Alopex process: visual receptive fields by response feedback.' *Biological Cybernetics*, **35**, 161–74.

29

Mathematical model and computer simulation of visual recognition in retina and tectum opticum of amphibians

UWE AN DER HEIDEN and GERHARD ROTH

29.1 The retina

29.1.1 Mathematical model of amphibian retina

The retina is composed of a variety of cell types including the photoreceptors, horizontal cells, bipolar cells, amacrine cells, and retina ganglion
cells (for a review see Grüsser & Grüsser-Cornehls, 1976). Only the
retina ganglion cells (RGCs) send axons to the brain of the animals.
Therefore any visual information the brain may rely on is mediated by
cells of this type.

According to their response properties the RGCs are usually divided
into four classes, which here for simplicity are called $R1, R2, R3$, and $R4$.
We have restricted our attention to the classes $R2$ and $R3$ because these
form the majority (about 93%) of cells projecting to the tectum opticum,
which is that area in the brain where recognition of prey objects is
supposed to be centered.

The recognition process starts in the retina. The overall operation of
the ganglion cells $(R2, R3)$ and their precursors (photoreceptors, etc.) on
some arbitrary visual scene can be decomposed into the following more
primitive operational components:

(1) Let $x(s, t)$ be any distribution of light in the visual field, where x
denotes light intensity (we do not consider colored scenes), $s = (s_1, s_2)$
some point in the visual field, and t is time.

(2) These ganglion cells do not respond to stationary, but only to
transitory, illumination. This feature is represented by a high pass filter
operation on $x(s, t)$ producing output $y(s, t)$:

$$y(s, t) = \int_0^\infty x(s, t')(\delta(t - t') - T^{-1} \exp(-(t - t')/T)) \, dt', \quad (1)$$

where δ denotes Dirac's function and T the time constant of the high pass filter.

(3) The receptive field of an RGC is composed of small patches showing either an ON-response or an OFF-response to brief point illuminations (compare Grüsser & Grüsser-Cornehls, 1976, in particular, their Fig. 13). This feature is modeled by the non-linear threshold operations (already suggested by Varjú, 1978):

$$z_{ON}(s, t) = \max\ (0, y(s, t)), \qquad (2a)$$

$$z_{OFF}(s, t) = \max\ (0, -y(s, t)), \qquad (2b)$$

where max (a, b) means the maximum of the values a and b.

(4) It is generally believed that the spatially local ON- and OFF-responses are mediated by retinal interneurons, predominantly by bipolar cells. Since each nerve cell also shows low pass filter characteristics (reflected in its membrane time constant m) it has to be assumed that the ganglion cells do not receive the signals z_{ON} and z_{OFF} directly but a low pass filtered weighted sum of these two quantities. Additionally it has been shown experimentally that retinal interneurons may act either inhibitory or excitatory on the ganglion cells. Altogether, the local excitatory input v_e to a ganglion cell is described by

$$m \cdot \partial v_e(s, t)/\partial t = b_{1e}z_{ON}(s, t) + b_{2e}z_{OFF}(s, t) - v_e(s, t) \qquad (3a)$$

and the local inhibitory input v_i by

$$m \cdot \partial v_i(s, t)/\partial t = b_{1i}z_{ON}(s, t) + b_{2i}z_{OFF}(s, t) - v_i(s, t), \qquad (3b)$$

with weight constants b_{rs}.

(5) The space variable s for the visual field is also used to denote positions in the retina (in a topographically canonical way). Let $e(s, t)$ denote the net excitation (measured in mV) of a ganglion cell, whose center of receptive field is located at the point s (as usual the receptive field of a visual cell is defined as that area of the visual field from which this cell may be excited or inhibited by small stimuli). The following operation takes into account the important and well-known fact that the receptive fields of $R2$- and $R3$-cells have a circular shape and are divided into an excitatory center and an inhibitory surround (the Mexican hat structure). The spatial integration constituting this structure is described by

$$e(s, t) = \iint (E_e v_e(\bar{s}, t) \exp\ (-k_e|s - \bar{s}|^2)$$
$$- E_i v_i(\bar{s}, t) \exp\ (-k_i|s - \bar{s}|^2))\ d\bar{s}, \qquad (4)$$

where the integration extends over the whole visual field. This equation presupposes that excitation and inhibition decay with distance from the receptive field center according to a Gaussian distribution. Because of the structure of the receptive field the constants must satisfy the inequalities

$$E_e > E_i \quad \text{and} \quad k_e > k_i. \tag{5}$$

(6) The membrane of the ganglion cell also acts as a low pass filter, hence its membrane potential $w(s, t)$ develops according to

$$m \cdot \partial w(s, t)/\partial t = e(s, t) - w(s, t). \tag{6}$$

(7) The membrane potential of the ganglion cell is transformed into the impulse frequency

$$w_+(s, t) = \max (0, w(s, t)), \tag{7}$$

where the threshold is normalized to 0.

Eqns (1)–(7) represent the total description of the spatio-temporal dynamics of a retina ganglion cell whose receptive field center is located at the point s in the visual field.

29.1.2 Simulation results for the retina ganglion cell model

The retinal network equations have been discretized and run on a digital computer. Constant parameters used in the simulations are listed in the figure captions below. The input light distributions are black rectangles on a white background moving (with a constant velocity of 7.6°/sec) horizontally and centrally through the receptive field of a retinal ganglion cell (more precisely of the RGC model). Fig. 29.1 shows the computed responses of the membrane potential $w(s, t)$ (with fixed centre of receptive field s in the centre region of the visual field) to rectangles whose longer axis is oriented perpendicular to the direction of movement (hence in this case the stimulus is oriented vertically). Let us call such stimuli 'perpendicular'.

Important remark: The model is constructed in such a way that its responses are invariant with respect to the absolute orientation of a stimulus (hence it is not a model for orientation sensitive cells!), but sensitive to the orientation relative to the direction of movement of a stimulus. Stationary stimuli do not elicit any response of the model. This is in accordance with experimental observations.

For each of the four curves in Fig. 29.1 the length of the short axis of the stimulus is 2° (angular degrees are taken as spatial units in visual field). Lengths of the long axes differ for each curve and are given in the diagram. With all four stimuli the membrane potential $w(s, t)$ is first hyperpolarized, which is caused by the entrance of the rectangular stimulus into the inhibitory surround of the receptive field. Afterwards, crossing of the excitatory receptive field center leads to a depolarization, followed by a second hyperpolarization through the re-entering of the stimulus into the inhibitory surround. Finally, the membrane potential returns to its resting value, which is necessary since with increasing eccentricity from the center s of the receptive field, excitation and inhibition fade away in a Gaussian fashion.

The mean impulse frequency resulting from these membrane potentials, i.e., the area above the abscissa in Fig. 29.1, divided by the time of super threshold depolarization, has been computed and plotted in the diagram of Fig. 29.4(a). Points on the horizontal axis represent lengths of the longer edge of the rectangular stimulus. The vertical axis represents impulse frequencies (imp s^{-1}). The small triangles mark the mean impulse frequencies generated in the retina ganglion cell by the corresponding four perpendicular rectangles. One observes that maximal (mean) impulse frequency is reached for the $2° \times 4°$ rectangle and that the response decreases dramatically for longer stimulus sizes.

Fig. 29.1. Simulated responses of the membrane potential w of the model retina ganglion cell (class $R2$) to moving rectangles whose long axis is oriented perpendicular to the direction of movement. Rectangles move at $7.6° s^{-1}$. For each of the four curves the length of the short axis of the stimulus is $2°$. Lengths of the longer axes are indicated in the diagram. Parameters used in the calculations: $T = 0.3$ s, $m = 5$ ms, $b_{1e} = 0$, $b_{1i} = 0.6$, $b_{2e} = b_{2i} = 1$, $E_e = 50$, $E_i = 14.7$, $k_e = 0.37$, $k_i = 0.06$.

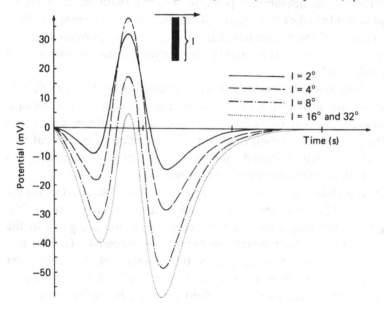

Similar computer simulations can be performed for square-like rectangles of various sizes. The resulting membrane potentials are plotted as functions of time in Fig. 29.2. The corresponding impulse frequencies are shown as functions of edge length by the curve in Fig. 29.4(*a*) labeled with small squares. Among the squares, that of size 4° × 4° leads to the strongest response.

In the third simulation sequence the stimuli were rectangles whose longer axis is oriented in the direction of movement. We call them 'parallel'. Fig. 29.3 shows the membrane potentials of the ganglion cell model for four of such stimuli with longer edge length again indicated in the diagram and the short axis always 2°. Despite large differences in stimulus extension the responses are nearly equal. This also shows up in the corresponding mean firing rates plotted in Fig. 29.4(*a*) with small circles. The mean impulse frequency is nearly independent of the length of parallel stimuli.

The picture of Fig. 29.4(*a*) is characteristic for a special class of retina ganglion cells, namely the *R*2-cells. For comparison data from real *R*2-cells are shown in Fig. 29.4(*b*).

Fig. 29.2. As in Fig. 29.1. Stimuli are now squares moving at 7.6° s⁻¹ through the visual field. Edge lengths are given in the diagram. Same parameters as in Fig. 29.1.

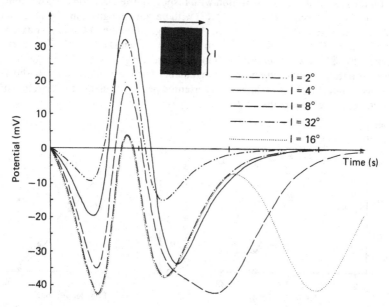

Fig. 29.3. As in Fig. 29.1. Stimuli are now rectangles whose longer axis is oriented parallel to the direction of movement. Length of short axis 2°, longer axes as indicated in the figure. Velocity of stimuli 7.6°/sec. Parameters as in Figs. 29.1 and 29.2.

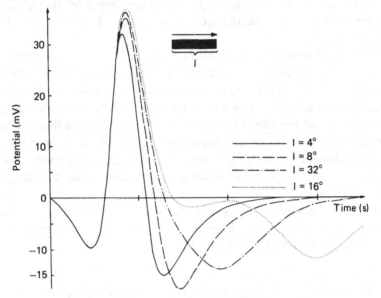

Fig. 29.4. Mean impulse frequencies of class 2 retina ganglion cells as a function of stimulus extension and orientation with respect to the direction of movement. (*a*) Model cell, described by eqns (1)–(7) with parameters given in Fig. 29.1. (*b*) real cell, after (Ewert & Hock, 1972). Abscissa gives length of the longer axis of the rectangular stimuli. Responses to squares are marked by ■. The curve marked by ● shows responses to elongated rectangles with the longer axis oriented parallel to the direction of movement. The curve marked by ▲ shows responses to rectangles with longer axis oriented perpendicular to the direction of movement. Short axis is always 2°.

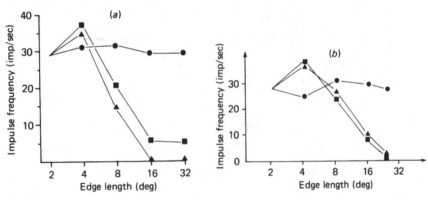

The data for real $R3$-cells are given in Fig. 29.5(b). In these cells the maximal responses both to squares and perpendicular stimuli occur at an edge length of 8°. This characteristic could also be obtained with the model network by choosing parameters E_i, k_e and k_i as indicated in the caption at Fig. 29.5 (leading to a broader Mexican hat than in the $R2$-model). All other parameters were the same as in the $R2$-simulations. Fig. 29.5(a) shows the result of the simulations with this set of parameter values.

To summarise: a model of the retina has been constructed on the basis of structural response properties of the retina; under suitable choice of parameters the model turned out to predict successfully the dynamic responses to a large class of rectangularly shaped moving stimuli for at least two types of retina ganglion cells, namely class 2 and 3, cells which supply the major retinal input to the tectum opticum. It is possible that other RGC types also may be modeled in this way. However, we did not perform corresponding simulations. Our model is two-dimensional in visual space, allowing to process visual stimuli of arbitrary size, form, and position in visual field.

29.2 The tectum opticum

29.2.1 Simple summatory model of amphibian tectum cells

The variety of different cell types in the tectum opticum of amphibians is even larger than that in the retina. For detailed descriptions see (Grüsser

Fig. 29.5. Mean impulse frequencies of class 3 retina ganglion cells as a function of stimulus extension and orientation with respect to the direction of movement. (a) Model cell, described by eqns (1)–(7), parameters as in Fig. 29.1 except that $E_i = 23.5$, $k_e = 0.07$, $k_i = 0.023$. (b) Real cells, after (Pfeiffer, 1975); description of stimuli as in Fig. 29.4.

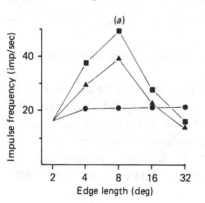
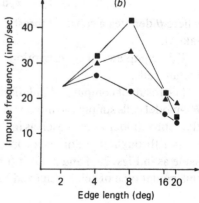

& Grüsser-Cornehls, 1976) and (Roth & Jordan, 1982). An additional complication arises from the fact that the wiring of the cells in the tectum is still less well known than that in the retina. Our strategy in modeling the dynamics of some of the observed tectal cell types was to assume neural operations on the tectal input (= retinal output of $R2$- and $R3$-cells) which are both as simple as possible and most likely to occur in this brain area.

The first operation we assumed is neuronal summation or integration of the output of retinal ganglion cells. We had the alternative of summation of $R2$-output only, summation of $R3$-output only, or mixed summation of $R2$- and $R3$-output. All of these cases are likely to occur since different retinal classes project to different layers in the tectum.

It is well known that this projection is topographic, hence the spatial variable s of the visual field can and will be also used to describe position in the tectal cell layers.

The summative process is mathematically described in the following way. Let $e_T(s, t)$ denote the retinal excitation of a tectum cell with s as the central point of its receptive field. Then

$$e_T(s, t) = a_T \iint w_+(\bar{s}, t) \exp\left(-k|s - \bar{s}|^2\right) d\bar{s}, \qquad (8)$$

where a_T is a proportionality constant. The Gaussian factor weights the influence of retinal cells depending on the distance $|s - \bar{s}|$ of their receptive field center to that of the tectal cell; w_+ means either the output of $R2$- or $R3$-cells or a weighted sum of these two output types.

The membrane potential $u(s, t)$ results from a low pass filtering of the input $e_T(s, t)$ with membrane time constant m:

$$m \cdot \partial u(s, t)/\partial t = e_T(s, t) - u(s, t). \qquad (9)$$

Finally, the membrane potential is transformed into the impulse frequency $u_+(s, t)$ according to

$$u_+(s, t) = a_+ \max\left(\theta, u(s, t)\right), \qquad (10)$$

where θ denotes a constant threshold value (in all simulations $\theta = 0$ was taken).

This completes the description of the simple summatory model of tectum cells.

The result of computer simulations of this model in the situation where $R2$-model cells supply the input is shown in Fig. 29.6(a). (Parameters for the retina model were chosen as in Section 29.1. Tectum parameters $a_T = a_+ = 1$ throughout.) Stimulus configuration and mode of plotting is the same as in Figs. 29.4 and 29.5. It turns out that the maximal response of this model type of cell is achieved to squares with edge length of 8°. The response to a parallel rectangle whose longer edge also measures 8° (shorter edge always 2°) is weaker and a perpendicular rectangle of the same size gives the weakest response. This is in line with observations of real tectum cells belonging to the type $T5.1$ according to the classification of Grüsser and Grüsser–Cornehls. Fig. 29.6(b) shows data from Ewert & von Wietersheim (1974) for this cell type. At least for square and perpendicular stimuli and for parallel stimuli not longer than 12° there is good agreement between the real and the model neuron type. The disagreement for long parallel rectangles may have something to do with the large distance between the leading and the trailing edge of these stimuli, leading sometimes to bursts in the response of retinal and tectum cells. In this case average impulse frequency possibly is not a good measure for neural activity.

If, alternatively, the input of the tectum cell model is assumed to consist of the activity of retinal $R3$-model cells (all other parameters being the same as in the previous case) then Fig. 29.7(a) is obtained. Here again, squares elicit the strongest responses. However, the relationship between responses to parallel and perpendicular stimuli is reversed as compared with the type $T5.1$. Now in the whole range of angles perpendicular stimuli are preferred to parallel stimuli.

Such cells indeed have been found in the tectum. They probably belong to the type $T5.3$ of Grüsser & Grüsser-Cornehls classification. Fig. 29.7(b) shows measurements obtained with this type in the laboratory of G. Roth. Note, that the abscissa here measures velocity. (In the

Fig. 29.6. Responses of tectum cells. Description of stimuli and coordinates as in Fig. 29.4. (a) Model tectum cell with input from model retina cells of class 2 and no lateral inhibition ($a_i = 0$). (b) Measurements from real tectum cells of type $T5.1$ (after Ewert & von Wietersheim, 1974).

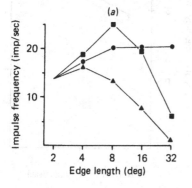
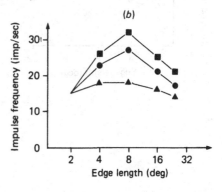

present paper we do not consider velocity dependence, but the model has this feature, too.) Since in these computer simulations we took velocity to equal $7.6° s^{-1}$, in Fig. 29.7(b), only the data belonging to this velocity are relevant for comparison with Fig. 29.7(a).

Clearly, by choosing suitably mixed input from $R2$- and $R3$- model cells all 'linearly' intermediate pictures between Fig. 29.6(a) and Fig. 29.7(a) may be obtained. This corresponds to the experimental finding of many cells whose responses lie inbetween the 'pure' types discussed in the early literature on this area.

29.2.2 Model of amphibian tectum cells including summation and lateral inhibition

We were not able to simulate, with the basic model of Section 29.2.1, another cell type which shows strongest responses to stimuli elongated parallel to the direction of movement, see Fig. 29.8(b). Such $T5.2$-cells have been considered to be important for the detection of prey objects whose longer axis is oriented parallel to their direction of movement, as

Fig. 29.7. Responses of tectum cells. Description of stimuli and coordinates as in Fig. 29.4. (a) Model tectum cell with input from model retina cells of class 3 and no lateral inhibition among tectal cells ($a_i = 0$). (b) Measurements from real tectum cells of type $T5.3$ (after Roth & Jordan, 1982). Here stimulus edge length is always 8°.

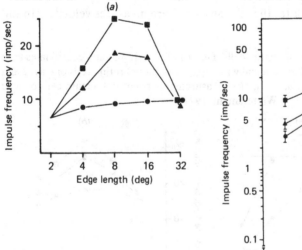
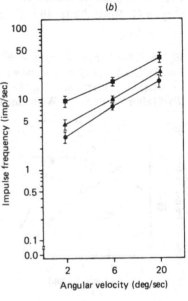

may be the case, e.g., with worms (Ewert & von Wietersheim, 1974). In fact, if toads are confronted with prey dummies of different geometric configurations they much prefer those which we have called parallel stimuli (Ewert, 1972, 1976). Earlier hypotheses including that of Ewert & von Seelen (1974) supposed that $T5.2$-cells have to receive input from other brain areas, e.g. from the thalamus–pretectum region, in order to constitute their specific responses.

We suggest here an intratectal mechanism which also leads to the $T5.2$ characteristic. It is well known that the tectum opticum contains inhibitory interneurons, the most probable candidates being the stellate cells. Via the interneurons tectum cells receiving input from the retina may inhibit each other.

Without going into the details of interneuronal dynamics we simply assume that a subclass of retina driven cells inhibit each other directly and mutually. This mechanism of lateral recurrent inhibition is added to eqn (9) in the following way:

$$m \cdot \partial u(s, t)/\partial t = e_T(s, t) - u(s, t) - a_i \iint u_+(\bar{s}, t) \, \mathrm{d}\bar{s}, \qquad (11)$$

with a constant inhibitory coefficient a_i.

The extended tectum cell model is thus described by eqns (8), (10), and (11). The simple summatory model is obtained as the special case $a_i = 0$.

Of course, for very weak lateral inhibition (i.e., a_i very small) the responses of the extended model are very similar to those of the simple model. However, if lateral inhibition is sufficiently strong (e.g., $a_i = 0.04$) then, as is shown in Fig. 29.8(a) the responses of the model tectum neuron

Fig. 29.8. Responses of tectum cells. Description of stimuli and coordinates as in Fig. 29.4. (a) Model tectum cell with input from model retina cells of class 2 and sufficiently large lateral inhibition ($a_i = 0.04$). (b) Measurements from real tectum cells of type $T5.2$ (after Ewert & von Wietersheim, 1974).

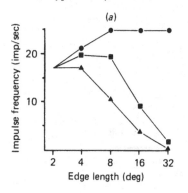
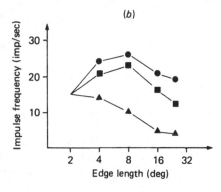

Uwe an der Heiden & Gerhard Roth

are strongest for parallel rectangles (worm like stimuli), the $T5.2$ type of cells is obtained. In these simulations retinal input to the model tectum cell originated only from class $R2$ model retina ganglion cells.

Increase of lateral inhibition thus inverts the relationship of responses to squares and parallel stimuli. A qualitative and heuristic argument for this effect is that squares activate a larger area of the tectum than parallel

Fig. 29.9. Responses of tectum cells. Description of stimuli and coordinates as in Fig. 29.4. (a) Model tectum cell with input from model retina cells of class 3 and medium lateral inhibition ($a_i = 0.16$). (b) Model tectum cell with input from model retina cells of class 3 and strong lateral inhibition ($a_i = 2$).

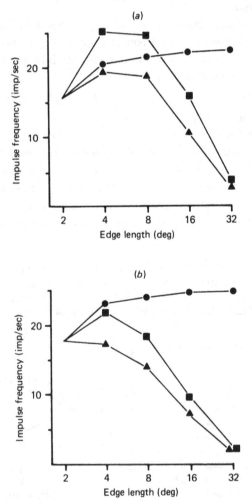

rectangles with corresponding edge length. As a consequence, in the first case more cells act inhibitorily, leading to a stronger decrease of the response as compared to the second case.

The situation is somewhat different if only $R3$-cells excite the model tectum cells. In the case of no or very weak inhibition the $T5.3$ characteristic is present as noted above. For a medium range of inhibition (e.g. for a_i = 0.16) the $T5.1$ characteristic is obtained, see Fig. 29.9(a). Thus this type can be constituted in two ways: either by $R2$ input and without lateral inhibition or by $R3$ input in combination with lateral inhibition of medium size.

If one takes larger values of the inhibitory coefficient (e.g., a_i = 2) then the $T5.2$ type of responses appears, see Fig. 29.9(b). Therefore, this type can also be generated in two ways: by sufficiently strong lateral inhibition in combination with input either from $R2$-cells or from $R3$-cells. Clearly, a mixed retinal input would also generate this tectum cell type.

29.3 Conclusion

We presented two mathematical models for neural networks in the visual system of amphibians. One of them described the spatio-temporal dynamics involved in the constitution of retina ganglion cell responses, in particular those of class 2 and class 3 retina ganglion cells. Output of the model retinal cells was used as input to a tectum cell model developed in Section 29.2. It was possible to generate the responses of three types of tectum cells: $T5.1$, $T5.2$, and $T5.3$ according to the classification of Grüsser and Grüsser-Cornehls. It is commonly believed that these cell types are involved in the recognition of prey by these animals.

Acknowledgement

This research was supported by Deutsche Forschungsgemeinschaft.

References

Ewert, J.-P. (1972). 'Zentralnervöse Analyse und Verarbeitung visueller Sinnesreize.' *Naturwissenschaftliche Rundschau*, **25**, 1–11.

Ewert, J.-P. (1976). 'The visual system of the toad: Behavioral and physiological studies on a pattern recognition system.' In *The Amphibian Visual System*, ed. K. V. Fite. New York, San Francisco, London: Academic Press.

Ewert, J.-P. & Hock, F. J. (1972). 'Movement sensitive neurons in the toad's retina.' *Experimental Brain Research*, **16**, 41–59.

Ewert, J.-P. & von Seelen, W. (1974). 'Neurobiologie und Systemtheorie eines visuellen Muster-Erkennungsmechanismus bei Kröten.' *Biological Cybernetics*, **14**, 167–83.

Ewert, J.-P. & von Wietersheim, A. (1974). 'Musterauswertung durch Tektum- und

Thalamus/Praetectum-Neurone im visuellen System der Kröte (*Bufo bufo L.*).' *Journal of Comparative Physiology*, **92**, 131–48.

Grüsser, O.-J. & Grüsser-Cornehls, U. (1976). 'Neurobiology of the anuran visual system.' In *Frog Neurobiology*, eds. R. Llinas & W. Precht. Berlin, Heidelberg, New York: Springer.

an der Heiden, U. (1980). *Analysis of Neural Networks*. Berlin, Heidelberg, New York: Springer.

an der Heiden, U. & Roth, G. (1983). 'Cooperative neural processes in amphibian visual prey recognition.' In *Synergetics of the Brain*, eds. E. Basar, H. Flohr, H. Haken & A. J. Mandell. Berlin, Heidelberg, New York, Tokyo: Springer.

an der Heiden, U. & Roth, G. (1988). 'Mathematical model and simulation of retina and tectum opticum of lower vertebrates.' *Acta Biotheoretica,* **36** (to appear).

Pfeiffer, E. (1975). Musterauswertung durch retinale Ganglienzellen beim Frosch (*Rana esculenta L.*). Diplomarbeit, Universität Darmstadt.

Roth, G. & Jordan, M. (1982). 'Response characteristics and stratification of tectal neurons in the toad *Bufo bufo (L.).*' *Experimental Brain Research*, **45**, 393–8.

Varjú, D. (1978). 'Excitatory and inhibitory processes giving rise to the delayed response in the retinal ganglion cell of the frog.' In *Theoretical Approaches to Complex Systems*, eds. R. Heim & G. Palm. Berlin, Heidelberg, New York: Springer.

Supported by Deutsche Forschungsgemeinschaft.

30

Pattern recognition with modifiable neuronal interactions

J. V. WINSTON

30.1 Introduction

Neural networks with plasticity (dynamic connection coefficients) can recognize and associate stimulus patterns. Previous studies have shown the usefulness of a simple algorithm called 'brain-washing' which leads to networks which can have many eligible neurons with large variations in activity and complex cyclic modes (Clark & Winston, 1984). Methods of modifying connection coefficients are discussed and evaluated.

Successful pattern recognition with quasirandom, rather than topographic, networks would be much more significant and general. There is no doubt that topographic networks could be more efficient in the brain but less adaptable to changing conditions. A quasirandom network could be trained to recognize temporal and spatial stimuli, while a topographic network would be limited to a particular type of stimuli.

Three types of neurons have been incorporated into the network. A group of 10 input (stimulus) neurons (N_i) send μ_i efferents to neurons in the main network (see Figs. 30.1 and 30.2). Neurons in the main network are interconnected by μ_a afferent connections and μ_e efferent connections. In addition a group of output neurons (N_o) can be included to monitor activity of the main network and to train the network.

Components of a successful, sensible and biologically feasible training algorithm will be discussed.

30.2 Physical limitations to training algorithms

A specified neuron obtains the majority of information from afferent and efferent neurons. Non-specific information certainly could be passed to groups of neurons via humeral transmitters (i.e. hormones) or by adjacent but non-interconnected neurons. Knowledge of the action at a distant

Fig. 30.1. Diagram of a model neuron. Incoming potentials to neuron
i $(u_i(t + \tau))$ is equal to the potential at the previous time period times δ plus the
sum of the active connection coefficients entering neuron i. If this potential is
greater than the threshold voltage and the neuron has not fired within the
refractory period then neuron i will be active $(s_i(t + \tau))$. Both an absolute (R_a)
and relative refractory period (R_r) are tested. If the neuron is beyond the absolute
refractory period and within the relative refractory period then a higher threshold
voltage is used (θ_r).

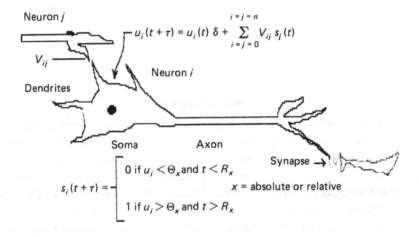

Diagram of model neuron

Neuron j

$$u_i(t + \tau) = u_i(t)\,\delta + \sum_{i=j=0}^{i=j=n} V_{ij}\,s_j(t)$$

V_{ij}

Neuron i

Dendrites

Soma   Axon

Synapse →

$$s_i(t + \tau) = \begin{cases} 0 \text{ if } u_i < \Theta_x \text{ and } t < R_x \\[6pt] 1 \text{ if } u_i > \Theta_x \text{ and } t > R_x \end{cases}$$

x = absolute or relative

Fig. 30.2. Structure of neural network with input (sensory) neurons (N_i) each
sending μ_i efferent connections randomly to neurons in the main network of N
neurons. Neurons in the main network are interconnected by μ_a randomly
distributed afferent connections and μ_e efferent connections. Each output (motor)
neuron (N_o) has μ_o afferent connections from the main network.

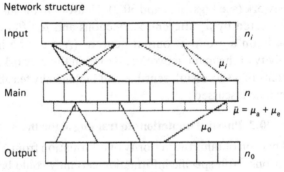

Network structure

Input n_i

μ_i

Main n

$\bar{\mu} = \mu_a + \mu_e$

μ_o

Output n_o

Pseudorandom connections in main net

non-interconnected neuron would not be available. Each synapse should know the activity of both the afferent and efferent neuron at the current and previous time step $(t - \tau)$.

An assumption will be made that only the magnitude of the V_{ij} will be retained between time intervals and that incremental changes will occur when specified conditions are met as determined by the algorithm. It is difficult to imagine that a neuron would have knowledge of previous activity other than the magnitude of V_{ij}. It would seem logical that humoral messages could inform groups of neurons when training is to occur and possibly which training algorithm to use.

30.3 Elements of training algorithms

Training algorithms are based on the knowledge of activity of the two connecting neurons at each synapse. The training algorithms can also take into account whether the synapse is inhibitory or exitatory. There are then eight possible categories. The magnitude of V_{ij} can be increased, decreased or unchanged.

The magnitude of the change must also be incorporated into the training algorithm. The simplest possibility is to increment by a constant incremental factor (f) as in eqn (1). Limits on the magnitude must also be checked when a linear system is used. Another method used is to multiply by f, which causes a larger change in larger connection coefficients (equation (2)). This works well for decreasing the magnitude when the factor is between 1 and 0, because the lower limit is zero. In this paper the V_{ij} is multiplied by a fraction of the difference between V_{ij} and the maximum magnitude (V_{max}) as in eqn (3). This prevents the connection from exceeding the V_{max} without having to test each time the connection is increased. Eqns (4), (5) and (6) show the three methods of decreasing the magnitude of connection coefficients.

Connection modification equations

Equation	Restrictions

Increase magnitude

$$|V_{ij}| = |V_{ij}| + f \qquad\qquad |V_{ij}| \leqslant V_{max} \text{ and } f \geqslant 0, \qquad (1)$$

$$V_{ij} = V_{ij} \times f \qquad\qquad |V_{ij}| \leqslant V_{max} \text{ and } f \geqslant 1, \qquad (2)$$

$$|V_{ij}| = |V_{ij}| + (V_{max} - |V_{ij}| \times f) \qquad 0 \leqslant f \leqslant 1, \qquad (3)$$

Decrease magnitude

$$|V_{ij}| = |V_{ij}| - f \qquad\qquad |V_{ij}| < V_{max} \text{ and } f \geqslant 0, \qquad (4)$$

$$V_{ij} = V_{ij}/f \qquad\qquad |V_{ij}| < V_{max} \text{ and } f \geqslant 1, \qquad (5)$$

$$V_{ij} = V_{ij} - (V_{ij} \times f) \qquad\qquad 0 \leqslant f \leqslant 1. \qquad (6)$$

If no attempt is made to try to decrease the magnitude of as many connections as are increased then excessive activity will occur. Normalization can be used to decrease the activity in the net by decreasing all V_{ij} intermittently. The sum of all connection coefficients is maintained constant by reducing all coefficients proportionally after training. A second method of preventing overactivity is to raise the threshold voltage or increase refractory period.

Determining the intensity of training is most difficult. Prolonged training can destroy the training of other stimulus patterns or progress to overactivity. Currently this is being done empirically by varying f or the number of time steps in which training occurs. Future training algorithms can incorporate tests to determine the correct amount of training.

30.4 Experience with one training algorithm

The first goal was to produce cyclic modes of low activity in response to specific repeating stimuli. A network consisting of 10 input neurons (N_i) with five efferent connections (u_i) to the main network of 50 neurons (N) with an average of 50 efferent connections to other neurons in the main net with a minimum of 25 afferent connections (u_a) and 25 efferent connections (u_e) assigned with quasirandom numbers. The magnitude of the initial connection coefficient strength for the main net is $1 \pm 0.5\varepsilon$, where ε is a quasirandom number between 0 and 1. The magnitude of the efferent input neuron connections is 10 with a threshold voltage of 9 so that each input connection can activate a neuron in the main net. The fraction of inhibitory neurons (h) is $\frac{3}{10}$. The absolute refractory period (R_a) is two time steps which allows a maximum firing rate of every other time step. Potentials are summed only during the current time step and are not saved for the next time step ($\delta = 0$). The threshold voltage (θ) is 9. The stimulus pattern consisted of input neuron 1 at time step 1, neuron 2 at time step 2 and neuron 3 at time step 3. This pattern was then repeated. Fig. 30.3 displays all ten stimulus patterns used in the experiments.

The training algorithm with modification of connection coefficients began on time step 9. Fig. 30.4 is a computer printout of a table of activity with stimulus pattern (P_i), input potential ($POT = 10$), training mode ($S = 2$) and incremental factor ($f = 0.039$). The goal of training algorithm 2 is to engram a repeating stimulus into the random network so that cyclic activity will quickly occur with a single presentation of any of the first three patterns. One would expect similar cyclic modes for each of the first three stimulus patterns after training. Prior to training the net dies with high threshold voltage. Note that there is a large stimulus potential of 10 and a large θ of 10 to prevent over activity during this intense stimuli. Only main net neurons directly connected to the stimulus neurons ($\mu_i = 5$) should be active. During training all connections between active neurons are strengthened by eqn (3). The absolute value of inhibitory connections are reduced. As training proceeds cyclic activity does not usually change. After 55 steps of training 15 excitatory connection coefficients were increased to between 7 and 8. At the completion of training, 3-step cyclic mode continued with low activities (active neurons/total neurons) of 0.10, 0.08 and 0.06.

30.5 Evaluation of trained network

With single presentation of P_1, a 3-step cyclic mode with activities of 0.16, 0.10 and 0.22 occurred with threshold voltage at 4. The same cyclic mode occurred with P_3. A single presentation of P_2 progressed to maximum activity with 2-step cycling with activities of 0.3 and 0.7 with threshold voltage at 4. P_2 failed to produce the same cyclic activity because two extra neurons were allowed to fire because they were no longer in their refractory period. P_2 produced a similar but less active cycling mode (0.08, 0.08 and 0.06) with a higher threshold voltage of 6.8.

Additional training was performed with a repeating stimulus P_4, P_5 and P_6. After training, a single presentation of stimulus P_4, P_5 or P_6, all produced the same cyclic pattern with a threshold voltage of 8. Presentation of stimulus patterns P_1 and P_3 produced a slightly different cyclic pattern with a period of 6. P_2 produced a different cyclic pattern with a

Fig. 30.3. Representation of ten stimulus patterns. Each pattern displays which input neurons are active (*) or inactive (O). Only neuron 1 is active in stimulus pattern 1. Multiple input neurons can be active in a stimulus pattern.

Stimulus patterns	
1	*000000000
2	0*00000000
3	00*0000000
4	000*000000
5	0000*00000
6	00000*0000
7	000000*000
8	0000000*00
9	00000000*0
10	000000000*

Fig. 30.4. Computer printout of table at each time step. The activity (ACT), stimulus pattern (P), input potential ($POT = 10$), training mode ($S = 2$) and incremental factor ($f = 0.039$) are listed for each time step. The asterisk displays the activity (active neurons/total neurons) along the horizontal graph. The lower part of the figure displays the firing patterns at each time step. The first number in each line is the time step followed by the activity of the network. Each character represents one of the 50 neurons. The asterisk represents an active excitatory neuron and a plus sign an active inhibitory neuron. The O represents an inactive excitatory neuron and the zero represents an inactive inhibitory neuron. Note that there is three state cycling during stimulation of repeating stimulus patterns P_1, P_2 and P_3. Training of the network with modification of connection coefficients begins at step 9.

Neural networks program

Table of neural network activity

STEP	ACT	P	POT	S	F	0 0.1 0.2 0.3 0.4 0.5 0.6 0.7
0	0.000	0	0.000	0	0.000	*
1	0.100	1	10.000	0	0.000	*
2	0.060	2	10.000	0	0.000	*
3	0.100	3	10.000	0	0.000	*
4	0.080	1	10.000	0	0.000	*
5	0.060	2	10.000	0	0.000	*
6	0.100	3	10.000	0	0.000	*
7	0.080	1	10.000	0	0.000	*
8	0.060	2	10.000	0	0.000	*
9	0.100	3	10.000	2	0.039	*
10	0.080	1	10.000	2	0.039	*
11	0.060	2	10.000	2	0.039	*
12	0.100	3	10.000	2	0.039	*
13	0.080	1	10.000	2	0.039	*
14	0.060	2	10.000	2	0.039	*
15	0.100	3	10.000	2	0.039	*
16	0.080	1	10.000	2	0.039	*
17	0.060	2	10.000	2	0.039	*
18	0.100	3	10.000	2	0.039	*
19	0.080	1	10.000	0	0.000	*
20	0.060	2	10.000	0	0.000	*
21	0.100	3	10.000	0	0.000	*

```
 0  0.000  0000000000000000000000000000000000000000000000000
 1  0.100  000000*000+00000000000*0000000000000000000000*0+000000
 2  0.060  00000000000000000000*00000000000000000*000000000*0000
 3  0.100  00000+00*00000000000+000000000000000000*0000000000*0
 4  0.080  000000*000+0000000000000000000000000000000000*0+000000
 5  0.060  00000000000000000000*0000000000000000*000000000*0000
 6  0.100  00000+00*00000000000+000000000000000000*0000000000*0
 7  0.080  000000*000+0000000000000000000000000000000000*0+000000
 8  0.060  00000000000000000000*0000000000000000*000000000*0000
 9  0.100  00000+00*00000000000+000000000000000000*0000000000*0
10  0.080  000000*000+0000000000000000000000000000000000*0+000000
11  0.060  00000000000000000000*0000000000000000*000000000*0000
12  0.100  00000+00*00000000000+000000000000000000*0000000000*0
13  0.080  000000*000+0000000000000000000000000000000000*0+000000
14  0.060  00000000000000000000*0000000000000000*000000000*0000
15  0.100  00000+00*00000000000+000000000000000000*0000000000*0
16  0.080  000000*000+0000000000000000000000000000000000*0+000000
17  0.060  00000000000000000000*0000000000000000*000000000*0000
18  0.100  00000+00*00000000000+000000000000000000*0000000000*0
19  0.080  000000*000+0000000000000000000000000000000000*0+000000
20  0.060  00000000000000000000*0000000000000000*000000000*0000
21  0.100  00000+00*00000000000+000000000000000000*0000000000*0
```

Fig. 30.5. Displays the cyclic modes after a single presentation of each of the ten stimulus patterns after training. P_1, P_2 and P_3 have identical cyclic modes as hoped because they were trained to produce identical cyclic modes. P_4, P_5 and P_6 were trained to have cyclic modes different from the first three groups. P_4 and P_6 successively produced the same 3-step cyclic mode of which was different from that produced by P_1. P_5 however produced a cyclic mode like P_1. P_7, P_8, P_9 and P_{10} were trained to produce a different cyclic mode, however only P_9 produced a different cyclic mode with a period of 2.

Neural networks program

```
*STIM-1

   4  0.080   OOOOOO*OOOOOOOOO*OOOOOOOOOOOOOOOOOOOOOO*OOOO+OOOOOO
   5  0.080   OOOOOOOOOOOOOOOOOOO*O+OO+OOOOOOOOOOOOOOOOOOOOOO*OOOO
   6  0.080   +OOOOOOO*OOOOOOOOOOOOOOOOOOOOOOOOOOOOOOO*OOOOOOOOOO*O
*STIM-2

   5  0.080   +OOOOOOO*OOOOOOOOOOOOOOOOOOOOOOOOOOOOOOO*OOOOOOOOOO*O
   6  0.080   OOOOOO*OOOOOOOOO*OOOOOOOOOOOOOOOOOOOOOO*OOOO+OOOOOO
   7  0.080   OOOOOOOOOOOOOOOOOOO*O+OO+OOOOOOOOOOOOOOOOOOOOOO*OOOO
*STIM-3

   4  0.080   +OOOOOOO*OOOOOOOOOOOOOOOOOOOOOOOOOOOOOOO*OOOOOOOOOO*O
   5  0.080   OOOOOO*OOOOOOOOO*OOOOOOOOOOOOOOOOOOOOOO*OOOO+OOOOOO
   6  0.080   OOOOOOOOOOOOOOOOOOO*O+OO+OOOOOOOOOOOOOOOOOOOOOO*OOOO
*STIM-4

   4  0.040   OOOOOOOOOOOOOOOOOOOO+OO+OOOOOOOOOOOOOOOOOOOOOOOOOOOO
   5  0.020   OOOOOOOO*OOOOOOOOOOOOOOOOOOOOOOOOOOOOOOOOOOOOOOOOOOO
   6  0.060   OOOOOOOOOO+OOOOO*OOOOOOOOOOOOOOOOOOOO*OOOOOOOOOO
*STIM-5

   5  0.080   OOOOOOOOOOOOOOOOOOO*O+OO+OOOOOOOOOOOOOOOOOOOOOO*OOOO
   6  0.080   +OOOOOOO*OOOOOOOOOOOOOOOOOOOOOOOOOOOOOOO*OOOOOOOOOO*O
   7  0.080   OOOOOO*OOOOOOOOO*OOOOOOOOOOOOOOOOOOOOOO*OOOO+OOOOOO
*STIM-6

   5  0.040   OOOOOOOOOOOOOOOOOOOO+OO+OOOOOOOOOOOOOOOOOOOOOOOOOOOO
   6  0.020   OOOOOOOO*OOOOOOOOOOOOOOOOOOOOOOOOOOOOOOOOOOOOOOOOOOO
   7  0.060   OOOOOOOOOO+OOOOO*OOOOOOOOOOOOOOOOOOOO*OOOOOOOOOO
*STIM-7

   5  0.040   OOOOOOOOOOOOOOOOOOOO+OO+OOOOOOOOOOOOOOOOOOOOOOOOOOOO
   6  0.020   OOOOOOOO*OOOOOOOOOOOOOOOOOOOOOOOOOOOOOOOOOOOOOOOOOOO
   7  0.060   OOOOOOOOOO+OOOOO*OOOOOOOOOOOOOOOOOOOO*OOOOOOOOOO
*STIM-8

  22  0.040   OOOOOOOOOOOOOOOOOOOO+OO+OOOOOOOOOOOOOOOOOOOOOOOOOOOO
  23  0.020   OOOOOOOO*OOOOOOOOOOOOOOOOOOOOOOOOOOOOOOOOOOOOOOOOOOO
  24  0.060   OOOOOOOOOO+OOOOO*OOOOOOOOOOOOOOOOOOOO*OOOOOOOOOO
*STIM-9

   6  0.260   +OOOOOOOO+OOOOO*OOO+OO+OOO+OOOOO*+OO**OO*O+OOOO*O
   7  0.140   OOOO*O*O*OOOOOOOOO*OOOOOOOOOOO+OOO*OOOOOOOOO*OOOO
*STIM-10

   5  0.040   OOOOOOOOOOOOOOOOOOOO+OO+OOOOOOOOOOOOOOOOOOOOOOOOOOOO
   6  0.020   OOOOOOOO*OOOOOOOOOOOOOOOOOOOOOOOOOOOOOOOOOOOOOOOOOOO
   7  0.060   OOOOOOOOOO+OOOOO*OOOOOOOOOOOOOOOOOOOO*OOOOOOOOOO
```

period of 2. At this point there were 22 connection coefficients with values greater than 7 and 11 with values close to the maximum of 10.

Additional training was then performed with a sequence of repeating stimulus patterns P_7, P_8, P_9 and P_{10}. Because of overlapping interconnecting neurons, the cyclic patterns in response to some of the previous stimuli were changed. The cyclic pattern generated by the repeating stimulus could not be reproduced by a single presentation of pattern 7. Fig. 30.5 displays the cyclic modes after a single presentation of each of the ten stimulus patterns after all of the above training.

30.6 Discussion

The example above illustrates that cyclic patterns can be produced after training in response to a single stimuli. Similar cyclic patterns can be produced from different stimuli which were presented sequentially during training. A second set of stimuli were presented and produced different cyclic modes. This corresponds to Boolean 'AND' and 'OR' functions. Complex logic could then be produced by linking various nets together. A final solution can then be produced by training output neurons to respond to specific cyclic modes as shown in previous pattern recognition experiments (Clark *et al.*, 1985). In those experiments four cyclic modes were produced by four different stimuli. Each of the two output neurons were trained to recognize two of the four stimuli by strengthening connections of output neurons to the appropriate output neuron.

There is no doubt that structured neural networks could be trained to recognize a greater number of stimuli more efficiently, but would not have the same degree of adaptability. It is well known that the sensory neocortex has a specific structure with cells oriented in columns from superficial to deep layers (Shepherd, 1979). Most afferent connections from input neurons are located in layer IV. Pyramidal cells are output neurons located in layers III and V. They receive these afferents and send their axons to other cortical areas, superior colliculus and the thalamus. Golgi and bipolar cells are present as intrinsic neurons whose axons and dendrites are located in columns. Adjacent columns in the sensory neocortex represent adjacent sensory fields.

This structure maintains two degrees of topographical organization. Vertically input and output neurons are located at different levels and are connected to different types of neurons. Adjacent vertical columns contain adjacent somatosensory areas. This structure maintains restrictions but is ideally suited for the purpose of monitoring sensory stimuli and responding appropriately with motor response.

30.7 Computer applications

New parallel processing machines such as the 'Connection Machine' designed by Daniel Hillis at Thinking Machines Corporation of Cambridge, Mass. (Elmer-DeWitt, 1986) would be ideal for rapid simulation of neural networks. This computer has 65 536 parallel processors with 4096 switching station connecting all of the processors. Each processor has its own small memory bank and all are synchronized by the operating system. Time magazine reports that AT&T Bell Laboratories is experimenting with computer circuits which mimic nerve cells.

Each microprocessor can have a program to emulate a nerve cell. When signaled by the operating system, each microprocessor can sum all incoming potentials, determine if this exceeds the threshold potential and if the neuron is beyond its refractory period. The operating system could then poll each microprocessor at intervals to determine which ones are active. Output neurons could give continuous feedback via display devices such as video terminal, light array or printout.

Future study with neural networks should incorporate structures of different neuron types with topographical connections and more complicated stimuli such as 2-dimensional figures. Neural networks could also be designed to simulate feedback circuits to monitor and control external conditions.

Appendix: parameter list and definitions

N	Number of neurons in main network.
μ_a	Number of afferent (incoming) connections to each neuron.
μ_e	Number of efferent (outgoing) connections to each neuron.
$\bar{\mu}$	Average number of connections to each neuron $= \mu_a + \mu_e$.
h	Fraction of inhibitory neurons in the main network.
N_i	Number of input (stimulus or sensory) neurons.
μ_i	Number of efferents from input neurons to network.
N_o	Number of output (motor) neurons.
μ_o	Number of afferent neurons from main net to output neurons.
R_a	Absolute refractory time.
R_r	Relative refractory time.
θ_r	Threshold voltage between R_a and R_r.
θ_a	Threshold voltage after the refractory periods.
$S_i(t)$	State of neuron i at time t. (0 if inactive: 1 if active).
$U_i(t)$	Sum of incoming potentials of neuron i at time t.
τ	Unit time step.
δ	Fraction attenuation of potential between time steps.

ε Pseudorandom number between 0 and 1.

V_{ij} Connection (coupling) coefficient for the connection between neuron j and neuron i. $V_{ij} = 0$ if no connection.

V_{max} Maximum connection coefficient.

f Training incremental factor ($0 \leqslant f \leqslant 1$).

P_i Stimulus pattern i.

References

Clark, J. W., Rafelski, J., Winston, J. V. (1985). 'Brain without mind: computer simulation of neural networks with modifiable neuronal interactions.' *Physics Reports*, **123**(4), 215–73.

Clark, J. W., Winston, J. V. (1984). 'Self-organization of neural networks.' *Physics Letters*, **102A**, (4), 207–11.

Elmer-DeWitt, P. (1986). 'Letting 1000 Flowers Bloom.' *TIME*, June 9, 64.

Shepherd, G. M. (1979). 'The Synaptic Organization of the Brain.' New York: Oxford University Press.

31

Texture description in the time domain

H. J. REITBOECK, M. PABST, and R. ECKHORN

31.1 Introduction

The detection of image regions and their borders is one of the basic
requirements for further (object domain-) image processing in a general-
purpose technical pattern recognition system and, very likely, also in the
visual system. It is a pre-requisite for object separation (figure–ground
discrimination, and separation of adjoining and intersecting objects),
which in turn is necessary for the generation of invariances for object
recognition (Reitboeck & Altmann, 1984).

Texture is a powerful feature for region definition. Objects and background usually have different textures; camouflage works by breaking
this rule. For texture characterization, Fourier (power) spectra are
frequently used in computer pattern recognition. Although the signal
transfer properties of visual channels can be described in the spatial (and
temporal) frequency domain, there has been no conclusive evidence that
pattern processing in the primary visual areas would be in terms of local
Fourier spectra.

In the following we propose a model for texture characterization in the
visual system, based on region labeling in the time domain via correlated
neural events. The model is consistent with several basic operational
principles of the visual system, and its texture separation capacity is in
very good agreement with the pre-attentive texture separation of humans.

31.2 Texture region definition via temporal correlations

When we look at a scene, we can literally generate a 'matched filter' and
use it to direct our attention to a specific object region. It appears as if this
region were somehow 'labeled', so that it is perceived as an entity. In the
proposed model, texture regions are labeled, and linked to regions that

belong to a given object, via correlated or even quasi-synchronous activity of those visual neurons that are activated by the object. In the retina, correlated activity is induced by the shifts of the retinal image. In normal vision, the retinal image is permanently moving across the retina; this results in temporal variations of the activity of the receptors and of subsequent visual neurons. Spatial differences, e.g. in local brightness, are thus transformed into (spatial and) temporal variations of neural activities. The discharge patterns of neurons that are activated by regions of similar texture should, therefore, be similar, whereas neural activities evoked by discriminable textures should be different. The differences should be detectable by appropriate temporal sampling. The proposed model of pre-attentive texture discrimination describes these early processing stages only. At the higher visual processing levels (possibly already in the lateral geniculate nucleus), efferent signals from various visual areas would selectively affect the temporal order in the neural assemblies that respond to specific object regions. Finally, interaction with memory is assumed to modify the temporal and spatial associations for object definition and object classification. An attractive property of the model is that neural assemblies in separate cortical areas can be linked via correlated activity without requiring dedicated lines.

31.3 Methods

The texture discrimination capability of the model was tested using a variety of pre-attentively discriminable and non-discriminable textures similar to those used by Julesz (Julesz 1981a,b; Julesz, 1986).

The line textures (Figs. 31.1–31.6) were constructed of texture elements of 16×16 pixels arranged in a square mosaic with 15 elements per side. A whole image thus consists of 240×240 pixels. Binary textures were used, i.e., the pixel brightness was assumed to be 0 or 1 only. The general principle is also applicable to images with grey values; in this case, a detectable brightness gradient has to be specified by a threshold. All line textures were 1 pixel wide. In the dot textures, pixels were allowed to cluster.

The image $h(x, y)$ is projected onto a topographically organized 'neural layer' $N1$. The neurons in $N1$ are assumed to respond to brightness transients in one direction only. While $h(x, y)$ is moving across $N1$, a specific neuron will produce a spike at the instant when a 0/1-transition shifts over its receptive field. The distances between 0/1-transitions in shift direction therefore determine the time intervals between the spikes. If the shift velocity v is constant, the spike interval Δt is proportional to the spatial interval d between two 0/1-transitions, $\Delta t = d/v$. Equidistant temporal sampling of the activity of the neurons in $N1$ is used in order to detect those regions in $h(x, y)$ where spatial intervals of length d occur; the sampling interval Δt determines the value of d to be detected. This temporal sampling is assumed to be realized in a subsequent neural layer $N2$ that consists of an array of AND gates with one common (strobed) input. The density (frequency) of intervals of specific lengths is plotted in global interval histograms. These histograms also contain higher order intervals, i.e., concatenations of basic intervals. $N2$, therefore, can be realized as outlined above, without additional circuitry to exclude higher order intervals.

For texture comparison, interval histograms are represented as a multi-dimensional pattern vector. The Euclidian distance between these vectors according to

$$E = \sqrt{\left[\sum_{d=1}^{n} (NA(d) - NB(d))^2 \right]},$$

is used as a criterion of texture similarity, where $NA(d)$, $NB(d) =$ number of intervals of length d for texture A and B, and $n =$ maximum interval length in pixels.

For improved separation, a pattern vector of higher dimensionality can be constructed, using interval distributions for several scan directions. In the examples, a simpler method was used: the distance d was calculated for the four shift directions (0°, 45°, 90° and 135°) and the inverse of their sum was used as a criterion of similarity:

$$S = 1/\Sigma E.$$

In the following section, texture separation via interval histograms will be compared with psychophysical results on pre-attentively discriminable and non-discriminable textures. The results are in good agreement with texture separation based on the texton concept (Julesz, 1981a).

31.4 Texture discrimination experiments

31.4.1 Texture discrimination via interval histograms

For each texture pair, the density of intervals between 0/1-transitions is computed for interval lengths ranging from 1 to 16 pixels. Four shift directions are used (horizontal, vertical and two oblique) yielding four interval histograms. For many texture pairs it is possible to achieve adequate discrimination with the histogram for just one shift direction.

31.4.2 Spatial distribution of intervals of specific length

For a fast and simple definition of texture regions, the location of neurons responding to a specific gating interval are marked in the space domain. This results in a characteristic spatial distribution of intervals of a specific length that is often sufficient to separate the texture regions without requiring a texture vector based on the complete interval histogram.

31.4.3 Results

31.3.1 Line textures. We have tested the method on 19 line texture pairs, 11 of which are pre-attentively discriminable whereas the other eight are not. All texture pairs that are pre-attentively discriminable show significantly different amplitude distributions in their interval histograms. Certain modifications of the texture elements (e.g., anisotropic stretching) which decreased visual discrimination yields to an increase of the similarity S (see above) and vice versa. As an example, four pre-attentively discriminable and two indiscriminable texture pairs are shown in Figs. 31.1–31.6.

Global interval distribution histograms have been used for overall texture description (Figs. 31.1–31.6(d,e)). For texture region separation, the complete histogram, generally, is not required. Region separation in Figs. 31.1–31.6(f) is based on a single characteristic interval, i.e. on one component of the local pattern vector. Pre-attentively discriminable textures seem to contain at least one interval length (corresponding to one sampling interval) for which there is a distinct difference in the density of these intervals. In textures that are pre-attentively not discriminable there is no interval for any shift direction that would generate a density difference in the plots. This method often emphasizes a border between texture regions (as in Fig. 31.5(f)).

31.4.3.2 Dot textures. In the interval histogram of 34 dot texture pairs (18 discriminable, 16 not discriminable) we found three textures where the discrimination of our model did not agree with psychophysical results on humans (Fig. 31.7).

Fig. 31.7(a) shows a random dot pattern with 50% black and 50% white pixels. In Fig. 31.7(b) white, and in Fig. 31.7(c) black triangles of equal orientation and varying size are randomly distributed, and the spaces in between are filled with random black dots. The total number of black and white pixels is equal. The resulting three texture pairs are pre-attentively discriminable, while discrimination via interval histograms is hardly possible (Fig. 31.7(d,e,f)).

Fig. 31.1. Pre-attentively discriminable texture pair (different first-order statistics, different size of elongated blobs). (*a*) Texture *A*. (*b*) Texture pair. (*c*) Texture *B*. (*d*) Interval histogram of texture *A* (horizontal intervals). (*e*) Interval histogram of texture *B* (horizontal intervals). (*f*) Spatial distribution of 6-pixel intervals of the texture pair.

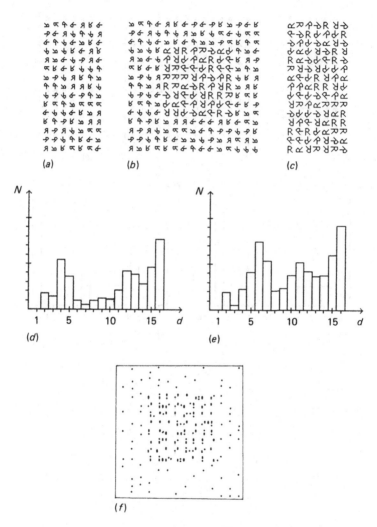

Fig. 31.2. Pre-attentively discriminable texture pair (different second-order statistics, different orientation of elongated blobs). (*a*) Texture *A*. (*b*) Texture pair. (*c*) Texture *B*. (*d*) Interval histogram of texture *A* (horizontal intervals). (*e*) Interval histogram of texture *B* (horizontal intervals). (*f*) Spatial distribution of 7-pixel intervals of the texture pair.

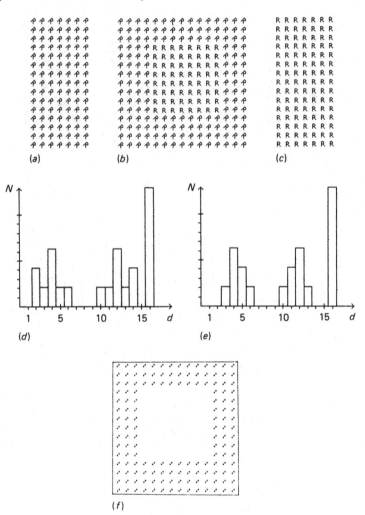

Fig. 31.3. Pre-attentively discriminable texture pair (identical second-order statistics, different number of line terminators). (*a*) Texture *A*. (*b*) Texture pair. (*c*) Texture *B*. (*d*) Interval histogram of texture *A* (diagonal intervals, +45°). (*e*) Interval histogram of texture *B* (diagonal intervals, +45°). (*f*) Spatial distribution of 8-pixel intervals of the texture pair.

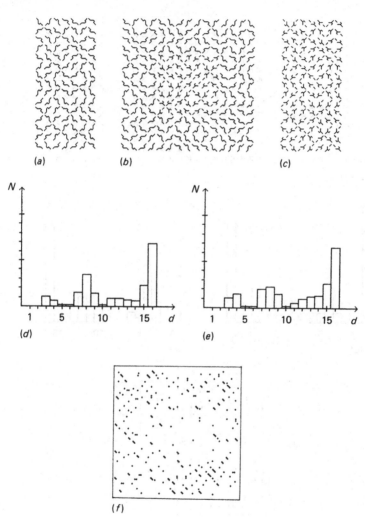

Fig. 31.4. Pre-attentively indiscriminable texture pair (identical second-order statistics, identical textons). (a) Texture A. (b) Texture pair. (c) Texture B. (d) Interval histogram of texture A (horizontal intervals). (e) Interval histogram of texture B (horizontal intervals). (f) Spatial distribution of 4-pixel intervals of the texture pair. There is no interval which occurs more often in one texture than in the other.

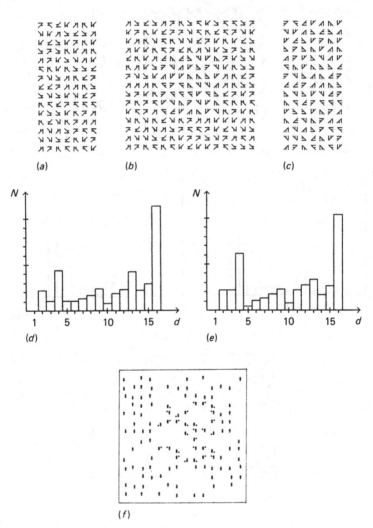

Fig. 31.5. Pre-attentively indiscriminable texture pair (identical second-order statistics, identical textons). (*a*) Texture *A*. (*b*) Texture pair. (*c*) Texture *B*. (*d*) Interval histogram of texture *A* (horizontal intervals). (*e*) Interval histogram of texture *B* (horizontal intervals). (*f*) Spatial distribution of 4-pixel intervals of the texture pair. There is no interval which occurs more often in one texture than in the other.

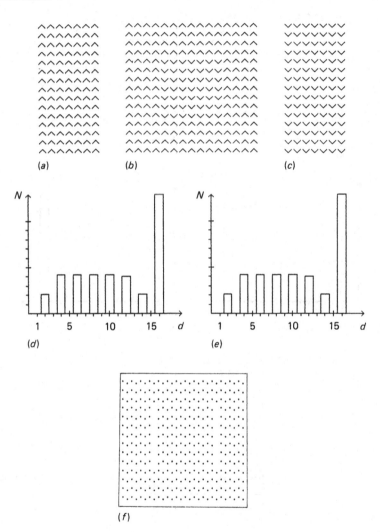

Fig. 31.6. Pre-attentively discriminable texture pair (different second-order statistics, identical textons). (*a*) Texture *A*. (*b*) Texture pair. (*c*) Texture *B*. (*d*) Interval histogram of texture *A* (horizontal intervals). (*e*) Interval histogram of texture *B* (horizontal intervals). (*f*) Spatial distribution of 4-pixel intervals of the texture pair.

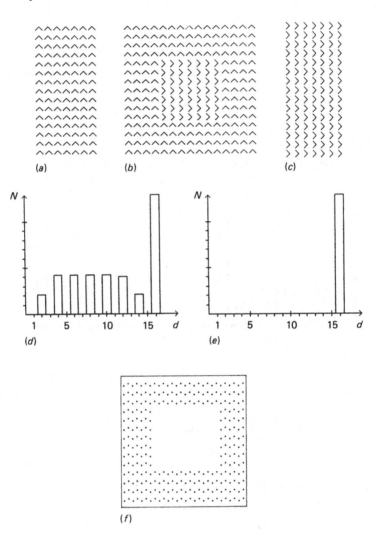

Fig. 31.7. Pre-attentively discriminable texture triplet (*a*, *b*, *c*) that cannot be discriminated via the interval histograms (*d*, *e*, *f*; horizontal intervals) generated by the simple model based on one retinal cell type (Y-ON response) only.

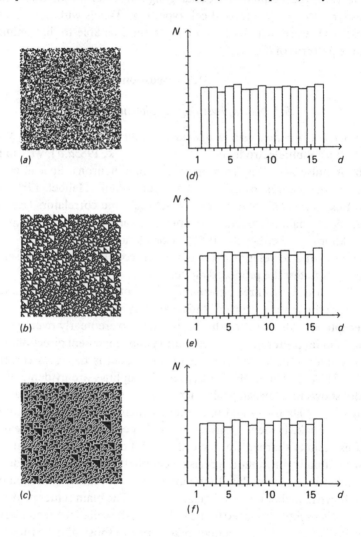

Although the patterns of Fig. 31.7 cannot be discriminated by the present model, it should be remembered, that this model was based on one cell type (similar to retinal ganglion Y-cells with transient ON-response) only. If a second cell type, e.g. X-cells with more sustained response, were included, the model should be able to discriminate the three patterns of Fig. 31.7.

31.5 Discussion

31.5.1 Neurophysiological plausibility of the model

31.5.1.1 Correlated activity of neurons in the visual cortex of cat. With the Marburg multielectrode technique (Reitboeck, 1983a,b), we can record the impulse activities from up to 19 single neurons. Special computer search procedures for appropriate group stimuli (Habbel, 1985; Habbel & Eckhorn, 1985) and multi-channel real time correlators (Eckhorn *et al.*, 1986) enable us to search for correlated activity during the experiment (Eckhorn & Reitboeck, 1986). Correlations due to common visual stimulus and correlations due to synaptic couplings have to be separated in order to test the proposed model.

Fig. 31.8 shows three different types of couplings between pairs of cells recorded from the primary and secondary visual cortex of the cat. The receptive fields (RFs) of the neuron pairs were nearly overlapping and had similar preferences for orientation and movement direction. Particularly interesting in the context of our model is the cross correlogram Fig. 31.8(*a*). Three different types of couplings are evident: the lower plot shows three broad peaks that are due to the phase-locked activations by the 1.7 Hz forth- and back-movements of the stimulus texture. The center peak, however, differs in its shape from both side peaks. It is considerably sharper, i.e. the cells exhibit correlated spike patterns that are mutually much more precisely coupled than the coupling due to the common visual stimulus. In the upper plots of Fig. 31.8, the center peak is shown in higher temporal magnification. The main center peak of 40 ms width is slightly displaced to the right, i.e., the cell of the secondary visual area discharges its correlated spikes prior to those of the primary visual area. At the center of this peak a sharp second peak is riding. This indicates that a second excitatory coupling path or a common pacing input of high temporal precision is active.

The correlograms in Fig. 31.8 were produced using a moving random dot stimulus. This results in a relatively broad peak in the stimulus-induced contributions to the cross correlogram. More structured textures

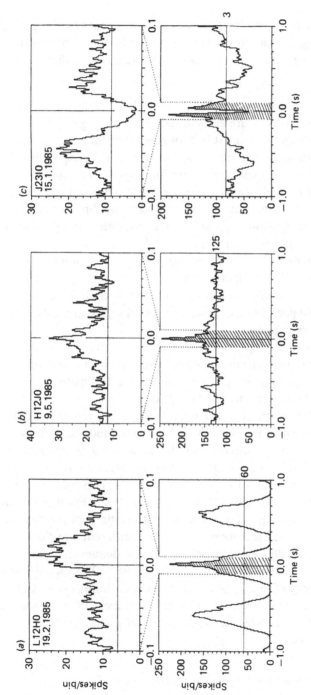

Fig. 31.8. Crosscorrelograms of three pairs of cat visual cortex neurons with overlapping receptive fields (RF). Stimulus: (a) and (b) Random dot texture moving sinusoidally in and against the cell's optimal direction (at 1.7 Hz). (b) Randomly jumping light spot. Cell types: (a) two simple cells from corresponding RF positions in primary and secondary visual area. (b) A simple and a complex cell from secondary visual area. (c) Two complex cells from secondary visual area. The upper plots are expanded from the lower central ± 100 ms. For more details see text.

do produce structured correlograms with narrower peaks (see, e.g., the correlation histograms of visual neurons in area 17 and 18 of the cat in response to moving random bar patterns (Schneider *et al.*, 1983)).

31.5.2 Occulomotor mechanisms

The proposed model of texture analysis requires a moving retinal image. Eye movements seem to be well suited for generating that image motion. Even during fixation the eye moves and causes retinal image shifts. In humans and higher vertebrates there are four types of eye movements: tremor, drifts, flicks† and saccades (Alpern, 1969). The discharge pattern of a visual neuron is determined by the velocity and direction of these movements, by the spatio-temporal transfer properties of the receptive units and by the spatial properties of the visual stimulus.

Image movements due to the eye tremor (maximal amplitude: 1′; maximal velocity: 20′ s^{-1}; Alpern, 1969) probably cannot play a significant role in texture interval detection, but tremor could be a suitable mechanism for the generation of precise temporal signals at the locations of sharp brightness transients.

Eye drifts (maximal amplitude: 5′, average velocity: 1′ s^{-1}, Alpern, 1969) would permit the detection of larger intervals but, because of their small drift velocity, they are primarily suited for the spatio-temporal transformation of fine structures within a texture.

For the transformation of a wider range of texture interval lengths, rapid eye flicks seem to be well suited. Their amplitudes are up to 20′ (Alpern, 1969), so that a suitable large image segment moves over the receptive fields. Intervals up to 20′ can thus be detected during a single flick. The average velocity of 10° s^{-1} (Alpern, 1969) corresponds to the velocity at which neurons in area 17 and 18 respond well. For the analysis of isotropic textures a single eye flick in an arbitrary direction is sufficient; anisotropic textures may require several flicks in different directions.

Eye saccades, finally, have velocities that predominately stimulate neurons in area 18 only (100–1000° s^{-1}, Hyde, 1959). The spatial resolution and sensitivity of the visual system is reduced during eye saccades. Nevertheless, recent investigations (Deubel & Elsner, 1986) indicate a facilitative effect of saccades on the detection of periodic stimuli (e.g., sine wave gratings).

---

† In the literature, eye flicks are frequently also called saccades.

31.5.3 Conclusions

The human visual system is able to pre-attentively discriminate certain textures, whereas it cannot discriminate others (Julesz 1981a,b, 1986). In the Julesz model, texture discrimination is assumed to depend on so-called textons, such as size and orientation of elongated blobs, number of line-endings, etc., and the pre-attentive system can discriminate textures only if they differ in one texton at least.

In our model, discrimination is based on texture intervals. In order to get an exact transformation of spatial intervals between image structures into temporal intervals between spikes, neurons with small receptive fields (simple cells in primary visual cortex area 17) would be best suited. The model requires coincidence detection (temporal sampling), a function that can be realized easily by neurons. Lateral interconnections are required, since gating pulses must be fed to all neurons of the filter layer $N2$. A possible brain structure that could serve as a central timing unit could be a subcortical structure outside the visual system, or groups of neurons receiving similar temporal activation. For a foveally located sampling circuit, that texture would be filtered out onto which the gaze is directed.

The inability of the model to discriminate the textures of Fig. 31.7 indicates that there must be some further mechanisms in texture perception. For example, the black and white triangles could be perceived as an entity because of the constant brightness within a triangle. Another possible solution is the assumption of the existence of sustained responding neurons (X-cells). Interval histograms of such responses seem to permit a discrimination of these textures.

Psychophysical experiments have shown that the discrimination of certain textures is enhanced if the size of texture elements and texture element distances are reduced. This is explained by the described method using rather small image shifts: interval lengths greater than the shift amplitude cannot be detected.

The movement of a textured area (e.g., object motion) in a non-moving surround yields strong region separation. The proposed model is able to explain this easily: the motion velocity and direction determines the spike intervals of the neurons in $N1$. Thus, the right sampling rate filters out the moving texture even if the non-moving (or with another velocity or direction moving) surround has identical texture.

References

Alpern, M. (1969). 'Types of movement.' In (ed. Hugh Davson) *The Eye*, vol. 3, pp. 65–174. Acad. Press, New York.

Altmann, L. (1982). Psychophysische Untersuchungen zur Rolle der Synchronität bei der Mustererkennung mit Hilfe einer mikroprozessorgesteuerten. LED-Matrix, M.S. Thesis, Marburg/Hamburg, F.R.G.

Deubel, H. & T. Elsner (1986). 'Threshold perception and saccadic eye movements.' *Biol. Cybern.*, **54**, 351–8.

Eckhorn, R., J. Schneider & R. Keidel (1986). 'Real-time covariance computer for cell assemblies is based on neuronal principles.' *J. Neurosc. Meth.*, **18**, 371–83.

Eckhorn, R. & H. J. Reitboeck (1986). 'Assessment of cooperative firing in groups of neurons: special concepts for multi-unit recordings from the visual system.' In (ed. E. Basar) Springer Series in *Brain Dynamics*, vol. 1, pp. 219–27. Springer-Verlag, Berlin, Heidelberg, New York.

Habbel, C. & R. Eckhorn (1985). 'Automatic search for effective stimuli for units in the cat's visual cortex.' *Neurosc. Lett., Suppl.*, **22**, 302.

Habbel, C. (1985). 'Anpassung von Bildsignalen an die Übertragungseigenschaften von visuellen rezeptiven Einheiten.' Ph.D. Thesis, Philipps-University, Marburg, F.R.G.

Hyde, J. E. (1959). 'Some characteristics of voluntary human occular movements in the horizontal plane.' *Am. J. Ophthal.*, **48**, 85–94.

Julesz, B. (1981a). 'Textons, the elements of texture perception and their interactions.' *Nature*, **290**, 91–7.

Julesz, B. (1981b). 'A theory of preattentive texture discrimination based on first-order statistics of textons.' *Biol. Cybern.*, **41**, 131–8.

Julesz, B. (1986). 'Texton gradients: the texton theory revisited.' *Biol. Cybern.*, **54**, 245–51.

Malsburg, von der, Ch. (1981). *The Correlation Theory of Brain Function*. Internal Report. University of Goettingen, F.R.G.

Nothdurft, H. C. & C. Y. Li (1985). 'Texture discrimination: representation of orientation and luminance differences in cells of the cat striate cortex.' *Vis. Res.*, **25**, 99–113.

Reitboeck, H. J. (1983a). 'Fiber electrodes for electrophysiological recordings.' *J. Neurosc. Meth.*, **8**, 249–62.

Reitboeck, H. J. (1983b). 'A 19-channel matrix drive with individually controllable fiber microelectrodes for neurophysiological applications.' *IEEE Trans. Syst., Man & Cybern. SMC*, **13**, 676–83.

Reitboeck, H. J. (1983c). In (eds. Basar *et al.*) *Synergetics of the Brain*. Springer-Verlag, pp. 174–82.

Reitboeck, H. J. & J. Altmann (1984). 'A model for size- and rotation-invariant pattern processing in the visual system.' *Biol. Cybern.*, **51**, 11–20.

Schneider, J., R. Eckhorn, & H. J. Reitboeck (1983). 'Evaluation of neuronal coupling dynamics.' *Biol. Cybern.*, **46**, 129–34.

Spangenberg, H. (1982). Ein Mustererkennungssystem, das gleichzeitig Analysen im Bildbereich und im Bereich der räumlichen Frequenzen durchführt. M.S. Thesis, Philipps-University, Marburg, F.R.G.

32

Computer-aided design of neurobiological experiments

INGOLF E. DAMMASCH

32.1 Motivation

A neuron's electrophysiological response to a disturbance is within the millisecond range and consists of action potentials which are produced when the threshold potential is being crossed. This response can be measured with microelectrodes and related to the stimulus. With neuroanatomical responses, this is a completely different task. Morphogenetic changes, such as reactive synaptogenesis or degeneration, take hours to days, so they cannot be directly observed by microelectrodes or the like. Besides, it would be very hard to relate the measured functional changes of electrical signals to changes in the synaptical 'hardware'. Therefore, animals have to be taken at different stages of time and the development of the central nervous system (with or without disturbances) has to be concluded from changes of their individual morphology. Moreover, to get reliable data, several animals have to be sacrificed at each time step. Sometimes, even that may not be enough, as the following example may show.

Measuring the development of the number of synapses in rat cortex from postnatal day 2 to adulthood (Balcar, Dammasch & Wolff, 1983), we expected to fit the data with a sigmoid curve corresponding to logistic growth, but the material appeared to be systematically disturbed. A population-kinetic model (Wagner & Wolff, subm.) developed at that time, could explain the disturbance as a temporary overshoot of free synaptic offers that were not distinguishable from bound synaptic elements. This stopped us declaring the data as faulty and repeating the experiment. Thus, a good model can help save animals.

32.2 Introduction

The theory underlying our morphogenetic models is the compensation theory of synaptogenesis (Wolff & Wagner, 1983). It describes the morphogenetic behavior of a nerve cell supposed to occur as a consequence of long-term disturbances of its excitation–inhibition equilibrium. Fundamentals are: (a) pre- and postsynaptic elements are separately formed; (b) the formation of presynaptic and postsynaptic elements is influenced by long-term changes of input, mediated either by synaptic or extrasynaptic receptors; (c) contact formation occurs according to the spatial density of pre- and postsynaptic contact partners.

Neurocytological results (Joó *et al.*, 1979; Wolff *et al.*, 1979) lead to the following hypotheses: long-term excitation leads to promoted formation (or reduced break down) of presynaptic elements and inhibitory postsynaptic elements, and to inhibited formation (or accelerated break down) of excitatory postsynaptic elements. Long-term inhibition has the opposite effect and leads to promoted formation of excitatory postsynaptic elements and to accelerated break down of presynaptic elements and inhibitory postsynaptic elements (therefore 'compensation' theory).

With this kind of behavior, the neurons interconnected in a network react individually to initial deviations. In an interactive, self-organizing process, they 'try' to gain equilibrium simultaneously, without knowing the overall network situation. The feed-back process works as follows: each neuron's afferent synapse spectrum influences – via transmission of signals from other neurons – its average membrane potential. Long-term excitation or inhibition leads to a 'morphogenetic state' outside a desirable range. It results in synaptical changes according to the compensation theory as mentioned above. This in turn leads – via degeneration of bound and recombination of free synaptic elements – to new afferent and efferent spectra. (For a detailed description of the algorithm, see Dammasch, Wagner & Wolff, 1986.)

The behavior of a neural system cannot be intuitively extrapolated from the compensatory behavior of its components, because of non-linearities and interactive effects. Therefore, the system's morphogenetic behavior was tested with two models: randomly connected networks and closed circuits.

32.3 Networks of logical neurons

A logical neuron as introduced by McCulloch & Pitts (1943) is a simplified cellular automaton (see Fig. 32.1(*a*)) with an output that can be either

Fig. 32.1. (*a*) The component of a network: a logical neuron capable of plasticity. (*b*) Experimental situation: the SCG cell increases its number of free postsynaptic elements because it is over-inhibited ('low'). The hypoglossal nerve has a number of free presynaptic elements. These two offers can recombine and form new synapses.

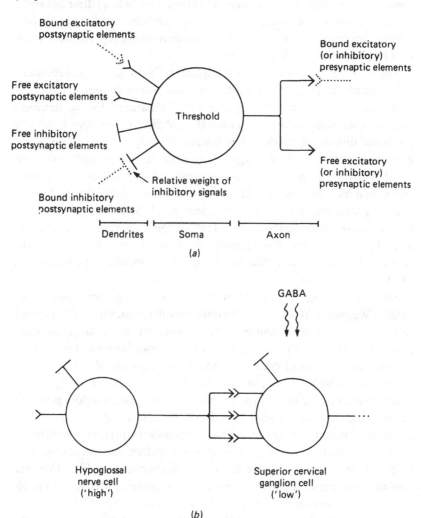

(*a*)

(*b*)

'active' or 'inactive'. When the postsynaptic potential (sum of active excitatory inputs minus weighted sum of active inhibitory inputs) reaches the threshold, the cell becomes active itself and influences others. In the networks we used, the synaptic strengths were randomly distributed on a connectivity matrix. Under certain conditions (see below) these networks are able to produce cyclic oscillations and maintain a medium integrated activity, avoiding situations where the whole network is permanently 'on' or 'off' (Dammasch & Wagner, 1984).

The task of the compensation algorithm is to save this functional behavior while moving all individual neurons into a 'desired' excitation–inhibition-equilibrium. This equilibrium – measured by the neuron's postsynaptic potential averaged over several different cycles – is initially disturbed due to the random distribution of synaptic connections: some neurons are more excited ('high' type), some are more inhibited ('low' type). During the morphogenetic process, all neurons in the network move their morphogenetic state towards the desired range by successively changing their pre- and postsynaptic elements. When this is achieved, the whole network is in equilibrium and morphogenesis comes to an end. As a result of this process, the input configurations (afferent spectra) of the neurons converge to a certain order, i.e., to a comparable ratio between excitatory and inhibitory inputs.

All this happens successfully under the following conditions (Dammasch, Wagner & Wolff, 1988): to obtain oscillations, we need (a) a small but powerful set of inhibitors, (b) a threshold low enough to allow sustained activity, (c) stochasticity in the input spectra, i.e., a non-uniform distribution of synaptic connections in the initial network, (d) a desired range wide enough to avoid too much order in the end phase of compensation, because an ordered network loses its oscillatory potential (Dammasch, 1986). For smooth convergence, we need (a) postsynaptic potentials instead of spikes to rule the compensation process, (b) different network states to start different oscillations before each morphogenetic step, (c) several cycles before each morphogenetic step, (d) a low time constant leading to a sensible speed for the search process. To enable convergence towards stability, (a) the net effect of growth and degeneration of synaptic elements should lead to an expected 10% decrease in the number of bound synapses, (b) the kinetics within excitatory and inhibitory elements have to be equally fast. The 'kinetic' parameters have to be chosen accordingly; these parameters govern the changes of synaptic elements proportionally to their numbers and their cell's deviation from the desired range.

The heart of the compensatory process is the combined synaptic rule, i.e., the rule describing the interactive effects of pre- and postsynaptical local decisions between the clusters of 'high' and 'low'-type neurons. At this level, our rule is not of the 'Hebb' type and therefore does not enforce structures or patterns. On the other hand, it leads to equilibrium merely on the basis of individual cell behavior, and no further assumptions have to be added to avoid instabilities (e.g., caused by exponential growth of the number of synapses). The combined rule results in the following morphogenetic consequences:

(1) Between 'high'-type neurons, the excitatory connections degenerate and the inhibitory connections increase by recombination of free offers.

(2) Between 'high'-type presynaptic and 'low'-type postsynaptic neurons, the excitatory connections increase while the inhibitory connections decrease.

(3) Between 'low'-type presynaptic and 'high'-type postsynaptic neurons, the excitatory connections degenerate significantly more.

(4) Between 'low'-type neurons, the inhibitory connections degenerate significantly more.

As a net effect, the deviation of the postsynaptic neuron is always compensated in the right direction (compare Table 32.1). From these four different morphogenetic consequences, the second one may explain the following experimental result (Dames *et al.*, 1985): It was found that local GABA-application into the intact superior cervical ganglion of the adult rat allows active innervation of a surgically implanted hypoglossal nerve in addition to the normal nerve supply of the ganglion. GABA is not only an inhibitory transmitter but has morphological effects too (Wolff, 1979). The result is the second case: 'high' hypoglossal presynaptic neuron meets 'low' SCG postsynaptic neuron, consequently leading to synaptogenesis by recombination of free pre- and postsynaptic offers (see Fig. 32.1(*b*)).

Similar experiments will be carried out in the future, e.g. we will observe the consequences of external afferences onto a subset of neurons in a simulated network and compare it with experimental data.

32.4 Closed circuits of logical neurons

For our second approach to plasticity, we used an even more simplified neuron model: Here, the activity is not produced in the form of spikes or oscillations, but a continuous flow is sent through the axon onto the following neuron. Two or three neurons of this type are grouped into a

Table 32.1. *The compensation theory of synaptogenesis.*

Cell reaction type	morphogenetic change
'high'	bound and free *excitatory* postsynaptic elements ↓
	free *inhibitory* postsynaptic elements ↑
	free *presynaptic* elements
'low'	free *excitatory* postsynaptic elements ↑
	bound and free *inhibitory* postsynaptic elements ↓
	bound and free *presynaptic* elements

Network reaction connection type	combined morphogenetic change
'high' on 'high'	excitatory synapses ↓ inhibitory synapses ↑
'high' on 'low'	excitatory synapses ↑ inhibitory synapses ↓ (!)
'low' on 'high'	excitatory synapses ↓ inhibitory synapses →
'low' on 'low'	excitatory synapses → inhibitory synapses ↓

Note: Several (simulated) network oscillations lead to deviations in the individual postsynaptic potentials: each neuron is either type 'high' or 'low'. This in turn results in individual morphogenetic reactions (cell level) and system reactions (network level). Note that pre- and postsynaptic elements are separately formed. 'Free' elements are contact offers, 'bound' elements are already engaged in a synaptic contact. The second type of network reaction may explain the situation in Fig. 32.1(*b*).

closed circuit (see Fig. 32.2), i.e., the activity builds up in a kind of feed-back loop. The equilibrium value of each neuron's activity level depends on its autonomous initial activity, the activity it receives from diffuse excitatory and inhibitory environments, and the activity it receives from its presynaptic neuron. The feed-back process is stable under a biologically plausible condition: Each neuron's equilibrium value is finite and unique, if the synaptic weights are such that less than 100% of the activity is transmitted from pre- to postsynaptic neuron.

This first equilibrium can be disturbed when the activity input from the environment is changed. Modeling a lesion of afferent excitatory fibers, the synaptic weight of the excitatory environment of one neuron is reduced and kept at this low level. As a direct consequence, the activity levels of all neurons will move to a new equilibrium. Now it is the task of the morphogenesis algorithm to restore the first equilibrium by changing the synaptic weights; again this is done according to the principles of the

Fig. 32.2. (*a*) The components of a two-neuron closed circuit. (*b*) Experimental situation: visual cortex cells, among them inhibitors projecting into outer borders, are isolated from thalamic afferences, therefore become 'low'-type and grow excitatory postsynaptic offers. These can be matched by presynaptic offers of disinhibited (and therefore 'high') excitatory cells from the outer borders of the visual cortex.

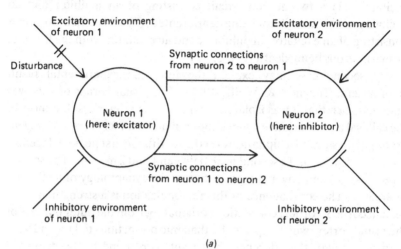

(*a*)

(*b*)

compensation theory. The question of interest is: What can the other neurons contribute to compensate the deficiency of the disturbed neuron?

We tested all combinations of excitatory and inhibitory components, looking for the cases with a significant reinnervation of the deafferented neuron by terminal sprouting. We found it only in cases with a disinhibited excitator: (1) a two-neuron circuit consisting of an inhibitor and an excitator, with the inhibitor being deafferented; (2) a three-neuron circuit consisting of an excitator, an inhibitor and an excitator, with the first one or two neurons being deafferented.

The second case may explain the following experimental result (Holzgraefe, Teuchert & Wolff, 1981): The visual cortex of rats was undercut such that it was isolated from thalamic afferences, but most of the callosal and associative connections remained intact. Terminal degeneration then showed a biphasic time course with the first peak of degeneration at 3–5 days, and a second peak between 1 and 2 months. The second phase may accompany a reorganization of the synaptology of lamina IV in area 17. The consequence of this reorganization is a strengthening of certain cortico–cortical connections originating from the outer borders of the visual cortex, which replace the thalamic projections to lamina IV.

In our model, the afferences being cut correspond to the disturbed excitatory environment of the first two neurons. The disturbance causes a low activity of these two neurons, leading to a disinhibition of the third one. Being overactive ('high' type), the excitator corresponding to the neurons from the outer borders of the visual cortex starts sprouting, i.e., producing free presynaptic offers. These can recombine with the excitatory postsynaptic offers of the deafferented first neuron. Thus, our model could explain the new cortico–cortical connections.

Other cases will be tested in the future. It will also be interesting to simulate cases with a periodical disturbance from the environment. First experiments indicate that after several changes, some connections degenerate significantly less than others, or even become stronger. A necessary condition is again the existence of an inhibitory interneuron. With a configuration like that, a 'Hebbian' kind of synaptogenesis may evolve as a system phenomenon.

References

Balcar, V. J., Dammasch, I. E. & Wolff, J. R. (1983). 'Is there a non-synaptic component in the K$^+$-stimulated release of GABA in the developing rat cortex? *Dev Brain Res*, **10**, 309–11.

Dames, W., Joó, F., Fehér, O., Toldi, J. & Wolff, J. R. (1985). 'γ-aminobutyric acid enables synaptogenesis in the intact superior cervical ganglion of the adult rat.' *Neurosc. Letters*, **54**, 159–64.

Dammasch, I. E. (1986). 'Morphogenesis and properties of neuronal model networks. In: Trappl, R. (ed.). *Cybernetics and Systems '86*. Reidel Publ. Co., Dordrecht, pp. 327–34.

Dammasch, I. E. & Wagner, G. P. (1984). 'On the properties of randomly connected McCulloch–Pitts networks: differences between input-constant and input-variant networks.' *Cybernetics and Systems*, **15**, 91–117. Hemisphere Publ. Co.

Dammasch, I. E., Wagner, G. P. & Wolff, J. R. (1986). 'Self-stabilization of neuronal networks I: The compensation algorithm for synaptogenesis.' *Biol Cybern*, **54**, 211–22.

Dammasch, I. E., Wagner, G. P. & Wolff, J. R. (1988). 'Self-stabilization of neuronal networks II: Stability conditions for synaptogenesis.' *Biol. Cybern.*, **58** (in press).

Holzgraefe, M., Teuchert, G. & Wolff, J. R. (1981). 'Chronic isolation of visual cortex induces reorganization of cortico-cortical connections.' In Flohr, H. & Precht, W. (eds): *Lesion-induced Neuronal Plasticity in Sensorimotor Systems*. Springer, Berlin, Heidelberg, New York, pp. 351–9.

Joó, F., Dames, W. & Wolff, J. R. (1979). 'Effect of prolonged sodium bromide administration on the fine structure of dendrites in the superior cervical ganglion of adult rat.' *Prog. Brain Res*, **51**, 109–15.

McCulloch, W. S. & Pitts, W. H. (1943). 'A logical calculus of ideas immanent in nervous activity.' *Bull Math Biophys*, **5**, 115–33.

Wagner, G. P. & Wolff, J. R. (submitted). 'A kinetic model of synaptogenesis based on morphogenetic consequences of excitation and inhibition.'

Wolff, J. R. (1979). 'Indications for a dual role of GABA as a synaptic transmitter and as a morphogenetic factor.' *Verh Dtsch Zool Ges*, **72**, 194–200.

Wolff, J. R., Joó, F., Dames, W. & Fehér, O. (1979). 'Induction and maintenance of free postsynaptic membrane thickenings in the adult superior cervical ganglion.' *J Neurocytol*, **8**, 549–63.

Wolff, J. R. & Wagner, G. P. (1983). 'Selforganization in synaptogenesis: interaction between the formation of excitatory and inhibitory synapses.' In Basar, E., Flohr, H., Haken, H. & Mandell, A. J. (eds): *Synergetics of the Brain*. Springer, Berlin, Heidelberg, New York, Tokyo, pp. 50–9.

33

Simulation of the prolactin level fluctuations during pseudopregnancy in rats

P. A. ANNINOS, G. ANOGIANAKIS,
M. APOSTOLAKIS and S. EFSTRATIADIS

33.1 Introduction

The use of pharmacological agents in neuroendocrine studies had a significant impact on our perception of the control mechanisms involved in prolactin secretion. In contrast to other anterior pituitary hormones, prolactin is thought to be regulated by the hypothalamus through a prolactin inhibiting factor (PIF) a peptide of MW < 5000 that is tonically released into the hypophysial portal vessels. The prolactin secretory cells themselves are assumed to be driven by a prolactin releasing factor (PRF), an unidentified as yet neurosecretory product. PRF neurosecretory cells are in turn thought to be driven by serotoninergic neurons located in the medial basal hypothalamus.

Of the major CNS neurotransmitters dopamine is a potent inhibitor of prolactin release, although the exact nature of the interaction between the PIF and dopamine is at best unclear at present. The original postulate that PIF secretion is stimulated by dopaminergic neurons located in the medial basal hypothalamus is challenged by the fact that dopamine receptors have been located on the prolactin secretory cells (Clemens, 1976). The emerging synthetic view of the problem postulates that the PIF secreting cells act in parallel and are at the same time driven by the dopaminergic neurons of the medial basal hypothalamus (Fig. 33.1).

Serotonin is the other major CNS neurotransmitter involved in the control of prolactin secretion. It is again as yet unclear whether serotonin stimulates prolactin secretion by inhibiting the PIF release or by stimulating PRF release. Indeed, simultaneous injections of serotonin and agents that selectively inhibit amine uptake into serotoninergic neurons result in remarkable increases over and above the basal serum prolactin levels, thus ruling out a non-specific influence of serotonin as the cause of the increase. However, it is almost certain that the serotonin action is mediated by a GABA interneuron since picrotoxin is able to block the serotonin induced rise in serum prolactin levels in estrogen primed rats, while strychnine, a glycine inhibitor, has a substantially less pronounced effect (Caligaris & Taleisnik, 1974).

On the basis of the neuropharmacological evidence available, a prolactin release neuronal control circuit has been proposed that can act as a monostable device, i.e., it must be reset every time it is triggered (Fig. 33.2). In previous experimental studies we attempted to explore the possibility that the hippocampus is involved in the prolactin release neuronal control circuit (Anogianakis, Apostolakis, Guiba-Tziampiri, Kaikis-Astara & Matziari, 1984). We found that there was an extremely high correlation between the low-θ EEG activity (4, 3–6, 3 Hz) derived from electrodes implanted in the CA_1 (Lorente de Nó) area of the hippocampus and the plasma prolactin levels during pseudopregnancy and proposed the medial corticohypothalamic tract which projects from the hippocampus to the arcuated nucleus, as the prime candidate for a negative feedback loop that would reset the prolactin release neuronal control circuit. In the present analysis we attempt to explore the dynamics of a theoretical neural nerve net model based on the interaction between two subsystems operating under the influence of externally activated inhibition as a potential model of the prolactin fluctuations during pseudopregnancy.

Fig. 33.1.

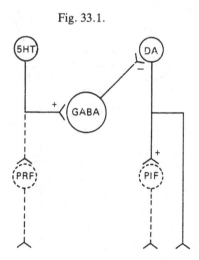

Notation

The subscript i is a marker label and refers to the properties of a subpopulation of neurons in the netlet characterized by the ith marker.

Structural parameters of the netlet

τ Synaptic delay.

A Total number of neurons in the netlet.

h_i Fraction of inhibitory neurons.

μ_i^+ The average number of neurons receiving excitatory postsynaptic potentials (EPSP's) from one excitatory neuron.

μ_i^- The average number of neurons receiving inhibitory postsynaptic potentials (IPSP's) from one excitatory neuron.

μ_0^+ The average number of synaptic contacts made by an external excitatory $(+)$ or inhibitory $(-)$ neuron in the netlet.

k_i^+ The size of PSP produced by an excitatory neuron of the netlet.

k_i^- The size of PSP produced by an inhibitory neuron of the netlet.

Fig. 33.2.

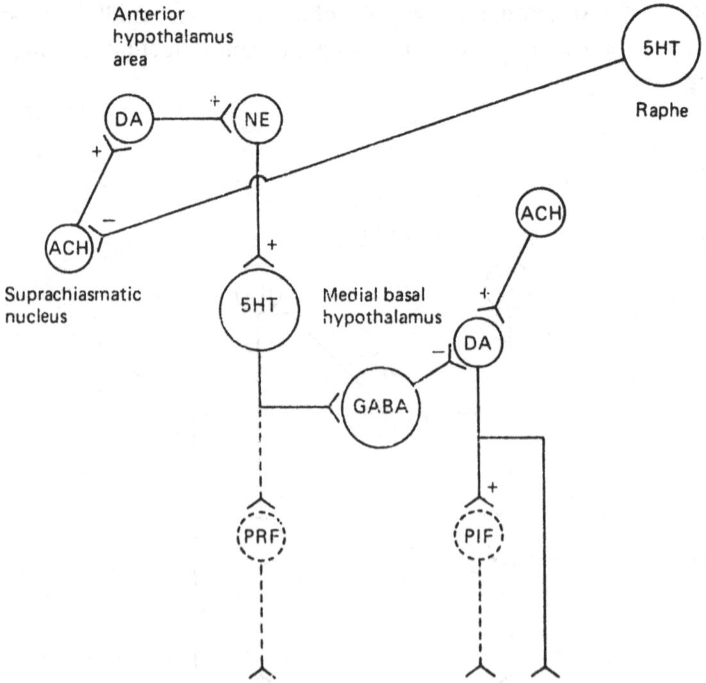

$k_0^{\pm}$ The average PSP produced by external excitatory $(+)$/inhibitory $(-)$ afferent fibers in the netlet.

m_i Fraction of neurons in the netlet carrying the ith marker.

θ_i Firing thresholds of neurons.

$\bar{\theta}_i$ Average neural firing threshold.

Statistical parameters of the netlet

δ_i Standard deviation of the Gaussian distribution of the neural firing thresholds.

r_i Refractory period.

Dynamical parameters of the netlet

n An integer giving the number of elapsed synaptic delays.

a_n The activity, i.e., the fractional number of active neurons in the netlet at time $t = nr$.

33.2 The model

The neural net model for the release of prolactin for the pseudopregnancy in rats is based on the model developed by Kokkinidis and Anninos (1985) which consists of two subsystems characterised by two chemical markers a and b. The activity a_n of such system at time $t = n\tau$ will depend exclusively on the firing record of the system at $t = (n - 1)\tau$ and on the level of the spontaneous activity in the netlet. For an isolated netlet with two markers a and b the expectation value of the activity is given by:

$$\langle a_{n+1}\rangle = (1 - a_n)\left\{ m_a \sum_{I=0}^{I_{max}} \sum_{L=0}^{L_{max}} P_L Q_I T_{\delta_a}(\theta_a) \right.$$
$$\left. + (1 - m_a) \sum_{I'=0}^{I'_{max}} \sum_{L'=0}^{L'_{max}} P'_{L'} Q'_{I'} T_{\delta_b}(\theta_b) \right\}, \qquad (1)$$

where P_L, Q_I and $P'_{L'}$, $Q'_{I'}$ are the probabilities that a given neuron will receive L-EPSP's, I-IPSP's or L'-EPSP's, I'-IPSP's at $t = (n + 1)\tau$ in the subsystems a or b respectively. These probabilities are given by the following equations:

$$\left.\begin{array}{l} P_L = \exp\left[-a_n\mu_a^+(1 - h_a)m_a\right]\left[a_n\mu_a^+(1 - h_a)m_a\right]^L/L! \\[4pt] Q_I = \exp\left[-a_n\mu_a^- h_a m_a\right]\left[a_n\mu_a^- h_a m_a\right]^I/I! \\[4pt] P'_{L'} = \exp\left[-a_n\mu_b^+(1 - h_b)(1 - m_a)\right] \\[4pt] \qquad \times \left[a_n\mu_b^+(1 - h_b)(1 - m_a)\right]^{L'}/L'! \\[4pt] Q'_{I'} = \exp\left[-a_n\mu_b^- h_b(1 - m_a)\right]\left[a_n\mu_b^- h_b(1 - m_a)\right]^{I'}/I'! \end{array}\right\}. \quad (2)$$

The upper limits in the sums in eqn (1) are obtained from the following equations:

$$\left.\begin{array}{l} L_{\max} = A a_n \mu_a^+ (1 - h_a) m_a \\ I_{\max} = A a_n \mu_a^- h_a m_a \\ L'_{\max} = A a_n \mu_b^+ (1 - h_b)(1 - m_a) \\ I'_{\max} = A a_n \mu_b^- h_b (1 - m_a) \end{array}\right\}. \tag{3}$$

The $T_{\delta_a}(\theta_a)$ and $T_{\delta_b}(\theta_b)$ are defined as the probabilities that the instantaneous neural thresholds are equal to or less than the values θ_a and θ_b in the subsystems a and b respectively:

$$\left.\begin{array}{l} T_{\delta_a}(\theta_a) = \dfrac{1}{\sqrt{2\pi}} \displaystyle\int_{x=(\hat{\theta}_a - \theta_a)/\delta_a}^{\infty} \exp\left(-\dfrac{x^2}{2}\right) dx \\[4mm] T_{\delta_b}(\theta_b) = \dfrac{1}{\sqrt{2\pi}} \displaystyle\int_{x=(\hat{\theta}_b - \theta_b)/\delta_b}^{\infty} \exp\left(-\dfrac{x^2}{2}\right) dx \end{array}\right\}. \tag{4}$$

In order to simulate the release of prolactin we consider that the above system is attached to a cable of afferent fibers. Then the expectation value of the activity under the influence of sustained inputs is given by (1, 2):

$$\langle a_{n+1} \rangle = (1 - a_n) \left\{ m_a \sum_{M=0}^{M_{\max}} \sum_{I=0}^{I_{\max}} \sum_{L=0}^{L_{\max}} P_L Q_I R_M T_{\delta_a}(\theta_a) \right.$$
$$\left. + (1 - m_a) \sum_{M'=0}^{M'_{\max}} \sum_{I'=0}^{I'_{\max}} \sum_{L'=0}^{L'_{\max}} P'_{L'} Q'_{I'} R'_{M'} T_{\delta_b}(\theta_b) \right\}, \tag{5}$$

where R_M and $R'_{M'}$ are the probabilities that a given neuron in the subsystems a or b will receive M or M' PSP's, respectively, from an external neuron carrying the same type of marker as its own. Let σ be the fraction of such active fibers, i.e., those carrying action potentials at a particular instant. R_M and $R'_{M'}$ are then given by:

$$\left.\begin{array}{l} R_M = \exp\left(-\sigma\mu_0^{\pm} m_a\right)(\sigma\mu_0^{\pm} m_a)^M/M! \\ R'_{M'} = \exp\left(-\sigma\mu_0'^{\pm}(1 - m_a)\right)(\sigma\mu_0'^{\pm}(1 - m_a))^{M'}/M'! \end{array}\right\}. \tag{6}$$

The upper limits in the sums in eqn (5) are:

$$M_{\max} = A_0 \sigma \mu_0^{\pm} m_a \quad M'_{\max} = A_0 \sigma \mu_0'^{\pm}(1 - m_a). \tag{7}$$

In the present model the afferent fibers are of inhibitory nature. It takes into account several experimental observations (3, 4) which suggest that inhibitory interactions may play an important role in the prolactin release level. We assume here that the inhibitory mechanism which is activated when the value of δ in the netlet becomes abnormally high is a very simple one. It is realized by external inhibitory inputs (σ^-) which increase linearly with time and gradually reduce the high level of neural activity in the system which was attained due to the increase of δ. Furthermore, it is assumed that these inputs cease only after neural activity is completely suppressed. This external inhibition to the system is allowed to reach its highest possible value $(\sigma^- = 1)$ and remain in this state until the activity in the netlet is reduced to α_{ss} a level corresponding to the lowest stable steady state for $\sigma^- = 1$. After the activity level is suppressed, the external inhibition ceases immediately, thus allowing the subsequent activity to rise again and the whole process is repeated as long as δ is abnormally high. With these assumptions, taking into account the effects of an initial activity α_n, the variation of σ^- with time can be described with the following equations:

$$\left.\begin{aligned}
\sigma^-(t) &= \begin{cases} \sigma_0^- t & \text{for} \quad 0 \le t \le D(1) \\ 1 & \text{for} \quad D(1) < t < t_0 \end{cases} \\
\sigma^-(t) &= \begin{cases} \sigma_0^{-\prime}(t - t_0) & \text{for} \quad t_0 \le t \le t_0 + D(1) \\ 1 & \text{for} \quad t_0 + D(1) < t < D + t_0 \end{cases} \\
\sigma^-(t) &= \sigma_0^{-\prime}(t - nD) \quad \text{for} \quad t_0 + nD \le t \le (n + 1)D + t_0
\end{aligned}\right\}, \quad (8)$$

where $n = 1, 2, 3, 4, \ldots$.

Fig. 33.3 describes the time course of σ^- immediately after δ acquires

Fig. 33.3. Time course of external inhibition (σ^-) which is activated by an increase in the spontaneous activity in the netlet. (a) Variation of σ^- when the initial value of the activity α_0 deviates from the value of α_{ss} for $\sigma^- = 1$. (b) Variation of σ^- for $\alpha_0 = \alpha_{ss}$ for $\sigma^- = 1$.

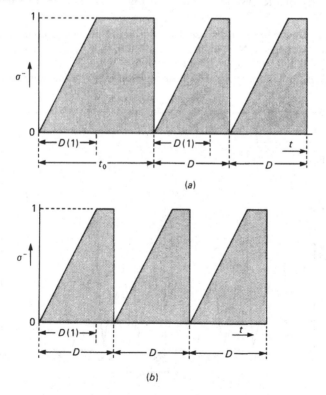

an abnormally high value; t_0 is the time required to suppress both the effects due to the increased δ and the initial activity of the system. These effects are regarded as suppressed when the α_n reaches the low value of α_{ss} for $\sigma^- = 1$.

$D(1)$ is the time required for σ^- to reach the value $\sigma^- = 1$. After the effects of initial activity are suppressed and the activity has first reached the α_{ss}, the activity is allowed to rise again due to the cessation of external inhibition. This, however, induces a new linear rise of σ^- towards the value of $\sigma^- = 1$. This value is reached within a time interval $D(1)$ due to the constant rate at which σ^- increases. After the maximum value is reached, the level of external inhibition is maintained (at $\sigma^- = 1$). This again results in a decrease of the neural activity back to the value of α_{ss}. If the δ is still abnormally high, the process described by eqn (8) will be periodically repeated. Here D is the period of the σ^- variation which is not arbitrarily predefined but, rather, results from the time course of the neural activity of the system.

33.3 Discussion

The effects of the proposed model on the release of prolactin as well as on the activity of the system is shown in Fig. 33.4. The high value of the

Fig. 33.4. Time course of the activity for a netlet under the influences of the inhibitory mechanism. Net parameters: $m_a = 0.8$; $\theta_a = 4$; $\mu_{0_a}^{\pm} = 8$; $\mu_a^{\pm} = 9$; $h_a = 0.03$; $m_b = 0.2$; $\theta_b = 4$; $\mu_0^{\pm} = 10$; $\mu_b^{\pm} = 190$; $h_b = 0.0$; $r_a = r_b = 0$; $\delta_a = \delta_b = 2.5$; $\kappa_0^{\pm} = 0.5$; $\sigma_0^- = 0.02$; $a_0 = 0.6$. The dotted lines are the external inhibition σ^-.

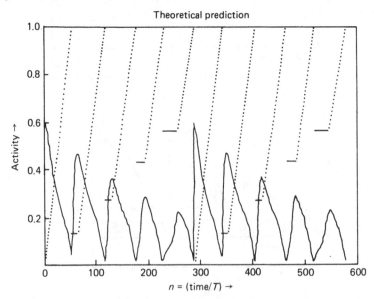

spontaneous activity in the system ($\delta = 2, 5$) and the $\sigma_0^{-\prime} = \sigma_0^{-}$ results first in a rapid increase of the activity of the system and a similar increase in the prolactin level. Parallel to this variation of activity, the initial activated external inhibition σ_0^{-} increases linearly with time up to the maximum possible level of $\sigma^{-\prime} = 1$. This value is then maintained until the activity of the system reaches the quiescent state or, to be more specific, until it reaches the value of α_{ss} corresponding to $\sigma^{-} = 1$. This variation which follows the law described in Fig. 33.4 is then periodically repeated after the variation of the external inhibition $\sigma_0^{-\prime}$ reaches $\sigma^{-} = 1$. As shown in Fig. 33.4 this variation may at first appear surprising since at the same time $\sigma_0^{-\prime}$ is also increasing. However, this behavior and the other features of the time course of the activity may be explained by Fig. 33.5, which shows the phase diagram of the system for a level of spontaneous activity corresponding to $\delta = 2, 5$ (Kokkinidis & Anninos, 1985). Here the steady states α_{ss} are plotted against σ^{-}, the level of inhibitory sustained inputs and it illustrates the initial rise. As is clearly shown in Fig. 33.5, α_n will first rise trying to reach the instantaneous α_{ss} value. At the same time, however, the value of α_{ss} is decreasing due to the shift of σ^{-} towards higher values. Thus after the α_n vs. σ^{-} curve intersects the curve of the phase diagram, α_n will be trapped in the high stable steady state of the phase diagram and will be forced to follow its path in the direction of

Fig. 33.5.

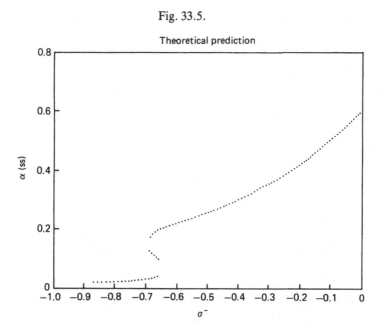

increasing σ^-. Consequently, the activity and the prolactin level will gradually decrease and will finally acquire the very small value corresponding to the value of the external $\sigma^- = 1$. After the external inhibition reaches the value $\sigma^- = 1$ it ceases and the activity will rise to a new lower level according to the initial values of the external inhibition $\sigma_0^-{}'$ and then due to the shift of $\sigma_0^-{}'$ to higher values the activity will decrease again to a level which corresponds to $\sigma^- = 1$. It turns out that the system chosen has a period of 96 h with 24 h for each peak in the cycle involved and with $\tau = 1329{,}23$ s and $n = 0, 65, 130, 195, 260$.

Acknowledgement

This research was supported by a grant from the Greek Ministry of Industry, Research and Technology.

References

Anninos, P. A. & Kokkinidis, M. (1984). *J. Theor. Biol.*, **109**, 95.

Anninos, P. A., Kokkinidis, M. & Skouras, A. (1984). *J. Theor. Biol.*, **109**, 581.

Anogianakis, G., Apostolakis, M., Guiba-Tziampiri, O., Kaikis-Astara, A. & Matziari, C. (1984). 5th Int. Meeting of the Inter. Soc. for Developmental Neuroscience, Chieti, Italy.

Caligaris, L. & Taleisnik, S. (1974). *J. Endocrin.*, **62**, 25–33.

Clemens, J. A. (1976). In F. Labrie, J. Meites & G. Pelletier (eds.) *Hypothalamus and Endocrine Functions*. Plenum Press, New York.

Kokkinidis, M. & Anninos, P. (1985). *J. Theor. Biol.*, **113**, 559.

34

Applications of biological intelligence to command, control and communications

LESTER INGBER

34.1 Introduction

It is quite evident that, while all sane people desire peace, all countries must practically provide for their self-defense. Thus, issues of procurement and implementation of combat systems must be objectively analyzed. When performing such analyses, it is useful and important to distinguish between specific combat components ('anatomy') and the Command, Control and Communications (C^3) functions ('physiology') of these systems. If enormous financial and human resources must indeed be spent on a specific weapons system, then C^3 models can offer procurement decision aids to spending these resources more efficiently. However, even before procuring specific weapon components, C^3 models should be used to develop battle-management decision aids to help determine if it is feasible to consider building planned large-scale systems at all.

Even without agreement on just what C^3 is, there is widespread criticism that we do not spend enough on C^3 relative to what we spend on specific weapons systems (Blair, 1985). The Eastport Study Group (Eastport Study Group, 1985) has made this issue its primary concern with regard to the Strategic Defense Initiative (SDI) program. There is also an everpresent problem of weighing the political and military aspects between the hierarchical and distributed designs of C^3, the former being politically desirable and appropriate for deterministic or modestly stochastic operations, and the latter being more appropriate for severely stochastic systems (Orr, 1983).

While there is much criticism and theoretical discourse on what C^3 should be concerned with, there is a lack of empirical data because of the lack of modern large-scale wars. Therefore, we must learn as much as possible from other similar but testable systems for which empirical data

514 Lester Ingber

exists, e.g., other large-scale systems such as neocortex. Combat simulations also provide a potential source of empirical data, but only when their limitations are clearly presented (Comptroller General, 1980).

Future battle management, e.g., as being investigated by the SDI program, must certainly consider distributive adaptive C^3 for severely stochastic systems (Eastport Study Group, 1985). Such objective considerations are the only practical means for scientists to influence governments who will determine if and how such programs as SDI will be implemented.

In this paper I will outline an interdisciplinary approach which is attempting to piece together a specific coherent C^3 model that may yield insights into those C^3 systems which are most appropriate for severely stochastic combat operations.

34.2 Biological intelligence (BI)

34.2.1 Introduction

Biological Intelligence (BI) demonstrates the physiology of neocortex at coarse columnar scales. Proper treatment of nonlinearities of these columnar interactions demonstrates how multiple hypotheses are generated and processed by short-term memory (STM). Similarly, if BI is relevant to C^3, it should be expected that useful decision aids to commanders, i.e., to generate alternative scenarios, will require robust C^3 nonlinear models of previous combat operations.

A series of publications has detailed a statistical mechanics approach to macroscopic regions of neocortex, derived from statistical aggregates of microscopic neurons, i.e., a statistical mechanics of neocortical interactions (SMNI) (Ingber, 1981a, 1982, 1983b, 1984b, 1985c,d,e). As has been found necessary for other nonlinear nonequilibrium systems, a mesoscopic scale is sought to develop a Gaussian–Markovian statistics for further macroscopic development (Haken, 1983; van Kampen, 1981). This mesoscopic scale is found in the observed physiology of columnar interactions. Long-term-memory (LTM) properties and the duration and capacity of STM, i.e., the '7 ± 2 rule', have been derived from multiple minima of a nonlinear Lagrangian (time-dependent and space-dependent 'cost function'); the alpha frequency and velocity of propagation of columnar information-processing, consistent with observed movements of attention across the visual field, have been derived in linearized ranges within these minima.

These technical methods are quite general, and I also have applied them to nuclear physics – detailing Riemannian contributions to the binding energy of nucleons interacting via exchanges of mesons (Ingber, 1968, 1983a, 1984a, 1986), and to financial markets – defining an approach to explain various phenomena such as leptokurtosis, the biasing of price data (Ingber, 1984c). These systems are all quite different in their natures, but they do share a common approach by these methods of nonlinear nonequilibrium statistical mechanics. The nuclear physics system illustrates how patterns of information can be represented by eigenfunctions of the probability distribution. The markets system illustrates how the mesoscopic scale can be formulated phenomenologically, without the luxury of deriving it from a microscopic system as was done for the neocortical system.

Coarse-graining is an important general method of treating nonlinear nonequilibrium statistical systems, e.g., in order to develop Gaussian–Markovian probability distributions. Also, less resources are required to process the coarser variables, which is efficient if that is all that is required for macroscopic function. The theory capable of treating these systems requires mathematical tools only developed in the late 1970s (Cheng, 1972; Dekker, 1979; DeWitt, 1957; Grabert & Green, 1979; Graham, 1977a,b; Langouche, Roekaerts & Tirapegui, 1982; Mizrahi, 1978; Schulman, 1981), including quite general nonlinear nonequilibrium structures into previous 'flat-space' treatments of Gaussian–Markovian systems (Feynman & Hibbs, 1965).

This theory is geared to explain macroscopic neocortical activity, retaining as much correct description of underlying microscopic synaptic activity as can be carried by modern mathematical physics, which turns out to be sufficient for several important circumstances. Only after this process is completed, are approximate numerical and algebraic methods applied to solve the resulting mathematics. It is at *this* stage that modeling is most useful. The 1980s have already demonstrated that many systems require the use of several complementary algebraic and numerical algorithms to detail several scales of interaction (National Research Council, 1984). Neocortex is not unique in requiring several approaches.

For example, without sufficient mathematical or physical justification, many models assume (quasi-)linear deterministic rate equations – analogous to conserved quadratic 'Hamiltonians' – to postulate 'average' neurons, thereby neglecting statistical and stochastic background interactions, nonlinearities induced by interactions among neurons, and spatio-temporal statistics of large ensembles of these interacting neurons. In fact, these nonlinearities and statistics are essential mechanisms of

STM (Ingber, 1984b, 1985d), and possibly of alpha rhythm observed in electroencephalographic (EEG) and magnetoencephalographic (MEG) (Williamson, Kaufman & Brenner, 1979) activity (Ingber, 1985c). These results are obtained by taking reasonable synaptic parameters, developing the statistical mechanics of neocortical interactions, and then discovering that indeed they are consistent with the empirical macroscopic data. Other models which have offered plausible brain mechanisms can be processed by this theory, extending their ranges of validity (Ingber, 1981a, 1982).

34.2.2 Description of theory

Microscopic neurons. When describing the activity of large ensembles of neocortical neurons, each one typically having many thousands of synaptic interactions, it is a reasonable assumption that simple algebraic summation of excitatory (E) depolarizations and inhibitory (I) hyperpolarizations at the base of the inner axonal membrane determine the firing depolarization response of a neuron within its absolute and relative refractory periods (Shepherd, 1979).

This is straightforwardly mathematically summarized by folding a distribution Ψ of inter-neuronal interactions modeling chemical transmission across synapses, with a distribution Γ of intra-neuronal interactions modelling net polarizations induced at axons of neurons which possess many different geometries and synaptic sites (Shaw & Vasudevan, 1974; Ingber, 1982). Within $\tau_j \sim 5$–10 ms, the conditional probability that neuron j fires, given its previous interactions with k neurons, is

$$p_{\sigma_j} \simeq \Gamma\Psi$$

$$\simeq \frac{\exp\,(-\sigma_j F_j),}{\exp\,(F_j)\,+\,\exp\,(-F_j)}$$

$$F_j = \frac{V_j - \sum_k a_{jk} v_{jk}}{\left[\pi \sum_{k'} a_{jk'} (v_{jk'}^2 + \phi_{jk'}^2)\right]^{1/2}},$$

$$a_{jk} = \tfrac{1}{2}A_{jk}(\sigma_k + 1) + B_{jk}. \tag{1}$$

This is reasonable for Γ Poisson, and for Ψ Poisson or Gaussian. V_j is the axonal depolarization threshold, v_{jk} is the induced synaptic polarization of E or I type at the axon, and ϕ_{jk} is its variance. The efficacy a_{jk}, related to the inverse conductivity across synaptic gaps, is composed of a contribution A_{jk} from the connectivity between neurons which is activated if the impinging k-neuron fires, and a contribution B_{jk} from spontaneous background noise. Here, $\sigma_j = +1$ designates the firing of neuron j, and $\sigma_j = -1$ designates its non-firing.

Mesoscopic domains. As is found for most nonequilibrium systems, a mesoscopic scale is required to formulate the statistical mechanics of the microscopic system, from which the macroscopic scale can be developed (Haken, 1983). Neocortex is particularly interesting in this context in that a clear scale for the mesoscopic system exists, both anatomically (structurally) and physiologically (functionally). 'Minicolumns' of about $N \simeq 100$ neurons (about 200 in visual cortex) comprise modular units vertically oriented relative to the warped and convoluted neocortical surface throughout most, if not all, regions of neocortex (Gilbert & Wiesel, 1983; Goldman & Nauta, 1977; Hubel & Wiesel, 1962; Imig & Reale, 1980; Jones, Coulter & Hendry, 1978; Mountcastle, 1978). Clusters of about 100 neurons have been deduced to be reasonable from other considerations as well (Bullock, 1980). The overwhelming majority of neuronal interactions are short-ranged, diverging out via efferent minicolumnar fibers to within ~1 mm, which is the extent of a 'macrocolumn' comprising ~10^3 minicolumns of $N^* \simeq 10^5$ neurons. Macrocolumns also exhibit rather specific information-processing features. This theory has retained the divergence–convergence of minicolumn–macrocolumn efferent–afferent interactions by considering domains of minicolumns as having similar synaptic interactions within the extent of a macrocolumn. This dynamically macrocolumnar-averaged minicolumn is designated in this theory as a 'mesocolumn'.

After statistically shaping the microscopic system, the parameters of the mesoscopic system are minicolumnar-averaged parameters, i.e., reflecting the statistics of millions of synapses with regard to their chemical and electrical properties. Explicit laminar circuitry, and more complicated synaptic interactions, e.g., dependent on all combinations of presynaptic and postsynaptic firings, can be included without loss of detailed analysis (Ingber, 1983*b*).

The mathematical development of the probability distribution of mesocolumnar firings P establishes a mesoscopic Lagrangian L, which may be considered as a 'cost function'. The Einstein summation convention is used for compactness, whereby any index appearing more than once among factors in any term is assumed to be summed over, unless otherwise indicated by vertical bars, e.g., $|G|$.

$$P = \prod_G P^G[M^G(r; \ t + \tau)|M^{\hat{G}}(r'; \ t)]$$

$$= \sum_{\sigma_j} \delta\left(\sum_{jE} \sigma_j - M^E(r; \ t + r)\right)\delta\left(\sum_{jI} \sigma_j - M^I(r; \ t + r)\right)\prod_j^N p_{\sigma_j}$$

$$\approx \prod_G (\pi i g^{GG})^{-1/2} \exp(-N\tau L^G),$$

$$P \approx (2i\pi\tau)^{-1/2}g^{1/2} \exp(-N\tau L),$$

$$L = (2N)^{-1}(\dot{M}^G - g^G)g_{GG'}(\dot{M}^{G'} - g^{G'}) + M^G J_G/(2N\tau) - V',$$

$$V' = \sum_G V''^G_{G'}(\varrho\nabla M^{G'})^2,$$

$$g^G = -\tau^{-1}(M^G + N^G \tanh F^G),$$

$$g^{GG'} = (g_{GG'})^{-1} = \delta^{G'}_G \tau^{-1}N^G \operatorname{sech}^2 F^G,$$

$$g = \det(g_{GG'}),$$

$$F^G = \frac{(V^G - a^{|G|}_{G'}v^{|G|}_{G'}N^{G'} - \frac{1}{2}A^{|G|}_{G'}v^{|G|}_{G'}M^{G'})}{(\pi[(v^{|G|}_{G'})^2 + (\phi^{|G|}_{G'})^2](a^{|G|}_{G'}N^{G'} + \frac{1}{2}A^{|G|}_{G'}M^{G'}))^{1/2}}$$

$$a^G_{G'} = \frac{1}{2}A^G_{G'} + B^G_{G'}, \tag{2}$$

where $A^G_{G'}$ and $B^G_{G'}$ are minicolumnar-averaged inter-neuronal synaptic efficacies, $v^G_{G'}$ and $\phi^G_{G'}$ are averaged means and variances of contributions to neuronal electric polarizations, and nearest-neighbor (NN) interactions V' are detailed in other SMNI papers. The Lagrange multipliers J_G model long-ranged fibers which act as constraints on short-ranged mesocolumnar firings.

Macroscopic regions. Inclusion of all the above microscopic and mesoscopic features of neocortex permits a true nonphenomenological Gaussian–Markovian formal development for macroscopic regions encompassing $\sim 5 \times 10^5$ minicolumns of spatial extent $\sim 5 \times 10^9 \ \mu m^2$, albeit one that is still highly nonlinear and in nonequilibrium. The development of mesocolumnar domains presents conditional probability distributions for mesocolumnar firings with spatially coupled NN interactions. The macroscopic spatial folding of these mesoscopic domains and their macroscopic temporal folding of tens to hundreds of τ, with a resolution of at least τ/N (Ingber, 1984b), yields a true path-integral formulation, in terms of a Lagrangian possessing a *bona fide* variational principle for most-probable firing states. At this point in formal development, no continuous-time approximation has yet been made; this is done, with clear justification, for some applications discussed in the next section. Much of this algebra is greatly facilitated by, but does not require, the use of Riemannian geometry (Misner, Thorne & Wheeler, 1973; Weinberg, 1972) to develop the non-linear means, variances, and 'potential' contributions to the Lagrangian (Langouche, Roekaerts & Tirapegui, 1982).

Many neuroscientists have criticized the use of simple local circuits to model the brain, suggesting the alternative concept of a 'neural throng' (Bullock, 1980) similar to social interactions. In this context, the theory for neocortex developed here is strikingly similar mathematically to nonlinear nonequilibrium models developed for social (Weidlich & Haag, 1983) and economic (Ingber, 1984c) systems.

The mathematical macroscopic development proceeds by 'folding' the mesoscopic probability distribution over and over, in time θ,

$$\dot{M}^G = [M^G(t + \theta) - M^G(t)]/\theta, \quad \theta < \tau, \tag{3}$$

and in a space of $\Lambda \sim 5 \times 10^5$ macrocolumns $\sim 5 \times 10^9 \ \mu m^2$. For momentary simplicity, consider the folding of just one variable M at just one spatial point over many time epochs: Labelling u intermediate time epochs by s, i.e., $t_s = t_0 + s\Delta t$, in the limits $\lim_{u \to \infty}$ and $\lim_{\Delta t \to 0}$, and assuming $M_{t_0} = M(t_0)$ and $M_t = M(t \equiv t_{u+1})$ are fixed,

$$P[M_t | M_{t_0}] = \int \ldots \int dM_{t-\Delta t} \, dM_{t-2\Delta t} \ldots dM_{t_0+\Delta t}$$

$$\times \, P[M_t | M_{t-\Delta t}] P[M_{t-\Delta t} | M_{t-2\Delta t}] \times \ldots P[M_{t_0+\Delta t} | M_{t_0}],$$

$$P[M_t | M_{t_0}] = \int \ldots \int DM \exp \left(-\sum_{s=0}^{u} \Delta t L_s \right),$$

$$DM = (2\pi \hat{g}_0^2 \Delta t)^{-1/2} \prod_{s=1}^{u} (2\pi \hat{g}_s^2 \Delta t)^{-1/2} \, dM_s,$$

$$\int dM_s \to \sum_{\alpha=1}^{N} \Delta M_{\alpha s}, \quad M_0 = M_{t_0}, \quad M_{u+1} = M_t, \tag{4}$$

where α labels the range of N values of M.

There are a number of non-trivial technical points which must be considered when dealing with multivariate nonlinear systems. Very fortunately for this theory, the necessary mathematical techniques for handling such systems were developed by physicists in the late 1970s, and this neuroscience problem is the first physical system that used these methods. For example, mesocolumns were derived in a 'prepoint' discretization, e.g.,

$$\dot{M}_s^G = [M^G(t + \theta) - M(t)]/\theta,$$
$$g_s^G = g^G[M^G(t), t]. \tag{5}$$

To capture a flavor of some of the mathematical technicalities, consider that there exists a transformation to the midpoint discretization, in which the standard rules of differential calculus hold for the *same* distribution in terms of a transformed L, defined as a Feynman Lagrangian L_F.

$$M^G(\bar{t}_s) = \tfrac{1}{2}(M^G_{s+1} + M^G_s), \quad \dot{M}^G(\bar{t}_s) = (M^G_{s+1} - M^G_s)/\theta,$$

$$\bar{P} = \prod_v P,$$

$$P = \int \cdots \int DM \, \exp\left(-\sum_{s=0}^{u} \Delta t L_{F_s}\right),$$

$$DM = g_0^{1/2}(2\pi\Delta t)^{-1/2} \prod_{s=1}^{u} g_s^{1/2} \prod_{G=1}^{\Theta} (2\pi\Delta t)^{-1/2} \, dM^G_s,$$

$$\int dM^G_s \rightarrow \sum_{a=1}^{N^G} \Delta M^G_{as}, \quad M^G_0 = M^G_{t_0}, \quad M^G_{u+1} = M^G_t,$$

$$L_F = \tfrac{1}{2}(\dot{M}^G - h^G)g_{GG'}(\dot{M}^{G'} - h^{G'}) + D\tfrac{1}{2}h^G_{;G} + R/6 - V$$

$$[\cdots]_{,G} = \frac{\partial[\cdots]}{\partial M^G},$$

$$h^G = g^G - \tfrac{1}{2}g^{-1/2}(g^{1/2}g^{GG'})_{,G'},$$

$$g_{GG'} = (g^{GG'})^{-1},$$

$$g_s[M^G(\bar{t}_s), \bar{t}_s] = \det(g_{GG'})_s, \quad g_s = g_s[M^G_{s+1}, \bar{t}_s],$$

$$h^G_{;G} = h^G_{,G} + \Gamma^F_{GF}h^G = g^{-1/2}(g^{1/2}h^G)_{,G},$$

$$\Gamma^F_{JK} \equiv g^{LF}[JK, L] = g^{LF}(g_{JL,K} + g_{KL,J} - g_{JK,L}),$$

$$R = g^{JL}R_{JL} = g^{JL}g^{JK}R_{FJKL},$$

$$R_{FJ,KL} = \tfrac{1}{2}(g_{FK,JL} - g_{JK,FL} - g_{FL,JK} + g_{JL,FK})$$
$$+ g_{MN}(\Gamma^M_{FK}\Gamma^N_{JL} - \Gamma^M_{FL}\Gamma^N_{JK}). \tag{6}$$

That is, expanding all prepoint-discretized functions about the midpoint $t + \theta/2$ introduces many additional terms, which are recognized as having the same structure of a Riemannian geometry induced on the M^G variables.

Using the midpoint discretization, the variational principle offers insight, but the prepoint discretization does not contain explicit Riemannian terms. The nonlinear variances considerably complicate the algebra required. Riemannian geometry facilitates, but is not necessary, to derive these results. The Riemannian geometry is a reflection that the probability distribution is invariant under general nonlinear transformations of these variables. In other words, the same information content can be expressed in a variety of ways. For example, sensory cortex may transmit information to motor cortex, although they have somewhat different neuronal structures or neuronal languages. Information can be transmitted between 'different-looking' regions, e.g., between motor cortex and sensory cortex:

$$I = \int D\tilde{M}\hat{P} \ln (\hat{P}/\check{P}).$$ (7)

It should be stressed that this Riemannian geometry arises as a natural consequence of invariance of Gaussian–Markovian systems under nonlinear transformations, and that in the neocortical problem this permits the explicit *derivation* of a Riemannian metric *within* a cortical region. This is quite different from *hypothesizing* a Riemannian metric *between* cortical regions (Pellionisz, 1984). However, before developing nearest-neighbor interactions, stochastic variables M^{Gv} may be considered, where v labels spatial sites (Ingber, 1985a). This defines a metric $g_{GvG'v'}$ which spans cortical regions, albeit the function dependencies on M^{Gv} in the drifts g^{Gv} and diffusions $g^{GvG'v'}$ must reflect the separation of these regions.

34.2.3 Applications

Several papers have described in detail how this theory can be used to advantage (Ingber, 1981a, 1982, 1983b, 1984b, 1985c,d,e). These applications provide a conceptual framework for treating other similar systems, e.g., those of C^3.

(1) *Intuitive view of statistical analyses.* Three-dimensional views over $E - I$ of the stationary Lagrangian offers an intuitive 'potential' description of neocortical interactions, detailing local minima and maxima (Ingber, 1982, 1983b). Such pairwise presentation of variables offers an intuitive and accurate estimate of relative probabilities and variances associated with multiple minima.

(2) *Processing of patterned information.* Firing states linearized about stationary firing states, give rise to simple eigenfunction expansions of the macroscopic probability distribution (Ingber, 1981a, 1982). These eigenfunctions are to be identified with the algebraic vector spaces utilized to great advantage by other investigators (Anderson, Silverstein, Ritz, & Jones, 1977; Cooper, 1973), but not derived by them from realistic synaptic interactions respecting the nonlinear statistical nature of this dynamic system. This identification will permit detailed numerical calculation of associative learning, retrieval and storage of memories, etc. For example, the accuracy of retrieval of a specific pattern is directly proportional to the overlap of a STM 'search'-eigenfunction with a long-term memory (LTM) stored eigenfunction. These eigenfunctions may encom-

pass various degrees of neural mass (Erickson, 1982), ranging from minicolumns, to aggregates of mesocolumns coupled by NN interactions, to regions coupled by long-ranged fibers. Such searches may be facilitated by long-ranged fibers acting as constraints on columnar processing.

More specifically, learning and retrieval mechanisms can be developed by first determining expansion coefficients of eigenfunction expansions of the differential Fokker–Planck distributions (Blackmore & Shizgal, 1985), e.g., considering stationary states as Hermite polynomials in neighborhoods of minima. Although this is a reasonably large computer calculation, similar calculations of greater computational difficulty are routinely performed, e.g., when calculating quantum states of Schrödinger wave-functions of nucleon–nucleon scattering and of nuclear matter, using realistic forces, i.e., quite nonlinear nucleon-nucleon forces derived from meson-exchange forces (Ingber, 1968). The Fokker–Planck equation is quite similar to the Schrödinger equation, and this analogy has recently been used to great advantage, to apply the modern methods used here for neocortex to determine Riemannian contributions to nuclear forces (Ingber, 1983*a*, 1984*a*, 1986).

(3) *Short-term-memory capacity.* The most detailed and dramatic application of this theory has been to predict a stochastic mechanism underlying the phenomena of human STM capacity (Ingber, 1984*b*, 1985*d*), transpiring on the order of tenths of a second to seconds, limited to the retention of 7 ± 2 items (Miller, 1956). This is true even for apparently exceptional memory performers who, while they may be capable of more efficient encoding and retrieval of STM, and while they may be more efficient in 'chunking' larger patterns of information into single items, nevertheless are also limited to a STM capacity of 7 ± 2 items (Ericsson & Chase, 1982). This 'rule' is verified for acoustical STM, but for visual or semantic STM, which typically require longer times for rehearsal in an hypothesized articulatory loop of individual items, STM capacity may be limited to as few as two or three chunks (Zhang & Simon, 1985). This STM capacity-limited chunking phenomena has also been noted with items requiring varying depths and breadths of processing (Ingber, 1972, 1976, 1981*b*,*c*, 1985*a*). Another interesting phenomena of STM capacity explained by this theory is the primacy vs. recency effect in STM serial processing, wherein first-learned items are recalled most error-free, with last-learned items still more error-free than those in the middle (Murdock, 1983).

STM is the mechanism by which neocortex holds multiple hypotheses for further processing. Multiple minima of Lagrangians modeling similar systems can be similarly analyzed.

Contour plots of the stationary Lagrangian $\bar{L}$, for typical synaptic parameters balanced between predominately inhibitory and predominately excitatory firing states, are examined at many scales when the background synaptic noise is only modestly shifted to cause both efferent M^G and afferent M^{*G} mesocolumnar firing states to have a common most-probable firing, centered at (Ingber, 1984b)

$$M^G = M^{*G} = 0. \tag{8}$$

Within the range of synaptic parameters considered, for values of $\tau\bar{L} \sim 10^{-2}$, this 'centering' mechanism causes the appearance of from 5 to 10–11 extrema for values of $\tau\bar{L}$ on the order of $\sim 10^{-2}$. In the absence of external constraints and this centering mechanism, no stable minima are found in the interior of M^G space. For example, the system either shuts down, with no firings, or it becomes epileptic, with maximal firings at the upper limits of excitatory or of excitatory and inhibitory firings. The appearance of these extrema due to the centering mechanism is clearly dependent on the nonlinearities present in the derived Lagrangian, stressing competition and cooperation among excitatory and inhibitory interactions at columnar as well as at neuronal scales.

A maximum of nine minima possessing jump times of first passage between each other within tenths of a second, as empirically observed, are determined when the resolution of the contours is commensurate with the resolution of columnar firings, i.e., on the order of 5–10 neuronal firings per columnar mesh point. Most important contributions to the probability distribution P come from ranges of the time slice θ and the 'action' NL, such that $\theta NL \lesssim 1$. By considering the contributions to the first and second moments of ΔM^G for small slices θ, conditions on the time and variable meshes can be derived (Wehner & Wolfer, 1983a,b).

$$\langle M^G(t + \theta) - M^G(t) \rangle \approx g^G(t)\theta,$$
$$\langle [M^G(t + \theta) - M^G(t)]^2 \rangle \approx g^{GG}(t)\theta. \tag{9}$$

The time slice is determined by $\theta \leqslant (N\bar{L})^{-1}$ throughout the ranges of M^G giving the most important contributions to the probability distribution P. The variable mesh, a function of M^G, is optimally chosen such that ΔM^G is measured by the covariance $g^{GG'}$ (diagonal in neocortex due to independence of E and I chemical interactions), or $\Delta M^G \sim (g^{GG}\theta)^{1/2}$ in the notation of the SMNI papers. For $N \sim 10^2$ and $\bar{L} \sim 10^{-2}/\tau$, it is reasonable to pick $\theta \sim \tau$. Then it is calculated that optimal meshes are $\Delta M^E \sim 7$ and $\Delta M^I \sim 4$, essentially the resolutions used in the coarse contour plots. Thus, although the firing rate for an 'average neuron', $\dot{M}^G/N$, can be as fine as θ/N, it suffices to take $\theta \sim \tau$ in the path integral to derive the continuous-time Fokker–Planck equation or Langevin rate-equation representation. As such, this path-integral representation can reflect asynchronous firings for 'average neurons'. This calculation also serves to specify the resolution of the mesoscopic system.

When the number of neurons/minicolumn is taken to be ~220, modeling visual neocortex (Ingber, 1984b), then the minima become deeper and sharper, consistent with sharper depth of processing, but several minima become isolated from the main group. This effect might be responsible for the lowering of STM capacity for visual processing, mentioned above. Here note that increasing the number of 'connected' neurons can actually decrease the number of most likely mesoscopic states.

(4) *Wave-propagation dispersion relations and alpha frequency.* Only after the multiple minima are established, may it be useful to perform linear expansions about specific minima, specified by the Euler–Lagrange variational equations. This permits the development of stability analyses and dispersion relations in frequency–wavenumber space (Ingber, 1982, 1983b, 1985c). This calculation requires the inclusion of global constraints, discussed in (2) above.

More specifically, the variational principle permits derivation of the Euler–Lagrange equations. These equations are then linearized about a given local minima to investigate oscillatory behavior. Here, long-ranged constraints in the form of Lagrange multipliers J_G were used to search efficiently for minima corresponding to roots of the Euler–Lagrange equations. Oscillatory frequencies are calculated for typical synaptic parameters,

$$\omega \sim 10^2 \text{ s}^{-1}, \tag{10}$$

which is equivalent to

$$\nu = \omega/(2\pi) = 16 \text{ cps (Hz)}, \tag{11}$$

as observed for the alpha frequency. The use of the Euler–Lagrange equations, essentially an average over mesocolumnar fluctuations, and of tuning J_G long-ranged constraints, is consistent with the observed nature of EEG and MEG measurements which collect data detailing the nonspecific alpha frequency.

The propagation velocity v is calculated from

$$v = d\omega/d\xi \simeq 1 \text{ cm s}^{-1}, \ \xi \sim 30\varrho, \tag{12}$$

which tests the NN interactions. Thus, within 10^{-1} s, short-ranged interactions over several minicolumns of 10^{-1} cm may simultaneously interact with long-ranged interactions over tens of cm, since the long-ranged interactions are speeded by myelinated fibers affording velocities of 600–900 cm s^{-1} (Nunez, 1981). In other words, interaction among different neocortical modalities, e.g., visual, auditory, etc., may simultaneously interact within the same time scales, as observed.

This propagation velocity is consistent with the observed movement of attention (Tsal, 1983) and with the observed movement of hallucinations across the visual field (Cowan, 1982), of $\sim\frac{1}{2}$ mm s^{-1}, about five times as slow as v (i.e., the observed movement is $\sim$8 ms/°, and a macrocolumn $\sim$ mm processes 180° of visual field). Therefore, NN interactions may play some part, i.e., within several interactions of interactions, in disengaging and orienting selective attention.

34.2.4 Yin–Yang processing of information

This theory demonstrates that, relatively independent of local information-processing at the sub-microscopic synaptic and microscopic neuronal scales, there is statistical global processing of patterns of information at the mesoscopic and macroscopic scales.

This picture represents neocortex as a pattern-processing computer. The underlying mathematical theory, i.e., the path-integral approach, specifies a parallel-processing algorithm which statistically finds those parameter-regions of firing which contribute most to the overall probability distribution: This is a kind of 'intuitive' algorithm, globally searching a large multivariate data base to find parameter-regions deserving more detailed local information-processing. The derived probability distribution can be thought of as a filter, or processor, of incoming patterns of information. This filter is adaptive, as it can be modified because it interacts externally or internally with previously stored patterns of information, changing the mesoscopic synaptic parameters.

34.3 Applications of BI to C^3

34.3.1 A generic system

In order to demonstrate how the mathematics developed for neocortex also arise naturally in other systems, consider a grid, defined within a given time epoch, where the grid is to be conceived as a generalized 'radar' screen, representing data being accumulated by multiple sensors. Each cell has information pertaining to relocatable sightings that may be moving between cells. For example, clusters of sightings may have a number of associated variables, e.g., coordinate position, velocity, acceleration, numbers of sightings within these categories, etc. The information collected within each time epoch serves to define changes in these variables between neighboring epochs, both within each cell and between neighboring cells.

The size and complexity of real physical systems, and their response-time and computational constraints, dictate that without always being able to make a best single decision, there exist elements of risk in any response algorithm. This risk must be quantified, at least in order to assess the chances to be taken by alternative responses. The 'expected gain' of any response is the sum of products of each possible response multiplied by its associated risk, assuming independence among responses; otherwise, cross-correlations must be assessed and folded into this analysis. Only if past events include these '2nd moment' fits, i.e., only by fitting *bona fide* probability distributions, can the future be optimally predicted, albeit only with some quantifiable degree of statistical uncertainty. These features typically are not included in many AI-type models of systems (Ingber, 1985a).

34.3.2 Method of solution

There are three equivalent representations of this stochastic system.

For simplicity, again consider the 'radar' grid, but now consider only one parameter, $M(t)$, in just one cell, representing just one of the variables discussed above. The problem of determining the change of M within time Δt can be described for many systems as

$$M(t + \Delta t) - M(t) = \Delta t f[M(t)], \tag{13}$$

where $f[M]$ is some function to be fit, which describes how M is changing. For small enough Δt, and assuming continuity of M, this is written as

$$\dot{M} = \frac{dM}{dt} = f. \tag{14}$$

If background noise, η, is present, assumed to be Gaussian–Markovian ('white' noise), then this affects the description of changing M by

$$\dot{M} = f + \hat{g}\eta,$$
$$\langle \eta(t) \rangle_\eta = 0,$$
$$\langle \eta(t)\eta(t') \rangle_\eta = \delta(t - t'), \tag{15}$$

where $\hat{g}^2$ is the variance of the background noise. Here η is assumed to have a zero mean. Eqn (15) is referred to as a Langevin rate-equation in the literature.

Physicists and engineers, e.g., in fluid mechanics, recognize an equivalent 'diffusion' equation to eqn (15), defining a differential equation for the conditional probability distribution, $P[M(t + \Delta t)|M(t)]$, of finding M at the time $t + \Delta t$, given its value at time t

$$\frac{\partial P}{\partial t} = \frac{\partial(-fP)}{\partial M} + \frac{1}{2}\frac{\partial^2(\hat{g}^2 P)}{\partial M^2} \tag{16}$$

is known as a Fokker-Planck equation.

Some physicists, e.g., in elementary-particle physics, are familiar with yet another representation of eqn (15). For small time epochs, the conditional probability P is

$$P[M_{t+\Delta t}|M_t] = (2\pi\hat{g}^2\Delta t)^{-1/2} \exp(-\Delta tL),$$
$$L = (\dot{M} - f)^2/(2\hat{g}^2), \tag{17}$$

where L is defined to be the Lagrangian. This representation for P permits a 'global' path-integral description of the evolution of P from time t_0 to a long time t, i.e., in contradistinction to the 'local' differential eqn (16). Labelling u intermediate time epochs by s, i.e., $t_s = t_0 + s\Delta t$, in the limits $\lim_{u\to\infty}$ and $\lim_{\Delta t\to 0}$, and assuming $M_{t_0} = M(t_0)$ and $M_t = M(t \equiv t_{u+1})$ are fixed,

$$P[M_t|M_{t_0}] = \int \cdots \int dM_{t-\Delta t}\, dM_{t-2\Delta t}\cdots dM_{t_0+\Delta t}$$
$$\times P[M_t|M_{t-\Delta t}]P[M_{t-\Delta t}|M_{t-2\Delta t}] \times \cdots P[M_{t_0+\Delta t}|M_{t_0}],$$

$$P[M_t|M_{t_0}] = \int \cdots \int DM \exp\left(-\sum_{s=0}^{u}\Delta tL_s\right),$$

$$DM = (2\pi\hat{g}_0^2\Delta t)^{-1/2} \prod_{s=1}^{u}(2\pi\hat{g}_s^2\Delta t)^{-1/2}\, dM_s,$$

$$\int dM_s \to \sum_{\alpha=1}^{N}\Delta M_{\alpha s}, \quad M_0 = M_{t_0}, \quad M_{u+1} = M_t, \tag{18}$$

where α labels the range of N values of M.

There are some advantages to the path-integral representation over its equivalent Fokker–Planck and rate-equation representations. For example, there exists a variational principle wherein a set of Euler–Lagrange differential equations exist for the Lagrangian L, directly yielding those values or trajectories of M which give the largest contribution to the probability distribution P. Because P is a *bona fide* probability distribution, there exist Monte Carlo numerical algorithms, sampling the M-space without having to calculate all values of M at all intermediate time epochs from t_0 to t to find P. This numerical algorithm also has the nice feature of avoiding traps in local minima when there are deeper minima to be had, representing more probable states. This is so useful that noise is sometimes artificially added to otherwise deterministic systems, e.g., as in simulated annealing (Kirkpatrick, Gelatt & Vecchi, 1983) to derive optimum circuitry on chips, by hypothesizing a cost function similar to a time independent Lagrangian.

In practice, some of these benefits are often illusory. Monte Carlo methods are notoriously poor for most nonstationary systems with multiple minima. However, a new method has been developed for explicitly solving the path integral, thereby obtaining the dynamic evolution of all states (minima) of the system (Wehner & Wolfer, 1983*a,b*). This cannot be done with the differential equation representations. Calculating *P* via the path integral facilitates the inclusion of boundary conditions, and the new methods can also take advantage of the Gaussian–Markovian nature of the system to produce an efficient numerical algorithm.

It is possible to formulate Langevin equations, Fokker–Planck equations, and path-integral equations that generalize to many nonlinear variables, labeled by G ($G = 2$ for the neocortical problem above), and to many cells, labeled by ν (Ingber, 1985*a*). This defines a time-dependent and space-dependent Lagrangian $\bar{L}$.

The Lagrangian can be fit to the data by assuming functional forms for $g_s^{G\nu}$ and $g_s^{GG'\nu\nu'}$.

$$
\begin{aligned}
g^G &= X^G + X_G^G \cdot M^{G'} + X_{G'G''}^G M^{G'} M^{G''} + \ldots, \\
g_{GG'} &= Y_{GG'} + Y_{GG'G''} M^{G''} + Y_{GG'G''G'''} M^{G''} M^{G'''} + \ldots, \\
M_s^{G\nu} &= M_s^{G\nu} - \langle\langle M_s^{G\nu} \rangle\rangle,
\end{aligned}
\tag{19}
$$

where it is understood that the *X*s and *Y*s are also labelled according to the number of minima. The convergence of $\bar{L}$ is expected to be quite good. That is, even polynomial forms for $g_s^{G\nu}$ and $g_s^{GG'\nu\nu'}$, with coefficients to be fit, define a Padé rational approximate to $\bar{L}$ usually giving better convergence than that obtained for $g_s^{G\nu}$ or $g_s^{GG'\nu\nu'}$ separately. Also, note that $\bar{L}_s$ is a single scalar function to be fit.

Once the parameters $\{X, Y, \langle\langle M \rangle\rangle\}$ are fit, the theory is ready to track or predict. Science is not only empiricism. Modeling and chunking of information is required, not only for aesthetics, but also to reduce required computational resources of brains as well as machines.

34.3.3 Combat simulations

An important class of problems confronting C^3 systems concerns how to pass enough, but not too much, timely information to decision-makers to permit them to assess the overall 'macroscopic' nature of detailed 'microscopic' operations unfolding in time. Similarly, there must also be a reasonable information-conduit through which their macroscopic decisions can be effectively implemented at the microscopic level.

Modern methods of nonlinear nonequilibrium statistical mechanics can be utilized to approach such problems, not just merely to model abstract scenarios. Basically, this approach seeks to define a 'mesoscopic' scale, established between the microscopic and macroscopic scales, specifically appropriate to each C^3 system: nonlinear multivariate functions describing drifts (trends) and diffusions (risks) must be sought. This requires trial and error, intelligence and creativity, and much experience is to be gained by dealing with at least several C^3 systems (a process similar to the development of the functional description of nuclear forces). These functional forms and their coefficients must be fit to real empirical data, e.g., initial, intermediate and final resources, to develop a time-dependent multivariable probability distribution of order parameters defining the mesoscopic scale. Then, after this algebraic and numerical development, there is the possibility that the resulting codes can be implemented on small computers in the field, affording useful software support for decision-making and intelligence-gathering, while being robust against perturbations in these functional fits.

At NPS, we are developing statistical mechanical C^3 models of combat simulations. Simulations can be an important source of empirical data only if their assumptions are clearly recognized. That is they are at best only as good as they can model actual combat (Comptroller General, 1980). It is hoped that by fitting nonlinear statistical mechanical models to simulation data, we may capture the essence of realistic operations.

34.3.4 Statistical BI decision-making

A typical scenario that might take advantage of previous analyses which has fit a Lagrangian to previous data follows. For example, assume that in the middle of an engagement, a commander (human or machine) has available data representing measures of readiness of his forces and those of his opponent. He makes a judgement as to which of several established classes of conflict he is engaged in, e.g., possibly severely or moderately stochastic, possibly overwhelming resources in, or not in, his favor, etc. He chooses one of the previously established Lagrangians which is a coarse description of his present engagement, and sets the initial time boundary condition according to his present data.

He chooses some time in the future when he feels he will be called upon to make a judgement with regard to the deployment of his resources. He uses a small computer to determine the distribution of his variables at the future time. Most likely, he will obtain several possible likely states, with varying degrees of first moments ('probability') and second moments ('risk').

He might do this for several alternative initial parameter settings, especially if he can exercise some immediate control of their values, thereby obtaining another possible set of future states of the engagement. He might also have to fold in some constraints, in the form of Lagrange multipliers, to accommodate orders he has received from a higher command. He could also use the associated Euler–Lagrange variational equations to determine the most likely trajectory that his resources would follow enroute from his present state to his selected future state.

Thus, the commander has obtained a valuable source of information to aid him in making decisions, and in determining sets of orders of constraints which he should pass down to his subordinates. Conversely, his subordinates, by aggregating their data into the specified order parameters, can communicate information to their commander in a language readily accessible to his decision-making process.

Acknowledgement

This chapter was prepared while the author was a National Research Council-NPS Senior Research Associate.

References

Anderson, J. A., Silverstein, J. W., Ritz, S. A. & Jones, R. S. (1977). 'Distinctive features, categorical perception and probability learning: some applications of a neural model.' *Psych. Rev.*, **84**, 413–51.

Blackmore, R. & Shizgal, B. (1985). 'Discrete-ordinate method of solution of Fokker–Planck equations with nonlinear coefficients.' *Phys. Rev. A*, **31**, 1855–68.

Blair, B. G. (1985). *Strategic Command and Control.* Washington, D.C.: Brooking Institution.

Bullock, T. H. (1980). 'Reassessment of neural connectivity and its specification.' In *Information Processing in the Nervous System*, eds. H. M. Pinsker & W. D. Willis, Jr. New York: Raven Press.

Cheng, K. S. (1972). 'Quantization of a general dynamical system by Feynman's path integration formulation.' *J. Math. Phys.*, **13**, 1723–6.

Comptroller General (1980). *Models, Data, and War: A Critique of the Foundation for Defense Analyses.* Washington, D.C.: U.S. General Accounting Office.

Cooper, L. N. (1973). 'A possible organization of animal memory and learning.' In *Collective Properties of Physical Systems*, eds. B. Lundqvist & S. Lundqvist, pp. 252–64. New York: Academic Press.

Cowan, J. D. (1982). 'Spontaneous symmetry breaking in large scale nervous activity.' *Int. J. Quant. Chem.*, **22**, 1059–82.

Dekker, H. (1979). 'Functional integration and the Onsager–Machlup Lagrangian for continuous Markov processes in Riemannian geometries.' *Phys. Rev. A*, **19**, 2102–11.

DeWitt, B. S. (1957). 'Dynamical theory in curved spaces. I. A review of the classical and quantum action principles.' *Rev. Mod. Phys.*, **29**, 377–97.

Eastport Study Group (1985). *A Report to the Director Strategic Defense Initiative Organization.* Washington, D.C.: SDIO.

Erickson, R. P. (1982). 'The across-fiber pattern theory: an organizing principle for molar neural function.' *Sensory Physiol.*, **6**, 79–110.

Ericsson, K. A. & Chase, W. G. (1982). 'Exceptional memory.' *Am. Scientist*, **70**, 607–15.

Feynman, R. P. & Hibbs, A. R. (1965). *Quantum Mechanics and Path Integrals.* New York: McGraw-Hill.

Gilbert, C. D. & Wiesel, T. N. (1983). 'Functional organization of the visual cortex.' *Prog. Brain Res.*, **58**, 209–18.

Goldman, P. S. & Nauta, W. J. H. (1977). 'Columnar distribution of cortico-cortical fibers in the frontal association, limbic, and motor cortex of the developing rhesus monkey.' *Brain Res.*, **122**, 393–413.

Grabert, H. & Green, M. S. (1979). 'Fluctuations and nonlinear irreversible processes.' *Phys. Rev. A*, **19**, 1747–56.

Graham, R. (1977*a*). 'Covariant formulation of non-equilibrium statistical thermodynamics.' *Z. Physik*, **B26**, 397–405.

Graham, R. (1977*b*). 'Lagrangian for diffusion in curved phase space.' *Phys. Rev. Lett.*, **38**, 51–3.

Haken, H. (1983). *Synergetics*, 3rd edn. New York: Springer.

Hubel, D. H. & Wiesel, T. N. (1962). 'Receptive fields, binocular interaction and functional architecture in the cat's visual cortex.' *J. Physiol.*, **160**, 106–54.

Imig, T. J. & Reale, R. A. (1980). 'Patterns of cortico–cortical connections related to tonotopic maps in cat auditory cortex.' *J. Comp. Neurol.*, **192**, 293–332.

Ingber, L. (1968). 'Nuclear forces.' *Phys. Rev.*, **174**, 1250–63.

Ingber, L. (1972). 'Editorial: Learning to learn.' *Explore*, **7**, 5–8.

Ingber, L. (1976). *The Karate Instructor's Handbook.* Solana Beach, CA: PSI-ISA.

Ingber, L. (1981*a*). 'Attention, physics and teaching.' *J. Social Biol. Struct.*, **4**, 225–35.

Ingber, L. (1981*b*). *Karate: Kinematics and Dynamics.* Hollywood, CA: Unique.

Ingber, L. (1981*c*). 'Towards a unified brain theory.' *J. Social Biol. Struct.*, **4**, 211–24.

Ingber, L. (1982). 'Statistical mechanics of neocortical interactions. I. Basic formulation.' *Physica D*, **5**, 83–107.

Ingber, L. (1983*a*). 'Riemannian corrections to velocity-dependent nuclear forces.' *Phys. Rev. C*, **28**, 2536–9.

Ingber, L. (1983*b*). 'Statistical mechanics of neocortical interactions. Dynamics of synaptic modification.' *Phys. Rev. A*, **28**, 395–416.

Ingber, L. (1984*a*). 'Path-integral Riemannian contributions to nuclear Schrödinger equation.' *Phys. Rev. D*, **29**, 1171–4.

Ingber, L. (1984*b*). 'Statistical mechanics of neocortical interactions. Derivation of short-term-memory capacity.' *Phys. Rev. A*, **29**, 3346–58.

Ingber, L. (1984*c*). 'Statistical mechanics of nonlinear nonequilibrium financial markets.' *Math. Modelling*, **5**, 343–61.

Ingber, L. (1985*a*). *Elements of Advanced Karate.* Burbank, CA: Ohara.

Ingber, L. (1985*b*). 'Statistical mechanics algorithm for response to targets (SMART).' In *Workshop on Uncertainty and Probability in Artificial Intelligence*, pp. 258–64. Menlo Park, CA: AAAI-RCA.

Ingber, L. (1985*c*). 'Statistical mechanics of neocortical interactions. EEG dispersion relations.' *IEEE Trans. Biomed. Eng.*, **32**, 91–4.

Ingber, L. (1985*d*). 'Statistical mechanics of neocortical interactions: stability and duration of the 7 ± 2 rule of short-term-memory capacity.' *Phys. Rev. A*, **31**, 1183–6.

Ingber, L. (1985*e*). 'Towards clinical applications of statistical mechanics of neocortical interactions.' *Innov. Tech. Biol. Med.*, **6**, 753–8.

Ingber, L. (1986). 'Riemannian contributions to short-ranged velocity-dependent nucleon–nucleon interactions.' *Phys. Rev. D*, **33**, 3781–4.

Jones, E. G., Coulter, J. D. & Hendry, S. H. C. (1978). 'Intracortical connectivity of architectonic fields in the somatic sensory, motor and parietal cortex of monkeys.' *J. Comp. Neurol.*, **181**, 291–348.

Kirkpatrick, S., Gelatt, C. D. Jr & Vecchi, M. P. (1983). 'Optimization by simulated annealing.' *Science*, **220**, 671–80.

Langouche, F., Roekaerts, D. & Tirapegui, E. (1982). *Functional Integration and Semiclassical Expansions*. Dordrecht: Reidel.

Miller, G. A. (1956). 'The magical number seven, plus or minus two.' *Psychol. Rev.*, **63**, 81–97.

Misner, C. W., Thorne, K. S. & Wheeler, J. A. (1973). *Gravitation*. San Francisco: Freeman.

Mizrahi, M. M. (1978). 'Phase space path integrals, without limiting procedure.' *J. Math. Phys.*, **19**, 298–307.

Mountcastle, V. B. (1978). 'An organizing principle for cerebral function: the unit module and the distributed system.' In *The Mindful Brain*, eds. G. M. Edelman & V. B. Mountcastle, pp. 7–50. Cambridge: Massachusetts Institute of Technology.

Murdock, B. B. Jr (1983). 'A distributed memory model for serial-order information.' *Psychol. Rev.*, **90**, 316–38.

National Research Council Committee on the Applications of Mathematics (1984). *Computational Modeling and Mathematics Applied to the Physical Sciences*. Washington, D.C.: National Academy Press.

Nunez, P. L. (1981). *Electric Fields of the Brain: The Neurophysics of EEG*. New York: Oxford Univ.

Orr, G. E. (1983). *Combat Operations C3: Fundamentals and Interactions*. Maxwell Air Force Bace, AL: Air University.

Pellionisz, A. J. (1984). 'Coordination: a vector-matrix description of transformations of overcomplete CNS coordinates and a tensorial solution using the Moore–Penrose generalized inverse.' *J. Ther. Biol.*, **110**, 353–75.

Schulman, L. S. (1981). *Techniques and Applications of Path Integration*. New York: J. Wiley & Sons.

Shaw, G. L. & Vasudevan, R. (1974). 'Persistent states of neural networks and the random nature of synaptic transmission.' *Math. Biosci.*, **21**, 207–18.

Shepherd, G. M. (1979). *The Synaptic Organization of the Brain*, 2nd edn, New York: Oxford Univ.

Tsal, Y. (1983). 'Movements of attention across the visual field.' *J. Exp. Psychol.*, **9**, 523–30.

van Kampen, N. G. (1981). *Stochastic Processes in Physics and Chemistry*. Amsterdam: North-Holland.

Wehner, M. F. & Wolfer, W. G. (1983*a*). 'Numerical evaluation of path-integral solutions to Fokker-Planck equations'. I. *Phys Rev. A*, **27**, 2663–70.

Wehner, M. F. & Wolfer, W. G. (1983*b*). 'Numerical evaluation of path-integral solutions to Fokker-Planck equations. II. Restricted stochastic processes'. *Phys Rev. A*, **28**, 3003–11.

Weidlich, W. & Haag, G. (1983). *Concepts and Models of a Quantitative Sociology.* Berlin: Springer.
Weinberg, S. (1972). *Gravitational Cosmology.* New York: Wiley.
Williamson, S. J., Kaufman, L. & Brenner, D. (1979). 'Evoked neuromagnetic field of the human brain'. *J. Appl. Phys.*, **50**, 2418–21.
Zhang, G. & Simon, H. A. (1985). 'STM capacity for Chinese words and idioms: Chunking and acoustical loop hypothesis'. *Memory and Cognition*, **13**, 193–201.

35

Josin's computational system for use as a research tool

GARY JOSIN

35.1 Introduction

In dealing with the problem of trying to describe mathematically neural tissue populations, known as neural nets, two approaches can be taken, the global and the microscopic. The global approach gives a phenomenological description of neural tissue populations. The microscopic, derived through appropriate simplifications, gives properties of the net from the properties of its constituents, the neurons, the connections and the synapses. While phenomenological theories appear to be easier to build and, overall, yield more results that are in agreement with experiments, it is impossible to build a realistic model of the brain without knowing the detailed functioning, interactions and interrelations of its constituents.

For the construction of an actual neural net machine, theories based on the properties of the fundamental constituents of the net will be more applicable to discovering the laws that govern the secrets of biological information processing. For instance, it is more relevant to simulate the activities of the brain from the underlying fundamental laws of nature. Examples taken from physics itself clarifies this point.

From a philosophical point of view it is more appealing to derive the laws of thermodynamics from the statistical behaviour of the particles that make up the system than to introduce thermodynamics as an independent branch of physics.

Analogously, it is more significant to derive the properties of superconductivity from the actual properties of the electrons and lattice than from phenomenological reasoning. Indeed, it is extremely important to understand how matter becomes organized, that is, how the laws of physics change when making the transition from a normal to a superconducting state.

Although the process of biological information processing is not fully understood at the present time, it is important to use neural network theories as tools to help push research disciplines forward, to reach the threshold where a change in theories becomes necessary. That will be when the transition will have to be made from neural net theories to biological information processing systems.

The aim of this paper is to present a microscopic theory of neural nets. This paper is divided into four parts. In the first part, a theory, as presented here, describes a neural net that is based on our knowledge of the actual functioning of the single constituents of the net, the neurons. In the second part, a heuristic mathematical proof illustrates the flexible structure, storage capacity and response time of neural network. In the third part, the theoretical results on the connectivity vs. functionality are proofed by computer simulations which show the system's versatility, efficiency and reliability. These simulations also demonstrate that the computational properties of the net may remain even when there is a minimal number of connections between processors. The computational system is then discussed in the last part, in light of its use as a research tool to help push research disciplines forward.

35.2 Josin's computational system

A neural net is physically an array of processors or a mathematical array within a processor. Ideally, these processors or nodes simulate neurons and through their connections emerges biological information processing. A neural net is designed to emulate a possible method by which information processing occurs within a living brain.

A theory of a neural net as presented here in this paper is described by the following equation:

$$U_{h,t_h+1} = \theta_h \left[\sum_{k=1}^{N} \sum_{r=0}^{l(h)} A_{hk}^{(r)} U_{k,t_k} - S_h \right], \tag{1}$$

where $\theta_h[x]$ is sigmoidal function defining the output of processor (h), $U_{h,t}$ is a function that admits one of two values $(1, 0)$, t_h is a random characteristic delay of a particular processor, $l(h)$ is the number of previous intervals of time on which a processor (h) depends, S_h is the threshold of processor (h), $A_{hk}^{(r)}$ are explicit functions of the processors that change over time,

$$A^{(r)}_{hk} = f_{hk}(U_1, U_2, \ldots, U_{N-Y}, U_{N-Y+1}, \ldots, U_N), \qquad (2)$$

where processors (k) can be different processors (k').

These connections form a zero-diagonal mathematical array whose values are believed (Caianiello, 1961; Hopfield, 1982; Josin, 1977) to hold memories and thoughts.

Each processor (h) takes on a value which depends explicitly on the values of the other processors (k) to which it is connected. A logical rule is, if processor (h) and processor (k) have the same values over time, that is, if both processors have positive values or both processors have negative values, then the connection between the processors is represented by a positive number. Whereas, if processor (h) and processor (k) have different values over time, that is, if one of the processors has a positive value and the other processor has a negative value or vice-versa, then the connection between processor (h) and processor (k) is ambiguous, and the connection between them is represented by a negative number. One can apply the same logical rule by replacing (k) with processors $(k)'$. Now this rule defines a mapping between two processors in neighbouring regions.

For N processors, each processor (h) independently sums the positive and negative values represented by its $C_h(t)$ connections. If the sum of the connection values from other processors to which it is connected is greater than the threshold of processor (h), then the processor takes on a value given by the functional form of $\theta_h[x]$. If this sum is less than or equal to the threshold, processor (h) changes its value based on its current value and the functional form of $\theta_h[x]$. Two such functions are given by:

$$\theta_h[V_h] = \frac{1}{1 + \exp{(-A)}} \quad \text{and} \quad \theta_h[V_h] = \begin{cases} 1 \\ 0 \end{cases} \text{if} \begin{array}{c} V_h > 0 \\ V_h \leq 0 \end{array} \qquad (3)$$

where $A = V_h/T_h(t)$, V_h is the sum of the connection values for processor (h) and is given by:

$$V_{h,t_h} = \sum_{k=1}^{N} \sum_{r=0}^{l(h)} f^{(r)}_{hk}(U_1, U_2, \ldots, U_{N-Y}U_{N-Y+1}, \ldots, U_N)\theta_k[V_{t_k}] - S_h$$

$$(4)$$

and $T_h(t)$ is an efficacy parameter.

As can be seen from eqn (1), the net operates in three stages. First the net is trained on a particular set of patterns–knowledge. The net distributes the patterns uniformly amongst its processors. When a particular input pattern is presented to the net, any behaviour is statistically characterized by the processors. The state of the net is given by the values of the N processors.

It will be shown in the results that the tag processors U_{N-Y+1}, U_{N-Y+2}, ..., U_N characterize the behaviour of the net.

To illustrate the flexible structure, storage capacity Y and response time of a net, consider a checkerboard pattern with $N = 9$ and a tag processor $Y = 1$,

$$U_0 = (1, 0, 1, 0, 1, 0, 1, 0, 1).$$

According to the previously described logical rule, after training, the array which defines the connections is given by:

$$A_{hk}^{(0)} = \begin{matrix}
0 & - & + & - & + & - & + & - & + \\
- & 0 & - & + & - & + & - & + & - \\
+ & - & 0 & - & + & - & + & - & + \\
- & + & - & 0 & - & + & - & + & - \\
+ & - & + & - & 0 & - & + & - & + \\
- & + & - & + & - & 0 & - & + & - \\
+ & - & + & - & + & - & 0 & - & + \\
- & + & - & + & - & + & - & 0 & - \\
+ & - & + & - & + & - & + & - & 0
\end{matrix}$$

Now consider the following heuristic proof:

Study the mathematical array A and the encoded pattern U which is represented within A. Since on average any random pattern will have $N/2$ 1's and $N/2$ 0's, the array can have $N/2$ columns with all values of its connections set equal to 0. The other $N/2$ columns need to have at least one connection in them. The total number of connections in the array is $N(N - 1)$. The ratio of the number of columns that have one connection, and there are $N/2$ of them, divided by the total number of connections, is directly proportional to the amount of the array that can be disconnected and a net having the capability of tagging the input pattern. Therefore

$$D = 1 - 1/2(N - 1) \tag{5}$$

of a neural net can be disconnected and the net can tag an input pattern.

Moreover, for one training pattern only 51% of the $N/2$ processors that have one connection are necessary to enable the net to tag an input pattern – to recognize.

Therefore the minimal number of connections that are absolutely necessary to decode a training pattern is

$$D = 1 - 51/200(N - 1), \tag{6}$$

which represents the 'critical' number necessary to recognize a particular pattern.

Eqns (5) and (6) are of some interest since they show that after training, the number of necessary connections per processor to characterize an input pattern is inversely proportional to the number of processors in the net.

The storage capacity Y can be derived. The number of connections necessary to store a pattern is equal to $N/2$, and the total number of connections is $N(N - 1)$, which shows that at most the number of tag processors or the storage capacity per pattern is proportional to N.

From an information theoretical point of view, the number of connections reduces to $\log N$. From this consideration eqn (5), becomes:

$$D = 1 - \frac{\log N}{N^2} \tag{7}$$

and the storage capacity, in the limit of large N, is proportional to:

$$Y = \frac{N^2}{\log N} = N^2. \tag{8}$$

This result shows that N^2 connections virtually represent N^3 connections – N of them are free. Therefore neural nets are a more efficient technical memory than conventional designs.

In fact, for highly interconnected nets the theorem holds true for any input pattern since the array that defines the connections characterizes its behaviour.

It is of interest, that as the number of processors approaches infinity for the nets presented here, the subsequent response time would appear instantaneous relative to nets that are highly connected because the number of computations is reduced.

In the sections that follow the results from a neural simulator based on a theory are presented and in the last section it is discussed in light of its relevance to biological information processing.

35.3 Results

A neural net simulator has been written to test a theory as presented here. First, the results of the test will be presented and then remarks will be made as to how a computational system may be of use as a research tool.

The network was trained on 40 variations of eight groups of patterns. Before the patterns were loaded from a text file to train the net, the tag processors were set to be either a 1 or a 0. Tagging each of the patterns depended on which group a pattern belonged to. This process is simple and 'biases' the net. The patterns are shown in Table 35.1. To train the net the user only has to be capable of assigning the right pattern to the right group. The tag processors are in row 9 of a training pattern and are specified before training the net.

The capability of the neural net simulator to correctly characterize a particular input pattern after biasing was tested by accumulating the statistics on how well the net performed in finding the correct training pattern while making the transition from highly connected to minimally connected nets.

Fig. 35.1 shows a typical training pattern from the set that was tested. The pattern represents one of the patterns learned by training the net whereas the other patterns represent a subpart of that information. First, the net was trained on the patterns shown in Table 35.1. Second, an input pattern was given to the net and the output patterns tag was re-entered to play back the most probable pattern. Fig. 35.1 shows this sequence of events.

Fig. 35.1 shows an input pattern that progressively gets further away from resembling a training pattern. Fig. 35.2 also shows $V_h(t)$ which, when inserted into eqn (3), conveys information and directly relates to the probability that an input pattern resembles a training pattern. A tag processor's integer values convey information on the resemblance of an input pattern to the training patterns.

The last input pattern in the sequence shows a pattern that is an equal fragment of two of the training patterns. In this case, both of the tags which correspond to two different training patterns receive the same integer values. This outcome shows that a net can go beyond its experience or training, that is, it has a capability for abstraction.

For all test simulations the net and tag processor always detected the input patterns even when they are unexpected or confusing. If the pattern is constructed of 60% of one pattern and 40% of another pattern the net matches it to the pattern containing the 60% – see Fig. 35.3.

For ambiguous input patterns that are constructed from 50% of one pattern and 50% of another the net matches it to no response – see Fig. 35.3. This feature is true only if the training patterns have been shown to the net an equal number of times. If a net has been trained on one pattern more than another one, a net develops a priority recognition capability. For ambiguous input patterns a net matches it to the pattern with the higher priority. For example, if a net has been trained on two patterns, and has been trained on one pattern twice as much as the other, the output is no response when an input pattern is constructed of 25% of the first pattern and 75% of the other one.

Gary Josin

Table 35.1. *Training patterns*

11000000	00000011	00011000	00000000	00100000
11000000	00000110	00110000	00000000	00010000
01100000	00001100	00011000	00000000	00010000
00011000	00011000	00011000	11111111	00001000
00001100	01100000	00011000	11111111	00010000
00000110	11000000	00011000	00000000	00001000
00000011	11000000	00011000	00000000	00001000
00000001	10000000	00011000	00000000	00010000
1.......	.1......	..1.....	...1....	..1.....
00000001	00000000	00000000	00000000	11000000
00000010	00000000	00000000	00000000	00100000
00000100	00000000	00111100	00111100	00100000
00001000	00010100	00111100	00101100	00011100
00010000	11101011	00111100	00101100	00001100
00100000	00000000	00111100	00111100	00001110
01000000	00000000	00000000	00000000	00000011
10000000	00000000	00000000	00000000	00000011
.1......	...1....	....1...	....1...	1.......
00010000	00000000	00101000	10000000	00000000
00001000	00000000	00010000	01100000	00000110
00010000	00000000	00011000	00100000	00001100
00001000	11101101	00001000	00110000	00011000
00010000	10110110	00010000	00001000	00110000
00010000	00000000	00001000	00001100	00100000
00001000	00000000	00001000	00000010	01000000
00010000	00000000	00010000	00000001	10000000
..1.....	...1....	..1.....	1.......	.1......
00000000	00000000	11000000	00000001	00110000
00000000	00000000	00100000	00000010	00010000
00110100	00111000	00110000	00001100	00001000
00110100	00101100	00010000	00010000	00010000
00010100	00110100	00001100	00010000	00001000
00111100	00101100	00000110	01100000	00011000
00000000	00000000	00000010	10000000	00010000
00000000	00000000	00000001	10000000	00011000
....1...	....1...	1.......	.1......	..1.....

```
00100000   10000000   00000001   00000000   00000000
00010000   01100000   00000110   00000000   00000000
00011000   00100000   00000100   00000000   00111100
00001000   00110000   00011000   01010100   00101000
00010000   00001100   00110000   10101011   00101100
00001000   00000100   00100000   00000000   00111100
00011000   00000110   01000000   00000000   00000000
00011000   00000001   11000000   00000000   00000000
..1.....   1.......   .1.....    ...1....   ....1...
00000011   11000000   00000011   11000000   00000011
00000011   01000000   00000010   10000000   00000010
00000011   10000000   00000001   11000000   00000011
00000011   11000000   00000011   01000000   00000001
00000011   01000000   00000011   11000000   00000011
00000011   11000000   00000010   10000000   00000010
00000011   10000000   00000011   11000000   00000011
00000011   11000000   00000010   11000000   00000001
......1.   .....1..   ......1.   .....1..   ......1.
10000000   00000011   00000000   00000000   11000000
01000000   00000010   00000000   00000000   11000000
00100000   00000110   00000000   00000000   11000000
00010000   00010000   01010101   11101101   11000000
00001000   00010000   10101010   10101010   11000000
00000100   01000000   00000000   00000000   11000000
00000010   11000000   00000000   00000000   11000000
00000001   10000000   00000000   00000000   11000000
1.......   .1......   ...1....   ...1....   .....1..
10000000   01000000   00000100   00010000   00000001
00000001   00000100   00100000   00001000   10000000
00100000   00010000   00000000   00000100   10100000
00000010   10000000   00001000   10000000   00000000
01000000   00000100   10000000   00100000   10000000
00000010   00000010   00000010   00010000   00010000
00010000   00010000   00000001   00000100   00000100
00001000   00001000   01000000   10000000   00000010
.......1   .......1   .......1   .......1   .......1
```

Gary Josin

Fig. 35.1. Input–output characteristics of a neural net.

Training pattern	Input patterns	Output patterns	Reinput tags	Output pattern
11000000	11000000	11111111	00000000	11000000
11000000	11000000	11111111	00000000	11000000
11000000	11000000	11111111	00000000	11000000
11000000	11000000	11110111	00000000	10000000
11000000	11000000	11100111	00000000	01000000
11000000	11000000	11111111	00000000	11000000
01100000	11000000	11111111	00000000	11000000
11000000	11000000	11111111	00000000	01000000
.....1..	00000000	.....1..	.....1..	00000000

$$V_6 = 40$$

	11000000	11111111	00000000	11000000
	11000000	10111110	00000000	10000000
	11000000	11111111	00000000	11000000
	11000000	11111111	00000000	11000000
	00000000	11101100	00000000	11000000
	00000000	01111110	00000000	01000000
	00000000	11111100	00000000	11000000
	00000000	11111111	00000000	11000000
	00000000	.....1..	.....1..	00000000

$$V_6 = 18$$

	11000000	11111110	00000000	11000000
	11000000	01111111	00000000	11000000
	01000000	11111111	00000000	11000000
	00000000	10111011	00000000	10000000
	00000000	11111111	00000000	11000000
	00000000	11111111	00000000	01000000
	00000000	11111111	00000000	11000000
	00000000	.....1..	.....1..	00000000

$$V_6 = 12$$

	00000000	11111111	00000000	
	00000000	11111111	00000000	
	11000000	11111111	00000000	
	11000000	11111111	00000000	
	00000000	11111111	00000000	
	00000000	11101111	00000000	
	00000000	11111111	00000000	
	00000000	...1.1..	...1.1..	

$$V_4 = 8$$
$$V_6 = 8$$

Fig. 35.2. Some input–output responses from a neural net.

11000011	11110001	11000000	11000011	11111010
11000011	11111111	11000000	11000011	11111111
11000011	11111111	10000000	11000011	11111111
11000010	11111111	11000000	11000011	11111111
11000000	11111111	11000000	11000011	11111111
11000000	11111111	11000000	11000011	11111111
11000000	11111111	11000000	11000011	11111111
11000000	11111111	11000000	11000011	11111111
00000000	00000010	00000000	00000000	00000000
Confused input	Output pattern	Output after re-entering tag	Ambiguous input	Output = no response

35.3.1 A hierarchical net

A natural extension of the neural simulator is to input the values of the tag processors values into the next layer of the net. In the next level, tags also exist which are inputs to the next level in the hierarchy, and so on, for example, primal features, characters, words, sentence type, etc. As shown by eqn (6), this may reduce the number of connections that are necessary in a highly interconnected next layer.

To test a hierarchical net it was trained on the five variations of three patterns – see Fig. 35.3 which shows one of the variations. The other patterns that are not shown in the diagram varied in size, angles of the lines defining the letter and thickness of line.

The tag processors were entered into another neural net made up of 28 processors plus four tag processors. The fourth tag was introduced to train the net on unintelligible letters – not shown in the diagram.

The same results were found for this hierarchical net as for the previously discussed net. The net performed reliably, always identifying a letter that could be identified by a human subject.

The character recognition tag processors were then entered into a net with five processors with a one-word tag processor to indentify a particular word XOY. At this level the inputs had usually been corrected at a lower level. Again, the net performed reliably for all test cases.

These results illustrate a method by which nets can be trained hierarchically for pattern recognition and suggest how they may be trained for developing a pattern recognition reasoning capability.

The efficacy parameter $T_h(t)$ affects the convergence rate – focusing the net.

Fig. 35.3. (*a*) One of the variations of three training patterns – to see the characters, view this diagram from a distance. (*b*) Three typical input patterns – tags are the outputs.

```
00000000    00000000    00000000    00000000    00000000    00000000
11000000    00000011    00000000    00000000    11000000    00000011
01100000    00000110    00000111    11100000    11000000    00000011
00110000    00001100    00011100    00011100    11000000    00000011
00011000    00011000    00011000    00001100    11000000    00000011
00001100    00110000    00011000    00001100    11000000    00000011
00000110    01100000    00011000    00001100    11000000    00000011
00000011    11000000    00011000    00001100    01100000    00000110
00000011    11000000    00011000    00001100    00110000    00001100
1.......    .1......    ..1.....    ...1....    .....1..    ......1.
00000011    11000000    00011000    00001100    00001100    00110001
00000110    01100000    00011000    00001100    00000110    01100000
00001100    00110000    00011000    00001100    00000011    11000000
00011000    00011000    00011000    00001100    00000011    11000000
00110000    00001100    00011000    00011000    00000011    11000000
01100000    00000110    00011100    00111000    00000011    11000000
11000000    00000011    00000111    11100000    00000011    11000000
11000000    00000011    00000000    00000000    00000011    11000000
.1......    1.......    ..1.....    ..1.....    ......1.    ......1..
```

(*a*)

```
11000000    00000000    00000000    00000000    10000000    00000001
01110000    00000000    00001111    11111000    01100000    00000110
00110000    00000000    01110000    00011100    00100000    00001100
00010000    00011000    01110000    00001110    00110000    00011000
00011000    00110000    01110000    00001110    00001100    00110000
00001100    01100000    00110000    00001110    00001100    00100000
00000110    11000000    00110000    00001100    00000010    01000000
00000011    11000000    00110000    00001100    00000001    10000000
...1....    ...1....    ..1.....    ..1.....    1.......    .1......
00000011    00000000    00011000    00011000    00000010    11000000
00001100    00000000    00011000    00110000    00000001    11000000
00011000    00000000    00011000    00110000    00000001    11000000
00110000    00000000    00001000    01100000    00000000    11000000
00000000    00000000    00000111    11000000    00000000    01100000
00000000    00000000    00000000    00000000    00000000    00110000
00000000    00000000    00000000    00000000    00000000    00011000
00000000    00000000    00000000    00000000    00000000    00011000
....1...    ........    .1......    ..1.....    .1......    ..1.....
```

(*b*)

35.4 Connectivity/functionality

To confirm a previously derived theoretical result expressed by eqn (5), a net was trained on the set of patterns shown in Table 35.1. Complete representations of the training patterns were input to the net. Each time the net correctly tagged all the input patterns, 10% of the total number of connections were randomly disconnected by setting them to zero. This process of altering the structure was continued until a unique tag could not be made. Simulations show nets can compensate for large changes in structure. For this particular problem 93.2% of the net was disconnected before the net became confused, that is, just before the net lost its capability of correctly responding to confused or ambiguous inputs patterns. At the critical value determined from eqn (5), the net still has the capability of tagging a complete input pattern.

For this particular simulation, the total number of connections the net had left was 355, which means that on average, each processor had approximately five remaining connections. From eqn (5), the theoretical value for the total number of connections necessary to tag an input pattern is 256 or approximately four connections per processor per pattern.

These simulations verify the previously heuristically derived theoretical results. The total number of connections for all eight patterns is 576, which is approximately 2 times the number of remaining connections. These results hold true for input patterns, proving a precise quantitative law on the capability of a network to characterize an input pattern reliably. Simulations were then carried out on the net to verify this result. If four of the 64 bits of an input pattern are correct the net and tag are at the threshold of reliably characterizing any input patterns.

These results can be interpreted in terms of spatial and rotational recognition invariance. When the net is minimally connected an input pattern has to completely resemble a training pattern, that is confined in space, whereas a highly connected net allows for spatial and rotational variance.

This principle was tested by writing the word XOY at different angles and different spatial positions. These tests were somewhat limited because of the image size, but again the results show that the net performed reliably. By the addition of a threshold to a word tag processor or by disconnecting the net, the net would turn on the tag processor if the hand-written characters were up to a certain predefined standard – quality control.

To verify eqn (8), a net of $N = 9$ processors was trained on 12 patterns. Each of the 12 patterns were entered in turn and the output pattern matched the input pattern even if the input processor had one wrong starting value. The result verifies the existence of virtual connections.

It is of interest that the subsequent response time of the net decreases for minimally connected nets.

These simulations show that as the net contains more and more connections, the property of association arises at a heuristically proved 'critical' number of connections. As the net comes closer to being fully connected, it becomes more sensitive to a particular biased pattern. For example, Fig. 35.2, reveals that with increasing connectivity a net is capable of responding to a continuous range of patterns. The first pattern was the only one recognized with minimal connectivity. The diagram shows some of the ones recognized with a highly interconnected net. This is generalization and differentiation. Moreover, the essential computational features can remain at low connectivity, that is, the net still responds properly to ambiguous and confused input patterns. However, this result depends on chance, or a predefined disconnection strategy.

For nets with large N, it is impossible with conventional computers to link a training pattern with a particular piece of a pattern. To make this point clear when $N = 156$, there are 10^{47} possible output patterns. To process that number of patterns by serial matching with anything made of matter would exceed the information processing rate of 10^{47} bits gm-s^{-1} found from the Heisenberg uncertainty principle. In contrast, by defining a 'tag' processor, even when $N = 156$ and it is impossible to predict which of the patterns will be selected, a neural network can match unexpected and confused patterns.

However, when a neural net evolves by the reappearance of the same set of patterns but with variations, these nets have to be 'biased' by specifying to which group in a set a pattern belongs. For some types of learning a teacher biases the net. In other cases the bias is learned automatically from repetition. Automatic learning has been presented in an earlier work. A theory that is presented here remains microscopic in origin by introducing a 'bias'.

35.5 Relevence to biology

Eqns (5) and (6), were derived without considering how topological mappings are assembled in the brain. For an orderly mapping to take place from one region to another (in eqn (1), k would equal k', which would be some neighbouring processors) region, neighbouring processors will remain connected and distant processors will be disconnected. This process could be an underlying mechanism for the way the brain forms topological mappings. A theory presented here could be judged as a general method by which nervous systems evolve to organize themselves, allowing biological information processing – connectivity/functionality.

The connectivity/functionality simulations will be used by researchers in many diverse fields to compare actual with expected behaviours to detect differences in real brain microstructures.

For example, animals with bilateral damage to the amygdala have a great deal of difficulty in finding a solution to simple visual problems. They can be trained to respond to a visual pattern, but they cannot associate, that is, they cannot respond to variations in training patterns.

In a theory of this type neurons play two different roles. The net as a whole is connected and the tag processor neurons correspond to biological neurons that have a genetically programmed bias. These biases self-organize the whole net, resulting in a biological microstructure enabling a functionality that transcends the microstructure.

If biological neurons are genetically biased, as discussed in the introduction, a theory will remain microscopic in origin and it will have reached the threshold of having to make a transition from neural network theories to biological information processing systems. If neurons are not genetically biased then we have to elicit a phenomenological theory that automatically learns the necessary bias based on environmental feedback. An example of one of these theories is expressed by the generalized delta rule (5), which modifies the connections by first inputting a pattern into the net, then the net learns the difference between a target bias and an actual output. If biological neurons use a rule of this type then when combined with the presented theory a significant improvement will be gained in the number of connections that have to be modified. In an engineering context this result is appealing from an applications view point but such a theory may not have any biological relevance. That is, a phenomenological theory may be able to predict structural differences in the microstructure of a living brain but in no way could such theories give information on the connectivity/functionality.

In contrast, it appears that the microscopic theory presented in this paper provides proof of connectivity–functionality theories, and suggests a novel way of introducing self-control in a neural net (Josin, 1977). It would be interesting to do experiments on learning in light of this theory to investigate connectivities/functionalities.

Furthermore, this theory shows that simple models of neural nets are versatile enough that they can solve different classes of computationally difficult problems. Figure 35.2 can be interpreted in many ways. For example, neural nets may be the way the brain solves many problems, such as priority recognition, edge detection, surface interpolation (Koch, Marroquin & Yuille, 1985), shape from shading, brightness perception, speech processing (Sejnowski & Rossenberg, 1986), knowledge-based reasoning, adaptive and knowledged based control, and perhaps even to develop concepts of quality, and space-time.

This theory will allow researchers in many diverse fields to develop their own uses to reach a threshold where the next progression begins.

35.6 Conclusion

A theory of neural nets and some of its most recent developments have been presented in this paper. This theory, despite its simplifications of natural behaviour, results in a quantitative law on connectivity–functionality. Computer simulations have shown that, given a threshold number of connections between the nodes of a network, a form of self-organization takes place, allowing the emergence of general differential, priority and fault tolerant capabilities – a critical facet of intelligence hitherto not observed in AI simulations.

Although this process of self-organization is not fully understood at the present time, it is clear that this line of research will lead ultimately to an increase in our understanding of the fundamental functions of intelligence – perhaps eventually to the first truly intelligent machines.

Furthermore, apart from the usefulness of future neural simulators for solving computationally difficult problems, neural network theory may lead to our understanding of the living brain, in terms of its microstructure connectivity–functionality.

Acknowledgement

The author would like to thank his father, Michael Josin, for partial financial support, and his mother, Bernadine Josin, for encouraging this work.

References

Caianiello, E. R. (1961). 'Outline of thinking machines and thought-processes'. *J. Theor. Biol.*, **1**.

Hopfield, J. J. (1982). 'Neural networks and physical systems with emergent collective computational abilities'. *Proc. Nat. Acad. Sci., USA*, **79**, 2554–8.

Josin, G. M. (1977). 'Self-control in neural nets'. *Biol. Cybernetics*, **27**, 185–7.

Koch, C., Marroquin, J. & Yuille, A. (1985). 'Analog "neuronal" networks in early vision'. *Proc. Nat. Acad. Sci., USA* (in press).

Sejnowski, T. & Rossenberg, C. (1986). *NETalk: a Parallel Network that Learns to Read Aloud*. Johns Hopkins University.

NAME INDEX

SUBJECT INDEX

Page numbers in italics indicate references to tables or figures.